CHALLENGES IN
Inflammatory Bowel Disease

CHALLENGES IN

Inflammatory Bowel Disease

EDITED BY

Derek P. Jewell

Neil J. Mortensen

A. Hillary Steinhart

John H. Pemberton

Bryan F. Warren

Second edition

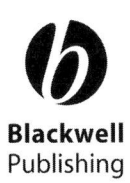

Blackwell
Publishing

© 2001, 2006 by Blackwell Publishing Ltd

Blackwell Publishing, Inc., 350 Main Street, Malden, Massachusetts 02148-5020, USA
Blackwell Publishing Ltd, 9600 Garsington Road, Oxford OX4 2DQ, UK
Blackwell Publishing Asia Pty Ltd, 550 Swanston Street, Carlton, Victoria 3053, Australia

The right of the Authors to be identified as the Authors of this Work has been asserted in accordance with the Copyright, Designs and Patents Act 1988.

All rights reserved. No part of this publication may be reproduced, stored in a retrieval system, or transmitted, in any form or by any means, electronic, mechanical, photocopying, recording or otherwise, except as permitted by the UK Copyright, Designs and Patents Act 1988, without the prior permission of the publisher.

First published 2001
Second edition 2006

1 2006

Catalogue records for this title are available from the British Library and Library of Congress

ISBN-13: 978-1-4051-2234-4
ISBN-10: 1-4051-2234-X

Set in 9.25/12 by TechBooks, India
Printed and bound in India by Replika Press Pvt., Ltd

Commissioning Editor: Alison Brown
Editorial Assistant: Saskia van der Linden
Development Editor: Fiona Pattison
Production Controller: Kate Charman

For further information on Blackwell Publishing, visit our website:
http://www.blackwellpublishing.com

The publisher's policy is to use permanent paper from mills that operate a sustainable forestry policy, and which has been manufactured from pulp processed using acid-free and elementary chlorine-free practices. Furthermore, the publisher ensures that the text paper and cover board used have met acceptable environmental accreditation standards.

Contents

List of Contributors and Editors vii
Preface xi

I Clues to aetiology and pathogenesis 1

1. RICHARD F. A. LOGAN AND EMMA L. ARMITAGE: Global changes in incidence 3

2. JOHN B. BECKLY, TARIQ AHMAD AND DEREK P. JEWELL: The role of genetics in inflammatory bowel disease 14

3. ROBIN G. LORENZ AND CHARLES O. ELSON: Microbial sensing in the intestine by pattern recognition receptors 33

4. ROBERT PENNER AND KAREN MADSEN: The role of bacteria 44

5. KENNETH CROITORU: The appendix – how might it influence susceptibility to ulcerative colitis: the legend of Qebehsenuef 57

II Diagnosis and assessment 65

6. BRYAN F. WARREN AND NEIL A. SHEPHERD: What are the controversies in histopathological diagnosis? 67

7. GARY C. CHEN AND SIMON K. LO: The challenges of using capsule endoscopy in the diagnosis and management of inflammatory bowel disease 85

8. STUART TAYLOR AND STEVE HALLIGAN: Cross-sectional imaging of inflammatory bowel disease 105

III Management of ulcerative colitis 117

9. MILES P. SPARROW, WEE-CHIAN LIM AND STEPHEN B. HANAUER: Mesalazine for maintenance therapy in ulcerative colitis – how much, how long? 119

10. SIMON TRAVIS: Refractory distal colitis 124

11. FERGUS SHANAHAN, JUDE RYAN AND SHOMIK SIBARTIE: Pharmabiotics and inflammatory bowel disease – on the verge of evidence-based medicine 144

12. R. JOHN NICHOLLS AND MARK J. CHEETHAM: Current controversies in the surgical management of ulcerative colitis 154

13. ALAN F. HORGAN, WILLIAM J. SANDBORN AND JOHN H. PEMBERTON: What are the causes and treatment of ileoanal pouch dysfunction? 167

IV Management of Crohn's disease 179

14. A. HILLARY STEINHART: Is mesalazine useful in Crohn's disease? 181

15. MIQUEL A. GASSULL: Steroids or nutrition? 194

16. SÉVERINE VERMEIRE AND PAUL RUTGEERTS: Do antibiotics have a role in Crohn's disease? 206

17 GEERT D'HAENS: The optimal use of infliximab in Crohn's disease 213

18 STEPHAN R. TARGAN AND LOREN C. KARP: Designer drugs: from bench to bedside 221

19 W.M. CHAMBERS, I. LINDSEY AND N.J. MORTENSEN: Current controversies in the surgical management of Crohn's disease 232

20 CARL J. BROWN AND ROBIN S. MCLEOD: Perianal Crohn's disease 246

21 KAREL GEBOES: What is dysplasia? 266

22 URBAN SJÖQVIST AND ROBERT LÖFBERG: Colonoscopic surveillance – if and when? 281

23 RALF KIESSLICH AND MARKUS F. NEURATH: Cancer: new colonoscopic techniques 293

24 JACINTHA N. O'SULLIVAN AND TERESA A. BRENTNALL: Molecular markers – a realistic hope? 303

25 MAHA GUINDI AND ROBERT H. RIDDELL: Adenomas versus dysplasia associated lesion or mass – recognition and management? 312

V Special management problems 327

26 THOMAS D. WALTERS AND ANNE M. GRIFFITHS: Growth impairment in children 329

27 SUBRATA GHOSH: Osteopenia 340

28 PHILIPPE MARTEAU: Pregnancy 360

29 ROBERT HILSDEN AND LLOYD SUTHERLAND: Can prognosis of ulcerative colitis be predicted? 369

Index 377

List of Contributors and Editors

EDITORS

Derek P. Jewell, *Gastroenterology Unit, Radcliffe Infirmary, Woodstock Road, Oxford, UK*

Neil J. Mortensen, *Department of Colorectal Surgery, John Radcliffe Hospital, Headley Way, Oxford, UK*

John H. Pemberton, *Professor of Surgery, Mayo Clinic College of Medicine, Division of Colon and Rectal Surgery, Mayo Clinic, Gonda 9-s, 200 First Street SW, Rochester, MN 55905, USA*

A. Hillary Steinhart, *Head, Combined Division of Gastroenterology, Mount Sinai Hospital/University Health Network, Associate Professor of Medicine, University of Toronto, Toronto, M5G 1X5 Canada*

Bryan F. Warren, *Department of Cellular Pathology, John Radcliffe Hospital, Headley Way, Oxford, UK*

CONTRIBUTORS

Tariq Ahmad, *Gastroenterology Unit, Radcliffe Infirmary, Woodstock Road, Oxford, UK*

Emma L. Armitage, *Specialist Registrar, Gastroenterology, GI Unit, Western General Hospital, Crewe Road, Edinburgh, UK*

John B. Beckly, *Gastroenterology Unit, Radcliffe Infirmary, Woodstock Road, Oxford, UK*

Teresa A. Brentnall, *Department of Medicine, University of Washington, Seattle, 98195, USA*

W. M. Chambers, *Department of Colorectal Surgery, John Radcliffe Hospital, Headley Way, Oxford, UK*

Carl J. Brown, *Resident in Colorectal Surgery, University of Toronto, Canada*

Gary C. Chen, *Department of Medicine Cedars-Sinai Medical Center, Los Angeles, California 90048, USA*

Mark J. Cheetham, *St Mark's Hospital, Watford Road, Harrow, Middlesex, UK*

Kenneth Croitoru, *Intestinal Diseases Research Program, Division of Gastroenterology, McMaster University, Hamilton, Ontario, Canada*

Charles O. Elson, *Department of Medicine, University of Alabama at Birmingham, Birmingham, AL 35294, USA*

Miquel A. Gassull, *Associate Professor of Medicine, Universitat Autonoma de Barcelona, Head of the Department of Gastroenterology, Hospital Universitari Germans Trias i Pujol., Badalona, Catalonia, Spain*

Karel Geboes, *Professor in Pathology, Department of Pathology, University Hospital Kul, Minderbroedersstraat 12, 3000 Leuven, Belgium*

Subrata Ghosh, *Professor of Gastroenterology, Imperial College London, Hammersmith Hospital, Ducane Road, London*

Anne M. Griffiths, *Associate Chief (Clinical), Division of GI Nutrition, 555 University Avenue, Hospital for Sick Children, University of Toronto, Toronto, Canada*

Maha Guindi, *Assistant Professor, Department of Laboratory Medicine and Pathobiology, University of Toronto, and Department of Pathology, University Health Network/Toronto General Hospital, Toronto, Ontario, Canada*

Geert D'Haens, *Gastroenterology Unit, Imelda GI Clinical Research Centre, Bonheiden, Belgium*

Steve Halligan *Professor of Gastrointestinal Radiologist Dept of Specialist X-Ray University College Hospital, London, UK*

Stephen B. Hanauer, *Professor of Medicine and Clinical Pharmacology, Director, Section of Gastroenterology and Nutrition, University of Chicago Medical Center*

Robert Hilsden, *Associate Professor, Department of Medicine and Community Health Sciences, University of Calgary, Calgary, Alberta, Canada*

Alan F. Horgan *Consultant Colorectal Surgeon Freeman Hospital, High Heaton, Newcastle, NE7 7DN, UK*

Loren C. Karp, *Division of Gastroenterology, Inflammatory Bowel Disease Center, and Immunobiology Institute, Cedars-Sinai Medical Center, 8700 Beverly Blvd., Suite D4063, Los Angeles CA 90048, USA*

Ralf Kiesslich, *I. Med. Klinik und Poliklinik, Johannes Gutenberg Universität Mainz, Mainz, Germany*

Wee-Chian Lim, *Section of Gastroenterology and Nutrition, University of Chicago Medical Center, Chicago, USA*

I. Lindsay, *Department of Coloretal Surgery, John Radcliffe Hospital, Oxford, UK*

Simon K. Lo, *Associate Clinical Director of GI Endoscopy, Professor of Medicine, David Geffen School of Medicine at UCLA, Cedars-sinai Medical Center, Los Angeles, California, USA*

Robert Löfberg, *Karolinska Institute, Huddinge University, Stockholm, Sweden*

Richard F. A. Logan, *Professor of Clinical Epideimiology, Division of Epidemiology and Public Health, University of Nottingham, Queen's Medical Centre, Nottingham, UK*

Robin G. Lorenz, *Department of *Pathology, The University of Alabama at Birmingham, Birmingham, AL 35294, USA*

Karen Madsen, *Associate Professor, Division of Gastroenterology, University of Alberta, Edmonton, Alberta, Canada*

Philippe Marteau, *Gastroenterology Department, Lariboisiere Hospital, Assistance Publique des Hôpitaux de Paris, and Paris V University, France*

Robin S. McLeod, *Professor of Surgery and Health Policy, Management and Evaluation, University of Toronto; Head, Division of General Surgery, Mount Sinai Hospital, Toronto, Ontario, Canada*

Markus F. Neurath, *I. Med. Klinik und Poliklinik, Johannes Gutenberg Universität Mainz, Mainz, Germany*

R. John Nicholls, *St Mark's Hospital, Watford Road, Harrow, Middlesex, UK*

Robert Penner, *Kelowna General Hospital, 564 Leon Avenue, Kelowna, British Columbia*

Jacintha N. O'Sullivan, *Senior Research Scientist, Centre for Colorectal Disease, Education and Research Centre, St Vincents University Hospital, Elm Park, Dublin 9, Ireland*

Robert H. Riddell, *Professor of Pathology, Department of Laboratory Medicine and Pathobiology, University of Toronto, and Department of Pathology, Mount Sinai Hospital, Toronto, Ontario, Canada*

Paul Rutgeerts, *Head of the IBD Research Unit, Department of Gastroenterology, University Hospital Gasthuisberg, Herestraat 49, 3000 Leuven, Belgium*

Jude Ryan, *Alimentary Pharmabiotic Centre and Department of Medicine, University College Cork, National University of Ireland, Ireland*

William J. Sandborn, *Professor of Medicine, Mayo Clinic College of Medicine, Division of Gastroenterology and Hepatology, Mayo Clinic, 200 First Street SW, Rochester, MN 55902, USA*

Fergus Shanahan, *Alimentary Pharmabiotic Centre and Department of Medicine, University College Cork, National University of Ireland, Ireland*

Neil A. Shepherd, *Department of Histopathology, Gloucestershire Royal Hospital, Great Western Road, Gloucester, UK*

Shomik Sibartie, *Alimentary Pharmabiotic Centre and Department of Medicine, University College Cork, National University of Ireland, Ireland*

Urban Sjöqvist, *Senior Consultant, Department of Medicine, Karolinske Institutet at Stockholm Söder Hospital, Stockholm, Sweden*

Miles P. Sparrow, *Section of Gastroenterology and Nutrition, University of Chicago Medical Center, Chicago, USA*

Lloyd Sutherland, *Departments of Medicine and Community Health Sciences, Univeristy of Calgary, Calgary Alberta Canada*

Stephan R. Targan, *Director, Division of Gastroenterology, Inflammatory Bowel Disease Center, and Immunobiology Institute, Cedars-Sinai Medical Center, 8700 Beverly Blvd., Suite D4063, Los Angeles CA 90048, USA*

Stuart Taylor, *Consultant Radiologist and Senior Lecturer Department of Specialist X-Ray University College Hospital, London, UK*

Simon Travis, *Consultant Gastroenterologist, John Radcliffe Hospital, Oxford, UK*

Séverine Vermeire, *Department of Gastroenterology, University Hospital Gasthuisberg, Herestraat 49, 3000 Leuven, Belgium*

Thomas D. Walters, *Fellow in Paediatric Gastroenterology and Nutrition, Division of Paediatric Gastroenterology and Nutrition, Hospital for Sick Children, University of Toronto, Toronto, Canada*

Preface

For many years the aetiology and management of inflammatory bowel disease seemed to have reached a steady state where only small but nonetheless important steps were made in our understanding of these potentially devastating diseases. Suddenly, with the molecular biology revolution, there is renewed interest in the mechanisms of inflammation, the genes that may determine them and the development of new powerful designer drugs. As never before, gastroenterologists are having to redefine the place of the established medical and surgical treatments alongside these novel treatments. This has led to unexpected problems in the diagnosis and definitions of disease as histopathologists have struggled with indeterminate colitis, pouchitis and perforating and stenosing varieties of Crohn's disease.

Although exacting and more robust epidemiological tests are available, it is still not clear whether the incidence of either ulcerative colitis or Crohn's disease is changing both within the western world and developing countries. The importance of infective agents within the gut lumen would seem to be intuitively relevant but their role remains undefined. Claims for the importance of specific organisms involved in the pathogenesis of either disease have had their fashionable 'rise and fall' so that no organism has been consistently implicated. Indeed, current evidence would suggest that these diseases represent a genetic susceptibility, mediated by many different genes, to a variety of environmental factors. This hypothesis allows for the very great heterogeneity that is seen by clinicians.

Since the 1950s, aminosalicylates and corticosteroids have provided the only effective treatments, but the final decade of the last millennium has seen the introduction of many new therapies, principally immunosuppressant and immunomodulatory drugs. It has been encouraging that their effectiveness has been tested in clinical trials and subsequent meta-analyses, continuing the evidence-based approach to these diseases which began with the early trials of corticosteroids and sulphasalazine and which has consistently underpinned the treatment of ulcerative colitis and Crohn's disease. Nevertheless, medical therapy is still imperfect: it may fail to control active disease. Maintenance therapy, especially for Crohn's disease, is very unsatisfactory and drug therapy frequently contributes to long-term morbidity; for example, corticosteroids may contribute to growth failure in children and to reduced bone density in adults. The rapid expansion in drug therapy has been matched with many surgical innovations such as restorative proctocolectomy for ulcerative colitis and the concept of minimal surgery for Crohn's disease. Thus, the number of surgical options now available to us inevitably raise questions concerning the choice of operation to be performed, when and by whom.

The purpose of this book is to address some of the challenges in our understanding of ulcerative colitis and Crohn's disease, the challenges of new diagnostic and therapeutic modalities and the clinical challenges of maintaining good health and hence quality of life for our patients. It is not intended to provide a further text book of inflammatory bowel disease, of which there are many, but rather to consider specific issues. Many readers will want to focus on individual chapters and therefore the editors make no apology for a degree of repetition which will allow maximum exposure to new knowledge and thought.

The editors are greatly appreciative of the time the authors have given to allow this book to gestate into a second edition. We are also most grateful to Mrs Toria McNeile for her help in assembling the manuscripts and to Ms Alison Brown and her staff at Blackwell for their patience and expertise.

DJ
NM
AHS
JHP
BW

I: Clues to aetiology and pathogenesis

1: Global changes in incidence

Richard F.A. Logan and Emma L. Armitage

Introduction

Variation in disease occurrence is the essence of epidemiology. When this variation is between place or person, and standardised measures are available, measurement of such variation can be relatively accurate, albeit often expensive and laborious, as demonstrated by the European collaborative study on inflammatory bowel disease (EC-IBD) [1]. In contrast, measurement of variation over time is usually fraught with difficulty and any trends revealed, unless substantial, are often surrounded by uncertainty. With regard to inflammatory bowel disease (IBD), more sensitive diagnostic techniques, widening case definitions, increasing availability of specialist investigation and greater public and professional awareness of both diseases will all serve to increase the numbers of new diagnoses and have the potential to contribute to an apparent rise in incidence. In this chapter we will review recent data on the incidence of IBD worldwide and, at the risk of over generalising, assess what they imply as to the aetiology of IBD.

The rise in incidences of ulcerative colitis and later Crohn's disease that was seen in many Western countries during the past century, preceded the growth of modern gastroenterology and was evident in both individual studies and routine morbidity and mortality data [2–4]. Over the last few years, however, there have been a number of conflicting reports of the incidence of both diseases either continuing to increase, or being stable or even declining. For example, Bernstein *et al.*, using health insurance data for Manitoba, Canada, reported an overall incidence of Crohn's disease of 146/million/year, the highest yet reported, whereas a few hundred miles to the south in Olmsted County, Minnesota, Loftus *et al.* found an incidence over a similar period of 69/million/year [5, 6]. An almost two-fold variation has also been reported from the United Kingdom, with Kyle finding the incidence of Crohn's disease continuing to rise in north-east Scotland at 98/million/year in 1985–87, while in the Cardiff area incidence was declining with the figure for 1986–90 being 62/million/year and 56/million/year for 1991–95 [7, 8]. There have been fewer reports of the time trends in incidences of ulcerative colitis, which may reflect the additional challenge for epidemiological studies of distinguishing it from non-recurrent, mainly infective forms of colitis. Even so, in the (EC) IBD study the incidence of ulcerative colitis in parts of Europe as far apart as Iceland and Crete was higher than previously recorded [1].

Are these differences real or can the disparate findings of these studies be explained by differences in study design or imperfections of the methods used? One possible explanation is that the differences reported reflect sampling and study size. For many diseases, cancer in particular, this problem can be overcome by examining mortality or morbidity routinely collected at a national or regional level.

Evidence from trends in routinely collected morbidity data

For IBD, mortality data are of little value in assessing its incidence over time. Death from IBD is now rare, with fewer than 400 deaths per year now being certified as due to IBD in the United Kingdom [9]. In addition, over 75% of these deaths occur in those over 70 years, whereas the incidence of IBD is greatest in those under age 40. Although mortality rates do show a broad correlation with incidence figures between countries, the relationship breaks down when comparing mortality and incidence within a country over time [10]. Thus, the rapid rise in incidence of Crohn's disease during the 1950s and 1960s in the United Kingdom and the United States was associated with a less than doubling of mortality rates [11]. At the same time, mortality from ulcerative colitis in these countries declined sharply when other data suggested incidence was unchanged or possibly increasing.

Routinely collected morbidity data has mainly consisted of data on hospital admissions, which has been collected over many years in several countries. Another source of data is that collected by health insurance or health maintenance organisations, typically from North America, which has the advantage of including data on outpatient (ambulatory) care as well as that for inpatient care. Using either source it is necessary to separate first admissions or contacts from repeat contacts. Hospital admission data are also affected by changing patterns of care, with patients being increasingly cared for as outpatients. With these considerations in mind it is notable that in Denmark the annual incidence of Crohn's disease, based on their national registry of inpatients, increased from 46 to 62/million/year in women between 1981–84 and 1989–92, and from 33 to 41/million/year in men over the same period [12]. The figures were similar to the overall crude incidence of 41/million/year reported elsewhere for Copenhagen County in 1979–87. In contrast, the incidence of ulcerative colitis over this period fell from 154 to 123/million/year in women and from 141 to 126/million/year in men.

Hospital admission data (now called hospital episode statistics) are collected in the United Kingdom, but except in the Oxford region and Scotland it is not possible to identify first admissions from repeat admissions [13, 14]. In England, hospital admission rates for Crohn's disease increased by approximately 4% annually during the period from 1970 to 1985, but when admissions in the Oxford region were linked to individuals, first admissions for men declined by 0.5% annually and for women rose by 0.1%, neither being statistically significant [13]. Over the same period hospital admission rates for ulcerative colitis in England showed no change, although first admission rates in the Oxford region showed a 1% average annual increase, which was not statistically significant [13].

Both these studies, like most studies on routinely collected data, relied on accurate coding of the discharge diagnosis. This is a particular problem for inflammatory bowel disease where there is often some uncertainty as to whether the diagnosis is Crohn's disease (CD) or ulcerative colitis (UC). To overcome this problem Bernstein *et al.* in their study using health insurance records for Manitoba, validated the diagnoses according to questionnaire responses obtained from a subset of patients directly approached [5]. They also ignored all cases with a first medical contact within the first 5 years of their study period to try to ensure that only incident cases were included. How successful they were is difficult to judge. Inclusion of a proportion of non-incident cases will disproportionately increase incidence in the older age groups. Their figures for the incidence of Crohn's disease are some of the highest reported at 169/million/year in women and 123/million/year in men. Incidence rates for ulcerative colitis were also high at 144/million/year in women and 143/million/year in men.

Thus, the routinely collected data give a mixed picture. The lack of increase in the figures from the Oxford region could reflect an increased proportion of patients having outpatient care only. The same restriction also applies to the Danish data, although a validation study on a subset showed the diagnostic accuracy to be high, and overall incidence was in keeping with a smaller hospital-based study [12]. The Canadian data are particularly remarkable, as generally the figures for IBD incidence reported from North America have tended to be lower than those from Europe. These three studies reflect some of the important limitations of routinely collected morbidity data – namely that it is usually difficult to make direct comparisons between data sets on account of differences in the health-care systems

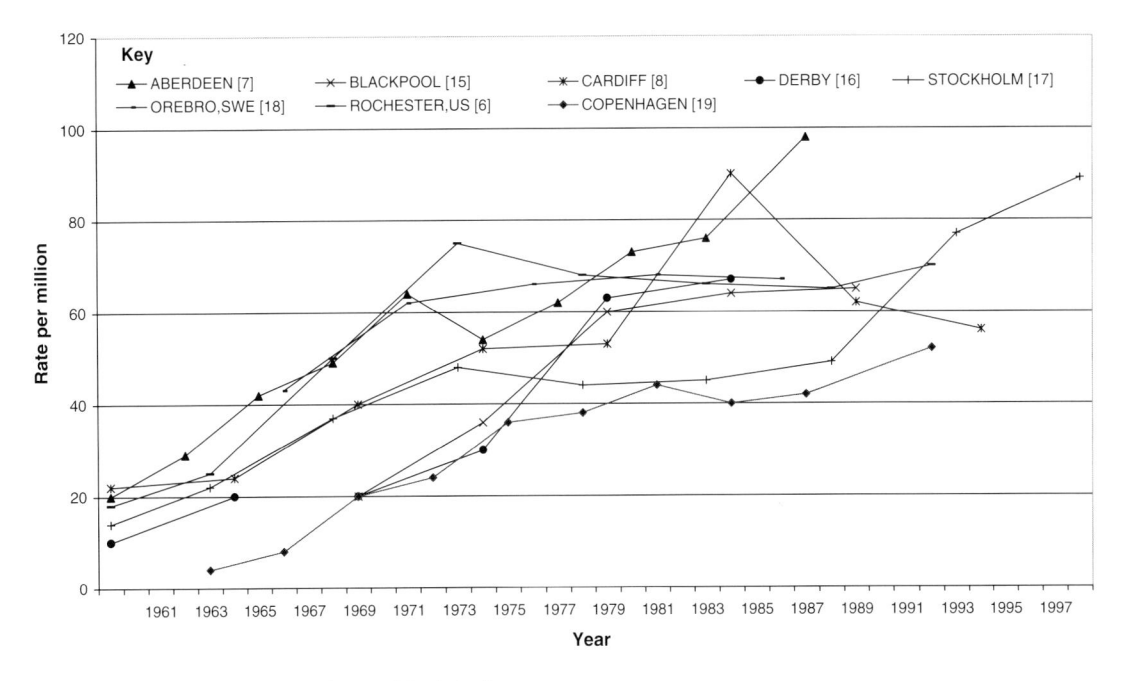

Fig 1.1 Recent time trends in incidence of Crohn's disease.

involved. Secondly, changes in how the data are collected often restrict analyses to time periods of less than 20 years. A third limitation is that it is usually not possible to validate the accuracy of diagnosis, which is of special importance when distinguishing Crohn's disease from ulcerative colitis.

Time trends in individual studies

The alternative to figures generated from routine data is to use the results of individual *ad hoc* studies. In many European countries with centralised state-funded health care, such studies appear deceptively straightforward. Population catchment areas are often well defined and specialist care is provided by a small number of gastroenterologists, who also usually provide whatever private care is available. However, IBD is relatively uncommon, and prospective studies need to be prolonged to provide reliable figures on time trends. Other issues that have not always been carefully addressed include the criteria for diagnosis, residence criteria and clear definitions for date of onset or diagnosis. In addition, as already mentioned, the effects of increasing awareness, better case ascertainment, greater use of more sensitive tests such as colonoscopy and evolving case definitions need to be considered.

Fortunately, in a few areas IBD incidence has been monitored either prospectively or by repeated retrospective studies over periods of more than 20 years, and these studies arguably provide the most reliable evidence on incidence trends (Figs 1.1 and 1.2). Rates have been plotted according to the last year of each time period reported and in most areas the rates have been age-standardised to correct for changes in their population age structures over time. Of the eight areas shown in Fig 1.1, only in the Aberdeen area and most recently in Stockholm has the incidence of Crohn's disease shown more than a small increase since 1980 [7, 25]. When the Aberdeen data are age-standardised there is some reduction in the rate of increase, although the final figure remains high at 88/million [26]. It is too soon to know whether this represents a sustained increase; a similar peak in incidence was previously found in Cardiff. Otherwise the remarkable feature is how little variation there is between places as different as Cardiff in the United Kingdom,

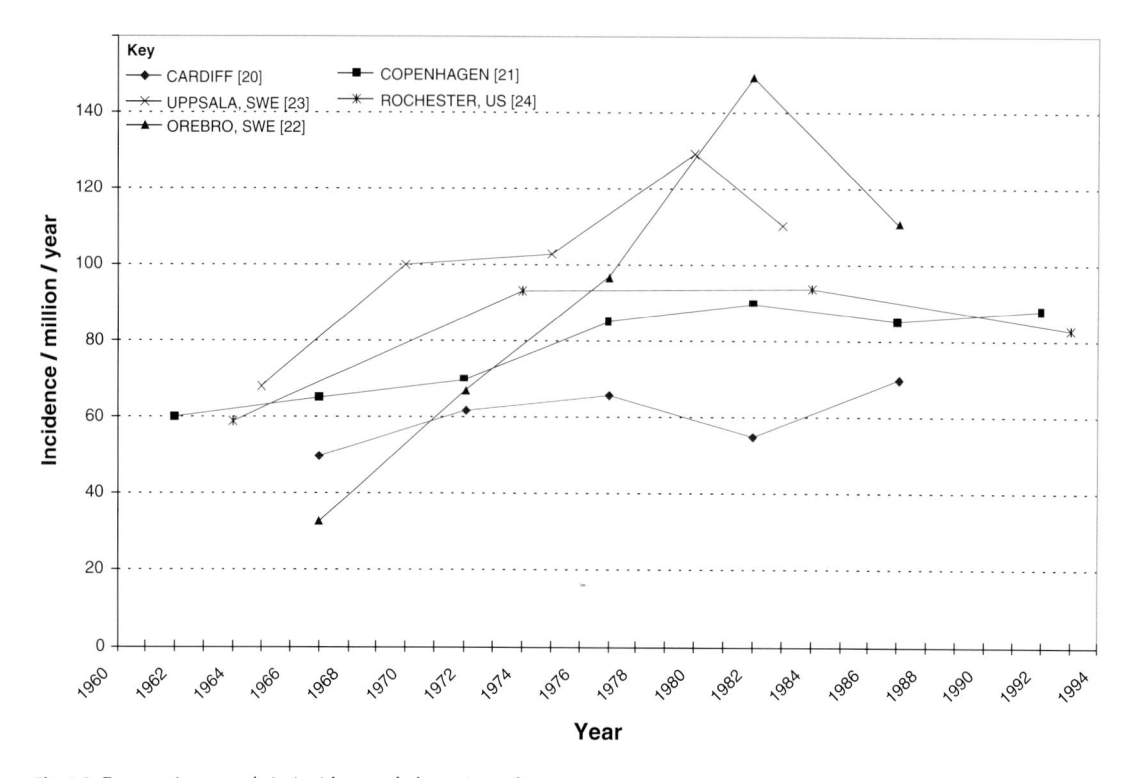

Fig 1.2 Recent time trends in incidence of ulcerative colitis.

Orebro in Sweden and Rochester in the United States.

These studies were all performed in an era when colonoscopy was not regarded as the standard investigation it has now become. For example, in northern France in the 1990s 92% of patients with Crohn's disease and 99% of those with ulcerative colitis had had a colonoscopy at diagnosis [17]. A recent updating of data from Stockholm found that 70% of Crohn's patients had a colonoscopy at diagnosis [25]. Equivalent figures for the 1980s and earlier have not been reported and it is unclear what proportion of IBD would have been labelled as ulcerative colitis in the absence of evidence, either macroscopic or microscopic, obtained at colonoscopy. Nevertheless, greater use of colonoscopy would account for the increasing proportion of patients found to have Crohn's disease affecting the colon, as reported in several recent studies [8, 17, 28].

There have been fewer studies of ulcerative colitis incidence. In the countries where IBD is common incidence rates for ulcerative colitis have tended to show more variation than those for Crohn's disease. Probably this reflects the additional problems posed by variable ascertainment of mildly symptomatic cases including those with proctitis only, and distinguishing single or transient episodes of colitis induced by infection or drugs. In Nottingham, the prevalence of previously undiagnosed ulcerative colitis in subjects offered faecal occult blood testing for colorectal cancer screening was 700/million [29]. Most were mildly symptomatic but had not sought medical advice. In the recent Norwegian study a diagnosis of ulcerative colitis could not be confirmed in 12% of patients when reinvestigated one year after diagnosis [30].

Given these considerations and the various changes in health care already mentioned, the increases in incidence over time (shown in Fig 1.2) are perhaps less than might have been expected. What does seem to have changed is the age-specific pattern, with an increase in incidence of ulcerative colitis at older ages in men but not in women. Thus, in the EC-IBD study and in the recent data from northern France the expected peak in incidence in the younger age groups was present for women but not for men [1, 27].

Geographic trends in incidence

Over the past 30 years a large number of other *ad hoc* studies have been reported from diverse locations worldwide. Table 1.1 shows the incidence rates reported from recent European studies. The incidence of both diseases appears to show around a 10-fold variation across Europe, but in general, the incidence of both is highest in countries in northern latitudes. The north-south gradient in IBD incidence was first described in Europe and was based on observations from these individual studies. However, the conclusions reached by comparison of these studies are once again hampered by variations in study design, notably case definition, methods of case ascertainment and time period of investigation. In addition, many studies reported only crude rather than age-standardised or age-specific incidence rates for their populations and in others, case ascertainment in children and the elderly was less complete than at other ages. The European collaborative study on IBD incidence was set up to overcome these problems by standardising methods throughout all participating centres. It concluded that the 'magnitude of the observed excess in north is less than expected on the basis of previous studies... this may reflect increases in incidence of IBD in Southern Europe whilst north may have stabilised' [1]. Incidence rates from centres participating in EC-IBD are shown in Table 1.1 in bold.

In North America significant geographic variation also appears to exist, and generally populations

Table 1.1 European studies of inflammatory bowel disease incidence in the 1990s (Centres from EC- IBD in bold).

First author	Year	Area	Time period	UC (n) Rates/100,000/year	CD (n)	Design
Shivananda EC-IBD [1]	1996	8 Northern European cities	1991–93	11.8 (869)	7.0 (477)	Prospective
Shivananda EC-IBD [1]	1996	12 Southern European cities	1991–93	8.7 (510)	3.9 (229)	Prospective
Bjornsson [28]	2000	Iceland	1990–94	16.5 (215)	5.5 (72)	Prospective
Moum [31, 32]	1997	South-east Norway	1990–93	12.8 (496)	6 (232)	Prospective
Salupere [33]	2001	Tartu, Estonia	1993–98	1.7 (16)	1.4 (13)	Prospective
Rubin [34]	2000	North Tees, UK	1990–94	13.9 (94)	8.3 (56)	Retrospective
Yapp [8]	2000	Cardiff, UK	1991–95		5.6 (84)	Retrospective
Russel [35]	1998	Netherlands	1991–95	10 (257)	6.9 (176)	Prospective
Latour [36]	1998	Leige, Belgium	1993–96	3.6 (111)	4.5 (137)	Prospective
Pagenault [37]	1997	Brittany, France	1994–95	2.9 (165)	2.8 (205)	Prospective
Flamenboum [38]	1997	Puy de Dome, France	1993–94	2.4 (29)	6.6 (79)	Prospective
Lakatos [39]	2004	Western Hungary	1977–01	5.8 (560)	2.2 (212)	Retrospective
Ranzi [40]	1996	Cremona, Italy	1990–93	7.0 (82)	3.4 (40)	Prospective
Trallori [41]	1996	Florence	1990–92	9.6	3.4	Retrospective
Tragnone [42]	1996	Italy (8 cities)	1989–92	5.2 (509)	2.3 (222)	Prospective
Manousos [43, 44]	1996	Crete	1990–94	11.3 (116)	3.5 (36)	Prospective
Tsianos [45]	2003	N W Greece	1982–97	6.6 (357)	0.5 (43)	Retrospective
Molinie [27]	2004	Northern France	1988–99	4.0 (2665)	6.0 (4013)	Prospective

UC: ulcerative colitis; CD: Crohn's disease.

with the highest incidence and prevalence rates have been located in northern latitudes [4, 5, 46, 47]. Once again, these findings are based on the results of individual studies and are therefore difficult to compare due to methodological differences. One study that overcomes these problems is a study in the United States of military veterans and Medicare beneficiaries, which shows that the incidence of IBD is higher in the north compared to the south [48, 49].

Further analysis of the large Scottish cohort of juvenile-onset IBD between 1981 and 1995 [50] has also found that northerly region of residence was an independent risk factor for developing CD but not UC [48]. The relative risk of CD in the south compared with the north was 0.73 (95% CI 0.58–0.92, $p < 0.001$), but UC did not show this north/south variation. This pattern has not been examined in other paediatric populations, but does support the hypothesis that CD incidence exhibits a latitudinal gradient with incidence increasing with more northern latitudes.

Rest of the world

Until the 1980s reports of IBD occurrence from outside Europe and North America consisted essentially of case reports or case series. The exception was South Africa where Wright *et al.* found the incidence of both diseases in the Cape Town area to be greatest in the Whites but with incidence less than half that found in equivalent European populations. Incidence of both diseases in the coloured population was lower again and lowest of all in the Blacks [51]. Recent well-researched studies from Japan and Korea have shown IBD to be much less common than in Europe with UC incidence being 10–20/million/year and CD less than 5/million/year [52–55].

In line with the data from Japan and the Far East, UC has traditionally been regarded as rare in the developing world. However, an impressive pair of population surveys in northern India has revealed an UC incidence of 60/million/year and a prevalence of symptomatic UC of 443/million – figures not much lower than those reported from several European countries [56]. It is unclear whether these figures reflect an increasing UC incidence, as this is the first formal study of IBD incidence from India.

Trends in incidence of juvenile-onset Crohn's disease

Incidence patterns for whole populations may conceal changes taking place in smaller subgroups of that population, such as children. Although Crohn's disease incidence may be stable overall, several groups have suggested that incidence in children is particularly increasing. The epidemiology of this subgroup is of particular importance because several current hypotheses as to the causes of CD and UC relate to events happening in infancy or childhood [57–61].

In assessing any increase in incidence in children, one needs to consider some additional factors that could account for a spurious increase (Table 1.2). Firstly, the steep increase in incidence at ages 15 and 16 coincides with the arbitrary division between childhood and adulthood. Thus, any reduction in the time between symptom onset and diagnosis could have a disproportionate effect on incidence in childhood. As Table 1.3 shows, researchers have been divided in choosing age 14, 15 or 16 as the upper limit of childhood. How this might affect the figures is difficult to gauge, but it is notable that in the study from Copenhagen where the low incidence below age 15 is based on only six cases, in a further 17 symptom onset was before age 15 but diagnosis occurred in adulthood. Secondly, time from symptom onset to diagnosis of Crohn's disease in children has shortened; in the United Kingdom this has gone from around 12 months in the early 1980s to around 5 months in the recent data collected [77]. Other factors include the increased intensity of investigation and changing criteria for diagnosis of Crohn's disease.

As noted above, diagnosis for all hospital admissions in Scotland are recorded in a linked fashion for the whole country in the 'Scottish Hospitals discharges linked database' [78]. The linkage of data allows the whole series of that patient's admissions to be identified at any one time, allowing identification of incident cases rather than just hospital admission episodes. Using this database Barton *et al.*

Table 1.2 Possible factors contributing to an increase in incidence of Crohn's disease in children.

Greater case ascertainment
Quicker diagnosis → diagnosis at age 15, not 16
Diagnostic transfer, atypical UC → CD
Widening case definitions e.g. inclusion of orofacial granulomatosis
Earlier onset in predisposed individuals
Real increase in incidence

UC: ulcerative colitis; CD: Crohn's disease.

looked at incidence rates for juvenile onset IBD from 1968 to 1983 [71]. They found a three-fold rise in incidence for CD, and a marginal fall in UC. The data for CD, after allowing for a short lag, would seem to parallel the increase seen in adults over the preceding few decades. Over the last decade with increasing interest in the aetiological role of perinatal and early childhood factors, other groups have now published comparable epidemiological studies of the juvenile-onset subgroup (Table 1.3).

The figures from the Scandinavian countries seem to show more variation, with the rates from Denmark and Finland being a half to a third of those from Sweden and Norway. In part, this reflects the different age bands used (Table 1.3). Nevertheless, the situation within Sweden is as varied, because the recent data from northern Stockholm (Table 1.4) suggests a doubling in incidence of Crohn's disease, predominantly accounted for by increasing colonic disease, and a decline in ulcerative colitis

Table 1.3 Recent incidence data for Crohn's disease (CD) and ulcerative colitis (UC) in childhood.

First author	Area	Period	Duration (years)	Age group	CD Rates per 100,000/year	n	UC Rates per 100,000/year	n
Europe								
Langholz [62]	Copenhagen	1962–87	15	0–14	0.2	6	2.0	63
Olafsdottir [63]	W Norway	1984–85	2	0–15	2.5	10	4.3	17
Bentsen [64]	SE Norway	1990–94	4	0–15	2.0	14	2.2	15
Lindberg [65]	SW Sweden	1984–86	3	0–15	1.9	211[†]	1.4	287[†]
		1993–95	3	0–15	2.0	–	3.2	–
Hildebrand [66]	N Stockholm	1990–01	12	0–15	4.9	102	2.4	50
Kolek [67]	Czech republic	1990–01	12	0–15	1.0	19	1.1	22
Van der Zaag-Loonen [68]	Netherlands	1999–01	2	0–17	2.1		1.6	
Tourtelier [69]	NW France	1994–97	4	0–16	1.6	43	0.6	14
UK								
Cosgrove [70]	S Wales	1983–93	11	0–15	2.2	21	0.7	7
Barton [71]	Scotland	1968	1	0–16	0.7	10	1.9*	18
		1983	1	0–16	2.3	28	1.6*	13
Armitage [72]	Scotland	1981–95	15	0–15	2.3	383	3.4	197
Hassan [73]	Wales	1995–97	1	0–16	1.4	20	0.8	11
Sawczenko [74]	UK	1998	1	0–15	3.1		1.4	
USA								
Kugathasan [75]	Wisconsin	2000–01	2	0–17	4.6	129	2.1	60
Australia								
Phavichitr [76]	Melbourne	1996–01	5	0–16	2.0	233	–	–

*Rate for 6–16 years.
[†]Numbers for both periods.

Table 1.4 Incidence of Crohn's disease in children – northern Stockholm [65].

	Rate per 100,000/year for ages 0–15 years (95% CI)	
	CD	UC
	N = 102	N = 48
1990–92	1.7 (0.7–3.3)	3.3 (1.9–5.4)
1993–95	3.5 (2.1–5.5)	1.8 (0.8–3.3)
1996–98	5.6 (3.8–8.1)	1.9 (0.9–3.5)
1999–01	8.4 (6.2–11.3)	1.8 (0.9–3.4)
Overall	4.9 (4.0–6.0)	2.2 (1.6–2.9)

UC: ulcerative colitis; CD: Crohn's disease.

in under 16-year-olds during the 1990s, while the larger study covering just over half the childhood population (< 16 years) of Sweden found no increase in Crohn's disease incidence but a two-fold rise in incidence of ulcerative colitis [65, 66].

In the paediatric age group, further research from Scotland has also shown a higher incidence of CD in the more affluent areas of Scotland, as defined by postcode sector [50]. This pattern was independent of temporal, gender or regional trends and was therefore not purely a reflection of the geographical distribution of deprivation. The relationship to affluence was seen in CD, but not in UC, thus it is unlikely that the association was simply due to a higher reporting of symptoms to primary care in affluent areas.

Conclusions

It would be a serious mistake to assume incidence trends should be similar even in developed countries. With these caveats, there is broad support for the following:

- In Westernised countries, where Crohn's disease is already common, there is no *consistent* evidence of a continuing rise with the most reliable data showing stable incidence since the 1980s.
- In areas reporting an increase in Crohn's disease (northern France and Stockholm) the increase has been predominantly in colorectal Crohn's disease.
- Overall incidence of ulcerative colitis in the same countries is not rising.
- In areas of Europe where historically IBD has been uncommon or rare the incidence of both diseases is rising, although some of the rise may reflect greater access to health care with the general pattern being of an increase in UC followed by Crohn's disease, within a generation or less.
- Both diseases are now appearing in Japan and the rest of Asia.
- The incidence of Crohn's disease in children is increasing but how much of the increase is accounted for by earlier diagnosis, varying definitions of childhood and changes in diagnostic criteria is still not clear.

Overall, this pattern is in keeping with some environmental factors associated with economic development or Westernised lifestyles. Focussing on the emergence of IBD in the developing world is likely to be a fruitful area for research.

References

1 Shivananda S, Lennard-Jones J, Logan R, *et al.* Incidence of inflammatory bowel disease across Europe: is there a difference between north and south? Results of the European collaborative study on inflammatory bowel disease (EC-IBD). *Gut* 1996; 39:690–7.
2 Miller DS, Keighley AC, Langman MJ. Changing patterns in epidemiology of Crohn's disease. *Lancet* 1974;2(7882):691–3.
3 Calkins BM, Mendeloff AI. Epidemiology of inflammatory bowel disease. *Epidemiol Rev* 1986;8: 60–91.
4 Sandler RS. Epidemiology of inflammatory bowel disease. In: Targan SR, Shanahan F, eds. *Inflammatory Bowel Disease: From Bench to Bedside*. Baltimore: Williams and Wilkins; 1994:5–32.
5 Bernstein CN, Blanchard JF, Rawsthorne P, Wajda A. Epidemiology of Crohn's disease and ulcerative colitis in a central Canadian province: a population-based study. *Am J Epidemiol* 1999;149(10):916–24.
6 Loftus EV Jr, Silverstein MD, Sandborn WJ, Tremaine WJ, Harmsen WS, Zinsmeister AR. Crohn's disease in Olmsted County, Minnesota, 1940–1993: incidence, prevalence, and survival. *Gastroenterology* 1998; 114(6):1161–8.
7 Kyle J. Crohn's disease in the northeastern and northern Isles of Scotland: an epidemiological review. *Gastroenterology* 1992;103:392–9.

8. Yapp TR, Stenson R, Thomas GA, Lawrie BW, Williams GT, Hawthorne AB. Crohn's disease incidence in Cardiff from 1930: an update for 1991–1995. *Eur J Gastroenterol Hepatol* 2000;12(8):907–11.

9. Gordon FH, Montgomery SM, Hamilton MI, Pounder RE. Mortality in inflammatory bowel disease: the case for a national confidential enquiry. *Gut* 1997;40(Suppl 1):A21.

10. Sonnenberg A. Geographic variation in the incidence of and mortality from inflammatory bowel disease. *Dis Colon Rectum* 1986;29(12):854–61.

11. Sonnenberg A. Mortality from Crohn's disease and ulcerative colitis in England–Wales and the U.S. from 1950 to 1983. *Dis Colon Rectum* 1986;29(10):624–9.

12. Fonager K, Sorensen HT, Olsen J. Change in incidence of Crohn's disease and ulcerative colitis in Denmark. A study based on the National Registry of Patients, 1981–1992. *Int J Epidemiol* 1997;26(5):1003–8.

13. Primatesta P, Goldacre MJ. Crohn's disease and ulcerative colitis in England and the Oxford record linkage study area: a profile of hospitalized morbidity. *Int J Epidemiol* 1995;24(5):922–8.

14. Sonnenberg A. Hospital discharges for inflammatory bowel disease. Time trends from England and the United States. *Dig Dis Sci* 1990;35(3):375–81.

15. Lee FI, Nguyen-Van-Tam JS. Prospective study of incidence of Crohn's disease in northwest England: no increase since the late 1970's. *Eur J Gastroenterol Hepatol* 1994;6:27–31.

16. Fellows IW, Freeman JG, Holmes GKT. Crohn's disease in the city of Derby, 1951–85. *Gut* 1990; 31:1262–5.

17. Lapidus A, Bernell O, Hellers G, Persson P-G, Loftberg R. Incidence of Crohn's disease in Stockholm County 1955–89. *Gut* 1997;41:480–6.

18. Lindberg E, Jarnerot G. The incidence of Crohn's disease is not decreasing in Sweden. *Scand J Gastroenterol* 1991;26:495–500.

19. Munkholm P, Langholz E, Nielsen OH, Kreiner S, Binder V. Incidence and prevalence of Crohn's disease in the County of Copenhagen, 1962–87: a six-fold increase in incidence. *Scand J Gastroenterol* 1992; 27:609–14.

20. Srivastava ED, Mayberry JF, Morris TJ, *et al.* Incidence of ulcerative colitis in Cardiff over 20 years: 1968–87. *Gut* 1992;33:256–8.

21. Binder V. Epidemiology. In: *Inflammatory Bowel Disease*. Falk Symposium No. 96. Dordrecht: Kluwer Academic; 1998:39–43.

22. Tysk C, Jarnerot G. Ulcerative proctocolitis in Orebro, Sweden. A retrospective epidemiologic study, 1963–1987. *Scand J Gastroenterol* 1992;27:945–50.

23. Ekbom A, Helmick C, Zack M, Adami H-O. The epidemiology of inflammatory bowel disease: a large, population-based study in Sweden. *Gastroenterology* 1991;100:350–8.

24. Loftus EV Jr, Silverstein MD, Sandborn WJ, Tremaine WJ, Harmsen WS, Zinsmeister AR. Ulcerative colitis in Olmsted County, Minnesota, 1940–1993: incidence, prevalence, and survival. *Gut* 2000;46: 336–43.

25. Lapidus, A. Crohn's disease in Stockholm County – an epidemiological update 1990–2001. *Gut* 2004; 53(Suppl 1):A139.

26. Morris DL, Kyle J, Montgomery SM, Wakefield AJ, Pounder RE. Crohn's disease in North-East Scotland: a real rise in incidence. *Gut* 1999; 44(Suppl 1):A28.

27. Molinie F, Gower-Rosseau C, Yzet T, *et al.* Opposite evolution in incidence of Crohn's disease and ulcerative colitis in Northern France (1988–1999). *Gut* 2004;53:843–8.

28. Bjornsson S, Johannsson JH. Inflammatory bowel disease in Iceland, 1990–1994: a prospective, nationwide, epidemiological study. *Eur J Gastroenterol Hepatol* 2000;12(1):31–8.

29. Howarth GF, Robinson MH, Jenkins D, Hardcastle JD, Logan RF. High prevalence of undetected ulcerative colitis: data from the Nottingham fecal occult blood screening trial. *Am J Gastroenterol* 2002;97(3):690–4.

30. Moum B, Ekbom A, Vatn MH, *et al.* Inflammatory bowel disease: re-evaluation of the diagnosis in a prospective population based study in southeastern Norway. *Gut* 1997;40(3):328–32.

31. Moum B, Vatn MH, Ekbom A, *et al.* Incidence of Crohn's disease in four counties in southeastern Norway, 1990–93. A prospective population-based study. The Inflammatory Bowel South-Eastern Norway (IBSEN) Study Group of Gastroenterologists. *Scand J Gastroenterol* 1996;31(4):355–61.

32. Moum B, Vatn MH, Ekbom A, *et al.* Incidence of ulcerative colitis and indeterminate colitis in four counties of southeastern Norway, 1990–93. A prospective population-based study. The Inflammatory Bowel South-Eastern Norway (IBSEN) Study Group of Gastroenterologists. *Scand J Gastroenterol* 1996; 31(4):362–6.

33. Salupere R. Inflammatory bowel disease in Estonia: a prospective epidemiologic study 1993–1998. *World J Gastroenterol* 2001;7(3):387–8.

34. Rubin GP, Hungin AP, Kelly PJ, Ling J. Inflammatory bowel disease: epidemiology and management in an English general practice population. *Aliment Pharmacol Ther* 2000;14(12):1553–9.

35. Russel MG, Dorant E, Volovics A, et al. High incidence of inflammatory bowel disease in The Netherlands: results of a prospective study. The South Limburg IBD Study Group. *Dis Colon Rectum* 1998;41(1):33–40.
36. Latour P, Louis E, Belaiche J. Incidence of inflammatory bowel disease in the area of Liege: a 3 years prospective study (1993–1996). *Acta Gastroenterol Belg* 1998;61(4):410–3.
37. Pagenault M, Tron I, Alexandre JL, et al. Incidence of inflammatory bowel diseases in Bretagne (1994–1995). ABERMAD [Association Bertonne d'Etude et de Recherche des Maladies de l'Appareil Digesif]. *Gastroenterol Clin Biol* 1997;21(6–7):483–90.
38. Flamenbaum M, Zenut M, Aublet-Cuvelier B, et al. Incidence of inflammatory bowel diseases in the department of Puy-de-Dome in 1993 and 1994. EPIMICI [Epidemiologie des Maladies Inflammatoires Cryptogenetiques de l'Intestin group]. *Gastroenterol Clin Biol* 1997;21(6–7):491–6.
39. Lakatos L, Mester G, Erdelyi Z, et al. Striking elevation in incidence and prevalence of inflammatory bowel disease in a province of western Hungary between 1977–2001. *World J Gastroenterol* 2004;10(3):404–9.
40. Ranzi T, Bodini P, Zambelli A, et al. Epidemiological aspects of inflammatory bowel disease in a north Italian population: a 4-year prospective study. *Eur J Gastroenterol Hepatol* 1996;8(7):657–61.
41. Trallori G, Palli D, Saieva C, et al. A population-based study of inflammatory bowel disease in Florence over 15 years (1978–92). *Scand J Gastroenterol* 1996;31(9):892–9.
42. Tragnone A, Corrao G, Miglio F, Caprilli R, Lanfranchi GA. Incidence of inflammatory bowel disease in Italy: a nationwide population-based study. Gruppo Italiano per lo Studio del Colon e del Retto (GISC). *Int J Epidemiol* 1996;25(5):1044–52.
43. Manousos ON, Giannadaki E, Mouzas IA, et al. Ulcerative colitis is as common in Crete as in northern Europe: a 5-year prospective study. *Eur J Gastroenterol Hepatol* 1996;8(9):893–8.
44. Manousos ON, Koutroubakis I, Potamianos S, Roussomoustakaki M, Gourtsoyiannis N, Vlachonikolis IG. A prospective epidemiologic study of Crohn's disease in Heraklion, Crete. Incidence over a 5-year period. *Scand J Gastroenterol* 1996;31(6):599–603.
45. Tsianos EV, Katsanos KH, Christodoulou D, Dimoliatis I, Kogevinas A, Logan RF, on behalf of Northwest Greece Inflammatory Bowel Disease Study Group. Continuing low incidence of Crohn's disease in Northwest Greece. *Dig Liver Dis* 2003;35:99–103.
46. Loftus EV Jr, Silverstein MD, Sandborn WJ, Tremaine WJ, Harmsen WS, Zinsmeister AR. Ulcerative colitis in Olmsted County, Minnesota, 1940–1993: incidence, prevalence, and survival. *Gut* 2000;46(3):336–43.
47. Pinchbeck BR, Kirdeikis J, Thomson AB. Inflammatory bowel disease in northern Alberta: an epidemiologic study. *J Clin Gastroenterol* 1988;10(5):505–15.
48. Sonnenberg A, McCarty DJ, Jacobsen SJ. Geographic variation of inflammatory bowel disease within the United States. *Gastroenterology* 1991;100:143–9.
49. Sonnenberg A, Wasserman IH. Epidemiology of inflammatory bowel disease among U.S. military veterans. *Gastroenterology* 1991;101(1):122–30.
50. Armitage EL, Aldhous MC, Anderson N, et al. Incidence of juvenile-onset Crohn's disease in Scotland: association with northern latitude and affluence. *Gastroenterolgy* 2004;127:1051–7.
51. Wright JP, Froggatt J, O'Keefe EA, et al. The epidemiology of inflammatory bowel disease in Cape Town 1980–1984. *S Afr Med J* 1986;70:10–15.
52. Lee YM, Fock KM, See SJ, Ng TM, Khor C, Teo EK. Racial differences in the prevalence of ulcerative colitis and Crohn's disease in Singapore. *J Gastroenterol Hepatol* 2000;15:622–5.
53. Morita N, Toki S, Hirohashi T, et al. Incidence and prevalence of inflammatory bowel disease in Japan: nationwide epidemiological survey during the year 1991. *J Gastroenterol* 1995;30:1–4.
54. Yang SK, Loftus EV Jr, Sandborn WJ. Epidemiology of inflammatory bowel disease in Asia. *Inflamm Bowel Dis* 1001;7:260–70.
55. Yang SK, Hong WS, Min YI, et al. Incidence and prevalence of ulcerative colitis in the Songpa-Kangdong District, Seoul, Korea, 1986–1997. *J Gastroenterol Hepatol* 2000;15:1037–42.
56. Sood A, Midha V, Sood N, Bhatia AS, Avasthi G. Incidence and prevalence of ulcerative colitis in Punjab, North India. *Gut* 2003;52:1587–90.
57. Gent AE, Hellier MD, Grace RH, Swarbrick ET, Coggon D. Inflammatory bowel disease and domestic hygiene in infancy. *Lancet* 1994;343(8900):766–7.
58. Montgomery SM, Pounder RE, Wakefield AJ. Infant mortality and the incidence of inflammatory bowel disease. *Lancet* 1997;349:472–3.
59. Bernstein CN, Kraut A, Blanchard JF, Rawsthorne P, Yu N, Walld R. The relationship between inflammatory bowel disease and socioeconomic variables. *Am J Gastroenterol* 2001;96:2117–25.

60 Gilat T, Hacohen D, Lilos P, Langman MJ. Childhood factors in ulcerative colitis and Crohn's disease. An international cooperative study. *Scand J Gastroenterol* 1987;22(8):1009–24.

61 Ekbom A, Adami HO, Helmick CG, Jonzon A, Zack MM. Perinatal risk factors for inflammatory bowel disease: a case-control study. *Am J Epidemiol* 1990;132(6):1111–19.

62 Langholz E, Munkholm P, Krasilnikoff PA, Binder V. Inflammatory bowel diseases with onset in childhood. Clinical features, morbidity, and mortality in a regional cohort. *Scand J Gastroenterol* 1997;32(2):139–47.

63 Olafsdottir EJ, Fluge G, Haug K. Chronic inflammatory bowel disease in children in western Norway. *J Pediatr Gastroenterol Nutr* 1989;8(4):454–8.

64 Bentsen BS, Moum B, Ekbom A. Incidence of inflammatory bowel disease in children in southeastern Norway: a prospective population-based study 1990–94. *Scand J Gastroenterol* 2002;37(5):540–5.

65 Lindberg E, Lindquist B, Holmquist L, Hildebrand H. Inflammatory bowel disease in children and adolescents in Sweden, 1984–1995. *J Pediatr Gastroenterol Nutr* 2000;30(3):259–64.

66 Hildebrand H, Finkel Y, Grahnquist L, Lindholm J, Ekbom A, Askling J. Changing pattern of paediatric inflammatory bowel disease in northern Stockholm 1990–2001. *Gut* 2003;52(10):1432–4.

67 Kolek A, Janout V, Tichy M, Grepl M. The incidence of inflammatory bowel disease is increasing among children 15 years old and younger in the Czech Republic. *J Pediatr Gastroenterol Nutr* 2004;38(3):362–3.

68 van der Zaag-Loonen HJ, Casparie M, Taminiau JA, Escher JC, Pereira RR, Derkx HH. The incidence of pediatric inflammatory bowel disease in the Netherlands: 1999–2001. *J Pediatr Gastroenterol Nutr* 2004;38(3):302–7.

69 Tourtelier Y, Dabadie A, Tron I, *et al*. Incidence of inflammatory bowel disease in children in Brittany (1994–1997). Breton association of study and research on digestive system diseases (Abermad). *Arch Pediatr* 2000;7(4):377–84.

70 Cosgrove M, Al Atia RF, Jenkins HR. The epidemiology of paediatric inflammatory bowel disease. *Arch Dis Child* 1996;74(5):460–1.

71 Barton JR, Gillon S, Ferguson A. Incidence of inflammatory bowel disease in Scottish children between 1968 and 1983; marginal fall in ulcerative colitis, three-fold rise in Crohn's disease. *Gut* 1989;30(5):618–22.

72 Armitage E, Drummond H, Ghosh S, Ferguson A. Incidence of juvenile-onset Crohn's disease in Scotland. *Lancet* 1999;353:1496–7.

73 Hassan K, Cowan FJ, Jenkins HR. The incidence of childhood inflammatory bowel disease in Wales. *Eur J Pediatr* 2000;159(4):261–3.

74 Sawczenko A, Sandhu BK, Logan RF, *et al*. Prospective survey of childhood inflammatory bowel disease in the British Isles. *Lancet* 2001;357:1093–4.

75 Kugathasan S, Judd RH, Hoffmann RG, *et al*. Epidemiologic and clinical characteristics of children with newly diagnosed inflammatory bowel disease in Wisconsin: a statewide population-based study. *J Pediatr* 2003;143(4):525–31.

76 Phavichitr N, Cameron DJ, Catto-Smith AG. Increasing incidence of Crohn's disease in Victorian children. *J Gastroenterol Hepatol* 2003;18(3):329–32.

77 Sawczenko A, Lynn R, Sandhu BK. Variations in initial assessment and management of inflammatory bowel disease across Great Britain and Ireland. *Arch Dis Child* 2003;88:990–4.

78 Heasman MA, Clarke JA. Medical record linkage in Scotland. *Health Bull (Edinb)* 1979;37:97–103.

2: The role of genetics in inflammatory bowel disease

John B. Beckly, Tariq Ahmad and Derek P. Jewell

Introduction

In the last 20 years there has been an exponential acceleration in our understanding of human molecular genetics. Important technical advances, such as the discovery of the polymerase chain reaction in the mid-1980s [1], have substantially improved both the precision and rapidity of processing DNA. This, coupled with the recent completion of the human genome project, has heralded a new era for molecular genetics and, in particular, has allowed the study of complex polygenic diseases.

The successful identification of disease-causing genes can follow a number of different pathways, which lead to the isolation of a manageable number of candidate genes. A common strategy, since the advent of micro-satellite marker maps [2], is to perform genome-wide scans of families multiply affected by a particular disease. Loci of interest can be identified by genotyping these individuals for markers distributed evenly across the genome. Linkage is achieved at a particular locus if the extent of allelic sharing between individuals is greater than would be expected by chance. However, these loci are relatively large and fine mapping is required. This can be achieved by using a higher density of markers, usually single nucleotide polymorphisms (SNPs), in the region of interest. Association studies can then be undertaken and candidate genes tested to identify differences in the disease population compared to controls. Functional experiments are then required to confirm a pathological role for the mutant gene identified. New micro-array technology has provided a method of simultaneously analysing the expression of many hundreds of selected genes or indeed the entire genome. This new field of so-called functional genomics promises to provide a more dynamic picture of gene expression in diseased tissue and sets the stage for inflammatory bowel disease (IBD) genetics in the new millennium.

Inflammatory bowel disease: a genetically determined condition?

The observation of familial clustering of IBD was first documented by Crohn *et al.* in the early 1930s. This ultimately led to the hypothesis that there might be a genetic component to the pathogenesis of IBD. A large number of epidemiological studies based on both hospital cohorts and unselected populations have supported this finding. Studies of first-degree relatives of patients with Crohn's disease (CD) have shown a relative risk of 10–35 for developing CD and a relative risk of 3–6 for developing ulcerative colitis (UC). The risk is lower in relatives of UC patients with a relative risk of 2–15 for developing UC and 2–3 for developing CD [3]. The risk of IBD is greater if more than one first-degree relative has the condition [3], and is of consistently increased prevalence in the Jewish population [4]. The relative risk of IBD is greatest for siblings [5], especially if the proband has CD [6, 7].

Segregation studies were used in the 1980s to model the mode of inheritance in IBD and were unable to support a simple Mendelian model [8–11]. This was confirmed by more recent genome-wide linkage studies supporting a polygenic model of

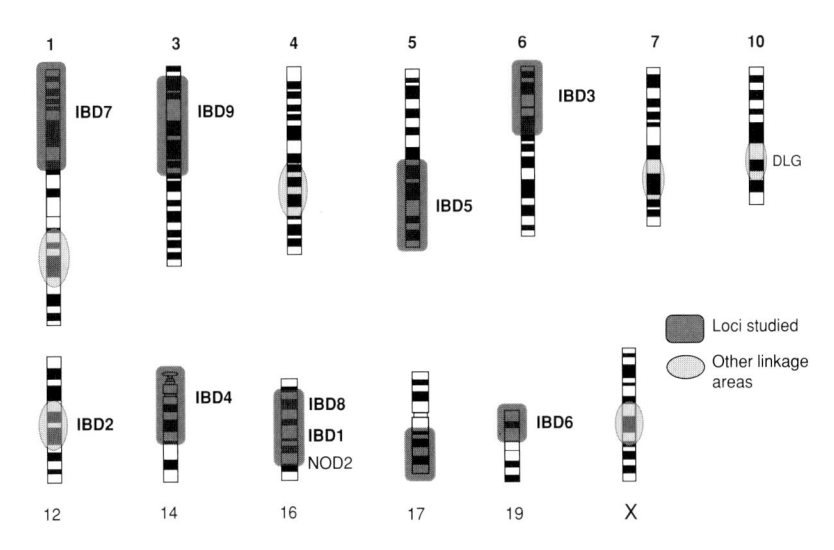

Fig 2.1 Inflammatory bowel disease linkage areas.

genetic susceptibility. Studies of twins have provided further evidence of the involvement of genes in IBD, with monozygotic twins showing greater concordance for IBD than dizygotic twins [12–15].

Disease phenotype is also genetically influenced with associations demonstrated for early disease onset, location and behaviour. It has become apparent that CD and UC are a clinical continuum influenced by an individual's underlying array of disease susceptibility and disease modifying genes. It has been proposed that these modifier genes, with no effect on disease susceptibility themselves, influence disease phenotype by interacting with a limited number of susceptibility genes, acting either alone or in combination [16]. It must be remembered that non-genetic factors also play a role in modifying disease phenotype, illustrated by the preferential CD phenotype in smokers from families susceptible to IBD [17].

These studies provide compelling evidence for the involvement of genes in the pathogenesis of IBD and also provide insight into the influence of genes on phenotype. The overlap of the CD and UC phenotypes within families challenges rigid concepts of distinct diseases and suggests a less polarised inter-play of multiple genes resulting in a given phenotype. This paves the way for a rather more robust molecular classification of IBD.

The disease susceptibility loci

Genome-wide linkage studies of multiply affected families have been a highly successful strategy in revealing a multitude of potentially relevant disease susceptibility loci, sometimes despite poor replication between studies. Since 1996 twelve genome-wide scans from Europe and North America have been published. These studies have resulted in the identification of a total of nine disease loci designated IBD1-9 (Fig 2.1). Five loci (IBD1, 2, 4–6) have met the stringent 'genome-wide' linkage criteria necessary for definite linkage [18]. IBD3 and IBD7 did not reach genome-wide significance initially, but after more focused studies there was sufficient supportive evidence for these regions to be designated as IBD loci [19, 20]. Interestingly, in a recent meta-analysis of genome-wide scans IBD3 was the only locus that met genome-wide significance whereas IBD1, IBD2 and IBD6 only demonstrated suggestive linkage [21]. There is growing evidence from the stratification of both genome-wide scans and association studies by CARD15 status and also by transmission disequilibrium testing (TDT) to support two further disease loci designated IBD8 (16p 25cMq telomeric to IBD1) [22, 23], and IBD9 (3p) [24], respectively. Two other regions are noteworthy, although they are yet to be replicated and designated as IBD loci. At the 10q23 locus, variants in the DLG5 gene that encodes an epithelial scaffolding protein, has been associated with IBD [25]. More recently, strong associations have been found on 7p14.3 between haplotypes (a series of linked alleles at different loci) in the terminal exons of NOD1 (nucleotide oligomerisation domain 1) and IBD [26]. NOD1, which is structurally similar to NOD2 (nucleotide oligomerisation domain 2) detects a tripeptide motif found in gram-negative bacterial peptidoglycan and like NOD2 activates NFκB and enhances apoptosis [27].

IBD1

In 1996 Hugot et al. identified the first IBD linkage area, designated IBD1 on the pericentromeric region of chromosome 16 [28]. This was subsequently replicated in seven further linkage studies prior to the identification of the causative gene [29–35]. It was not until 2001 that three independent groups, using rather different strategies, isolated mutations in the NOD2 gene [36–38], later renamed CARD15 (caspase-activation recruitment domain), as being significantly associated with CD. Nuñez and Cho's group initially cloned CARD15 and found that it subsequently mapped to the IBD1 locus. Sequencing of the gene in CD families revealed a frameshift mutation caused by a cytosine insertion (3020insC). A combination of transmission disequilibrium testing and case-control studies were then performed and showed significant association with CD [37]. Hampe et al. [38] followed a similar strategy aided by the knowledge of the recently cloned CARD15. In contrast, Hugot et al. [36] used pure linkage analysis methodology and found associations for the frame shift 3020insC mutation as well as two non-synonymous (amino-acid altering) SNPs (Arg702Trp and Gly908Arg), resulting in mis-sense variants of CARD15. Further, CARD15 variants have been identified but 82% of mutated alleles are accounted for by these three mutations [39].

In 2001 the IBD International Genetics Consortium [40] pooled data sets from studies that did not alone show significant linkage to IBD1 and found highly significant association with CD (logarithm of the odds (LOD) score 5.79). These apparently conflicting results merely reflect the relative underpowering of the individual studies. This is a common problem of many IBD genetic studies and accounts for much of the inter-study variability in results.

Other IBD linkage regions

A second genome-wide scan in 1996 identified genome-wide linkage, spanning part of the p and q arms on chromosome 12 (IBD2 locus) [41]. This locus has been replicated in several [32, 42, 43], but not all, studies [29, 44–46]. On current evidence, the IBD2 locus seems to be associated more with UC than with CD [40, 47]. Attempts to identify the precise gene have so far been unsuccessful.

Immune dysregulation plays a central role in the pathogenesis of IBD [48], which has resulted in considerable interest in the human leukocyte antigen complex (HLA) on chromosome 6p (IBD3). This region is highly polymorphic and gene-dense and includes the HLA class I, II and III genes. Although there have been numerous serological studies showing associations between class I and II HLA antigens and IBD, many of these early studies were underpowered. In an early molecular study by Satsangi and colleagues [49] linkage was demonstrated for UC with the HLA class II DRB1 locus and the DRB1 DQB haplotype. This group then went on to show in a case-control study significant associations for UC and the DRB1* 0103 and DRB1*12 alleles, a finding replicated in several other studies [50, 51]. For CD an American genome-wide scan provided suggestive evidence of linkage to chromosome 6p [52]. However, perhaps the most compelling evidence for linkage to this region comes from a collaborative Northern European study. In an initial genome-wide scan suggestive, but not significant, linkage to IBD3 was achieved [29]. In a subsequent follow-on study by the same group, using a higher density of markers, highly significant linkage for both CD and UC was demonstrated [20]. This finding was later independently replicated [53].

A study from Pittsburgh showed genome-wide significance to chromosome 14q (IBD4) for CD [43]. This supported previous data from two other North

American studies: Ma et al. [52] who found suggestive linkage to this locus for CD, and Cho et al. who showed nominal linkage in mixed CD and UC families [42]. A European study also provided support for the IBD4 locus [54].

In addition to the IBD4 linkage in the genome-wide scan by Ma et al. [52], suggestive linkage to a region on chromosome 5q (IBD5) was also found. A Canadian study of 158 sib-pair families also found suggestive linkage to this region [45]. High density mapping of the 5q locus resulted in significant linkage for CD [45] and subsequent linkage disequilibrium mapping revealed a common haplotype spanning 250 kb across the cytokine gene cluster [55]. This haplotype imparts a CD relative risk of 2 for heterozygotes and 6 for homozygotes [55]. These findings were then replicated by the same group in a second cohort [56] and by other independent groups [57, 58]. Giallourakis and colleagues [56] demonstrated that the IBD5 locus acts independently from CARD15 in conferring risk to CD, but epistatically (interaction between different genes) with CARD15 for conferring risk to UC. This association with UC was supported by a single-centre UK study that also found epistasis between CARD15 and the IBD5 risk haplotype for this phenotype [59], although only for the Arg702Trp mutation. Recently, variants in two genes (SLC22A4 and SLC22A5) encoding the organic cationic transporter proteins OCTN1 and OCTN2 have been identified as possibly being the relevant genes within the IBD5 linkage region. A two-allele (SLC22A4/SLC22A5) risk haplotype (SLC22A–TC) of these variants has been shown to be significantly associated with CD [60]. No association has been seen for this haplotype with UC even after stratification by CARD15 variants [61]. However, there is marked linkage disequilibrium within this region and these genes may therefore be only linked to the causative gene as part of an extended haplotype. Further replication and higher density mapping of this region is required before firm conclusions can be drawn.

Genome-wide significance to a region on 19p (IBD6) has also been demonstrated for the combined CD and UC phenotypes [45]. The IBD6 locus contains several gene candidates, but the most replicated is the association between ICAM-1 variants and IBD [62–64]. A study by van Heel and colleagues [22] stratified a genome-wide scan of 137 CD affected relative pairs by the common CARD15 mutations and the IBD5 haplotype. This approach provides a method by which genetic heterogeneity can be reduced, thus increasing the power of genome-wide scans to find minor susceptibility loci. In addition, epistatic relationships can be determined. Using this method, linkage to the chromosome 19 (IBD6) locus was only seen in CARD15 negative CD pairs. Further evidence for linkage to this locus was seen for CD pairs stratified for one or two copies of the IBD5 risk haplotype, demonstrating epistasis between IBD5 and 6 [22]. However, the lack of linkage to IBD6 in an earlier genome-wide scan by Hampe et al. [65] remained after stratification by CARD15 variants.

A North American genome-wide scan of Ashkenazi and non-Ashkenazi Jewish families demonstrated suggestive linkage to the 1p (IBD7) locus [34]. However, after stratification by ethnicity, linkage to IBD7 was found to be exclusive to non-Ashkenazi Caucasian families. The same group performed both linkage and linkage disequilibrium analysis on a genetically isolated population of unrelated American Chaldeans with IBD. They hypothesised that the degree of linkage disequilibrium around disease-causing mutations should be increased in this isolated population. Linkage and linkage disequilibrium at the same 1p locus as that found in the out bred population was subsequently demonstrated providing sufficient evidence for a major IBD susceptibility locus [19].

The IBD8 locus on 16p has, as previously mentioned, been identified by CARD15 stratification of linkage studies. A study by Hampe et al. [23] performed high-density micro-satellite marker mapping to further define the broad IBD1 linkage region from previous genome-wide scans. This strategy revealed three linkage peaks within the IBD1 region with the highest central peak located at the CARD15 position. Stratification by CARD15 variant negative patients resulted in a diminished CARD15 peak, but maintenance of the other flanking peaks. This suggested the presence of two further IBD susceptibility genes. Further association studies revealed a common haplotype that was significantly associated with CD only in the CARD15 variant negative patients [23]. The more recent stratified genome-wide scan of CD patients by van Heel and colleagues [22] confirmed a second locus in CARD15 variant negative patients 25cM q telomeric to IBD1.

In Satsangi et al.'s [41] 1996 genome-wide scan there was suggestive linkage for the combined IBD phenotype to chromosome 3p21. This finding was not significantly replicated in subsequent genome-wide scans. However, in 2001 Hampe and colleagues performed fine mapping of the region and replicated the earlier linkage to 3p21 as well as demonstrating a second p telomeric linkage peak [66]. A North American study further analysed this region by first performing TDT analysis (a method that circumvents the problem of population stratification) of a previous genome-wide scan and then an extended linkage analysis [24]. These data revealed significant linkage to 3p26 in IBD patients, approximately 10cM, from the second linkage peak seen in Hampe et al.'s study. These are likely to represent the same locus and provide sufficient evidence for this to be designated IBD9.

CARD15: ethnic heterogeneity

The international interest in CARD15 has resulted in sufficient data to gain some insight into the contribution of CARD15 polymorphisms in different populations. A recent large meta-analysis [67] looked at 42 international study cohorts, 37 of which were from Caucasian and 5 from Asian descent. No associations were seen in the Asian populations. In the Caucasian populations of non-Jewish descent, carriage of one high-risk CARD15 allele overall conferred a 3.15 times greater risk of CD (Arg702Trp: OR 2.20, Gly908Arg: OR 2.99 and 3020insC: OR 4.09). In the Jewish Caucasian population data was sparser, but the common CARD15 variants conferred a lower risk than in the non-Jewish population (Arg702Trp: OR 1.74, Gly908Arg: OR 1.93 and 3020insC: OR 2.45). Those carrying two or more risk alleles had an odds ratio of 17.1 for CD compared to people without high-risk alleles. The overall CD attributable fraction for the risk alleles was 12.7%. After exclusion of patients of Jewish descent this increased to 21.8% [67].

There is a trend towards higher rates of IBD in Northern European compared to Southern European populations, although the European Collaborative study on IBD was unable to show a clear delineation [68]. This delineation is similarly unclear in relation to the common CARD15 variants with a reduced contribution to CD phenotype demonstrated in Irish [69, 70], Scottish [70, 71] and Finnish populations [72]. However, strong associations between the CARD15 variants and CD have been seen in other Northern European populations. In a collaborative study of German and British cohorts (excluding Scottish) Hampe et al. [38] estimated that the 3020insC frameshift mutation accounted for approximately 18% of genetic risk of CD. This was further supported by a collaborative study in a similar cohort of British, German and Dutch patients, which also showed strong associations with the common CARD15 mutations and CD [73]. The authors estimated that heterozygotes for CARD15 mutations have a three-fold increased risk and that homozygotes and compound heterozygotes have a 20-fold increased risk of CD. In a single centre British cohort Ahmad and colleagues confirmed the increased risk of the three common CARD15 mutations and showed a relative risk of 6.5 for the 3020insC frameshift and a relative risk of 2.3 and 2.6 for the 908Arg and 702Trp mis-sense mutations respectively [74]. Studies from Denmark [75], Belgium [76, 77], Netherlands [78], Spain [79, 80] and Italy [81–83] have all confirmed the association of some but not all of the common CARD15 variants with CD. The most consistently replicated association is that of the 3020insC mutation. However, a study from Greece [84] was unable to demonstrate associations with this mutation and CD indicating that genetic heterogeneity of CARD15 mutations in Europe is not solely limited to the Northern populations.

Positive associations for CD and CARD15 mutations outside of Europe include studies from the United States [37, 85–87], Canada [88], Israel [89] and Australia [90]. The higher rates of CD in the Jewish population, and in particular Ashkenazi versus non-Ashkenazi Jews, are well described [91, 92]. Fidder et al. [89] showed lower CARD15 mutations in the Jewish Israeli population compared to the non-Jewish European studies. A North American study [87] stratified their CD patients and controls into Ashkenazi Jewish and white non-Jewish. They showed that patients had similar allele frequencies for the 3020insC frameshift mutation between the two ethnic groups. Case-control analysis also revealed significant associations for this mutation and CD in both ethnic groups. Similarly, a positive association between the 908Arg mutation and CD was found in both groups, but interestingly the allele frequency of the 908Arg mutation was higher in the Jewish compared to non-Jewish patients [87]. This is perhaps not surprising for a risk allele in a population with a high prevalence of CD [93]. However, the converse was true for the 702Trp mutation with no association seen with CD in the Jewish patients. However, as with the 908Arg mutation, higher allele frequencies were seen in this group [87]. Data from two separate studies have suggested that the increased prevalence of CD in the Jewish population may be from CARD15 mutations other than the three common ones [94, 95].

CARD15 mutations impart risk of CD primarily to Caucasian populations. African Americans have a significantly reduced allele frequency of the common mutations compared to their Caucasian counterparts, although unique variants have been detected [96]. The CARD15 mutations are absent in Asian populations studied; specifically no mutations have been found in Japanese [97, 98], Chinese [99] and Korean [94] studies.

CARD15 and phenotype

The most comprehensive study of phenotype/genotype associations have been in relation to CARD15 mutations. Although all CD phenotypes are represented in both CARD15 positive and negative patients, a consistent association is that of CARD15 mutations and ileal disease [72–74, 88, 100–102]. Ahmad and colleagues [74] genotyped 244 meticulously phenotyped CD patients with a median follow-up of 16 years and found that all patients with the CARD15 3020insC frameshift mutation and all compound heterozygotes and homozygotes of the other two common mutations had ileal disease. Economou et al.'s 2004 meta-analysis [67] gave an odds ratio of 2.53 for the development of small bowel CD if at least one high-risk variant was present. In the Jewish populations studied no clear associations could be found.

Disease behaviour is less consistent across studies. This is in part a reflection of the problem of accurate phenotyping as well as the changing pattern of disease over time [16]. Ahmad et al.'s study [74] showed that the CARD15 frameshift mutation protected against fistulating disease but was associated positively with stenotic disease. This association with stenotic disease was also demonstrated in Economou et al.'s meta-analysis [67]. However, the association for stenotic disease is not independent of ileal disease and perhaps is only a consequence of inflammation at that site [74, 77]. Indeed, Louis et al. [77] showed that in patients with no stricturing or perforating disease at diagnosis, 11% developed stricturing and 22% penetrating disease at 5 years. This was independent of CARD15 status [77]. Likewise, the reported higher rate of surgery in patients with CARD15 variants may also just reflect the preponderance of ileal disease [74]. However, there have been several studies that have shown independent associations of CARD15, ileal disease and fibrostenotic disease behaviour [100, 102]. Familial disease [67] and early age of disease onset has also been associated with CARD15 variants [39, 74]. There have been no consistent associations between the CARD15 variants and extra-intestinal manifestations of IBD [39, 88].

CARD15: pathogenesis

CARD15 is a member of the Apaf-1 transcription factors. It functions as an intra-cellular cytoplasmic receptor for muramyl dipeptide (MDP) [103, 104], which is a component of peptidoglycan found in the walls of both gram-positive and gram-negative bacteria and results in the activation of the intra-cellular signalling molecule nuclear factor-κB (NF-κB) (Fig. 2.2) [105]. The MDP combines with the leucine-rich region (LRR) of the CARD15 protein [103, 104, 106], which is the region where the three common mutations associated with CD are found [36]. How these mutations are involved in

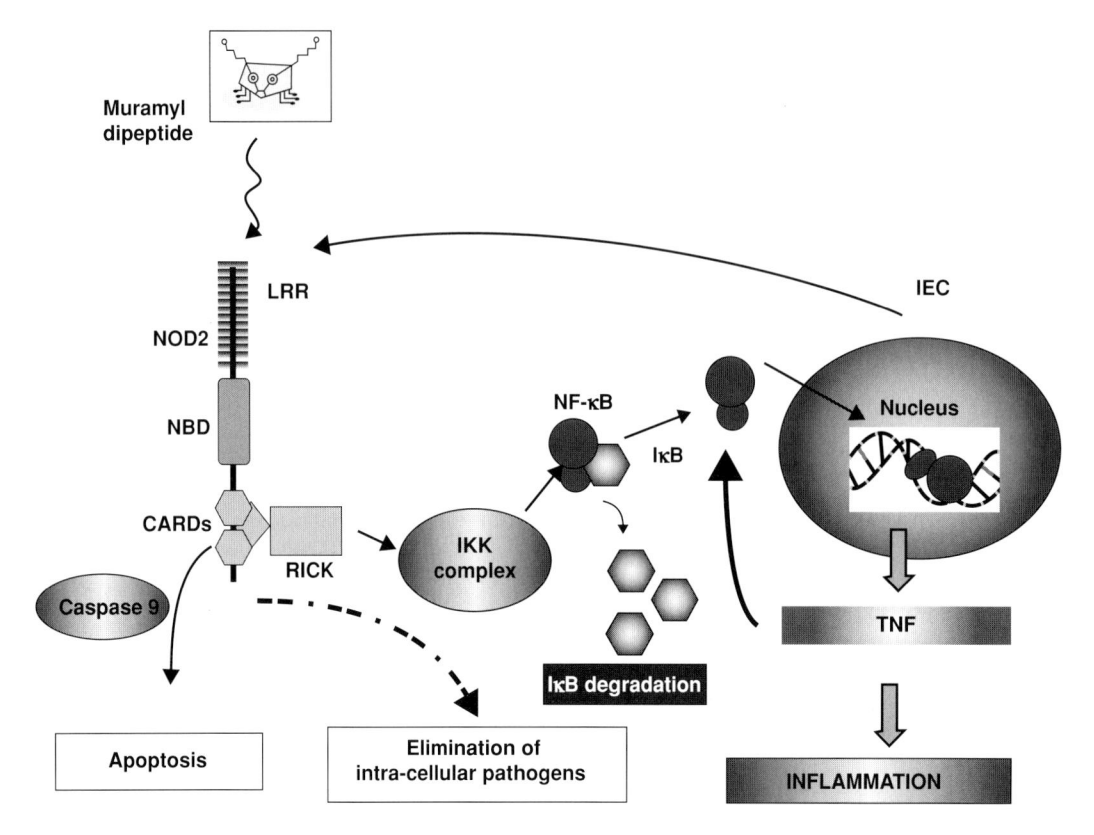

Fig 2.2 CARD15 intra-cellular signalling.

the pathogenesis of CD is not clear. The mutations are able to influence the function of the CARD15 protein but the results are highly dependent on the model system used. Data from experimental cell lines have shown that the common CARD15 variants, in particular the 3020insC frameshift mutation, result in reduced NFκB activation following stimulation with MDP [87, 107]. This defective NFκB activation seems to be at odds with the finding of raised NF-κB seen in IBD tissues [108]. CARD15 was initially thought to be solely expressed in monocytes [105], but was subsequently also found to be expressed in dendritic cells and intestinal epithelial cells (IECs) [109, 110]. Hisamatsu and colleagues demonstrated that in IECs CARD15 was vital for effective killing of *S. typhimurium* and that IECs transfected with the CARD15 3020insC frameshift variant lost the ability to affect this bacterial killing [110]. This abnormality of intra-cellular bacterial clearance provides a potential mechanism by which enteric bacteria may be involved in establishing chronic intestinal inflammation in CD.

In CARD15 knockout mice models there is no enhancement of either spontaneous or chemically induced colitis [111, 112]. In contrast to the earlier experimental cell line models, a recent study by Maeda *et al.* [113] demonstrated that in mice harbouring the 3020insC frameshift mutation, treatment of bone marrow derived macrophages with MDP resulted in a greater rise in NFκB compared to wild-type mice. Several NFκB target genes, in particular IL-1β were also increased in the CARD15 variant macrophages compared to wild-type. A similar effect of augmented NFκB activity and expression of pro-inflammatory cytokines was seen in the colons of dextran sodium sulphate (DSS) treated 3020insC mutated mice [113]. DSS disrupts the epithelial barrier allowing bacterial exposure of resident lamina propria macrophages. Concurrent DSS and antibiotic treatment of the mice negates any differences between CARD15 variant and wild-type mice and overall inflammation is much attenuated [113]. Co-administration of DSS and IL-1 receptor antagonist also resulted in attenuation of the inflammatory response [113]. This is consistent with the finding of raised intestinal IL-1 in IBD and a relative deficiency of the naturally occurring IL-1 receptor antagonist, suggesting a potentially important role of this cytokine in CD [114]. Kobayashi and colleagues [112], in the same edition of *Science*, generated CARD15 knockout mice and challenged them consecutively with intravenous, intra-peritoneal and intra-gastric *Listeria monocytogenes*. No differences were seen between the knockout and wild-type mice for the intravenous and intraperitoneal routes. However, intragastric *L. monocytogenes* resulted in a significantly increased number of bacteria recovered from the liver and spleens of the knockout mice suggesting a central role for CARD15 in preventing enteric bacterial infection [112]. It has recently been demonstrated that in MDP-stimulated primary human peripheral blood mononuclear cells, CARD15 mutations result in defective CARD15/toll-like receptor pathways and CARD15/IL-8 neutrophil recruitment [115], providing a putative mechanism for this abnormal bacterial clearance.

A recent report in the haematology literature demonstrated the involvement of CARD15 mutations in graft-versus-host disease (GvHD) following allogeneic bone marrow transplantation. Clinically gastrointestinal GvHD is associated with a poor prognosis [116]. Experimental data suggests that the gastrointestinal tract is central to the pathogenesis of GvHD and that translocated bacteria through the damaged epithelial barrier result in massive cytokine release from macrophages and an augmentation of systemic disease [117]. Holler et al. [116] showed that the cumulative incidence of GvHD was greatest if both donor and recipient harboured CARD15 mutations with the lowest incidence if both were wild-type. If one or other of the donor or recipient harboured the mutations then the cumulative incidence was at a middle point between wild-type and combined donor and recipient mutants.

CARD15 expression has been demonstrated in Paneth cells [118], which are specialised intestinal epithelial cells found throughout the small intestine but most highly concentrated in the terminal ileum [119]. They secrete a variety of antibacterial products, including α-defensins, and play an important role both in gut flora homeostasis as well as providing protection against enteric pathogens [119, 120]. In mice, CARD15 is also expressed in terminal ileal Paneth cells [112]. In Kobayashi and colleague's mouse knockout model, gene expression using micro-array analysis was measured before and after intra-gastric *Listeria* infection. The most striking finding was a constitutively low expression of a subgroup of cryptidins (α-defensins in humans) in the knockout mice compared to wild-type, which further reduced following *Listeria* infection [112]. This supports human data demonstrating that Paneth cells from NOD2 mutated CD patients show decreased α-defensin 5 expression [121]. The role of the Paneth cell in the aetiopathology of CD is becoming increasingly apparent and provides a convincing explanation for the preponderance of CD in the terminal ileum.

The exact mechanism by which CARD15 mutations are involved in the pathogenesis of CD remains to be elucidated. However, recent functional data has significantly advanced our understanding. These studies suggest that abnormal bacterial sensing through impaired MDP/CARD15 interaction results in defective enteric bacterial clearance. This increased susceptibility to enteric infection is mediated through abnormal innate immune responses and subsequent defective adaptive immunity. This abnormal immune response to pathogenic bacteria may also hold true for non-pathogenic bacteria. A breakdown in immune tolerance to the normal enteric flora by defective bacterial sensing and epithelial invasion could result in the chronic inflammation seen in CD.

IBD3: the HLA and IBD

There have been a large number of serological and molecular association studies implicating the classical HLA class I and II molecules in the pathogenesis of IBD. A meta-analysis of a combination of

29 serological and genetic HLA studies demonstrated significant positive associations between DR2 (subtype DRB1*1502), DR9 and DRB1*0103 with UC and DRB3*0301, DR7 and DQ4 with CD. Negative associations were demonstrated for CD with DR2 and DR3 [122]. A later study by Ahmad et al. [50] supported these findings and demonstrated a protective effect of the HLA haplotype DRB1*0401–DQB1*0301 for UC.

The HLA class III region harbours many genes that are important in the immune response and includes several excellent IBD candidate genes. Rather tantalisingly, in a linkage analysis of a Northern European cohort the tumour necrosis factor-α (TNF-α) gene was close to the peak of linkage [20]. Five functional SNPs in the TNF-α and the related lymphotoxin-α (LTA) (important in the development of oral tolerance [123]) genes were therefore tested in an association analysis [20]. Disappointingly, no associations were found despite the good evidence for the involvement of TNF-α in the pathogenesis of IBD [124–127]. The authors speculated that variations in TNF-α act as modulators in the inflammatory response rather than predisposing to IBD [20]. A variety of other studies have looked for associations between TNF, LTA and the heat shock proteins (known to be upregulated in IBD), although results have generally been inconsistent. A family based association study by van Heel et al. [128] looked at the common TNF promoter polymorphisms TNF-1031T/C, -863C/A, -857C/T and -308G/A. An association was found with the common TNF-857C allele and both UC and the combined IBD phenotype but not with the other mutations. Interestingly, after stratification there was significant association between this mutation and CD in patients who were CARD15 negative [128]. This finding is rather contradicted by an Australian study that found the strongest association of TNF-857C and CD in patients with CARD15 risk alleles [129]. Functional studies have shown that the TNF-857C mutation reduces inhibitory OCT1 binding to NFκB thereby providing a possible mechanism for its role in IBD [128]. In contrast to van Heel and colleagues' study, others have shown significant associations between the TNF-1031T/C [130, 131], -308G/A [132] mutations and CD.

Although the classical HLA regions have been the most intensely studied, there is a growing body of evidence of important IBD associations with the non-classical HLA class I region. Of particular interest in this region is the MIC gene family. MICA and MICB encode stress inducible glycoproteins expressed on various epithelial cells and intestinal cells and are important in the activation of both the innate and adaptive immune system [133]. A small Japanese study by Seki et al. [134] showed an association between the MICA A6 variant and UC. However, this finding was not replicated in a slightly larger German study [135]. Although differences in statistical power between the two studies might be responsible for this lack of replication, ethnic differences may play an important role. There is certainly significant ethnic variation in IBD associations across the HLA region. This is exemplified by the classical DRB1*1502 allele, which is most strongly associated with UC in Japanese populations [136, 137]. A study by Ahmad et al. [133] genotyped UC, CD and ethnically matched controls for 46 of the 54 MICA alleles, all 17 MICB alleles as well as micro-satellite genotyping of the exon 5 variable number of tandem repeats. No significant disease associations were found [133].

Progress towards finding disease-associated genes in this region is a challenge and is hampered by the low genotype relative risk of IBD-associated HLA alleles reducing statistical power [138], the complex linkage disequilibrium in the region [139] and the fact that there may be more than one susceptibility gene [140].

IBD3: HLA variants and phenotype

A variety of genotype/phenotype associations have been described both for individual allelic variants and for haplotypes. The relatively rare HLA-DRB1*0103 allele is associated with pure colonic disease in CD patients [74, 141] and extensive and severe disease requiring colectomy in UC patients [50, 51, 142–144]. However, its low allele frequency in the population limits its usefulness in disease prediction but does raise the interesting idea of a common molecular mechanism for colonic IBD. Ahmad and colleagues showed that a classical HLA autoimmune haplotype (A1-B8-DR3), associated with immunopathology in other diseases, was associated with colonic CD [74]. The TNF-308A risk polymorphism found in this haplotype was also associated with colonic CD in a study from Belgium [145]. Homozygotes for a TNF promoter polymorphism haplotype (TNF -1031T, -863C, -380G, -238G) that results in reduced gene transcription is associated with stable distal UC [50]. The MICA*010 and DRB*0103 alleles have both been associated with perianal disease [74].

There have been several associations between HLA variants and extra-intestinal manifestations (EIMs) of disease. Type I peripheral arthropathy (migratory, pauciarticular, large joint arthritis linked to IBD relapse and other EIMs) is associated with HLA-B*27 and the linked alleles B*35 and DRB1*0103, whilst type II peripheral arthropathy (chronic symmetric, small joint arthritis unrelated to disease activity) is associated with HLA-B*44 [146]. Positive associations have also been found for HLA-B*27 and DRB1*0103 with uveitis, and TNF-1031C with erythema nodosum [147]. Many other genotype/phenotype associations have been described, although all lack convincing replication reflecting the problem of identifying genes in a region where there is marked linkage disequilibrium.

IBD5: ethnic heterogeneity and phenotypic associations

A variety of studies from North America and Europe have replicated the association between the IBD5 risk haplotype and CD [55–58, 148]. However, there is evidence of ethnic heterogeneity at this locus. The IBD-risk haplotype is extremely rare in the Japanese [58] and Newman and colleagues [61] recently showed that the SLC22A-TC haplotype was less associated with CD in Jewish compared to non-Jewish patients.

There have been several studies that have shown genotype/phenotype associations with the IBD5 locus. Armuzzi and colleagues [57] looked for a variety of associations between the IBD5 risk haplotype in both CD and UC cohorts. An association was demonstrated between this haplotype and perianal CD with a three-fold increase seen in homozygotes. Homozygosity for this risk-haplotype has also been associated with early onset of disease [148] although this was a finding not replicated by Armuzzi et al. [57]. Newman et al. [61] recently reported, in patients homozygous for the SLC22A-TC haplotype, a significantly increased risk of terminal ileal disease (OR 2.42). This effect was lost in patients heterozygous for this haplotype. The combination of the SLC22A-TC haplotype and CARD15 mutations substantially increased the risk of terminal ileal disease (OR 4.61) to a level greater than each risk genotype alone. No association was seen for perianal disease and this haplotype [61].

IBD genetics: translation to clinical practice

The rapidly moving field of IBD genetics has undoubtedly improved our understanding of a number of aspects of the pathogenesis of CD and UC, although perhaps more questions have been raised than answered. From a clinical standpoint the field is still in its infancy with the impact of many of these molecular discoveries unlikely to be felt in mainstream practice for several years. It is intriguing to speculate how the common CARD15 mutations may play a role in disease prediction and outcome. Apart from robustly predicting both early disease onset and localisation to the ileum other associations such as disease behaviour, outcome of therapy, need for surgery and occurrence of EIMs have been inconsistent. Vermiere and colleagues [149] looked at the usefulness of CARD15 mutations in patients with indeterminate colitis and their ability to predict final disease phenotype. Their data revealed a disappointingly low specificity (77.6) and positive predictive value (7.1%) for patients with CARD15 variants eventually developing the CD phenotype, although numbers were rather small to draw definite conclusions [149]. Despite a variety of genotype/phenotype associations within the HLA region the lack of consistency and relatively low allele frequencies of disease-associated mutations are at present a barrier to any clinical application.

Pharmacogenetics

A field that does show some promise in current clinical practice is that of pharmacogenetics. The development of new therapeutic targets as a result of understanding the molecular mechanisms underpinning IBD is the pharmacogenetic goal. However, by far the greatest clinical impact at present and for the foreseeable future is in predicting response and side effects of current pharmacotherapies. This is exemplified by thiopurine S-methyltransferase (TPMT) polymorphisms and azathioprine (AZA)/ 6-mercaptopurine (6-MP) toxicity. The therapeutically active metabolites of these compounds are the 6-thioguanine nucleotides (6-TGNs) whose production is limited by xanthine oxidase and TPMT. Xanthine oxidase is absent in haematological tissue and therefore there is no secondary pathway to prevent high levels of myelotoxic 6-TGNs if the TPMT pathway is defective. Several TPMT variants that cause reduced enzymatic activity have been identified of which TPMT*2 and TPMT*3A are the most common [150–152]. Genotyping patients for alleles that confer reduced TPMT activity provides a way of identifying homozygotes who are likely to develop severe myelotoxicity on receiving AZA/6-MP and heterozygotes who may require a reduced dose. However, the majority of patients who develop myelotoxity do not have an enzyme altering TPMT polymorphism, suggesting that other unrelated mechanism have a greater influence on haematological side effects [153]. Because only 0.3% of the general population are homozygotes, for these polymorphisms it is questionable whether routine genotyping for these variants prior to starting thiopurine therapy should become standard clinical practice [154].

Methotrexate (MTX) provides an alternative to AZA/6-MP in patients who have either not been able to tolerate them or have shown poor response. Although the therapeutic mechanism of action of MTX is poorly understood, its metabolism is better delineated. A variety of polymorphisms have been identified in genes encoding components of the metabolic pathway. A study by Laverdiere et al. [155] showed that a polymorphism in the reduced folate carrier gene (RFC1) was associated with higher plasma MTX concentrations. Polymorphisms in the folypolyglutamase hydrolase (FPGH) gene, an enzyme that is important in the cellular efflux of MTX, has been associated with reduced enzyme activity [156]. MTX may exert therapeutic effect partly by diminishing reduced folate stores. Methylenetetrahydrofolate reductase (MTHFR) is vital in folate homeostasis and polymorphisms in the MTHFR are associated with MTX efficacy [157–159] and toxicity [159, 160]. A recent association study from Oxford looked at polymorphisms in the RFC1, FPGH and MTHFR genes and their effect on MTX efficacy and toxicity in IBD patients. A significant association was found between the MTHFR 1298C variant and MTX toxicity, particularly nausea and vomiting, but no association between any of these polymorphisms and efficacy was observed (Herrlinger K., 2005. Unpublished data).

Remission of active IBD is often effectively achieved with glucocorticoid therapy. However, some patients either do not respond to steroids or become dependent on them to prevent disease re-activation. Several mechanisms have been implicated in steroid responsiveness. There has been great interest in the multi-drug resistance 1 (MDR1) and the related transporter of antigenic peptide 2 (TAP2) genes. MDR1 encodes a drug efflux pump found on both lymphocytes and intestinal epithelial cells that actively transports glucocorticoids and several other drugs out of the cell [161]. Farrell and colleagues [162] found that increased MDR expression in peripheral blood lymphocytes was associated with the need for surgery in both CD and UC. A variety of polymorphisms have been identified in the MDR1 gene of which the C3435T variant has been the most thoroughly investigated and has been associated with UC [163]. However, studies investigating both this and other polymorphisms in the MDR1 gene have been disappointingly inconsistent. An interesting study by Heresbach et al. [164] showed that steroid unresponsiveness in CD patients was associated with SNPs in the TAP2 gene. Another important site of glucocorticoid resistance is the glucocorticoid receptor β. Steroid refractory UC is associated with a splice variant of the receptor that results in reduced signal transduction [165].

5-Aminosalicylates (5-ASA) have an important role in the maintenance of remission of UC. The acetylation of 5-ASA is catalysed by N-acetyltransferase 1 (NAT1) in the intestinal mucosa. Sulfapyridine is a toxic metabolite of sulphasalazine following breakdown by gut bacteria and is metabolised by NAT2 in the liver. Several polymorphisms have been identified in the genes of both of these enzymes but to date no associations have been found between these mutations and 5-ASA efficacy or sulfasalazine side effects [166].

The relatively novel anti-TNF monoclonal antibody infliximab has become rapidly established in the therapeutic armoury of CD with the original study by Targan et al. [127] showing a remission rate of 33% following a single dose. Infliximab's primary mechanism of action may be the induction of apoptosis by binding to transmembrane TNF on activated immune cells. This apoptotic effect is not seen with etanercept and perhaps explains its lack of efficacy in CD [167]. Unsurprisingly, molecular studies of infliximab efficacy have focused on the TNF gene and closely approximated regions. A North American study [168] found that the TNF micro-satellite haplotype 11-4-1-3-3 showed a trend towards a reduced response to infliximab. The same group then genotyped SNPs in the LTA and promoter of the TNF gene and found that patients who were homozygous for the Nco1-TNFc-aa13L-aa26 1-1-1-1 haplotype did not respond to infliximab [168]. Despite the attraction of TNF polymorphisms playing a pivotal role in infliximab efficacy there have been very few studies with positive associations. A large multicentre study looked at multiple SNPs in the TNF promoter and TNF receptor genes and showed a lack of association with infliximab response [131]. The lack of association at the TNF-308 position found in this study was replicated in a Belgian cohort [169]. This failure to demonstrate an association between clinical response and TNF polymorphisms is perhaps not surprising due to infliximab's predominately apoptotic effect on lymphocytes rather than as an anti-TNF agent. There have been more than 70 other biologic agents evaluated in IBD. Recently, promise has been shown for the fully humanised anti-TNFα monoclonal antibody, Adalimubab. Shen and colleagues demonstrated both monocyte apoptosis and IL-10 and IL-12 down-regulation with this agent [170]. It appears that there is a role for Adalimubab in CD patients who either cannot tolerate or have had a loss of response to infliximab [171]. It waits to be seen how genetic polymorphisms influence these newer agents.

Conclusions

Molecular genetics is rapidly gaining centre stage in many fields of medicine and IBD is no exception. Since the first IBD genome-wide scan in 1996 and the subsequent discovery of CARD15 there have been numerous studies revealing a multitude of disease associations. The identification of many susceptibility loci has both confirmed the polygenic nature of IBD and has provided broad regions for further detailed studies. Despite the limitations of case-control studies several important genotype/phenotype associations have been discovered with the promise of a more valid molecular rather than clinical classification of disease. The ultimate goal will be to individualise patient care based on a genetic profile providing accurate information for diagnosis, prognosis and treatment. The unravelling of this complex field is still in its formative years, but at the current pace real clinical application should not be far off.

References

1 Mullis K, Faloona F, Scharf S, et al. Specific enzymatic amplification of DNA in vitro: the polymerase chain reaction. *Cold Spring Harb Symp Quant Biol* 1986; 51(Pt 1):263–73.
2 Weissenbach J, Gyapay G, Dib C, et al. A second-generation linkage map of the human genome. *Nature* 1992;359(6398):794–801.
3 RK Russel JS. IBD: a family affair. *Best Pract Res Clin Gastroenterol* 2004;18(3):525–39.
4 Yang H, McElree C, Roth MP, et al. Familial empirical risks for inflammatory bowel disease: differences between Jews and non-Jews. *Gut* 1993;34(4):517–24.
5 van Heel DA, Satsangi J, Carey AH, Jewell DP. Inflammatory bowel disease: progress toward a gene. *Can J Gastroenterol* 2000;14(3):207–18.

6 Orholm M, Munkholm P, Langholz E, et al. Familial occurrence of inflammatory bowel disease. *N Engl J Med* 1991;324(2):84–8.

7 Probert CS, Jayanthi V, Hughes AO, et al. Prevalence and family risk of ulcerative colitis and Crohn's disease: an epidemiological study among Europeans and south Asians in Leicestershire. *Gut* 1993;34(11):1547–51.

8 Forabosco P, Collins A, Latiano A, et al. Combined segregation and linkage analysis of inflammatory bowel disease in the IBD1 region using severity to characterise Crohn's disease and ulcerative colitis. On behalf of the GISC. *Eur J Hum Genet* 2000;8(11):846–52.

9 Orholm M, Iselius L, Sorensen TI, et al. Investigation of inheritance of chronic inflammatory bowel diseases by complex segregation analysis. *BMJ* 1993;306(6869):20–4.

10 Monsen U, Iselius L, Johansson C, Hellers G. Evidence for a major additive gene in ulcerative colitis. *Clin Genet* 1989;36(6):411–4.

11 Kuster W, Pascoe L, Purrmann J, Funk S, Majewski F. The genetics of Crohn disease: complex segregation analysis of a family study with 265 patients with Crohn disease and 5,387 relatives. *Am J Med Genet* 1989;32(1):105–8.

12 Orholm M, Binder V, Sorensen TI, Rasmussen LP, Kyvik KO. Concordance of inflammatory bowel disease among Danish twins. Results of a nationwide study. *Scand J Gastroenterol* 2000;35(10):1075–81.

13 Thompson NP, Driscoll R, Pounder RE, Wakefield AJ. Genetics versus environment in inflammatory bowel disease: results of a British twin study. *BMJ* 1996;312(7023):95–6.

14 Tysk C, Lindberg E, Jarnerot G, Floderus-Myrhed B. Ulcerative colitis and Crohn's disease in an unselected population of monozygotic and dizygotic twins. A study of heritability and the influence of smoking. *Gut* 1988;29(7):990–6.

15 Halfvarson J, Bodin L, Tysk C, Lindberg E, Jarnerot G. Inflammatory bowel disease in a Swedish twin cohort: a long-term follow-up of concordance and clinical characteristics. *Gastroenterology* 2003;124(7):1767–73.

16 Ahmad T, Marshall S, Jewell D. Genotype-based phenotyping heralds a new taxonomy for inflammatory bowel disease. *Curr Opin Gastroenterol* 2003;19(4):327–35.

17 Bridger S, Lee JC, Bjarnason I, Jones JE, Macpherson AJ. In siblings with similar genetic susceptibility for inflammatory bowel disease, smokers tend to develop Crohn's disease and non-smokers develop ulcerative colitis. *Gut* 2002;51(1):21–5.

18 Lander E, Kruglyak L. Genetic dissection of complex traits: guidelines for interpreting and reporting linkage results. *Nat Genet* 1995;11(3):241–7.

19 Cho JH, Nicolae DL, Ramos R, et al. Linkage and linkage disequilibrium in chromosome band 1p36 in American Chaldeans with inflammatory bowel disease. *Hum Mol Genet* 2000;9(9):1425–32.

20 Hampe J, Shaw SH, Saiz R, et al. Linkage of inflammatory bowel disease to human chromosome 6p. *Am J Hum Genet* 1999;65(6):1647–55.

21 van Heel DA, Fisher SA, Kirby A, et al. Inflammatory bowel disease susceptibility loci defined by genome scan meta-analysis of 1952 affected relative pairs. *Hum Mol Genet* 2004;13(7):763–70.

22 van Heel DA, Dechairo BM, Dawson G, et al. The IBD6 Crohn's disease locus demonstrates complex interactions with CARD15 and IBD5 disease-associated variants. *Hum Mol Genet* 2003;12(20):2569–75.

23 Hampe J, Frenzel H, Mirza MM, et al. Evidence for a NOD2-independent susceptibility locus for inflammatory bowel disease on chromosome 16p. *Proc Natl Acad Sci USA* 2002;99(1):321–6.

24 Duerr RH, Barmada MM, Zhang L, et al. Evidence for an inflammatory bowel disease locus on chromosome 3p26: linkage, transmission/disequilibrium and partitioning of linkage. *Hum Mol Genet* 2002;11(21):2599–606.

25 Stoll M, Corneliussen B, Costello CM, et al. Genetic variation in DLG5 is associated with inflammatory bowel disease. *Nat Genet* 2004;36(5):476–80.

26 McGovern DP, Hysi P, Ahmad T, et al. Association between a complex insertion/deletion polymorphism in NOD1(CARD4) and susceptibility to inflammatory bowel disease. *Hum Mol Genet* 2005.

27 Chamaillard M, Hashimoto M, Horie Y, et al. An essential role for NOD1 in host recognition of bacterial peptidoglycan containing diaminopimelic acid. *Nat Immunol* 2003;4(7):702–7.

28 Hugot JP, Laurent-Puig P, Gower-Rousseau C, et al. Mapping of a susceptibility locus for Crohn's disease on chromosome 16. *Nature* 1996;379(6568):821–3.

29 Hampe J, Schreiber S, Shaw SH, et al. A genomewide analysis provides evidence for novel linkages in inflammatory bowel disease in a large European cohort. *Am J Hum Genet* 1999;64(3):808–16.

30 Brant SR, Fu Y, Fields CT, et al. American families with Crohn's disease have strong evidence for linkage to chromosome 16 but not chromosome 12. *Gastroenterology* 1998;115(5):1056–61.

31 Ohmen JD, Yang HY, Yamamoto KK, et al. Susceptibility locus for inflammatory bowel disease on

chromosome 16 has a role in Crohn's disease, but not in ulcerative colitis. *Hum Mol Genet* 1996;5(10): 1679–83.

32. Curran ME, Lau KF, Hampe J, *et al.* Genetic analysis of inflammatory bowel disease in a large European cohort supports linkage to chromosomes 12 and 16. *Gastroenterology* 1998;115(5):1066–71.

33. Cavanaugh JA, Callen DF, Wilson SR, *et al.* Analysis of Australian Crohn's disease pedigrees refines the localization for susceptibility to inflammatory bowel disease on chromosome 16. *Ann Hum Genet* 1998; 62(Pt 4):291–8.

34. Cho JH, Nicolae DL, Gold LH, *et al.* Identification of novel susceptibility loci for inflammatory bowel disease on chromosomes 1p, 3q, and 4q: evidence for epistasis between 1p and IBD1. *Proc Natl Acad Sci USA* 1998;95(13):7502–7.

35. Annese V, Latiano A, Bovio P, *et al.* Genetic analysis in Italian families with inflammatory bowel disease supports linkage to the IBD1 locus – a GISC study. *Eur J Hum Genet* 1999;7(5):567–73.

36. Hugot JP, Chamaillard M, Zouali H, *et al.* Association of NOD2 leucine-rich repeat variants with susceptibility to Crohn's disease. *Nature* 2001; 411(6837):599–603.

37. Ogura Y, Bonen DK, Inohara N, *et al.* A frameshift mutation in NOD2 associated with susceptibility to Crohn's disease. *Nature* 2001;411(6837):603–6.

38. Hampe J, Cuthbert A, Croucher PJ, *et al.* Association between insertion mutation in NOD2 gene and Crohn's disease in German and British populations. *Lancet* 2001;357(9272):1925–8.

39. Lesage S, Zouali H, Cezard JP, *et al.* CARD15/NOD2 mutational analysis and genotype-phenotype correlation in 612 patients with inflammatory bowel disease. *Am J Hum Genet* 2002;70(4):845–57.

40. Cavanaugh J. International collaboration provides convincing linkage replication in complex disease through analysis of a large pooled data set: Crohn disease and chromosome 16. *Am J Hum Genet* 2001;68(5):1165–71.

41. Satsangi J, Parkes M, Louis E, *et al.* Two stage genome-wide search in inflammatory bowel disease provides evidence for susceptibility loci on chromosomes 3, 7 and 12. *Nat Genet* 1996;14(2): 199–202.

42. Cho J H, Nicolae DL, Gold LH, *et al.* Identification of novel susceptibility loci for inflammatory bowel disease on chromosomes 1p, 3q and 4q: evidence for epistasis between 1p and IBD1. *Proc Natl Acad Sci USA* 1998;95:7502–7.

43. Duerr RH, Barmada MM, Zhang L, Pfutzer R, Weeks DE. High-density genome scan in Crohn disease shows confirmed linkage to chromosome 14q11-12. *Am J Hum Genet* 2000;66(6):1857–62.

44. Rioux JD, Daly MJ, Green T, *et al.* Absence of linkage between inflammatory bowel disease and selected loci on chromosomes 3, 7, 12, and 16. *Gastroenterology* 1998;115(5):1062–5.

45. Rioux JD, Silverberg MS, Daly MJ, *et al.* Genomewide search in Canadian families with inflammatory bowel disease reveals two novel susceptibility loci. *Am J Hum Genet* 2000;66(6):1863–70.

46. Vermeire S, Peeters M, Vlietinck R, *et al.* Exclusion of linkage of Crohn's disease to previously reported regions on chromosomes 12, 7, and 3 in the Belgian population indicates genetic heterogeneity. *Inflamm Bowel Dis* 2000;6(3):165–70.

47. Parkes M, Barmada MM, Satsangi J, *et al.* The IBD2 locus shows linkage heterogeneity between ulcerative colitis and Crohn disease. *Am J Hum Genet* 2000; 67(6):1605–10.

48. Shanahan F. Host-flora interactions in inflammatory bowel disease. *Inflamm Bowel Dis* 2004;10(Suppl 1): S16–24.

49. Satsangi J, Welsh KI, Bunce M, *et al.* Contribution of genes of the major histocompatibility complex to susceptibility and disease phenotype in inflammatory bowel disease. *Lancet* 1996;347(9010):1212–7.

50. Ahmad T, Armuzzi A, Neville M, *et al.* The contribution of human leucocyte antigen complex genes to disease phenotype in ulcerative colitis. *Tissue Antigens* 2003;62(6):527–35.

51. Roussomoustakaki M, Satsangi J, Welsh K, *et al.* Genetic markers may predict disease behavior in patients with ulcerative colitis. *Gastroenterology* 1997;112(6):1845–53.

52. Ma Y, Ohmen JD, Li Z, *et al.* A genome-wide search identifies potential new susceptibility loci for Crohn's disease. *Inflamm Bowel Dis* 1999;5(4):271–8.

53. Dechairo B, Dimon C, van Heel D, *et al.* Replication and extension studies of inflammatory bowel disease susceptibility regions confirm linkage to chromosome 6p (IBD3). *Eur J Hum Genet* 2001;9(8):627–33.

54. Vermeire S, Rutgeerts P, Van Steen K, *et al.* Genome wide scan in a Flemish inflammatory bowel disease population: support for the IBD4 locus, population heterogeneity, and epistasis. *Gut* 2004;53(7): 980–6.

55. Rioux JD, Daly MJ, Silverberg MS, *et al.* Genetic variation in the 5q31 cytokine gene cluster confers susceptibility to Crohn disease. *Nat Genet* 2001; 29(2):223–8.

56. Giallourakis C, Stoll M, Miller K, *et al.* IBD5 is a general risk factor for inflammatory bowel disease: replication of association with Crohn disease and

identification of a novel association with ulcerative colitis. *Am J Hum Genet* 2003;73(1):205–11.
57 Armuzzi A, Ahmad T, Ling KL, et al. Genotype-phenotype analysis of the Crohn's disease susceptibility haplotype on chromosome 5q31. *Gut* 2003;52(8):1133–9.
58 Negoro K, McGovern DP, Kinouchi Y, et al. Analysis of the IBD5 locus and potential gene–gene interactions in Crohn's disease. *Gut* 2003;52(4):541–6.
59 McGovern DP, Van Heel DA, Negoro K, Ahmad T, Jewell DP. Further evidence of IBD5/CARD15 (NOD2) epistasis in the susceptibility to ulcerative colitis. *Am J Hum Genet* 2003;73(6):1465–6.
60 Peltekova VD, Wintle RF, Rubin LA, et al. Functional variants of OCTN cation transporter genes are associated with Crohn disease. *Nat Genet* 2004; 36(5):471–5.
61 Newman B, Gu X, Wintle R, et al. A risk haplotype in the solute carrier family 22A4/22A5 gene cluster influences phenotypic expression of Crohn's disease. *Gastroenterology* 2005;128(2):260–9.
62 Braun C, Zahn R, Martin K, Albert E, Folwaczny C. Polymorphisms of the ICAM-1 gene are associated with inflammatory bowel disease, regardless of the p-ANCA status. *Clin Immunol* 2001;101(3): 357–60.
63 Matsuzawa J, Sugimura K, Matsuda Y, et al. Association between K469E allele of intercellular adhesion molecule 1 gene and inflammatory bowel disease in a Japanese population. *Gut* 2003;52(1):75–8.
64 Low JH, Williams FA, Yang X, et al. Inflammatory bowel disease is linked to 19p13 and associated with ICAM-1. *Inflamm Bowel Dis* 2004;10(3):173–81.
65 Shaw SH, Hampe J, White R, et al. Stratification by CARD15 variant genotype in a genome-wide search for inflammatory bowel disease susceptibility loci. *Hum Genet* 2003;113(6):514–21.
66 Hampe J, Lynch NJ, Daniels S, et al. Fine mapping of the chromosome 3p susceptibility locus in inflammatory bowel disease. *Gut* 2001;48(2):191–7.
67 Economou M, Trikalinos TA, Loizou KT, Tsianos EV, Ioannidis JP. Differential effects of NOD2 variants on Crohn's disease risk and phenotype in diverse populations: a metaanalysis. *Am J Gastroenterol* 2004;99(12):2393–404.
68 Shivananda S, Lennard-Jones J, Logan R, et al. Incidence of inflammatory bowel disease across Europe: is there a difference between north and south? Results of the European collaborative study on inflammatory bowel disease (EC-IBD). *Gut* 1996;39(5):690–7.
69 Bairead E, Harmon DL, Curtis AM, et al. Association of NOD2 with Crohn's disease in a homogenous Irish population. *Eur J Hum Genet* 2003;11(3):237–44.
70 Arnott ID, Nimmo ER, Drummond HE, et al. NOD2/CARD15, TLR4 and CD14 mutations in Scottish and Irish Crohn's disease patients: evidence for genetic heterogeneity within Europe? *Genes Immun* 2004;5(5):417–25.
71 Crichton D, Arnott IDR, Watts D, et al. NOD2/CARD15 mutations in a Scottish Crohn's disease population. *Gastroenterology* 2002;122:A298.
72 Helio T, Halme L, Lappalainen M, et al. CARD15/NOD2 gene variants are associated with familially occurring and complicated forms of Crohn's disease. *Gut* 2003;52(4):558–62.
73 Cuthbert AP, Fisher SA, Mirza MM, et al. The contribution of NOD2 gene mutations to the risk and site of disease in inflammatory bowel disease. *Gastroenterology* 2002;122(4):867–74.
74 Ahmad T, Armuzzi A, Bunce M, et al. The molecular classification of the clinical manifestations of Crohn's disease. *Gastroenterology* 2002;122(4):854–66.
75 Murillo L, Crusius JB, van Bodegraven AA, Alizadeh BZ, Pena AS. CARD15 gene and the classification of Crohn's disease. *Immunogenetics* 2002;54(1):59–61.
76 Vermeire S, Louis E, Rutgeerts P, et al. NOD2/CARD15 does not influence response to infliximab in Crohn's disease. *Gastroenterology* 2002;123(1):106–11.
77 Louis E, Michel V, Hugot JP, et al. Early development of stricturing or penetrating pattern in Crohn's disease is influenced by disease location, number of flares, and smoking but not by NOD2/CARD15 genotype. *Gut* 2003;52(4):552–7.
78 Linde K, Boor PP, Houwing-Duistermaat JJ, et al. Card15 and Crohn's disease: healthy homozygous carriers of the 3020insC frameshift mutation. *Am J Gastroenterol* 2003;98(3):613–7.
79 Mendoza JL, Murillo LS, Fernandez L, et al. Prevalence of mutations of the NOD2/CARD15 gene and relation to phenotype in Spanish patients with Crohn disease. *Scand J Gastroenterol* 2003;38(12):1235–40.
80 Nunez C, Barreiro M, Dominguez-Munoz JE, et al. CARD15 mutations in patients with Crohn's disease in a homogeneous Spanish population. *Am J Gastroenterol* 2004;99(3):450–6.
81 Palmieri O, Toth S, Ferraris A, et al. CARD15 genotyping in inflammatory bowel disease patients by multiplex pyrosequencing. *Clin Chem* 2003;49(10):1675–9.
82 Annese V, Palmieri O, Latiano A, et al. Frequency of NOD2/CARD15 variants in both sporadic and familial cases of Crohn's disease across Italy. An

Italian group for inflammatory bowel disease study. *Dig Liver Dis* 2004;36(2):121–4.
83 Giachino D, van Duist MM, Regazzoni S, et al. Analysis of the CARD15 variants R702W, G908R and L1007fs in Italian IBD patients. *Eur J Hum Genet* 2004;12(3):206–12.
84 Roussomoustakaki M, Koutroubakis I, Vardas EM, et al. NOD2 insertion mutation in a Cretan Crohn's disease population. *Gastroenterology* 2003;124(1):272–3; author reply 273–4.
85 Abreu MT, Taylor KD, Lin YC, et al. Mutations in NOD2 are associated with fibrostenosing disease in patients with Crohn's disease. *Gastroenterology* 2002;123(3):679–88.
86 Sugimura K, Taylor KD, Lin YC, et al. A novel NOD2/CARD15 haplotype conferring risk for Crohn disease in Ashkenazi Jews. *Am J Hum Genet* 2003;72(3):509–18.
87 Bonen DK, Ogura Y, Nicolae DL, et al. Crohn's disease-associated NOD2 variants share a signaling defect in response to lipopolysaccharide and peptidoglycan. *Gastroenterology* 2003;124(1):140–6.
88 Vermeire S, Wild G, Kocher K, et al. CARD15 genetic variation in a Quebec population: prevalence, genotype-phenotype relationship, and haplotype structure. *Am J Hum Genet* 2002;71(1):74–83.
89 Fidder HH, Olschwang S, Avidan B, et al. Association between mutations in the CARD15 (NOD2) gene and Crohn's disease in Israeli Jewish patients. *Am J Med Genet A* 2003;121(3):240–4.
90 Cavanaugh JA, Adams KE, Quak EJ, et al. CARD15/NOD2 risk alleles in the development of Crohn's disease in the Australian population. *Ann Hum Genet* 2003;67(Pt 1):35–41.
91 Monk M, Mendeloff AI, Siegel CI, Lilienfeld A. An epidemiological study of ulcerative colitis and regional enteritis among adults in Baltimore: II. Social and demographic factors. *Gastroenterology* 1969;56(5):847–57.
92 Acheson ED. The distribution of ulcerative colitis and regional enteritis in United States veterans with particular reference to the Jewish religion. *Gut* 1960;1:291–3.
93 Roth MP, Petersen GM, McElree C, et al. Familial empiric risk estimates of inflammatory bowel disease in Ashkenazi Jews. *Gastroenterology* 1989;96(4):1016–20.
94 Croucher PJ, Mascheretti S, Hampe J, et al. Haplotype structure and association to Crohn's disease of CARD15 mutations in two ethnically divergent populations. *Eur J Hum Genet* 2003;11(1):6–16.
95 Zhou Z, Lin XY, Akolkar PN, et al. Variation at NOD2/CARD15 in familial and sporadic cases of Crohn's disease in the Ashkenazi Jewish population. *Am J Gastroenterol* 2002;97(12):3095–101.
96 Bonin DK ND, Moran T, Turkyilmaz MA, et al. Racial differences in NOD2 variation: characterization of NOD2 in African–Americans with Crohn's disease. *Gastroenterology* 2002;122(Suppl):A-29.
97 Inoue N, Tamura K, Kinouchi Y, et al. Lack of common NOD2 variants in Japanese patients with Crohn's disease. *Gastroenterology* 2002;123(1):86–91.
98 Yamazaki K, Takazoe M, Tanaka T, Kazumori T, Nakamura Y. Absence of mutation in the NOD2/CARD15 gene among 483 Japanese patients with Crohn's disease. *J Hum Genet* 2002;47(9):469–72.
99 Leong RW, Armuzzi A, Ahmad T, et al. NOD2/CARD15 gene polymorphisms and Crohn's disease in the Chinese population. *Aliment Pharmacol Ther* 2003;17(12):1465–70.
100 Vavassori P, Borgiani P, D'Apice MR, et al. 3020insC mutation within the NOD2 gene in Crohn's disease: frequency and association with clinical pattern in an Italian population. *Dig Liver Dis* 2002;34(2):153.
101 Hampe J, Grebe J, Nikolaus S, et al. Association of NOD2 (CARD15) genotype with clinical course of Crohn's disease: a cohort study. *Lancet* 2002;359(9318):1661–5.
102 Brant SR, Picco MF, Achkar JP, et al. Defining complex contributions of NOD2/CARD15 gene mutations, age at onset, and tobacco use on Crohn's disease phenotypes. *Inflamm Bowel Dis* 2003;9(5):281–9.
103 Girardin SE, Boneca IG, Viala J, et al. Nod2 is a general sensor of peptidoglycan through muramyl dipeptide (MDP) detection. *J Biol Chem* 2003;278(11):8869–72.
104 Inohara N, Ogura Y, Fontalba A, et al. Host recognition of bacterial muramyl dipeptide mediated through NOD2. Implications for Crohn's disease. *J Biol Chem* 2003;278(8):5509–12.
105 Ogura Y, Inohara N, Benito A, et al. Nod2, a Nod1/Apaf-1 family member that is restricted to monocytes and activates NF-κB. *J Biol Chem* 2001;276(7):4812–8.
106 Chamaillard M, Girardin SE, Viala J, Philpott DJ. Nods, Nalps and Naip: intracellular regulators of bacterial-induced inflammation. *Cell Microbiol* 2003;5(9):581–92.
107 Chamaillard M, Philpott D, Girardin SE, et al. Gene-environment interaction modulated by allelic

108 Neurath MF, Fuss I, Schurmann G, et al. Cytokine gene transcription by NF-κB family members in patients with inflammatory bowel disease. *Ann NY Acad Sci* 1998;859:149–59.
109 Gutierrez O, Pipaon C, Inohara N, et al. Induction of Nod2 in myelomonocytic and intestinal epithelial cells via nuclear factor-kappa B activation. *J Biol Chem* 2002;277(44):41701–5.
110 Hisamatsu T, Suzuki M, Reinecker HC, et al. CARD15/NOD2 functions as an antibacterial factor in human intestinal epithelial cells. *Gastroenterology* 2003;124(4):993–1000.
111 Pauleau AL, Murray PJ. Role of nod2 in the response of macrophages to toll-like receptor agonists. *Mol Cell Biol* 2003;23(21):7531–9.
112 Kobayashi KS, Chamaillard M, Ogura Y, et al. Nod2-dependent regulation of innate and adaptive immunity in the intestinal tract. *Science* 2005; 307(5710):731–4.
113 Maeda S, Hsu LC, Liu H, et al. Nod2 mutation in Crohn's disease potentiates NF-κB activity and IL-1beta processing. *Science* 2005;307(5710):734–8.
114 Fiocchi C. Inflammatory bowel disease: etiology and pathogenesis. *Gastroenterology* 1998;115(1): 182–205.
115 van Heel DA, Gosh S, M Butler, et al. Amplification of toll-like receptor sensitivity by muramyl dipeptide is impaired in Crohn's disease associated NOD2 mutations. *Gut* 2005;54(Suppl):A1.
116 Holler E, Rogler G, Herfarth H, et al. Both donor and recipient NOD2/CARD15 mutations associate with transplant-related mortality and GvHD following allogeneic stem cell transplantation. *Blood* 2004; 104(3):889–94.
117 Hill GR, Ferrara JL. The primacy of the gastrointestinal tract as a target organ of acute graft-versus-host disease: rationale for the use of cytokine shields in allogeneic bone marrow transplantation. *Blood* 2000;95(9):2754–9.
118 Lala S, Ogura Y, Osborne C, et al. Crohn's disease and the NOD2 gene: a role for paneth cells. *Gastroenterology* 2003;125(1):47–57.
119 Porter EM, Bevins CL, Ghosh D, Ganz T. The multifaceted paneth cell. *Cell Mol Life Sci* 2002;59(1):156–70.
120 Wilson CL, Ouellette AJ, Satchell DP, et al. Regulation of intestinal alpha-defensin activation by the metalloproteinase matrilysin in innate host defense. *Science* 1999;286(5437):113–7.
121 Wehkamp J, Harder J, Weichenthal M, et al. NOD2 (CARD15) mutations in Crohn's disease are associated with diminished mucosal alpha-defensin expression. *Gut* 2004;53(11):1658–64.
122 Stokkers PC, Reitsma PH, Tytgat GN, van Deventer SJ. HLA-DR and -DQ phenotypes in inflammatory bowel disease: a meta-analysis. *Gut* 1999;45(3): 395–401.
123 Neurath MF, Fuss I, Pasparakis M, et al. Predominant pathogenic role of tumor necrosis factor in experimental colitis in mice. *Eur J Immunol* 1997; 27(7):1743–50.
124 Kontoyiannis D, Pasparakis M, Pizarro TT, Cominelli F, Kollias G. Impaired on/off regulation of TNF biosynthesis in mice lacking TNF AU-rich elements: implications for joint and gut-associated immunopathologies. *Immunity* 1999;10(3): 387–98.
125 Present DH, Rutgeerts P, Targan S, et al. Infliximab for the treatment of fistulas in patients with Crohn's disease. *N Engl J Med* 1999;340(18):1398–405.
126 Targan SR, Hanauer SB, van Deventer SJ, et al. A short-term study of chimeric monoclonal antibody cA2 to tumor necrosis factor alpha for Crohn's disease. Crohn's disease cA2 study group. *N Engl J Med* 1997;337(15):1029–35.
127 Yoshida H, Naito A, Inoue J, et al. Different cytokines induce surface lymphotoxin-alphabeta on IL-7 receptor-alpha cells that differentially engender lymph nodes and Peyer's patches. *Immunity* 2002;17(6): 823–33.
128 van Heel DA, Udalova IA, De Silva AP, et al. Inflammatory bowel disease is associated with a TNF polymorphism that affects an interaction between the OCT1 and NF(-kappa)B transcription factors. *Hum Mol Genet* 2002;11(11):1281–9.
129 O'Callaghan NJ, Adams KE, van Heel DA, Cavanaugh JA. Association of TNF-α-857C with inflammatory bowel disease in the Australian population. *Scand J Gastroenterol* 2003;38(5): 533–4.
130 Negoro K, Kinouchi Y, Hiwatashi N, et al. Crohn's disease is associated with novel polymorphisms in the 5'-flanking region of the tumor necrosis factor gene. *Gastroenterology* 1999;117(5):1062–8.
131 Mascheretti S, Hampe J, Kuhbacher T, et al. Pharmacogenetic investigation of the TNF/TNF-receptor system in patients with chronic active Crohn's disease treated with infliximab. *Pharmacogenomics J* 2002;2(2):127–36.
132 Louis E, Peeters M, Franchimont D, et al. Tumour necrosis factor (TNF) gene polymorphism in Crohn's disease (CD): influence on disease behaviour? *Clin Exp Immunol* 2000;119(1):64–8.
133 Ahmad T, Marshall SE, Mulcahy-Hawes K, et al. High resolution MIC genotyping: design and application to

the investigation of inflammatory bowel disease susceptibility. *Tissue Antigens* 2002;60(2):164–79.

134 Seki SS, Sugimura K, Ota M, et al. Stratification analysis of MICA triplet repeat polymorphisms and HLA antigens associated with ulcerative colitis in Japanese. *Tissue Antigens* 2001;58(2):71–6.

135 Glas J, Martin K, Brunnler G, et al. MICA, MICB and C1_4_1 polymorphism in Crohn's disease and ulcerative colitis. *Tissue Antigens* 2001;58(4):243–9.

136 Futami S, Aoyama N, Honsako Y, et al. HLA-DRB1*1502 allele, subtype of DR15, is associated with susceptibility to ulcerative colitis and its progression. *Dig Dis Sci* 1995;40(4):814–8.

137 Yoshitake S, Kimura A, Okada M, Yao T, Sasazuki T. HLA class II alleles in Japanese patients with inflammatory bowel disease. *Tissue Antigens* 1999;53(4, Pt 1):350–8.

138 Yap LM, Ahmad T, Jewell DP. The Contribution of HLA genes to IBD susceptibility and phenotype. *Best Pract Res Clin Gastroenterol* 2004;18(3):577–96.

139 Ahmad T, Neville M, Marshall SE, et al. Haplotype-specific linkage disequilibrium patterns define the genetic topography of the human MHC. *Hum Mol Genet* 2003;12(6):647–56.

140 Ahmad T, Tamboli CP, Jewell D, Colombel JF. Clinical relevance of advances in genetics and pharmacogenetics of IBD. *Gastroenterology* 2004;126(6):1533–49.

141 Silverberg MS, Mirea L, Bull SB, et al. A population- and family-based study of Canadian families reveals association of HLA DRB1*0103 with colonic involvement in inflammatory bowel disease. *Inflamm Bowel Dis* 2003;9(1):1–9.

142 Bouma G, Crusius JB, Garcia-Gonzalez MA, et al. Genetic markers in clinically well defined patients with ulcerative colitis (UC). *Clin Exp Immunol* 1999;115(2):294–300.

143 Yamamoto-Furusho JK, Uscanga LF, Vargas-Alarcon G, et al. Clinical and genetic heterogeneity in Mexican patients with ulcerative colitis. *Hum Immunol* 2003;64(1):119–23.

144 Parkes M, Satsangi J, Lathrop GM, Bell JI, Jewell DP. Susceptibility loci in inflammatory bowel disease. *Lancet* 1996;348(9041):1588.

145 Louis E, Belaiche J. Genetics of Crohn's disease behaviour. *Acta Gastroenterol Belg* 2000;63(4):377–9.

146 Orchard TR, Thiyagaraja S, Welsh KI, et al. Clinical phenotype is related to HLA genotype in the peripheral arthropathies of inflammatory bowel disease. *Gastroenterology* 2000;118(2):274–8.

147 Orchard TR, Chua CN, Ahmad T, et al. Uveitis and erythema nodosum in inflammatory bowel disease: clinical features and the role of HLA genes. *Gastroenterology* 2002;123(3):714–8.

148 Mirza MM, Fisher SA, King K, et al. Genetic evidence for interaction of the 5q31 cytokine locus and the CARD15 gene in Crohn disease. *Am J Hum Genet* 2003;72(4):1018–22.

149 Vermeire S, Chapman RW, Joossens S, et al. NOD2/CARD15 genotyping in patients with indeterminate colitis (IC): helpful towards definite diagnosis? *Gastroenterology* 2002;A(Suppl):M1416.

150 Krynetski EY, Schuetz JD, Galpin AJ, et al. A single point mutation leading to loss of catalytic activity in human thiopurine S-methyltransferase. *Proc Natl Acad Sci USA* 1995;92(4):949–53.

151 Tai HL, Krynetski EY, Yates CR, et al. Thiopurine S-methyltransferase deficiency: two nucleotide transitions define the most prevalent mutant allele associated with loss of catalytic activity in Caucasians. *Am J Hum Genet* 1996;58(4):694–702.

152 Tai HL, Krynetski EY, Schuetz EG, Yanishevski Y, Evans WE. Enhanced proteolysis of thiopurine S-methyltransferase (TPMT) encoded by mutant alleles in humans (TPMT*3A, TPMT*2): mechanisms for the genetic polymorphism of TPMT activity. *Proc Natl Acad Sci USA* 1997;94(12):6444–9.

153 Colombel JF, Ferrari N, Debuysere H, et al. Genotypic analysis of thiopurine S-methyltransferase in patients with Crohn's disease and severe myelosuppression during azathioprine therapy. *Gastroenterology* 2000;118(6):1025–30.

154 Weinshilboum RM, Sladek SL. Mercaptopurine pharmacogenetics: monogenic inheritance of erythrocyte thiopurine methyltransferase activity. *Am J Hum Genet* 1980;32(5):651–62.

155 Laverdiere C, Chiasson S, Costea I, Moghrabi A, Krajinovic M. Polymorphism G80A in the reduced folate carrier gene and its relationship to methotrexate plasma levels and outcome of childhood acute lymphoblastic leukemia. *Blood* 2002;100(10):3832–4.

156 Cheng Q, Wu B, Kager L, et al. A substrate specific functional polymorphism of human gamma-glutamyl hydrolase alters catalytic activity and methotrexate polyglutamate accumulation in acute lymphoblastic leukaemia cells. *Pharmacogenetics* 2004;14(8):557–67.

157 van der Put NM, Gabreels F, Stevens EM, et al. A second common mutation in the methylenetetrahydrofolate reductase gene: an additional risk factor for neural-tube defects? *Am J Hum Genet* 1998;62(5):1044–51.

158 Weisberg I, Tran P, Christensen B, Sibani S, Rozen R. A second genetic polymorphism in

158. methylenetetrahydrofolate reductase (MTHFR) associated with decreased enzyme activity. *Mol Genet Metab* 1998;64(3):169–72.
159. Urano W, Taniguchi A, Yamanaka H, *et al*. Polymorphisms in the methylenetetrahydrofolate reductase gene were associated with both the efficacy and the toxicity of methotrexate used for the treatment of rheumatoid arthritis, as evidenced by single locus and haplotype analyses. *Pharmacogenetics* 2002;12(3):183–90.
160. Ulrich CM, Yasui Y, Storb R, *et al*. Pharmacogenetics of methotrexate: toxicity among marrow transplantation patients varies with the methylenetetrahydrofolate reductase C677T polymorphism. *Blood* 2001;98(1):231–4.
161. Dilger K, Schwab S, Fromm MF. Identification of budesonide and prednisone as substrates of the intestinal drug efflux pump p-glycoprotein. *Inflamm Bowel Dis* 2004;10(5):573–8.
162. Farrell RJ, Murphy A, Long A, *et al*. High multidrug resistance (P-glycoprotein 170) expression in inflammatory bowel disease patients who fail medical therapy. *Gastroenterology* 2000;118(2):279–88.
163. Schwab M, Schaeffeler E, Marx C, *et al*. Association between the C3435T MDR1 gene polymorphism and susceptibility for ulcerative colitis. *Gastroenterology* 2003;124(1):26–33.
164. Heresbach D, Alizadeh M, Bretagne JF, *et al*. TAP gene transporter polymorphism in inflammatory bowel diseases. *Scand J Gastroenterol* 1997;32(10):1022–7.
165. Honda M, Orii F, Ayabe T, *et al*. Expression of glucocorticoid receptor beta in lymphocytes of patients with glucocorticoid-resistant ulcerative colitis. *Gastroenterology* 2000;118(5):859–66.
166. Ricart E, Taylor WR, Loftus EV, *et al*. N-acetyltransferase 1 and 2 genotypes do not predict response or toxicity to treatment with mesalamine and sulfasalazine in patients with ulcerative colitis. *Am J Gastroenterol* 2002;97(7):1763–8.
167. Sandborn WJ, Hanauer SB, Katz S, *et al*. Etanercept for active Crohn's disease: a randomized, double-blind, placebo-controlled trial. *Gastroenterology* 2001;121(5):1088–94.
168. Taylor KD, Plevy SE, Yang H, *et al*. ANCA pattern and LTA haplotype relationship to clinical responses to anti-TNF antibody treatment in Crohn's disease. *Gastroenterology* 2001;120(6):1347–55.
169. Louis E, Vermeire S, Rutgeerts P, *et al*. A positive response to infliximab in Crohn disease: association with a higher systemic inflammation before treatment but not with -308 TNF gene polymorphism. *Scand J Gastroenterol* 2002;37(7):818–24.
170. Shen C, Assche GV, Colpaert S, *et al*. Adalimumab induces apoptosis of human monocytes: a comparative study with infliximab and etanercept. *Aliment Pharmacol Ther* 2005;21(3):251–8.
171. Sandborn WJ, Hanauer S, Loftus EV Jr, *et al*. An open-label study of the human anti-TNF monoclonal antibody adalimumab in subjects with prior loss of response or intolerance to infliximab for Crohn's disease. *Am J Gastroenterol* 2004;99(10):1984–9.

3: Microbial sensing in the intestine by pattern recognition receptors

Robin G. Lorenz and Charles O. Elson

Introduction

The human intestine (small and large) is composed not only of mammalian epithelial cells and leukocytes, but also a complex community of microbiota. These three components have developed complex inter-relationships that are not well understood [1]. Recent studies on germ-free mice and zebrafish have shown that the intestinal microbiota modulate a wide range of gastrointestinal functions, such as nutrient processing and absorption, maturation of the intestine and stimulation of the mucosal immune system [2–5]. However, until recently it has been unclear how the host is able to sense the presence of these microbiota and trigger the many genes required for intestinal development. The answer appears to lie in the recent discovery of several families of molecules known as pattern recognition receptors. Both intestinal epithelial cells, as well as mucosal immune cells express a number of such pattern recognition receptors (PRR) [6]. These receptors recognise conserved patterns of molecules unique to microbes, termed microbe- (or pathogen)-associated molecular patterns (MAMPs). There are multiple types of PRRs, including the family of transmembrane toll-like receptors (TLRs), the family of cytosolic nucleotide-binding oligomerisation domain proteins (NOD) and phagocytic receptors (scavenger receptors, mannose receptors and beta-glucan receptors). In animal models TLRs appear to play a critical role in intestinal epithelial homeostasis and protect the intestine from epithelial injury, although NODs appear to detect intracellular bacterial products [7–11]. Stimulation of TLRs and NODs by microbial components triggers signalling via a number of adaptor molecules, resulting in the activation of NF-κB, which in turn induces expression of inflammatory cytokines (Fig 3.1) [12]. This chapter will focus on the expression and function of TLRs and NODs in human and murine intestine and discuss how these molecules may play a role in the resistance or susceptibility to intestinal inflammation.

TLR-intestinal expression and function

The intestinal epithelial cell not only presents a physical barrier to luminal microbiota, but also has the ability to sense the presence of microbiota through TLRs [13] (Table 3.1). Although the functional role of TLRs on intestinal epithelial cells is not understood, intestinal epithelial cells express several microbial sensors *in vivo* and *in vitro*, such as TLR2, -4, -5 and -9, which may play a role in the epithelial response to intestinal microbiota [17–21]. In the normal intestine, expression of these microbial sensors appears to be restricted to niches where exposure to microbiota would be controlled. TLR4 expression is restricted to epithelial cells at the bottom of crypts and TLR5 expression may be limited to the basolateral surface of intestinal epithelia, although that is disputed [21–23]. In addition, it has been reported that human intestinal epithelial cells are unresponsive to TLR2 ligands [24]. However, this limited exposure to microbiological products appears to be lost in the inflamed intestine. The levels and pattern of expression of TLR4 have clearly

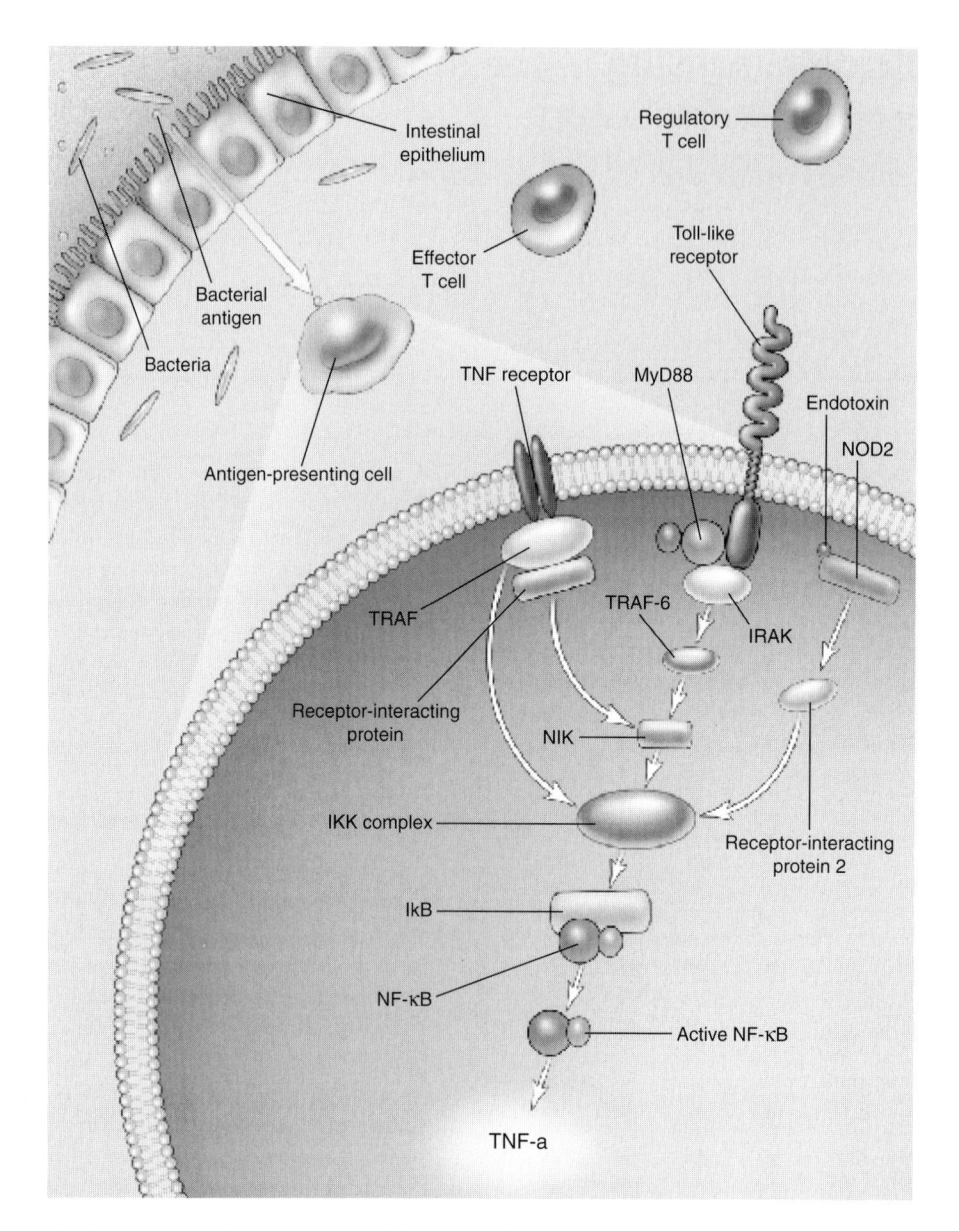

Fig 3.1 Intestinal pattern recognition receptors and their probable pathways. Microbial products (small circles) traversing the epithelium are detected by a variety of cell surface receptors for microbial products, such as the toll-like receptors (TLR) and by intracellular microbial pattern recognition receptors (PRR) such as NOD1 and NOD2. Ligand binding to PRR receptors induces a cascade via a variety of adaptor proteins, resulting in the activation of the nuclear factor-kappa B (NF-κB) complex. Cytokines such as IL-1β and TNFα use a similar but distinct signalling pathway.

TNFα, tumour necrosis factor alpha; TNF-R, tumour necrosis factor alpha-receptor; IRAK, IL-1 receptor associated kinase; TRAF6, TNF receptor associated factor 6; MyD88, myeloid differentiation factor 88; RIP2, receptor-interacting protein 2; IKK, inhibitor of kappa B kinase kinase; IkB, inhibitor of kappa B; NF-κB, nuclear factor of kappa B; NOD2, nuclear binding and oligomerisation domain protein 2 (reprinted with permission from Elson CO. *New Engl J Med* 2002;346:614–6).

Table 3.1 Pattern recognition receptors and their ligands.

PRR	Ligand(s) [6, 14, 15]	Expression in primary colonic epithelial cells [16]
TLR1	Bacterial lipopeptides	+
TLR2	Bacterial peptioglycans, zymosan and lipopeptides	+
TLR3	Viral dsRNA	+
TLR4	Bacterial lipopolysaccharide (LPS), heat shock protein 60	+
TLR5	Flagellin	+
TLR6	Mycoplasma lipopeptide	+
TLR7 (murine)	Viral ssRNA	+/−
TLR8 (human)	Viral ssRNA	+
TLR9	Unmethylated CpG DNA (bacterial and viral)	+
TLR10	?	−
TLR11	Uropathogenic bacteria	?
NOD1	GM-tri$_{DAP}$	+
NOD2	Muramyldipeptide (MDP)	+

been demonstrated to change dramatically in the inflamed intestine, where TLR4 RNA levels are increased and expression is no longer limited to crypt cells [18, 21, 25]. In addition, the response to TLR5 ligands is enhanced in multiple murine models of IBD, as well as in human patients [26]. The mechanisms that drive these changes in the expression and response of epithelial microbial sensors are not clear. TLR4 clearly traffics to cytoplasmic compartments in polarised intestinal epithelium and the importance of internalised LPS has been recently recognised in intestinal epithelial cells, because prevention of LPS internalisation significantly impairs its recognition by epithelial cells [20, 23]. In addition, the recent identification of epithelial NOD2, an intracellular protein that recognises muramyl dipeptide, further implicates intracellular recognition of microbial products by sensors in epithelial cells as critical in IBD [27–31].

TLRs are also expressed on innate immune cells, as human neutrophils express TLR1, TLR2 and TLR4 through TLR10 [32]. In addition, TLRs have distinct expression patterns on monocytes and dendritic cell (DC) subsets, with human monocytes primarily expressing TLRs 1, 2, 4 and 5, while human myeloid DCs express TLRs 1, 2, 3 and 5 [7]. Mouse DCs express TLRs 1, 2, 4, 6, 8 and 9, but not TLR3, a notable difference from the human system.

In addition, both mouse and human DCs are unresponsive to LPS, suggesting that the immunoinflammatory properties of LPS are mediated by alternative cell populations [7]. Stimulation of DCs through TLRs results in cytokine secretion and renders them able to activate T cells.

TLR2. Several TLRs are constitutively expressed at low levels on intestinal epithelial cells *in vivo*, including TLR2 in the proximal colon. However, expression does not directly translate into functional recognition of bacterial products by intestinal epithelial cells. For example, intestinal epithelial cells have been shown to be unresponsive to TLR2 ligands, probably due to the low expression of the TLR2 co-receptor TLR6 [24].

TLR4. TLR4 is expressed in colonocytes in the distal colon and has previously been demonstrated on the surface of macrophages and dendritic cells and in crypt epithelial cells of the murine small intestine [21, 33]. The latter anatomical site is relatively protected from the luminal microbiota and such sequestration might be one mechanism by which the TLR4 ligand LPS does not continuously cause activation in the intestine. However, it has now been demonstrated that intestinal epithelial TLR4 is predominantly found in the Golgi apparatus, in contrast to cell surface expressed TLR4 in myeloid cells [20]. LPS stimulation of the TLR4 in this intracellular location is critical for the function of TLR4 in intestinal epithelial cells, because prevention of LPS internalisation prevents TLR4 signalling [23]. Under inflammatory conditions, intestinal epithelial responses to LPS are enhanced. One mechanism of this enhanced sensitivity could be an increased expression of TLR4 [18, 21, 25]. But studies with human intestinal epithelial cells have demonstrated a second mechanism, which is augmentation of LPS uptake and the subsequent increased signalling through intracellular TLR4 [34].

TLR5. TLR5 recognises flagellin and is present in the ileum and colon, but the expression pattern of epithelial TLR5 is currently debated in the literature. In human T-84 colonic epithelial cell monolayers, TLR5 expression is restricted to the basolateral membrane, therefore implying that only microbes that can cross the epithelial barrier can stimulate TLR5 [19]. However, this pattern appears to be different in the normal intestine, where TLR5 has been reported to also be expressed on the apical surface of epithelial cells [35]. The reasons for this discrepancy are not clear; however, there does appear to be some mechanism for controlling immune reactivity to the TLR5 ligand flagellin. Normal mice do not display T-cell or antibody reactivity to flagellin, whereas three strains of colitic mice were found to have elevated serological and Th1 T-cell responses to flagellin [26]. These models were strains having different MHC haplotypes and very different mechanisms underlying the predisposition to develop IBD. For example, the colitis in C3H/HeJBir mice is an IL-12-driven, Th1-mediated inflammation that can be transferred by CD4$^+$ T cells [36]. This is in contrast to IL-10$^{-/-}$ mice, which have a defect in regulatory T cells and FVB.mdr1a$^{-/-}$ mice, which are believed to have epithelial barrier dysfunction. Intriguingly, this same reactivity to flagellins was seen in patients with Crohn's disease, implicating the TLR5 ligand flagellin as an immunodominant antigen in both human and animal models of IBD [26].

TLR9. TLR9 recognises a CpG oligodeoxynucleotide motif (CpG ODN) unique to bacterial DNA [17, 18, 20, 21]. In contrast to the diminished capacity of normal epithelial TLR2, TLR4 and TLR5 to respond to luminal microbiota, there is growing evidence that probiotic bacteria and DNA can signal through TLR9 on intestinal epithelial cells and that the latter can thereby mediate anti-inflammatory immune functions [37, 38]. CpG ODN are best known for their ability to induce the secretion of pro-inflammatory cytokines (e.g. IL-12 and IFNs) from haematopoietic cells [39]. However, it has recently been demonstrated that CpG ODN can also elicit the production of prostaglandins, such as PGE$_2$ [40, 41]. This increase in prostaglandin production occurs through transcriptional regulation of *COX-2* gene expression and is dependent on the endosomal acidification/processing of CpG DNA, the TLR9/MyD88 signalling pathway and NFκB and p38 MAP kinase [42, 43]. The expression of TLR9 mRNA differs between humans and mice. It has been reported that functional TLR9 is only expressed on B-cells and plasmacytoid dendritic cells (DC) in humans, although mRNA has been detected in NK-, NKT-, T-cells and macrophages [39, 44]. In mice, the expression pattern is similar, but functional TLR9 has also been reported on monocytes and myeloid DC [45]. TLR9 was originally identified in 2000 as a receptor that recognised bacterial DNA [46]. The precise optimal sequence motifs are host-species specific and in humans it is now clear that TLR9 can recognise at least three distinct classes of unmethylated CpG ODN [47]. For example CpG ODN of the B-class can stimulate strong B cell responses, while plasmacytoid DC are strongly stimulated by A-class ODN. The responses of epithelial TLR9 to CpG ODN classes have not been extensively studied; however, TLR9 stimulation in B-cells and DCs directly upregulates a cytokine/chemokine cascade that directs the maturation and differentiation of NK cells, T cells and monocytes.

TLR9 mediated down-regulation of pro-inflammatory responses has now been demonstrated in several animal models of colitis. The administration of either CpG ODN or DNA isolated from probiotic bacteria inhibited the production of pro-inflammatory cytokines and ameliorated clinical and histological colonic inflammation in

DSS-colitis, TNBS-colitis and in IL-10$^{-/-}$ mice [37, 38, 48]. Signalling through TLR9 is essential in mediating the anti-inflammatory effects of probiotic DNA; however, it is unclear which TLR9-expressing cell type is critical [38].

TLR mutations, infections and inflammatory bowel disease. TLR4 mutations have been associated with hypo-responsiveness to LPS in both humans and in animal models [49–54]. The TLR4 Asp299Gly polymorphism is associated with impaired LPS signalling and increased susceptibility to gram-negative infections [55, 56]. This mutation is associated with both Crohn's disease and ulcerative colitis with a relative risk of 2.6 [57]. In addition, a second polymorphism in TLR4, which results in impaired LPS signalling, Thr399Ile, has also been found with increased frequency in ulcerative colitis patients [58]. The importance of host recognition of microbial products in the control of inflammation is also reinforced by the recent report of an increased frequency of polymorphisms of the TLR9 gene (-1237 C/T) in patients with Crohn's disease [59]. Conversely, TLR2 polymorphisms predispose people to staphylococcal infections, leprosy and tuberculosis and a TLR5 polymorphism is associated with susceptibility to legionnaires' disease, but no association with inflammatory bowel disease has been reported for either TLR2 or TLR5 [60–64].

NOD-intestinal expression and function

NOD1 and NOD2 represent a second group of pattern recognition receptor molecules [65–67]. NOD1 and NOD2 share a common feature, namely the presence of a nucleotide-binding oligomerisation domain (NOD), which is also shared by a number of molecules of diverse function, the so-called 'NOD family'. NOD1 and NOD2 resemble the R factors in plants that confer resistance to infection and thus are biologically ancient, although relatively new to us. NOD2 has two copies of an amino terminal CARD domain (caspase activation and recruitment domain), whereas NOD1 has one CARD domain (Fig 3.2). CARD domains are found in some proteins that mediate apoptosis, although it remains to be seen whether NOD1 or NOD2 function in an apoptotic pathway. The official nomenclature has named NOD1 as CARD4 and NOD2 as CARD15 but the NOD designation is still commonly used. Activation of either NOD1 or NOD2 causes them to physically associate with an adapter protein RIP2 via CARD–CARD interactions. RIP2 then interacts with IKKγ triggering the NF-κB signalling pathway.

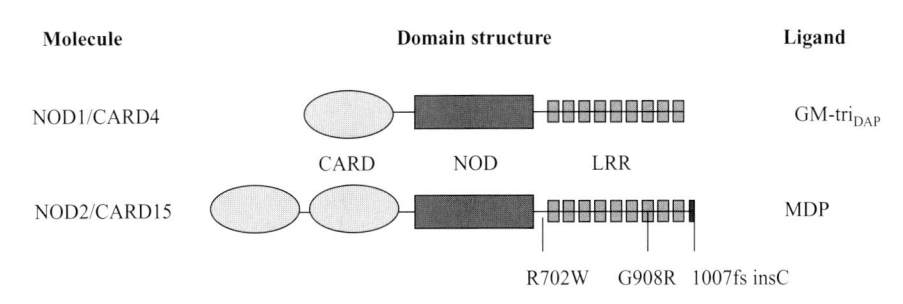

Fig 3.2 Domain structure and ligands of NOD1 and NOD2. The major differences are that NOD1 has one CARD domain whereas NOD2 has two. In addition NOD1 has 9 LRR regions whereas NOD2 has 10. The mutations in NOD2 resulting in enhanced susceptibility to Crohn's disease are all in or adjacent to the LRR domain as shown; the most distal mutation results in truncation of the tenth LRR region. Both NOD1 and NOD2 recognise similar but distinct muropeptides, which are bacterial peptidoglycan degradation products. The ligand specificity of NOD1 is for GM-tri$_{DAP}$ that is present in gram-negative bacteria plus some bacillus species, but not most gram-positives. The minimal ligand recognised by NOD2 is muyramyl dipeptide or MDP, which is present in both gram-positive and gram-negative bacteria. GM-tri$_{DAP}$, N-acetylglucosaminyl- N-acetyl muramyl- L-alanine-γ-D-Glu-meso- diaminopimelic acid; MDP, N-acetyl muramyl- L-alanyl- D- isoglutamine.

Thus, the end result of the bacterial ligand–NOD interaction is similar to that of the TLRs, albeit using different adapter proteins (Fig 3.1). In fact, the NOD and TLR pathways may interact via RIP2 in that TLR ligands elicit lower responses in RIP2 knockout mice [68].

What is the function of NODs? The presence of a leucine-rich repeat region in NOD1 and NOD similar to that seen in the TLRs initially raised the suspicion that these molecules might serve as pattern recognition receptors. NOD1 and NOD2 are expressed in the cytosol, rather than the cell surface and thus are localised optimally to detect intracellular bacterial products. Indeed, the original description of NOD2 demonstrated that a crude preparation of lipopolysaccharide introduced into the cytosol was detected by NODs, which then activated NF-κB [69]. Subsequent studies have shown convincingly that the ligand is not lipopolysaccharide but rather is bacterial peptidoglycan, another cell wall constituent present in bacteria. The NODs appear to recognise small muropeptides that are breakdown products of peptidoglycan [9, 10]. The minimal ligand for NOD1 is GM-tri$_{DAP}$ that is present in gram-negative bacteria plus some gram-positive bacillus species. In contrast, the minimal ligand for NOD2 is muramyldipeptide, which is expressed in both gram-positive and gram-negative bacteria (Fig 3.2). Both these ligands are known to have adjuvant function for the induction of immune responses and this action is presumably mediated by activation of NOD1 or NOD2 in antigen presenting cells. NOD1 has been shown to play a key role in detecting invasive gram-negative bacteria in epithelial cell lines *in vitro* [11]. Interestingly, the expression of NOD2 in intestinal epithelial cells confers resistance to Salmonella infection of those cells [70]; the mechanisms by which NOD2 accomplishes this remain to be defined. Although the NODs are expressed intracellularly and the TLRs on the cell surface, NOD1 has been shown to be able to detect extracellular bacteria such as *H. pylori* which can inject bacterial products into cells via a type 4 secretion apparatus [71]. In turn, TLRs can detect bacterial ligand within endosomes or phagolysosomes within the cells [72]. Thus, this distinction between extracellular and intracellular sensing is not absolute.

Cellular distribution of NOD1 and NOD2. In addition to the differences in binding specificity, NOD1 and NOD2 differ in their cellular distribution. NOD1 is expressed in a wide variety of cells, including intestinal epithelial cells and immune cells. NOD1, NOD2 and a number of TLRs are expressed by intestinal myofibroblasts that sit just below the epithelial layer; these cells may also participate in innate defence of the intestine [73]. NOD2 expression is more restricted. NOD2 is expressed in high amounts in blood monocytes and in intestinal Paneth cells and in lower amounts in dendritic cells and IEC. The importance of these different levels of expression are not clear in that the amount of NOD2 needed for bacterial sensing in a given cell type is unknown. The expression of high amounts of NOD2 in Paneth cells was unexpected and is intriguing [74]. Paneth cells are localised mainly in the base of the crypts in the ileum and caecum and these cells are known to produce and release bacteriocidal peptides known as defensins.

NOD2 mutations and Crohn's disease. NOD2/CARD15 is of particular interest to gastroenterology because mutations in its gene confer susceptibility to the development of Crohn's disease. Three mutations are particularly important at conferring susceptibility and all are in or near the leucine-rich repeat domain (Fig 3.2). Individuals homozygous for these mutations or individuals carrying any of the three mutations on both NOD2 alleles, called compound heterozygotes, have a 20–40-fold increase in susceptibility to Crohn's disease. The mechanisms by which mutations in NOD2 are able to induce Crohn's disease remain unknown. The major working hypothesis is that the mechanism involves a loss of bacterial sensing by the mutant NOD2. Indeed, the three major mutations occur in or near the leucine-rich repeat region and do appear to result in a loss of bacterial sensing. Why NOD1 or the other TLRs would not compensate for such a mutation has yet to be explained. It is quite possible that NOD2 has functions other than bacterial sensing that have yet to be elucidated. Indeed, a recent report implicates NOD2 as a negative regulator of the TLR2 pathway [75]. These studies utilised cells from NOD2-deficient mice, which, interestingly, have no reported intestinal pathology [76]. Macrophages from NOD2-deficient mice, however, failed to respond to muramyldipeptide stimulation. Yet a third possibility is that the NODs may turn out to play some role in apoptosis that is not yet defined [77]. Lastly, one possible interpretation of the localisation in Paneth cells is that NOD2 may play a role in the release of defensins by Paneth cells and that the mutant NOD2 may have an impaired release leaving the ileocaecum more vulnerable to microbes [31]. This idea is difficult to reconcile with the report that there is a deficiency of Paneth cell alpha defensins HD5 and HD6 mRNA in the ileum of patients with Crohn's disease and that this deficiency was more pronounced in patients with mutations in NOD2 [78].

Is the NOD2 genotype of patients clinically helpful? Studies on the phenotype of individuals with NOD2 mutations have shown that these mutations are associated with Crohn's disease of the ileum, a younger age at onset and perhaps the presence of stricturing disease. There is controversy over whether the stricturing disease is an independent variable or whether it is simply a concomitant of the ileal localisation. There is no evidence that NOD2 mutations predict disease severity or the long-term course and behaviour of Crohn's disease. Patients with NOD2 mutations respond in the same way to infliximab as do patients without NOD2 mutations. There are no data as yet on NOD2 mutations and other therapies, but there is no reason to suspect that the result would be different. Because NOD2 mutations account for a minority of cases with Crohn's disease and the absolute risk of developing Crohn's disease if one is homozygote for NOD2 mutations is only 3%, at the present time there is no clinical utility for measuring NOD2 genotype in patients, patient families or persons suspected of having Crohn's disease [79].

The identification of NOD2 as a microbial pattern recognition receptor and is coherent with a large body of research in experimental animal models of inflammatory bowel disease [80]. Many of these models have been generated by experiments in which a gene has either been deleted or transgenically inserted. A common feature is the observation that the enteric bacterial flora drives intestinal inflammation in virtually all of these models. Many of these models have features that mimic those of human Crohn's disease and this infers that the bacterial flora may also drive human IBD. The discovery that immune reactivity to bacterial flagellins is present in multiple experimental models and in about half of patients with Crohn's disease supports this notion [26].

Summary

Host interactions with microbes at the intestinal surface are complex and poorly understood. A concept that is emerging from current research is that normal intestinal homeostasis depends on interactions between microbes, the intestinal epithelium and intestinal immune cells. Each of these components appears to communicate with the other two and these interactions may well form a self-reinforcing circuit. It seems likely that the TLR and NOD pattern recognition receptors participate in this dialogue between the commensal flora, the intestinal epithelium and immune cells. There will undoubtedly be much additional research on this topic in the coming years.

References

1 McCracken VJ, Lorenz RG. The gastrointestinal ecosystem: a precarious alliance among epithelium, immunity and microbiota. *Cell Microbiol* 2001;3: 1–11.
2 Sonnenburg JL, Angenent LT, Gordon JI. Getting a grip on things: how do communities of bacterial symbionts become established in our intestine? *Nat Immunol* 2004;5:569–73.
3 Rawls JF, Samuel BS, Gordon JI. Gnotobiotic zebrafish reveal evolutionarily conserved responses to the gut microbiota. *Proc Natl Acad Sci USA* 2004;101: 4596–601.
4 Hooper LV, Gordon JI. Commensal host-bacterial relationships in the gut. *Science* 2001;292:1115–8.
5 Hooper LV, Wong MH, Thelin A, Hansson L, Falk PG, Gordon JI. Molecular analysis of commensal

host-microbial relationships in the intestine. *Science* 2001;291:881–4.
6. Mukhopadhyay S, Herre J, Brown GD, Gordon S. The potential for Toll-like receptors to collaborate with other innate immune receptors. *Immunology* 2004;112:521–30.
7. Iwasaki A, Medzhitov R. Toll-like receptor control of the adaptive immune responses. *Nat Immunol* 2004;5:987–95.
8. Rakoff-Nahoum S, Paglino J, Eslami-Varzaneh F, Edberg S, Medzhitov R. Recognition of commensal microflora by toll-like receptors is required for intestinal homeostasis. *Cell* 2004;118:229–41.
9. Girardin SE, Travassos LH, Herve M, Blanot D, Boneca IG, Philpott DJ, Sansonetti PJ, Mengin-Lecreulx D. Peptidoglycan molecular requirements allowing detection by Nod1 and Nod2. *J Biol Chem* 2003;278:41702–8.
10. Girardin SE, Boneca IG, Viala J, Chamaillard M, Labigne A, Thomas G, Philpott DJ, Sansonetti PJ. Nod2 is a general sensor of peptidoglycan through muramyl dipeptide (MDP) detection. *J Biol Chem* 2003;278:8869–72.
11. Kim JG, Lee SJ, Kagnoff MF. Nod1 is an essential signal transducer in intestinal epithelial cells infected with bacteria that avoid recognition by toll-like receptors. *Infect Immun* 2004;72:1487–95.
12. Takeda K, Akira S. Toll-like receptors in innate immunity. *Int Immunol* 2005;17:1–14.
13. Janssens S, Beyaert R. Role of Toll-like receptors in pathogen recognition. *Clin Microbiol Rev* 2003;16:637–46.
14. Akhtar M, Watson JL, Nazli A, McKay DM. Bacterial DNA evokes epithelial IL-8 production by a MAPK-dependent, NF-kappaB-independent pathway. *Faseb J* 2003;17:1319–21.
15. Cario E, Podolsky DK. Differential alteration in intestinal epithelial cell expression of toll-like receptor 3 (TLR3) and TLR4 in inflammatory bowel disease. *Infect Immun* 2000;68:7010–7.
16. Gewirtz AT, Navas TA, Lyons S, Godowski PJ, Madara JL. Cutting edge: bacterial flagellin activates basolaterally expressed TLR5 to induce epithelial proinflammatory gene expression. *J Immunol* 2001;167:1882–5.
17. Cario E, Brown D, McKee M, Lynch-Devaney K, Gerken G, Podolsky DK. Commensal-associated molecular patterns induce selective toll-like receptor-trafficking from apical membrane to cytoplasmic compartments in polarized intestinal epithelium. *Am J Pathol* 2002;160:165–73.
18. Ortega-Cava CF, Ishihara S, Rumi MA, Kawashima K, Ishimura N, Kazumori H, Udagawa J, Kadowaki Y, Kinoshita Y. Strategic compartmentalization of Toll-like receptor 4 in the mouse gut. *J Immunol* 2003;170:3977–85.
19. Bambou JC, Giraud A, Menard S, Begue B, Rakotobe S, Heyman M, Taddei F, Cerf-Bensussan N, Gaboriau-Routhiau V. In vitro and ex vivo activation of the TLR5 signaling pathway in intestinal epithelial cells by a commensal Escherichia coli strain. *J Biol Chem* 2004;279:42984–92.
20. Hornef MW, Normark BH, Vandewalle A, Normark S. Intracellular recognition of lipopolysaccharide by toll-like receptor 4 in intestinal epithelial cells. *J Exp Med* 2003;198:1225–35.
21. Melrned G, Thomas LS, Lee N, Tesfay SY, Lukasek K, Michelsen KS, Zhou Y, Hu B, Arditi M, Abreu MT. Human intestinal epithelial cells are broadly unresponsive to Toll-like receptor 2-dependent bacterial ligands: implications for host-microbial interactions in the gut. *J Immunol* 2003;170:1406–15.
22. Cario E, Rosenberg IM, Brandwein SL, Beck PL, Reinecker HC, Podolsky DK. Lipopolysaccharide activates distinct signaling pathways in intestinal epithelial cell lines expressing Toll-like receptors. *J Immunol* 2000;164:966–72.
23. Lodes MJ, Cong Y, Elson CO, Mohamath R, Landers CJ, Targan SR, Fort M, Hershberg RM. Bacterial flagellin is a dominant antigen in Crohn disease. *J Clin Invest* 2004;113:1296–306.
24. Ogura Y, Bonen DK, Inohara N, Nicolae DL, Chen FF, Ramos R, Britton, H, Moran T, Karaliuskas R, Duerr RH, Achkar JP, Brant SR, Bayless TM, Kirschner BS, Hanauer SB, Nunez G, Cho JH. A frameshift mutation in NOD2 associated with susceptibility to Crohn's disease. *Nature* 2001;411:603–6.
25. Hugot JP, Chamaillard M, Zouali H, Lesage S, Cezard JP, Belaiche J, Almer S, Tysk C, O'Morain CA, Gassull M, Binder V, Finkel Y, Cortot A, Modigliani R, Laurent-Puig P, Gower-Rousseau C, Macry J, Colombel JF, Sahbatou M, Thomas G. Association of NOD2 leucine-rich repeat variants with susceptibility to Crohn's disease. *Nature* 2001;411:599–603.
26. Hampe J, Cuthbert A, Croucher PJ, Mirza MM, Mascheretti S, Fisher S, Frenzel H, King K, Hasselmeyer A, MacPherson AJ, Bridger S, van Deventer S, Forbes A, Nikolaus S, Lennard-Jones JE, Foelsch UR, Krawczak M, Lewis C, Schreiber S, Mathew CG. Association between insertion mutation in NOD2 gene and Crohn's disease in German and British populations. *Lancet* 2001;357:1925–8.
27. Ogura Y, Saab L, Chen FF, Benito A, Inohara N, Nunez G. Genetic variation and activity of mouse Nod2, a susceptibility gene for Crohn's disease. *Genomics* 2003;81:369–77.

28. Ogura Y, Lala S, Xin W, Smith E, Dowds TA, Chen FF, Zimmermann E, Tretiakova M, Cho JH, Hart J, Greenson JK, Keshav S, Nunez G. Expression of NOD2 in Paneth cells: a possible link to Crohn's ileitis. *Gut* 2003;52:1591–7.

29. Hayashi F, Means TK, Luster AD. Toll-like receptors stimulate human neutrophil function. *Blood* 2003;102:2660–9.

30. Akashi S, Shimazu R, Ogata H, Nagai Y, Takeda K, Kimoto M, Miyake K. Cutting edge: cell surface expression and lipopolysaccharide signaling via the toll-like receptor 4-MD-2 complex on mouse peritoneal macrophages. *J Immunol* 2000;164:3471–5.

31. Suzuki M, Hisamatsu T, Podolsky DK. Gamma interferon augments the intracellular pathway for lipopolysaccharide (LPS) recognition in human intestinal epithelial cells through coordinated up-regulation of LPS uptake and expression of the intracellular Toll-like receptor 4-MD-2 complex. *Infect Immun* 2003;71:3503–11.

32. Didierlaurent A, Sirard JC, Kraehenbuhl JP, Neutra MR. How the gut senses its content. *Cell Microbiol* 2002;4:61–72.

33. Cong Y, Brandwein SL, McCabe RP, Lazenby A, Birkenmeier EH, Sundberg JP, Elson CO. CD4+ T cells reactive to enteric bacterial antigens in spontaneously colitic C3H/HeJBir mice: increased T helper cell type 1 response and ability to transfer disease. *J Exp Med* 1998;187:855–64.

34. Jijon H, Backer J, Diaz H, Yeung H, Thiel D, McKaigney C, De Simone C, Madsen K. DNA from probiotic bacteria modulates murine and human epithelial and immune function. *Gastroenterology* 2004;126:1358–73.

35. Rachmilewitz D, Katakura K, Karmeli F, Hayashi T, Reinus C, Rudensky, B, Akira S, Takeda K, Lee J, Takabayashi K, Raz E. Toll-like receptor 9 signaling mediates the anti-inflammatory effects of probiotics in murine experimental colitis. *Gastroenterology* 2004;126:520–8.

36. Krieg AM. CpG motifs in bacterial DNA and their immune effects. *Annu Rev Immunol* 2002;20:709–60.

37. Ghosh DK, Misukonis MA, Reich C, Pisetsky DS, Weinberg JB. Host response to infection: the role of CpG DNA in induction of cyclooxygenase 2 and nitric oxide synthase 2 in murine macrophages. *Infect Immun* 2001;69:7703–10.

38. Chen Y, Zhang J, Moore SA, Ballas ZK, Portanova JP, Krieg AM, Berg DJ. CpG DNA induces cyclooxygenase-2 expression and prostaglandin production. *Int Immunol* 2001;13:1013–20.

39. Yeo SJ, Yoon JG, Yi AK. Myeloid differentiation factor 88-dependent post-transcriptional regulation of cyclooxygenase-2 expression by CpG DNA: tumor necrosis factor-alpha receptor-associated factor 6, a diverging point in the Toll-like receptor 9-signaling. *J Biol Chem* 2003;278:40590–600.

40. Yeo SJ, Gravis D, Yoon JG, Yi AK. Myeloid differentiation factor 88-dependent transcriptional regulation of cyclooxygenase-2 expression by CpG DNA: role of NF-kappaB and p38. *J Biol Chem* 2003;278:22563–73.

41. Ashkar AA, Rosenthal KL. Toll-like receptor 9, CpG DNA and innate immunity. *Curr Mol Med* 2002;2:545–56.

42. Krieg AM. CpG motifs: the active ingredient in bacterial extracts? *Nat Med* 2003;9:831–5.

43. Hemmi H, Takeuchi O, Kawai T, Kaisho T, Sato S, Sanjo H, Matsumoto M, Hoshino K, Wagner H, Takeda K, Akira S. A Toll-like receptor recognizes bacterial DNA. *Nature* 2000;408:740–5.

44. Vollmer J, Weeratna R, Payette P, Jurk M, Schetter C, Laucht M, Wader T, Tluk S, Liu M, Davis HL, Krieg AM. Characterization of three CpG oligodeoxynucleotide classes with distinct immunostimulatory activities. *Eur J Immunol* 2004;34:251–62.

45. Rachmilewitz D, Karmeli F, Takabayashi K, Hayashi T, Leider-Trejo L, Lee J, Leoni LM, Raz E. Immunostimulatory DNA ameliorates experimental and spontaneous murine colitis. *Gastroenterology* 2002;122:1428–41.

46. Qureshi ST, Lariviere L, Leveque G, Clermont S, Moore KJ, Gros P, Malo D. Endotoxin-tolerant mice have mutations in Toll-like receptor 4 (Tlr4). *J Exp Med* 1999;189:615–25.

47. Poltorak A, He X, Smirnova I, Liu MY, Van Huffel C, Du X, Birdwell D, Alejos, E, Silva M, Galanos C, Freudenberg M, Ricciardi-Castagnoli P, Layton B, Beutler B. Defective LPS signaling in C3H/HeJ and C57BL/10ScCr mice: mutations in Tlr4 gene. *Science* 1998;282:2085–8.

48. Schmitt C, Humeny A, Becker CM, Brune K, Pahl A. Polymorphisms of TLR4: rapid genotyping and reduced response to lipopolysaccharide of TLR4 mutant alleles. *Clin Chem* 2002;48:1661–7.

49. Hoshino K, Takeuchi O, Kawai T, Sanjo H, Ogawa T, Takeda Y, Takeda K, Akira S. Cutting edge: Toll-like receptor 4 (TLR4)-deficient mice are hyporeponsive to lipopolysaccharide: evidence for TLR4 as the Lps gene product. *J Immunol* 1999;162:3749–52.

50. Okayama N, Fujimura K, Suehiro Y, Hamanaka Y, Fujiwara M, Matsubara T, Maekawa T, Hazama S, Oka M, Nohara H, Kayano K, Okita K, Hinoda Y.

Simple genotype analysis of the Asp299Gly polymorphism of the Toll-like receptor-4 gene that is associated with lipopolysaccharide hyporesponsiveness. *J Clin Lab Anal* 2002;16:56–8.

51 Arbour NC, Lorenz E, Schutte BC, Zabner J, Kline JN, Jones M, Frees K, Watt JL, Schwartz DA. TLR4 mutations are associated with endotoxin hyporesponsiveness in humans. *Nat Genet* 2000;25: 187–91.

52 Lorenz E, Mira JP, Frees KL, Schwartz DA. Relevance of mutations in the TLR4 receptor in patients with gram-negative septic shock. *Arch Intern Med* 2002;162:1028–32.

53 Kiechl S, Lorenz E, Reindl M, Wiedermann CJ, Oberhollenzer F, Bonora E, Willeit J, Schwartz DA. Toll-like receptor 4 polymorphisms and atherogenesis. *N Engl J Med* 2002;347:185–92.

54 Franchimont D, Vermeire S, El Housni H, Pierik M, Van Steen K, Gustot T, Quertinmont E, Abramowicz M, Van Gossum A, Deviere J, Rutgeerts P. Deficient host-bacteria interactions in inflammatory bowel disease? The toll-like receptor (TLR)-4 Asp299gly polymorphism is associated with Crohn's disease and ulcerative colitis. *Gut* 2004;53:987–92.

55 Torok HP, Glas J, Tonenchi L, Mussack T, Folwaczny C. Polymorphisms of the lipopolysaccharide-signaling complex in inflammatory bowel disease: association of a mutation in the Toll-like receptor 4 gene with ulcerative colitis. *Clin Immunol* 2004;112:85–91.

56 Torok HP, Glas J, Tonenchi L, Bruennler G, Folwaczny M, Folwaczny C. Crohn's disease is associated with a toll-like receptor-9 polymorphism. *Gastroenterology* 2004;127:365–6.

57 Lorenz E, Mira JP, Cornish KL, Arbour NC, Schwartz DA. A novel polymorphisms in the toll-like receptor 2 gene and its potential association with staphylococcal infection. *Infect Immun* 2000;68:6398–401.

58 Cook DN, Pisetsky DS, Schwartz DA. Toll-like receptors in the pathogenesis of human disease. *Nat Immunol* 2004;5:975–9.

59 Ogus AC, Yoldas B, Ozdemir T, Uguz A, Olcen S, Keser I, Coskun M, Cilli A, Yegin O. The Arg753GLn polymorphism of the human toll-like receptor 2 gene in tuberculosis disease. *Eur Respir J* 2004;23:219–23.

60 Bochud PY, Hawn TR, Aderem A. Cutting edge: a Toll-like receptor 2 polymorphism that is associated with lepromatous leprosy is unable to mediate mycobacterial signaling. *J Immunol* 2003;170: 3451–4.

61 Hawn TR, Verbon A, Lettinga KD, Zhao LP, Li SS, Laws RJ, Skerrett SJ, Beutler B, Schroeder L, Nachman A, Ozinsky A, Smith KD, Aderem A. A common dominant TLR5 stop codon polymorphism abolishes flagellin signaling and is associated with susceptibility to legionnaires' disease. *J Exp Med* 2003;198:1563–72.

62 Inohara N, Ogura Y, Nunez G. Nods: a family of cytosolic proteins that regulate the host response to pathogens. *Curr Opin Microbiol* 2002;5:76–80.

63 Chamaillard M, Girardin SE, Viala J, Philpott DJ. Nods, Nalps and Naip: intracellular regulators of bacterial-induced inflammation. *Cell Microbiol* 2003;5:581–92.

64 Girardin SE, Hugot JP, Sansonetti PJ. Lessons from Nod2 studies: towards a link between Crohn's disease and bacterial sensing. *Trends Immunol* 2003;24: 652–8.

65 Kobayashi K, Inohara N, Hernandez LD, Galan JE, Nunez G, Janeway CA, Medzhitov R, Flavell RA. RICK/Rip2/CARDIAK mediates signalling for receptors of the innate and adaptive immune systems. *Nature* 2002;416:194–9.

66 Ogura Y, Inohara N, Benito A, Chen FF, Yamaoka S, Nunez G. Nod2, a Nod1/Apaf-1 family member that is restricted to monocytes and activates NF-kappaB. *J Biol Chem* 2001;276:4812–8.

67 Hisamatsu T, Suzuki M, Reinecker HC, Nadeau WJ, McCormick BA, Podolsky DK. CARD15/NOD2 functions as an antibacterial factor in human intestinal epithelial cells. *Gastroenterology* 2003;124:993–1000.

68 Viala J, Chaput C, Boneca IG, Cardona A, Girardin SE, Moran AP, Athman R, Memet S, Huerre MR, Coyle AJ, DiStefano PS, Sansonetti PJ, Labigne A, Bertin J, Philpott DJ, Ferrero RL. Nod1 responds to peptidoglycan delivered by the Helicobacter pylori cag pathogenicity island. *Nat Immunol* 2004;5:1166–74.

69 Underhill DM, Ozinsky A, Hajjar AM, Stevens A, Wilson CB, Bassetti M, Aderem A. The Toll-like receptor 2 is recruited to macrophage phagosomes and discriminates between pathogens. *Nature* 1999;401: 811–5.

70 Otte JM, Rosenberg IM, Podolsky DK. Intestinal myofibroblasts in innate immune responses of the intestine. *Gastroenterology* 2003;124:1866–78.

71 Lala S, Ogura Y, Osborne C, Hor SY, Bromfield A, Davies S, Ogunbiyi O, Nunez G, Keshav S. Crohn's disease and the NOD2 gene: a role for paneth cells. *Gastroenterology* 2003;125:47–57.

72 Watanabe T, Kitani A, Murray PJ, Strober W. NOD2 is a negative regulator of Toll-like receptor 2-mediated T helper type 1 responses. *Nat Immunol* 2004;5: 800–8.

73 Pauleau AL, Murray PJ. Role of nod2 in the response of macrophages to toll-like receptor agonists. *Mol Cell Biol* 2003;23:7531–9.

74 Beutler B. Autoimmunity and apoptosis: the Crohn's connection. *Immunity* 2001;15:5–14.

75 Wehkamp J, Harder J, Weichenthal M, Schwab M, Schaffeler E, Schlee M, Herrlinger KR, Stallmach A, Noack F, Fritz P, Schroder JM, Bevins CL, Fellermann K, Stange EF. NOD2 (CARD15) mutations in Crohn's disease are associated with diminished mucosal alpha-defensin expression. *Gut* 2004;53: 1658–64.

76 Colombel JF. The CARD15 (also known as NOD2) gene in Crohn's disease: are there implications for current clinical practice? *Clin Gastroenterol Hepatol* 2003;1:5–9.

77 Elson CO, Weaver CT. Experimental mouse models of inflammatory bowel disease: new insights into pathogenic mechanisms. In: Targan SR, Shanahan F, Karp LC, eds. *Inflammatory Bowel Disease: From Bench to Bedside*. Dordrecht: Kluwer Academic Publishers; 2003:67–99.

78 Heil F, Hemmi H, Hochrein H, Hochrein H, Ampenberger F, Kirschning C, Akira S, Lipford G, Wagner H, Bauer S. Species-specific recognition of single-stranded RNA via toll-like receptor 7 and 8. *Science* 2004;303:1526–9.

79 Zhang D, Zhang G, Hayden MS, Greenblatt MB, Bussey C, Flavell RA, Ghosh S. A toll-like receptor that prevents infection by uropathogenic bacteria. *Science* 2004;303:1522–6.

80 Otte JM, Cario E, Podolsky DK. Mechanisms of cross hyporesponsiveness to Toll-like receptor bacterial ligands in intestinal epithelial cells. *Gastroenterology* 2004;126:1054–70.

4: The role of bacteria

Robert Penner and Karen Madsen

Acknowledgements: Alberta Heritage Foundation for Medical Research Crohn's and Colitis Foundation of Canada Canadian Institutes for Health Research

Introduction

The pathogenesis of Crohn's disease (CD) and ulcerative colitis (UC), the two major forms of inflammatory bowel disease (IBD), involves a complex interaction between genetic, environmental and immunological factors, with luminal bacteria appearing to be a significant factor in the onset and chronicity of inflammation in both diseases. There is substantial evidence that luminal microbial factors play a critical role in the aetiology of these diseases. IBD primarily occurs in areas of the intestine with the highest bacterial concentration [1]. Patients with Crohn's disease respond to diversion of the faecal stream and suffer relapsing injury when luminal contents are re-introduced [2, 3]. Under normal conditions, mucosal tolerance exists towards the high numbers of bacteria found in the gut, that is, an immune response is not mounted against these bacteria. Patients with IBD exhibit a loss of tolerance to commensal micro-flora, as evidenced by enhanced T-cell and humoral immune responses [4, 5]. To support this concept of a breakdown of tolerance to gut bacteria, van der Waaij et al. [6] have shown that in healthy individuals, only a small fraction of luminal bacteria are coated with IgA, IgG or IgM, whereas IBD patients with active disease have an increased percentage of immunoglobulin-coated faecal anaerobic bacteria. This loss of tolerance may occur as a result of several contributing factors, including alterations in regulatory T-cell function, defects in bacterial antigen recognition, a breakdown in gut barrier function and/or dysbiosis in the balance between beneficial and inflammatory microbes within the lumen of the gut.

It is becoming evident that genes regulating mucosal immune responses and microbial recognition and defence mechanisms define the host response to enteric micro-flora and subsequent susceptibility to developing inflammatory bowel disease. The recent case report of a patient with Hodgkin's lymphoma developing Crohn's disease following allogenic stem cell transplantation when the donor exhibited no signs of clinical disease [7], is evidence that development of clinical disease requires both genetic susceptibility and a particular local environment within the gut. The identification of NOD2 (CARD15) as a susceptibility gene for Crohn's disease [8] has led to a new appreciation of the role of the innate immune system in the pathogenesis of inflammatory bowel disease. NOD2(CARD15) is an intra-cellular protein that recognises and activates intra-cellular signalling pathways in response to muramyl dipeptide (MDP), a basic component of the cell wall of both gram-positive and gram-negative bacteria [9]. NOD2 variants associated with Crohn's disease demonstrate altered NF-κB activation and defensin expression, resulting in a defective clearance of invasive bacteria [10, 11]. Recent studies showing an association between IBD and polymorphisms in the toll-like receptors responsible for recognising and responding to bacterial lipopolysaccharide (TLR4) [12] and bacterial DNA (TLR9) [13] further support

Table 4.1 Pathogenic microbes associated with inflammatory bowel disease.

Microbe	Reference
Bacteroides	[14–18]
Enterobacteria	[19, 16]
Butyrivibrio, Rosburia, Thermotoga, Clostridium	[20]
Adherent/Invasive *E. coli*	[15, 21, 22, 23, 24, 25]
Enterococcus faecalis	[26]
Fusobacterium varium	[27, 28]
Listeria monocytogenes	[29, 30]
Helicobacter	[31, 32]
Pseudomonas fluorescens	[24, 25]
Clostridia	[16]
Chlamydia pneumoniae	[33]

the concept of a link between a defective innate immune response to micro-flora and the development of IBD. It has been hypothesised that these defective responses by the innate immune system to luminal micro-flora could result in a failure to clear microbes from the mucosa and cause a subsequent chronic inflammatory state characterised by heightened acquired immune responses. However, the possible presence of pathogenic microbial strains in patients with inflammatory bowel disease still cannot fully be discounted, especially considering 30–40% of the colonic micro-flora still cannot be cultured and belongs to undefined phylogenic groups (Table 4.1) [29, 33].

Commensal micro-flora

Bacteria are found throughout the entire intestine, but are concentrated in the colon. The stomach and small intestine have a sparse micro-flora of approximately 10^5 colony-forming units (CFU)/mL contents of primarily *Lactobacilli* sp. In the ileum, micro-flora concentrations increase to 10^8–10^9, finally reaching 10^{11}–10^{12} CFU in the colon [34]. It is estimated that more than 400–500 bacterial species are inhabitants of the human colon, with five genera accounting for the majority of anaerobic bacteria: *Bacteroides, Eubacterium, Bifidobacterium, Peptostreptococcus* and *Fusobacterium* [34]. However, the recent use of molecular techniques based on nucleic acid sequence comparisons suggests that these numbers, which are based on conventional culture, could be significantly underestimating both numbers and species diversity [35]. The typical intestinal flora in humans eating a western-style diet consists of the following organisms, in decreasing order of concentration: (1) *Bacteroides, Eubacteria, Peptostreptococci* and *Bifidobacteria* (10^{10}–10^{11} cfu/gm faeces; (2) *Enterobacteria* and *Streptococci* (10^8–10^9 cfu/gm faeces), the former includes mainly *Escherichia coli*, with some *Klebsiella* and *Proteus* species; (3) *Lactobacilli* (10^5–10^8 cfu/gm) and (4) *Clostridia* and *Staphylococci*. Various other facultative and aerobic bacterial strains are also found sporadically throughout the small and large intestine. There exist several different habitats within the gastrointestinal tract, which micro-organisms have adapted to. The endogenous flora differs between the small and large intestine and between right and left colon and rectum. Micro-organisms within the mucus layer of the colon are different from those in the lumen and from those living in close proximity to the surface of epithelial cells [1]. Each individual has his or her own unique combination of micro-flora, which remains stable over time. However, this large physiological inter-individual variation in micro-flora creates a challenge to the identification of organisms potentially involved in diseases processes.

Micro-organisms are critical for the proper development of a competent immune system and exert influence over the structural and functional development of the gut. Bacteria colonise the intestine within hours of birth, with the first organisms being *Enterobacteria* and *Enterococci*, followed by colonisation with *Bifidobacterium* [36]. The introduction of solid food causes a major shift in bacterial strains colonising the colon, with a rise of *Enterobacteria* and *Enterococci*, followed by colonisation with *Bacteroides* spp, *Clostridia* and anaerobic *Streptococci*. There is evidence that early colonisation of the gut may be influenced by genetic make-up of the host [37] and also that the early colonisers can influence gene expression in the host to generate a beneficial environment for themselves [38]. In weaned infants, children and adults, the composition remains relatively stable, unless disturbed by frequent use of antibiotics [39–41].

Overall, evidence is accumulating that the composition and activity of the intestinal micro-flora has a significant impact on the health of the host, due to its influence on the mucosal immune system and physiology of the intestinal tract [42, 43].

Factors affecting colonic micro-flora

Numerous environmental factors influence the intestinal micro-flora. Diet, infections and the use of antibiotics and/or other drugs can significantly alter the types and numbers of bacterial species present. In addition, several bacteria, such as *Bacteroides*, *Enterobacter* and *Enterococcus*, can release compounds that act as growth stimulators, or, conversely, growth inhibitors, for other species [44]. Thus, the levels of particular bacterial strains in the colon may be regulated, in part, by the presence or absence of other bacterial species. Furthermore, factors such as gastric acidity, intestinal motility, redox potential, immune status of the host and the presence of adherence factors can alter colonisation. Although ethnic origin and climate do not appear to be major determinants of intestinal micro-flora [45], geographical differences are seen in colonic micro-flora, although it is thought that differences are linked with the diets associated with the different regions [46].

Evidence from animal models

Animal models were crucial in early experimentation on infectious diseases, where they demonstrated fulfillment of Koch's postulates for disease-causing organisms. Although inflammatory bowel disease cannot at this time be explained by a simple one-agent-one-disease infectious model, the development of genetically altered animal models and the use of naturally occurring animal models of IBD have demonstrated that the luminal flora is essential to disease expression. However, these studies have also shown that the interaction between the mucosal immune system and its often troublesome guests is far more complex than a traditional infectious model.

The first of Koch's postulates states that an infectious agent should be present in all individuals with disease but not in healthy subjects. Micro-flora are present in the intestinal lumen of all normal individuals and studies in animal models of IBD demonstrate that the absence of luminal micro-flora will prevent disease expression. The absence of intestinal inflammation in germ-free animals genetically predisposed to inflammatory bowel disease has been demonstrated in multiple animal models, including the IL-10 and IL-2 deficient mouse models [47–49], the inbred SAMP1/Yit mouse [50], the HLA-B27 rat transgenic model [14] and various chemically induced models [1, 51]. In addition, some studies have demonstrated a dose-response correlation between the load of intestinal bacteria and the magnitude of inflammatory bowel disease expression [52]. Although luminal flora are necessary for disease onset in these animal models, the severity and location of lesions, as well as the rate of disease progression, is influenced by the genetic background of the host and by the composition of the micro-flora [53, 54]. It is clear that not all bacterial species are able to induce inflammation [55] and, in fact, some bacterial strains are immunosuppressive [56, 57]. Interestingly, effects of bacteria also appear to be specific to various regions of the gut [55, 58]. In IL-10-deficient mice, *Enterococcus faecalis* [26] and some *Helicobacter* species [31, 32] but not others [59], induce colitis, while *Lactobacillus reuteri* [57], *L. plantarum* [60], *L. salivarius* [61], *Bifidobacterium infantis* [61] and VSL3 [62], a combination of eight bacterial strains, exert beneficial effects. In the HLA-B27 transgenic rat model, a mixture of six bacterial strains induced colitis [14], but the same mixture had relatively minimal effect in IL-10-deficient mice [47]. In a similar fashion, *Bacteroides vulgatus* induced severe colitis in HLA-B27 rats [52], but only very mild disease in IL-10-deficient mice [47]. In addition to variation between mouse and rat models in response to defined micro-flora, there is also considerable variation in the development of colitis in different inbred mouse strains with the same genetic variance, even to the same micro-flora, indicating a major contribution from genetic background modifiers [53, 54]. Thus, although the exact nature of the interaction between the intestinal immune system and its resident micro-flora is far from understood, these and other experiments in animal models have suggested several conclusions. First, certain strains of bacteria appear to be more likely to induce disease than others; second, no single bacterial strain will consistently induce disease in all models and third, the host genetic background significantly influences disease severity and progression even in the presence of the same bacterial strains.

Koch's second postulate requires that an infectious organism be isolated and grown in pure culture. However, the enteric flora contains many different species of bacteria, an estimated 30–40% of these species have not been cultured or identified, and none have yet proven to be individual causative agents in humans. In fact, it is not known yet if live bacteria are necessary, or whether non-viable bacterial products may be sufficient to initiate and perpetuate inflammatory bowel diseases. Recent work has shown that naked bacterial DNA can both suppress [63–65] and exacerbate inflammation [66, 67], depending upon which bacterial strain the DNA is isolated from, suggesting that live organisms may not even be necessary. Koch's third and fourth postulates required that the inoculation of an isolated organism into a healthy animal produce disease, and that the organism must be re-isolated from the newly diseased animal. Early animal experimentation in Crohn's disease once again suggested that inflammatory bowel disease would be a more complex model, when the inoculation of faecal flora from patients suffering from Crohn's disease into germ-free rats failed to produce colitis or ileitis [68]. In addition, in many rodent models, mucosal inflammation can be transferred by injecting either isolated CD4+ T cells or lamina propria lymphocytes derived from diseased animals into immune-deficient mice, without the presence of live micro-organisms [1].

Alterations in microbial flora in IBD

Although no specific microbe has been conclusively linked with either Crohn's disease or ulcerative colitis, numerous studies using both culture-dependent and independent molecular techniques have shown that significant differences exist in both diversity and location of bacterial species in IBD patients compared with healthy individuals [15, 19, 21, 27, 28, 69–72]. Earlier studies using immunohistochemical methodology demonstrated the presence of antigens of *E. coli* and *Streptococci* in lamina propria macrophages under ulcers and fissures in Crohn's disease patients [24, 25]. In more recent studies, it has been reported that certain invasive *E. coli* strains with adhesive-like qualities are more likely to be found associated with the ileal mucosal of Crohn's disease patients [22, 23]. In some studies, IBD patients demonstrated increased levels of *Bacteroides* and *Enterococci* and decreased *Lactobacillus* and *Bifidobacterium* sp., especially during periods of active disease [19, 22, 71]. A common finding in both human IBD patients [16, 73, 74] and animal models of IBD [57] is a higher number of bacteria found closely associated with or adherent to the mucosa. Studies using 16S rDNA-based single-strand conformation polymorphism and real-time PCR have demonstrated a reduction in bacterial diversity in both Crohn's disease and ulcerative colitis patients due primarily to the loss of anaerobic bacteria [69]. However, in that up to 30% of the micro-flora in IBD patients has been shown to belong to undefined phylogenic groups [19]; substantially more work needs to be carried out in this area to conclusively identify all IBD-associated micro-flora.

Systemic immune responses to micro-flora

Although CD4+ T cells play a central role in the immune perturbations of IBD, human and animal studies suggest that only a small number of bacterial antigens appear to stimulate pathogenic T-cell responses [75, 76]. Using molecular techniques, specific reactivity to an antigen (I2) from *Pseudomonas fluorescens* [77, 78] and to the outer membrane porin protein C of *Escherichia coli* (anti-OmpC) have been described with a sero-prevalence for anti-OmpC of 55% and anti-I2 of 50% in Crohn's disease [79]. Reactivity to specific bacterial flagellins from the genera *Butyrivibrio*, *Rosburia*, *Thermotoga* and *Clostridium* have also been reported in Crohn's disease, but not ulcerative colitis [20]. These newly described sero-reactivities complement and extend previous studies examining the prevalence of antibodies directed against the oligomannan component of *Saccharomyes cerevisiae* (ASCA) and the perinuclear component of neutrophils (pANCA) and their usefulness as diagnostic tools for inflammatory bowel disease [80]. It appears that IBD patients display individual patterns of sero-reactivity against these bacterial antigens and can be grouped into subsets based upon microbial sero-reactivity. Given the complexity of the intestinal micro-flora and the heterogeneous nature of inflammatory bowel disease, it is not surprising that these different patterns of sero-reactivity are appearing. A strong relationship between phenotypic disease expression and progression, and the presence and magnitude of systemic immune responses to these microbial antigens has been shown to exist in patients with Crohn's disease [81, 82] and it will be interesting to determine if response to treatment also correlates with microbial reactivities.

Harnessing the bacteria: pre-, pro- and antibiotics

The most practical proof of principle that inflammatory bowel disease represents a deranged relationship with the enteric flora lies in the observations that therapies aimed at modifying luminal microflora are beneficial. Antibiotics have been in widespread use for many years, so it is no surprise that they were some of the earlier drugs to receive attention as possible treatments for inflammatory bowel disease. Indeed, because a luminal bacterial flora must be present for IBD to be expressed, it is intuitive that long-term complete bowel sterilisation with antibiotics could result in clinical remission. Although treatment of that intensity is probably not realistic, selective reduction of colonic bacterial loads with a variety of antibiotic agents, in a variety of clinical settings, has been attempted. For example, metronidazole, whose specificity is predominantly anaerobic, has demonstrated some efficacy as primary therapy for active Crohn's disease alone [83, 84], or in combination with ciprofloxacin [85]. It has also been effective in the setting of post-surgical prophylaxis for Crohn's disease and pouchitis following ileoanal pouch anastomosis [86, 87]. Ciprofloxacin, whose specificity is predominantly aerobic, has also had promising results in active Crohn's disease [88] and pouchitis [89]. Unfortunately, research on antibiotics in inflammatory bowel disease has often been of poor quality and yielded inconclusive results, but, despite these weaknesses, antibiotics remain a part of the therapeutic armamentarium for IBD [90]. Selective antibiotics for IBD treatment might hold more promise if they were able to selectively target relatively pathogenic strains while sparing beneficial bacteria. Such a strategy remains currently in the theoretical realm.

Probiotic therapy seeks to improve the disease course by replenishing or generating a protective bacterial flora. Several mechanisms have been proposed by which probiotic bacteria might exert a beneficial influence. First, probiotics might successfully compete with more pathogenic bacteria for a niche in the human bowel [91, 92]. This could occur by direct competition for a limited number of surface receptors, by secretion of factors toxic to pathogenic bacteria or by alteration of the chemical environment – for example, the luminal pH [93]. Second, probiotics might exert a beneficial effect on luminal immune regulation by decreasing production of pro-inflammatory cytokines like TNFα and IFNγ and increasing production of cytokines with a mediating effect, like IL-10 and TGFβ [57, 94–98]. Third, probiotics may improve epithelial defences against more pathogenic bacteria by enhancing epithelial barrier function and stimulating IgA secretion [62] (Table 4.2).

The exact mechanism through which probiotics exert their effects may vary depending on the organism being harnessed for therapy. This can complicate understanding of the literature, because a wide range of organisms are under study. Research using various probiotic substances in diverse clinical settings has had understandably variable conclusions, but has been particularly promising in maintaining antibiotic-induced remission of pouchitis [56, 137]. Probiotic therapies have often been inventive, as illustrated by one study in which faecal enemas derived from healthy donors were administered to active UC patients [138]. Although the existing literature on probiotics remains too inconsistent for routine use in clinical practice [139], positive experiences leave little doubt that there are physiologic benefits that can be gained through the use of faecal flora modification.

Table 4.2 Biologic effects of probiotic bacteria.

Mechanism of action	Biologic effect	References
Epithelial barrier	Enhanced epithelial resistance	[62]
	Enhanced phosphorylation of actinin and occluding	[99]
	Upregulation of MUC3 mRNA and secretion	[100]
	Maintenance of F-actin and transport and enzymatic activity	[101]
	Reduced colonic permeability	[102]
	Enhanced epithelial cell glycosylation	[103]
Antibody production	Enhanced Ab production	[104–116]
Cell mediated immunity	Enhanced phagocytic activity	
Antigen presentation	Enhanced NK activity	
	Modulation of dendritic cell phenotype and function	
Cell signalling	Modulation of NF-κB pathway	[63]
		[117, 118]
Apoptosis	Prevention of apoptosis	[119]
	Induction of apoptosis	[120]
Anti-oxidative	Enhanced survival in oxidative environment	[121]
	Inhibited linoleic acid peroxidation	
	Scavenge DPPH-free radicals	
Adhesive properties	Prevention of pathogenic strains from adhering to epithelial cells	[92]
	Disease-specific adhesion	[91]
	Strain-specific adhesion	[122–124]
Anti-microbial	Production of organic acids	[111, 125–130]
	Hydrogen peroxide	
	Bacteriocins	
	Reduction of luminal pH	
Cytokine production	Increased pro-inflammatory and/or	[57, 63, 95, 96, 131–136]
	Decreased pro-inflammatory	[61, 98]

The newest, and perhaps most elegant experimental therapy applying faecal flora modification for the treatment of IBD involves prebiotics. Prebiotics are substances, generally undigested carbohydrates, which selectively alter the faecal flora in favour of beneficial organisms, most commonly *Lactobacillus* and *Bifidobacterium*. They are theoretically tempting because they are relatively innocuous, promote the growth of favourable colonic bacteria and provide that flora with the building blocks required to produce beneficial substances such as short-chain fatty acids [140, 141]. Human studies in ulcerative colitis have been promising, demonstrating that germinated barley foodstuffs can alter the faecal flora in a theoretically beneficial way, while perhaps inducing clinical improvement, but the data remain preliminary in nature [142–144].

In summary, although many therapies targeting the luminal flora remain experimental, adequate evidence exists to conclude that the luminal flora plays a crucial role in inflammatory bowel disease expression. The continued use of molecular tools to identify and characterise gut micro-flora will greatly aid the quest to find the triggers for the development of disease. Furthermore, investigations aimed at determining the mechanisms underlying the alterations in the micro-biota associated with inflammatory bowel disease will likely yield new answers, and have the potential to open up new and exciting avenues for therapy based on modifying the luminal environment.

References

1. Sartor R. Microbial influences in inflammatory bowel disease: role in pathogenesis and clinical implications. In: Sartor RB SW, ed. *Kirsner's Inflammatory Bowel Diseases*. Edinburgh: Elsevier; 2003:138–62.
2. Harper PH, Lee EC, Kettlewell MG, Bennett MK, Jewell DP. Role of the faecal stream in the maintenance of Crohn's colitis. *Gut* 1985;26(3): 279–84.
3. D'Haens GR, Geboes K, Peeters M, Baert F, Penninckx F, Rutgeerts P. Early lesions of recurrent Crohn's disease caused by infusion of intestinal contents in excluded ileum [see comment]. *Gastroenterology* 1998;114(2):262–7.
4. Duchmann R, Kaiser I, Hermann E, Mayet W, Ewe K, Meyer zum Buschenfelde KH. Tolerance exists towards resident intestinal flora but is broken in active inflammatory bowel disease (IBD) [see comment]. *Clin Exp Immunol* 1995;102(3):448–55.
5. Macpherson A, Khoo UY, Forgacs I, Philpott-Howard J, Bjarnason I. Mucosal antibodies in inflammatory bowel disease are directed against intestinal bacteria. *Gut* 1996;38(3):365–75.
6. van der Waaij LA KF, Visser A, Nelis GF, Westerveld BD, Jansen PL, Hunter JO. Immunoglobulin coating of faecal bacteria in inflammatory bowel disease. *Eur J Gastroenterol Hepatol* 2004;16(7):669–74.
7. Sonwalkar SA, James RM, Ahmad T, Zhang L, Verbeke CS, Bernard DL, Jewell DP, Hull MA. Fulminant Crohn's colitis after allogeneic stem cell transplantation [see comment]. *Gut* 2003;52(10): 1518–21.
8. Bonen DK, Cho JH. The genetics of inflammatory bowel disease. *Gastroenterology* 2003;124(2): 521–36.
9. Inohara N, Ogura Y, Fontalba A, Gutierrez O, Pons F, Crespo J, Fukase K, Inamura S, Kusumoto S, Hashimoto M, Foster SJ, Moran AP, Fernandez-Luna JL, Nunez G. Host recognition of bacterial muramyl dipeptide mediated through NOD2. Implications for Crohn's disease. *J Biol Chem* 2003;278(8): 5509–12.
10. Hisamatsu T, Suzuki M, Reinecker HC, Nadeau WJ, McCormick BA, Podolsky DK. CARD15/NOD2 functions as an antibacterial factor in human intestinal epithelial cells [see comment]. *Gastroenterology* 2003;124(4):993–1000.
11. Wehkamp J HJ, Weichenthal M, Schwab M, Schaffeler E, Schlee M, Herrlinger KR, Stallmach A, Noach F, Prtz P, Schroder JM, Bevins CL, Fellerman K, Stange EF. NOD2 (CARD15) mutations in Crohn's disease are associated with diminished mucosal a-defensin expression. *Gut* 2004;53: 1658–64.
12. Franchimont D, Vermeire S, El Housni H, Pierik M, Van Steen K, Gustot T, Quertinmont E, Abramowicz M, Van Gossum A, Deviere J, Rutgeerts P. Deficient host-bacteria interactions in inflammatory bowel disease? The toll-like receptor (TLR)-4 Asp299gly polymorphism is associated with Crohn's disease and ulcerative colitis. *Gut* 2004;53(7):987–92.
13. Torok HP, Glas J, Tonenchi L, Bruennler G, Folwaczny M, Folwaczny C. Crohn's disease is associated with a toll-like receptor-9 polymorphism [comment]. *Gastroenterology* 2004;127(1):365–6.
14. Eckburg PB, Bik EM, Bernstein CN, Purdom E, Dethlefsen L, Sargent M, Gill SR, Nelson KE, Relman DA. Diversity of the human intestinal microbial flora. *Science* 2005;308(5728):1635–8.
15. Simon GL, Gorbach SL. Intestinal flora in health and disease. *Gastroenterology* 1984;86(1):174–93.
16. Harmsen HJ, Gibson GR, Elfferich P, Raangs GC, Wildeboer-Veloo AC, Argaiz A, Roberfroid MB, Welling GW. Comparison of viable cell counts and fluorescence *in situ* hybridization using specific rRNA-based probes for the quantification of human fecal bacteria. *FEMS Microbiol Lett* 2000;183(1): 125–9.
17. Lejeune C, Bourrillon A, Boussougant Y, de Paillerets F. Sequential development of the intestinal flora in newborn infants: a quantitative differential analysis. *Dev Pharmacol Ther* 1984; 7(Suppl 1):138–43.
18. Vaughan EE, de Vries MC, Zoetendal EG, Ben-Amor K, Akkermans AD, de Vos WM. The intestinal LABs. *Antonie van Leeuwenhoek* 2002;82(1–4):341–52.
19. Bry L, Falk PG, Midtvedt T, Gordon JI. A model of host-microbial interactions in an open mammalian ecosystem [see comment]. *Science* 1996; 273(5280): 1380–3.
20. Tannock GW. Analysis of the intestinal microflora using molecular methods. *Eur J Clin Nutr* 2002; 56(Suppl 4):S44–9.
21. Kimura K, McCartney AL, McConnell MA, Tannock GW. Analysis of fecal populations of *Bifidobacteria* and *Lactobacilli* and investigation of the immunological responses of their human hosts to the predominant strains. *Appl Environ Microbiol* 1997;63(9):3394–8.

22 McCartney AL, Wenzhi W, Tannock GW. Molecular analysis of the composition of the bifidobacterial and lactobacillus microflora of humans. *Appl Environ Microbiol* 1996;62(12):4608–13.

23 Hooper LV, Gordon JI. Commensal host-bacterial relationships in the gut. *Science* 2001;292(5519): 1115–18.

24 Hooper LV, Midtvedt T, Gordon JI. How host-microbial interactions shape the nutrient environment of the mammalian intestine. *Annu Rev Nutr* 2002;22:283–307.

25 Naidu AS, Bidlack WR, Clemens RA. Probiotic spectra of lactic acid bacteria (LAB). *Crit Rev Food Sci Nutr* 1999;39(1):13–126.

26 Hill MJ, Drasar DS. Bacteria and the aetiology of human cancer. *Br J Cancer* 1973;28(1):94.

27 Mai V. Dietary modification of the intestinal microbiota. *Nutr Rev* 2004;62(6, Pt 1):235–42.

28 Sellon RK, Tonkonogy S, Schultz M, Dieleman LA, Grenther W, Balish E, Rennick DM, Sartor RB. Resident enteric bacteria are necessary for development of spontaneous colitis and immune system activation in interleukin-10-deficient mice. *Infect Immun* 1998;66(11):5224–31.

29 Madsen KL, Malfair D, Gray D, Doyle JS, Jewell LD, Fedorak RN. Interleukin-10 gene-deficient mice develop a primary intestinal permeability defect in response to enteric microflora. *Inflamm Bowel Dis* 1999;5(4):262–70.

30 Sadlack B, Merz H, Schorle H, Schimpl A, Feller AC, Horak I. Ulcerative colitis-like disease in mice with a disrupted interleukin-2 gene [see comment]. *Cell* 1993;75(2):253–61.

31 Matsumoto S, Okabe Y, Setoyama H, Takayama K, Ohtsuka J, Funahashi H, Imaoka A, Okada Y, Umesaki Y. Inflammatory bowel disease-like enteritis and caecitis in a senescence accelerated mouse P1/Yit strain. *Gut* 1998;43(1):71–8.

32 Rath HC, Herfarth HH, Ikeda JS, Grenther WB, Hamm Jr. TE, Balish E, Taurog JD, Hammer RE, Wilson KH, Sartor RB. Normal luminal bacteria, especially *Bacteroides* species, mediate chronic colitis, gastritis, and arthritis in HLA-B27/human beta2 microglobulin transgenic rats. *J Clin Invest* 1996;98(4):945–53.

33 Onderdonk AB, Bartlett JG. Bacteriological studies of experimental ulcerative colitis. *Am J Clin Nutr* 1979; 32(1):258–65.

34 Rath HC, Ikeda JS, Linde HJ, Scholmerich J, Wilson KH, Sartor RB. Varying cecal bacterial loads influences colitis and gastritis in HLA-B27 transgenic rats. *Gastroenterology* 1999;116(2): 310–19.

35 Mahler M, Leiter EH. Genetic and environmental context determines the course of colitis developing in IL-10-deficient mice. *Inflamm Bowel Dis* 2002;8(5): 347–55.

36 Mahler M, Bristol IJ, Leiter EH, Workman AE, Birkenmeier EH, Elson CO, Sundberg JP. Differential susceptibility of inbred mouse strains to dextran sulfate sodium-induced colitis. *Am J Physiol* 1998;274(3, Pt 1):G544–51.

37 Rath HC, Schultz M, Freitag R, Dieliman LA, Li F, Linde HJ, Scholmerich J, Sartor RB. Different subsets of enteric bacteria induce and perpetuate experimental colitis in rats and mice. *Infect Immun* 2001;69(4):2277–85.

38 Madsen KL, Doyle JS, Jewell LD, Tavernini MM, Fedorak RN. Lactobacillus species prevents colitis in interleukin 10 gene-deficient mice [see comment]. *Gastroenterology* 1999;116(5):1107–14.

39 Kim SC, Tonkonogy SL, Albright CA, Tsang J, Balish EJ, Braun J, Huycke MM, Sartor RB. Variable phenotypes of enterocolitis in interleukin 10-deficient mice monoassociated with two different commensal bacteria. *Gastroenterology*, 2005;128(4): 891–906.

40 Balish E, Warner T. *Enterococcus faecalis* induces inflammatory bowel disease in interleukin-10 knockout mice. *Am J Pathol* 2002;160(6):2253–7.

41 Kullberg MC, Ward JM, Gorelick PL, Caspar P, Hieny S, Cheever A, Jankovic D, Sher A. *Helicobacter hepaticus* triggers colitis in specific-pathogen-free interleukin-10 (IL-10)-deficient mice through an IL-12- and gamma interferon-dependent mechanism. *Infect Immun* 1998;66(11):5157–66.

42 Dieleman LA, Arends A, Tonkonogy SL, Goerres MS, Craft DW, Grenther W, Sellon RK, Balish E, Sartor RB. *Helicobacter hepaticus* does not induce or potentiate colitis in interleukin-10-deficient mice. *Infect Immun* 2000;68(9):5107–13.

43 Schultz M, Veltkamp C, Dieleman LA, Grenther WB, Wyrick PB, Tonkonogy SL, Sartor RB. *Lactobacillus plantarum* 299V in the treatment and prevention of spontaneous colitis in interleukin-10-deficient mice. *Inflamm Bowel Dis* 2002;8(2):71–80.

44 McCarthy J, O'Mahony L, O'Callaghan L, Sheil B, Vaughan EE, Fitzsimons N, Fitzgibbon J, O'Sullivan GC, Kiely B, Collins JK, Shanahan F. Double blind, placebo controlled trial of two probiotic strains in interleukin 10 knockout mice and mechanistic link with cytokine balance. *Gut* 2003;52(7):975–80.

45 Madsen K, Cornish A, Soper P, McKaigney C, Jijon H, Yachimec C, Doyle J, Jewell L, De Simone C. Probiotic bacteria enhance murine and human

intestinal epithelial barrier function [see comment]. *Gastroenterology* 2001;121(3):580–91.

46 Jijon H, Backer J, Diaz H, Yeung H, Thiel D, McKaigney C, De Simone C, Madsen K. DNA from probiotic bacteria modulates murine and human epithelial and immune function. *Gastroenterology* 2004;126(5):1358–73.

47 Rachmilewitz D, Katakura K, Karmeli F, Hayashi T, Reinus C, Rudensky B, Akira S, Takeda K, Lee J, Takabayashi K, Raz E. Toll-like receptor 9 signaling mediates the anti-inflammatory effects of probiotics in murine experimental colitis [see comment]. *Gastroenterology* 2004;126(2):520–8.

48 Rachmilewitz D, Karmeli F, Takabayashi K, Hayashi T, Leider-Trejo L, Lee J, Leoni LM, Raz E. Immunostimulatory DNA ameliorates experimental and spontaneous murine colitis. *Gastroenterology* 2002;122(5):1428–41.

49 Obermeier F, Dunger N, Strauch UG, Grunwald N, Herfarth H, Scholmerich J, Falk W. Contrasting activity of cytosin-guanosin dinucleotide oligonucleotides in mice with experimental colitis. *Clin Exp Immunol* 2003;134(2):217–24.

50 Obermeier F, Dunger N, Deml L, Herfarth H, Scholmerich J, Falk W. CpG motifs of bacterial DNA exacerbate colitis of dextran sulfate sodium-treated mice. *Eur J Immunol* 2002;32(7):2084–92.

51 Bergstrand LO, Gustafsson BE, Holmstrom B, Norin KE. Ileal Crohn tissue and concomitant flora inoculated into germfree rats. *Acta Chir Scand* 1981;147(8):697–701.

52 Gorbach SL, Nahas L, Plaut AG, Weinstein L, Patterson JF, Levitan R. Studies of intestinal microflora. V. Fecal microbial ecology in ulcerative colitis and regional enteritis: relationship to severity of disease and chemotherapy. *Gastroenterology* 1968;54(4):575–87.

53 Keighley MR, Arabi Y, Dimock F, Burdon DW, Allan RN, Alexander-Williams J. Influence of inflammatory bowel disease on intestinal microflora. *Gut* 1978;19(12):1099–104.

54 Giaffer MH, Holdsworth CD, Duerden BI. The assessment of faecal flora in patients with inflammatory bowel disease by a simplified bacteriological technique. *J Med Microbiol* 1991;35(4):238–43.

55 Bullock NR, Booth JC, Gibson GR. Comparative composition of bacteria in the human intestinal microflora during remission and active ulcerative colitis. *Curr Issues Intest Microbiol* 2004;5(2):59–64.

56 Dickinson RJ, Varian SA, Axon AT, Cooke EM. Increased incidence of faecal coliforms with *in vitro* adhesive and invasive properties in patients with ulcerative colitis. *Gut* 1980;21(9):787–92.

57 Ohkusa T, Okayasu I, Ogihara T, Morita K, Ogawa M, Sato N. Induction of experimental ulcerative colitis by *Fusobacterium varium* isolated from colonic mucosa of patients with ulcerative colitis. *Gut* 2003;52(1):79–83.

58 Ohkusa T, Sato N, Ogihara T, Morita K, Ogawa M, Okayasu I. *Fusobacterium varium* localized in the colonic mucosa of patients with ulcerative colitis stimulates species-specific antibody. *J Gastroenterol Hepatol* 2002;17(8):849–53.

59 Cartun RW, Van Kruiningen HJ, Pedersen CA, Berman MM. An immunocytochemical search for infectious agents in Crohn's disease. *Mod Pathol* 1993;6(2):212–9.

60 Liu Y, van Kruiningen HJ, West AB, Cartun RW, Cortot A, Colombel JF. Immunocytochemical evidence of *Listeria, Escherichia coli*, and *Streptococcus* antigens in Crohn's disease [see comment]. *Gastroenterology* 1995;108(5):1396–404.

61 Neut C, Bulois P, Desreumaux P, Membre JM, Lederman E, Gambiez L, Cortot A, Quandalle P, van Kruiningen H, Colombel JF. Changes in the bacterial flora of the neoterminal ileum after ileocolonic resection for Crohn's disease. *Am J Gastroenterol* 2002;97(4):939–46.

62 Darfeuille-Michaud A, Boudeau J, Bulois P, Neut C, Glasser AI, Barnich N, Bringer MA, Swidsinski A, Beaugerie L, Colombel JF. High prevalence of adherent-invasive *Escherichia coli* associated with ileal mucosa in Crohn's disease. *Gastroenterology* 2004;127(2):412–21.

63 Schultsz C, Van Den Berg FM, Ten Kate FW, Tytgat GN, Dankert J. The intestinal mucus layer from patients with inflammatory bowel disease harbors high numbers of bacteria compared with controls. *Gastroenterology* 1999;117(5):1089–97.

64 Kleessen B, Kroesen AJ, Buhr HJ, Blaut M. Mucosal and invading bacteria in patients with inflammatory bowel disease compared with controls. *Scand J Gastroenterol* 2002;37(9):1034–41.

65 Swidsinski A, Ladhoff A, Pernthaler A, Swidsinski S, Loening-Baucke V, Ortner M, Weber J, Hoffmann U, Schreiber S, Dietal M, Lochs H. Mucosal flora in inflammatory bowel disease [see comment]. *Gastroenterology* 2002;122(1):44–54.

66 Ott SJ, Musfeldt M, Wenderoth DF, Hampe J, Brant O, Folsch UR, Timmis KN, Schreiber S. Reduction in diversity of the colonic mucosa associated bacterial microflora in patients with active inflammatory bowel disease. *Gut* 2004;53(5):685–93.

67 Seksik P, Rigottier-Gois L, Gramet G, Sutren M, Pochart P, Marteau P, Jian R, Dore J. Alterations of the dominant faecal bacterial groups in patients with Crohn's disease of the colon. *Gut* 2003;52(2):237–42.

68 Cong Y, Brandwein SL, McCabe RP, Lazenby A, Birkenmeier EH, Sundberg JP, Elson CO. CD4+ T cells reactive to enteric bacterial antigens in spontaneously colitic C3H/HeJBir mice: increased T helper cell type 1 response and ability to transfer disease. *J Exp Med* 1998;187(6):855–64.

69 Brandwein SL, McCabe RP, Cong Y, Waites KB, Ridwan BU, Dean PA, Ohkusa T, Birkenmeier EH, Sundberg JP, Elson CO. Spontaneously colitic C3H/HeJBir mice demonstrate selective antibody reactivity to antigens of the enteric bacterial flora. *J Immunol* 1997;159(1):44–52.

70 Wei B, Huang T, Dalwadi H, Sutton CL, Bruckner D, Braun J. *Pseudomonas fluorescens* encodes the Crohn's disease-associated I2 sequence and T-cell superantigen. *Infect Immun* 2002;70(12):6567–75.

71 Dalwadi H, Wei B, Kronenberg M, Sutton CL, Braun J. The Crohn's disease-associated bacterial protein I2 is a novel enteric t cell superantigen. *Immunity* 2001;15(1):149–58.

72 Landers CJ, Cohavy O, Misra R, Yang H, Lin YC, Braun J, Targan SR. Selected loss of tolerance evidenced by Crohn's disease-associated immune responses to auto- and microbial antigens. *Gastroenterology* 2002; 123(3):689–99.

73 Lodes MJ, Cong Y, Elson CO, Mohamath R, Landers CJ, Targan SR, Fort M, Hershberg RM. Bacterial flagellin is a dominant antigen in Crohn disease. *J Clin Invest* 2004;113(9):1296–306.

74 Reumaux D, Sendid B, Poulain D, Duthilleul P, Dewit O, Colombel JF. Serological markers in inflammatory bowel diseases. *Best Pract Res Clin Gastroenterol* 2003;17(1):19–35.

75 Arnott I, Landers CJ, Nimmo E, Drummond H, Smith B, Targan S, Satsangi J. Sero-reactivitiy to microbial components in Crohn's disease is associated with disease severity and progression, but not NOD2/CARD15 genotype. *Am J Gastro* 2004;99:2376–84.

76 Mow WS, Vasiliauskas EA, Lin YC, Fleshner PR, Papadakis KA, Taylor KD, Landers CJ, Abreu-Martin MT, Rotter JI, Yang H, Targan SR. Association of antibody responses to microbial antigens and complications of small bowel Crohn's disease [see comment]. *Gastroenterology* 2004;126(2):414–24.

77 Sutherland L, Singleton J, Sessions J, Hanauer S, Krawitt E, Rankin G, Summers R, Mekhjian H, Greenberger N, Kelly M. Double blind, placebo controlled trial of metronidazole in Crohn's disease. *Gut* 1991; 32(9):1071–5.

78 Ursing B, Alm T, Barany F, Bergelin I, Ganrot-Norlin K, Hoevels J, Huitfeldt B, Jarnerot G, Krause U, Krook A, Lindstrom B, Nordle O, Rosen A. A comparative study of metronidazole and sulfasalazine for active Crohn's disease: the cooperative Crohn's disease study in Sweden: II. Result. *Gastroenterology* 1982;83(3):550–62.

79 Greenbloom SL, Steinhart AH, Greenberg GR. Combination ciprofloxacin and metronidazole for active Crohn's disease. *Can J Gastroenterol* 1998;12(1):53–6.

80 Rutgeerts P, Hiele M, Geboes K, Peeters M, Penninckx F, Aerts R, Kerremans R. Controlled trial of metronidazole treatment for prevention of Crohn's recurrence after ileal resection. *Gastroenterology* 1995;108(6):1617–21.

81 Madden MV, McIntyre AS, Nicholls RJ. Double-blind crossover trial of metronidazole versus placebo in chronic unremitting pouchitis. *Dig Dis Sci* 1994;39 (6):1193–6.

82 Arnold GL, Beaves MR, Pryjdun VO, Mook WJ. Preliminary study of ciprofloxacin in active Crohn's disease. *Inflamm Bowel Dis* 2002;8(1):10–5.

83 Shen B, Achkar JP, Lashner BA, Ormsby AH, Remzi FH, Brzezinski A, Bevins CL, Bambrick ML, Seidner DL, Fazio VW. A randomized clinical trial of ciprofloxacin and metronidazole to treat acute pouchitis. *Inflamm Bowel Dis* 2001;7(4):301–5.

84 Greenberg GR. Antibiotics should be used as first-line therapy for Crohn's disease. *Inflamm Bowel Dis* 2004; 10(3):318–20.

85 He F, Ouwehand AC, Isolauri E, Hashimoto H, Benno Y, Salminen S. Comparison of mucosal adhesion and species identification of *Bifidobacteria* isolated from healthy and allergic infants. *FEMS Immunol Med Microbiol* 2001;30(1):43–7.

86 Lee YK, Puong KY. Competition for adhesion between probiotics and human gastrointestinal pathogens in the presence of carbohydrate. *Br J Nutr* 2002;88(Suppl 1):S101–8.

87 Eijsink VG, Axelsson L, Diep DB, Havarstein LS, Holo H, Nes IF. Production of class II bacteriocins by lactic acid bacteria; an example of biological warfare and communication. *Antonie van Leeuwenhoek* 2002;81(1–4):639–54.

88 Kato I, Endo-Tanaka K, Yokokura T. Suppressive effects of the oral administration of *Lactobacillus casei* on type II collagen-induced arthritis in DBA/1 mice. *Life Sci* 1998;63(8):635–44.

89. Haller D, Bode C, Hammes WP, Pfeifer AM, Schiffrin EJ, Blum S. Non-pathogenic bacteria elicit a differential cytokine response by intestinal epithelial cell/leucocyte co-cultures. *Gut* 2000;47(1):79–87.

90. Maassen CB, van Holten-Neelen C, Balk F, den Bak-Glashouwer MJ, Leer RJ, Laman JD, Boersma WJ, Claassen E. Strain-dependent induction of cytokine profiles in the gut by orally administered *Lactobacillus* strains. *Vaccine* 2000;18(23):2613–23.

91. Kalliomaki M, Salminen S, Arvilommi H, Kero P, Koskinen P, Isolauri E. Probiotics in primary prevention of atopic disease: a randomised placebo-controlled trial [see comment]. *Lancet* 2001;357(9262):1076–9.

92. Schultz M, Linde HJ, Lehn N, Zimmermann K, Grossmann J, Falk W, Scholmerich J. Immunomodulatory consequences of oral administration of *Lactobacillus rhamnosus* strain GG in healthy volunteers. *J Dairy Res* 2003;70(2):165–73.

93. Gionchetti P, Amadini C, Rizzello F, Venturi A, Campieri M. Review article: treatment of mild to moderate ulcerative colitis and pouchitis. *Aliment Pharmacol Ther* 2002;16(Suppl 4):13–9.

94. Mimura T, Rizzello F, Helwig U, Poggioli G, Schreiber S, Talbot IC, Nicholls RJ, Gionchetti P, Campieri M, Kamm MA. Once daily high dose probiotic therapy (VSL#3) for maintaining remission in recurrent or refractory pouchitis. *Gut* 2004;53(1):108–14.

95. Borody TJ, Warren EF, Leis S, Surace R, Ashman O. Treatment of ulcerative colitis using fecal bacteriotherapy. *J Clin Gastroenterol* 2003;37(1):42–7.

96. Fedorak RN, Madsen KL. Probiotics and the management of inflammatory bowel disease. *Inflamm Bowel Dis* 2004;10(3):286–99.

97. Jacobasch G, Schmiedl D, Kruschewski M, Schmehl K. Dietary resistant starch and chronic inflammatory bowel diseases. *Int J Colorectal Dis* 1999;14(4–5):201–11.

98. Kanauchi O, Mitsuyama K, Homma T, Takahama K, Fujiyama Y, Andoh A, Araki Y, Suga T, Hibi T, Naganuma M, Asakura H, Nakano H, Shimoyama T, Hida N, Haruma K, Koga H, Sata M, Tomiyasu N, Toyonaga A, Fukuda M, Kojima A, Bamba T. Treatment of ulcerative colitis patients by long-term administration of germinated barley foodstuff: multi-center open trial. *Int J Mol Med* 2003;12(5):701–4.

99. Bamba T, Kanauchi O, Andoh A, Fujiyama Y. A new prebiotic from germinated barley for nutraceutical treatment of ulcerative colitis. *J Gastroenterol Hepatol* 2002;17(8):818–24.

100. Mitsuyama K, Toyonaga A, Sata M. Intestinal microflora as a therapeutic target in inflammatory bowel disease. *J Gastroenterol* 2002;37(Suppl 14):73–7.

101. Kanauchi O, Suga T, Tochihara M, Hibi T, Naganuma M, Homma T, Asakura H, Nakano H, Takahama K, Fujiyama Y, Andoh A, Shimoyama T, Hida N, Haruma K, Koga H, Mitsuyama K, Sata M, Fukuda M, Kojima A, Bamba T. Treatment of ulcerative colitis by feeding with germinated barley foodstuff: first report of a multicenter open control trial. *J Gastroenterol* 2002;37(Suppl 14):67–72.

102. Onderdonk AB, Bronson R, Cisneros R. Comparison of bacteroides vulgatus strains in the enhancement of experimental ulcerative colitis. *Infect Immun* 1987;55(3):835–6.

103. Onderdonk AB, Cisneros RL, Bronson RT. Enhancement of experimental ulcerative colitis by immunization with bacteroides vulgatus. *Infect Immun* 1983;42(2):783–8.

104. Huijsdens XW, Linskens RK, Taspinar H, Meuwissen SG, Vandenbroucke-Grauls CM, Savelkoul PH. Listeria monocytogenes and inflammatory bowel disease: detection of *Listeria* species in intestinal mucosal biopsies by real-time PCR. *Scand J Gastroenterol* 2003;38(3):332–3.

105. Chen W, Li D, Paulus B, Wilson I, Chadwick VS. Detection of Listeria monocytogenes by polymerase chain reaction in intestinal mucosal biopsies from patients with inflammatory bowel disease and controls. *J Gastroenterol Hepatol* 2000;15(10):1145–50.

106. Fox JG, Gorelick PL, Kullberg MC, Ge Z, Dewhirst FE, Ward JM. A novel urease-negative *Helicobacter* species associated with colitis and typhlitis in IL-10-deficient mice. *Infect Immun* 1999;67(4):1757–62.

107. Resta-Lenert S, Barrett KE. Live probiotics protect intestinal epithelial cells from the effects of infection with enteroinvasive *Escherichia coli* (EIEC). *Gut* 2003;52(7):988–97.

108. Ouwehand AC, Lagstrom H, Suomalainen T, Salminen S. Effect of probiotics on constipation, fecal azoreductase activity and fecal mucin content in the elderly. *Ann Nutr Metab* 2002;46(3–4):159–62.

109. Lievin-Le Moal V, Amsellem R, Servin AL, Coconnier MH. *Lactobacillus acidophilus* (strain LB) from the resident adult human gastrointestinal microflora exerts activity against brush border damage promoted by a diarrhoeagenic *Escherichia coli* in human enterocyte-like cells. *Gut* 2002;50(6):803–11.

110 Garcia-Lafuente A, Antolin M, Guarner F, Crespo E, Malagelada JR. Modulation of colonic barrier function by the composition of the commensal flora in the rat [see comment]. *Gut* 2001;48(4):503–7.

111 Freitas M, Tavan E, Cayuela C, Diop L, Sapin C, Trugnan G. Host-pathogens cross-talk. Indigenous bacteria and probiotics also play the game. *Biol Cell* 2003;95(8):503–6.

112 Majamaa H, Isolauri E, Saxelin M, Vesikari T. Lactic acid bacteria in the treatment of acute rotavirus gastroenteritis. *J Pediatr Gastroenterol Nutr* 1995;20(3):333–8.

113 Fang H, Elina T, Heikki A, Seppo S. Modulation of humoral immune response through probiotic intake. *FEMS Immunol Med Microbiol* 2000;29(1):47–52.

114 Gill HS, Rutherfurd KJ. Immune enhancement conferred by oral delivery of *Lactobacillus rhamnosus* HN001 in different milk-based substrates. *J Dairy Res* 2001;68(4):611–6.

115 Gill HS, Shu Q, Lin H, Rutherfurd KJ, Cross ML. Protection against translocating *Salmonella typhimurium* infection in mice by feeding the immuno-enhancing probiotic *Lactobacillus rhamnosus* strain HN001. *Med Microbiol Immunol* 2001;190(3):97–104.

116 Gill HS, Rutherfurd KJ Cross ML, Gopal PK. Enhancement of immunity in the elderly by dietary supplementation with the probiotic *Bifidobacterium lactis* HN019. *Am J Clin Nutr* 2001;74(6):833–9.

117 Gill HS, Rutherfurd KJ, Cross ML. Dietary probiotic supplementation enhances natural killer cell activity in the elderly: an investigation of age-related immunological changes. *J Clin Immunol* 2001;21(4):264–71.

118 Gill HS, Rutherfurd KJ. Viability and dose-response studies on the effects of the immunoenhancing lactic acid bacterium *Lactobacillus rhamnosus* in mice. *Br J Nutr* 2001;86(2):285–9.

119 Park JH, Um JI, Lee BJ, Goh JS, Park SY Kim WS, Kim PH. Encapsulated *Bifidobacterium bifidum* potentiates intestinal IgA production. *Cell Immunol* 2002;219(1):22–7.

120 Shimada T, Cheng L, Ide M, Fukuda S, Enomoto T, Shirakawa T. Effect of lysed *Enterococcus faecalis* FK-23 (LFK) on allergen-induced peritoneal accumulation of eosinophils in mice. *Clin Exp Allergy* 2003;33(5):684–7.

121 Shimada T, Cheng L, Yamasaki A, Ide M, Motonaga C, Yasueda H, Enomoto K, Enomoto T, Shirakawa T. Effects of lysed *Enterococcus faecalis* FK-23 on allergen-induced serum antibody responses and active cutaneous anaphylaxis in mice. *Clin Exp Allergy* 2004; 34(11):1784–8.

122 Braat H, van den Brande J, van Tol E, Hommes D, Peppelenbosch M, van Deventer S. *Lactobacillus rhamnosus* induces peripheral hyporesponsiveness in stimulated CD4+ T cells via modulation of dendritic cell function. *Am J Clin Nutr* 2004;80(6):1618–25.

123 Leblanc J, Fliss I, Matar C. Induction of a humoral immune response following an *Escherichia coli* O157:H7 infection with an immunomodulatory peptideic fraction derived from *Lactobacillus helveticus*-fermented milk. *Clin Diagn Lab Immunol* 2004;11(6):1171–81.

124 Hart A, Lammers K, Brigidi P, Vitali B, Rizzello F, Gionchetti P, Campieri M, Kamm MA, Knight SC, Stagg A. Modulation of human dendritic cell phenotype and function by probiotic bacteria. *Gut* 2004;53(11):1602–9.

125 Neish AS, Gewirtz AT, Zeng H, Young AN, Hobert ME, Karmali V, Rao AS, Madara JL. Prokaryotic regulation of epithelial responses by inhibition of IkappaB-alpha ubiquitination [comment]. *Science* 2000;289(5484):1560–3.

126 Petrof E, Kojima K, Ropeleski MJ, Musch MW, Tao Y, De Simone C, Chang EB. Probiotics inhibit nuclear factor-kappaB and induce heat shock proteins in colonic epithelial cells through proteasome inhibition. *Gastroenterology* 2004;127(5):1474–87.

127 Yan F, Polk DB. Probiotic bacterium prevents cytokine-induced apoptosis in intestinal epithelial cells. *J Biol Chem* 2002;277(52):50959–65.

128 Di Marzio L, Russo FP, D'Alo S, Biordi L, Ulisse S, Amicosante G, De Simone C, Cifone MG. Apoptotic effects of selected strains of lactic acid bacteria on a human T leukemia cell line are associated with bacterial arginine deiminase and/or sphingomyelinase activities. *Nutr Cancer* 2001;40(2):185–96.

129 Kullisaar T, Zilmer M, Mikelsaar M, Vihalemm T, Annuk H, Kairane C, Kilk A. Two antioxidative lactobacilli strains as promising probiotics. *Int J Food Microbiol* 2002;72(3):215–24.

130 Boudeau J, Glasser AL, Julien S, Colombel JF, Darfeuille-Michaud A. Inhibitory effect of probiotic *Escherichia coli* strain Nissle 1917 on adhesion to and invasion of intestinal epithelial cells by adherent-invasive E. coli strains isolated from patients with Crohn's disease. *Aliment Pharmacol Ther* 2003;18(1):45–56.

131 Huang Y, Adams MC. An *in vitro* model for investigating intestinal adhesion of potential dairy propionibacteria probiotic strains using cell line C2BBe1. *Lett Appl Microbiol* 2003;36(4):213–6.

132. Kos B, Suskovic J, Vukovic S, Simpraga M, Frece J, Matosic S. Adhesion and aggregation ability of probiotic strain *Lactobacillus acidophilus* M92. *J Appl Microbiol* 2003;94(6):981–7.

133. Coconnier MH, Lievin V, Lorrot M, Servin AL. Antagonistic activity of *Lactobacillus acidophilus* LB against intracellular Salmonella enterica serovar Typhimurium infecting human enterocyte-like Caco-2/TC-7 cells. *Appl Environ Microbiol* 2000;66(3):1152–7.

134. Lievin V, Peiffer I, Hudault S, Rochat F, Brassart D, Neeser JR, Servin AL. Bifidobacterium strains from resident infant human gastrointestinal microflora exert antimicrobial activity. *Gut* 2000;47(5):646–52.

135. Caridi A. Selection of *Escherichia coli*-inhibiting strains of *Lactobacillus paracasei* subsp. paracasei. *J Ind Microbiol Biotechnol* 2002;29(6):303–8.

136. Flynn S, van Sinderen D, Thornton GM, Holo H, Nes IF, Collins JK. Characterization of the genetic locus responsible for the production of ABP-118, a novel bacteriocin produced by the probiotic bacterium *Lactobacillus salivarius* subsp. salivarius UCC118. *Microbiology* 2002;148(Pt 4):973–84.

137. Park SH, Itoh K, Fujisawa T. Characteristics and identification of enterocins produced by *Enterococcus faecium* JCM 5804T. *J Appl Microbiol* 2003;95(2):294–300.

138. Xiao H, Chen X, Chen M, Tang S, Zhao X, Huan L. Bovicin HJ50, a novel lantibiotic produced by *Streptococcus bovis* HJ50. *Microbiology* 2004;150(Pt 1):103–8.

139. von der Weid T, Bulliard C, Schiffrin EJ. Induction by a lactic acid bacterium of a population of CD4(+) T cells with low proliferative capacity that produce transforming growth factor beta and interleukin-10. *Clin Diagn Lab Immun* 2001;8(4):695–701.

140. He F, Morita H, Ouwehand AC, Hosoda M, Hiramatsu M, Kurisaki J, Isolauri E, Benno Y, Salminen S. Stimulation of the secretion of pro-inflammatory cytokines by *Bifidobacterium* strains. *Microbiol Immunol* 2002;46(11):781–5.

141. Smits HH, van Beelen AJ, Hessle C, Westland R, de Jong E, Soeteman E, Wold A, Wierenga EA, Kapsenberg ML. Commensal gram-negative bacteria prime human dendritic cells for enhanced IL-23 and IL-27 expression and enhanced Th1 development. *Eur J Immunol* 2004;34(5):1371–80.

142. Menard S, Candalh C, Bambou JC, Terpend K, Cerf-Bensussan N, Heyman M. Lactic acid bacteria secrete metabolites retaining anti-inflammatory properties after intestinal transport. *Gut* 2004;53(6):821–8.

143. Lammers KM, Helwig U, Swennen E, Rizzello F, Venturi A, Caramelli E, Kamm MA, Brigidi P, Gionchetti P, Campieri M. Effect of probiotic strains on interleukin 8 production by HT29/19A cells. *Am J Gastroenterol* 2002;97(5):1182–6.

144. Morita H, He F, Fuse T, Ouwehand AC, Hashimoto H, Hosoda M, Mizumachi K, Kurisaki J. Adhesion of lactic acid bacteria to caco-2 cells and their effect on cytokine secretion. *Microbiol Immunol* 2002;46(4):293–7.

5: The appendix – how might it influence susceptibility to ulcerative colitis: the legend of Qebehsenuef

Kenneth Croitoru

Introduction

The cause of ulcerative colitis (UC) or Crohn's disease (CD) is unknown. It is generally accepted that the inflammatory disease is a result of a genetically determined unbridled immune response to an environmental agent. The environmental agent may well be components of the normal gut flora or a 'pathogen' that has been difficult to identify. On the other hand, the exact nature of the abnormality in the immune response also remains to be defined. Recently a number of case control studies searching for risk factors associated with the development of IBD have identified a negative association between previous appendectomy and ulcerative colitis. The implications of these observations have received further support from studies in mouse models of colitis. The normal function of the appendix is not well understood, and is often considered a redundant non-essential mammalian vestige of the Bursa of Fabricius found in birds; yet the immune function of the mammalian appendix is also not clear. Yet the removal of the appendix early in life appears to decrease the risk of developing UC. In this chapter we will explore the epidemiological evidence supporting an association between appendectomy and the protection against ulcerative colitis, and then explore some of the work attempting to define the underlying mechanism of such an association.

Epidemiological observations

Cohort studies suggesting a negative association between appendectomy and ulcerative colitis

In order to determine if there is a possible association between appendectomies and the future development of UC, one would design a randomised control trial. This not being possible, we are left to consider data from cohort studies. Indeed, the concept that a negative association exists between appendectomies and UC was first suggested in cohort studies designed to identify risk factors for the development of CD and UC. One of the first such studies was an international case control study of 197 UC and 302 CD patients who were less than 20 years old at the time of diagnosis. This study showed that only 3% of UC patients had a previous history of having had an appendectomy, although the age-matched control patient population had a 10% incidence of previous appendectomies and this was statistically significant. Interestingly, this study also showed that CD patients had a 16% incidence rate of appendectomies suggesting either no association or an increased risk ($p < 0.015$) [1].

This study was followed by a number of case control studies such as the study of hygiene practices in British children where it was shown that there was an association between 'hot running water' and CD but not UC. This study also showed that children who had a previous appendectomy had a relative risk of developing UC of 0.3 (i.e. a negative association) [2]. Other studies reported odds ratio of 59.1 for the development of UC if no previous appendectomy versus 2.95 if a non-smoker [3].

Attempts were then made to distinguish between primary appendectomies (surgery for appendicitis) versus incidental appendectomies (removal of the appendix for other reasons). In a case control study where UC ($n = 197$) and CD ($n = 117$) patients were compared to dermatology outpatients ($n = 243$) there was a reduced rate of primary appendectomy in the UC group (adjusted odds ratio 0.20, $p < 0.0005$) but not in the Crohn's disease patients (adjusted odds ratio 0.93). These data suggest that 'appendicitis' may occur less commonly than would be expected in individuals who go on to develop UC [4].

A repeat case control study using control patients undergoing elective surgery and aimed at evaluating suspected risk factors for IBD, showed that 4.5% of UC patients reported a previous appendectomy compared with 19% of controls (OR 0.20, $p < 0.0001$). This inverse association was stronger for appendectomy performed before age 20 (OR 0.14) [5].

A formal meta-analysis of 13 studies published between 1987 and 1999 was published in 2000. The 13 case-control studies involved 2770 patients with UC and 3352 controls. Combining the results gave an overall odds ratio of 0.307 (95% CI 0.249–0.377) in favour of appendectomy ($p < 0.0001$). This suggests that appendectomy gives a 69% reduction in the risk of developing UC [6]. This group has recently updated their analysis to include four new studies and reported an overall odds ratio of 0.312 (95% CI 0.261–0.373) in favour of appendectomy ($p < 0.0001$) [7].

Since these meta-analysis studies, Hallas et al. published a large-scale cohort study that attempted to define if the appendix itself has biologic effects that promote the development of UC. Towards this end, they examined a population-based cohort of all 234,559 persons who had an appendectomy performed in Denmark from 1977 to 1999. They calculated the standardised incidence rate of UC both before and after the appendectomy. If the hypothesis of a constant, confounding factor were true (e.g. a genetic factor), incidence rates of UC would be equal before and after appendectomy. If the incidence of ulcerative colitis were lower after appendectomy than before, it would support the contention that there is a true protective effect of appendectomy on UC. Their results showed that of 234,559 persons who had an appendectomy, 559 developed UC during a mean follow-up of 17.5 years. The standardised incidence rate of ulcerative colitis was lower in the post-appendectomy period than in the pre-appendectomy period (incidence rate ratio = 0.74). Their conclusion was that appendectomy might have a genuine protective effect against the development of UC [8].

In an interesting and provocative study, the effect of appendectomy was studied in patients with primary sclerosing cholangitis (PSC) and UC. The phenotype of UC is different in patients with PSC. In this study from the Brisbane IBD Research Group database with controls from the Australian twin registry patients with PSC-inflammatory bowel disease (PSC-IBD, $n = 78$) were studied alongside (12 patients with pure PSC, 294 UC patients without PSC who were matched with 1466 controls). The results showed that appendectomy rates in the PSC groups were not different from the control groups, in sharp contrast with UC where the rate was four times less ($p = 0.0001$). Prior appendectomy appeared to be associated with an approximate 5-year delay in the onset of intestinal (PSC-IBD or UC) or hepatic (PSC) disease. Appendectomy did not independently alter the extent or severity of disease in PSC; but, prior appendectomy in UC was associated with more extensive disease, but with a lesser requirement for immunosuppression or colectomy for the treatment of colitis. There were trends for high-grade dysplasia or colorectal cancer with appendectomy in both PSC-IBD and UC. Although, these trends were not statistically significant, colorectal cancer appeared more frequent with appendectomy in a meta-analysis of the available UC data from this and another Australian study, raising a possible concern if appendectomies were to be considered for treatment of prevention. Nonetheless, appendectomy did not influence the prevalence of the PSC groups, or the extent of colitis in PSC-IBD, but as with UC, did appear to delay their onset [9].

In spite of this impressive cumulative evidence supporting a negative association between appendectomies and the development of UC and possibly even an influence on the natural history of the disease, several authors have raised a number of caveats. For example, in a Swedish study, the 10-year annual rate of appendectomy has decreased from 13,000 to 10,000 [10] and yet there has been no increase in the rate of UC during that time period [11].

Studies suggesting that appendicitis may represent the risk protector

As discussed above, Smithson et al. showed that the negative association between appendectomies performed for appendicitis had a stronger negative association with UC [4]. As a follow-up to this observation, Andersson et al. studied a large cohort of 212,963 patients who underwent appendectomy before the age of 50 (between 1964 and 1993). These patients were identified from the Swedish Inpatient Register and the nationwide census. The cohort was followed until 1995. Patients who underwent appendectomy for appendicitis and mesenteric lymphadenitis had a low risk of UC (for patients with perforated appendicitis, the adjusted hazard ratio was 0.58; for those with non-perforated appendicitis it was 0.76; and for those with mesenteric lymphadenitis it was 0.57). Interestingly, patients who underwent appendectomy for non-specific abdominal pain did not show a lowered rate of UC (adjusted hazard ratio, 1.06). For the patients who had appendicitis, an inverse relation with the risk of UC was found only for those who underwent surgery before the age of 20 years [11]. These findings, although supportive of the observations reported by Smithson et al., further suggest that the age at which appendicitis occurs may have a significant effect on the likelihood of subsequently developing UC.

In an effort to determine if appendicitis was on its own a marker of a more diffuse mucosal inflammatory disorder or specifically related to UC, Scott et al. examined surgical pathology over the period from 1980 to 1994. There was a 48% prevalence of appendiceal inflammation in ulcerative colitis. This was significantly more that the 8% incidence found in controls, but similar to that found in Crohn's disease (52%). Of note was the finding that the inflamed appendices from IBD patients tended to show histological features typical of UC or CD rather than acute appendicitis. Therefore, it was concluded that in UC and in CD, appendiceal inflammation can occur as a skip lesion and histologically resembled the colonic disease rather than acute appendicitis. How this serves to explain the lower prevalence of appendectomies in UC patients is not clear unless the appendiceal inflammation actually reflects an infective process that once removed prevents 'spread' to the remainder of the colon. This would not explain why there is no such negative association or protection with appendectomies and the development of CD [12].

Appendectomies may influence the natural history of ulcerative colitis

In addition to the observed negative association more recent studies have begun to examine if appendectomies might influence the severity of UC in those patients who go on to develop the disease. One of the first such studies was an Australian study of patients from the Brisbane Inflammatory Bowel Disease database. This study first confirmed the negative association between appendectomy and UC (OR 0.23). Interestingly, this study found a similar result for CD once the bias of appendectomy at diagnosis was addressed (OR 0.34). Most interesting was the finding that prior appendectomy also delayed the age of presentation for both UC and CD. Furthermore, patients with UC and prior appendectomy had clinically milder disease with reduced requirement for immunosuppressants and proctocolectomy [13].

In a second study, 638 UC patients were interviewed between 1997 and 2000 to assess the severity of their disease. The study showed that the 10-year risk of colectomy was 16% in previously appendectomised patients ($n = 49$) compared with 33% in non-appendectomised patients ($n = 589$). This difference was statistically significant and further Cox regression analysis showed that previous appendectomy and current smoking were independent factors protecting against colectomy (adjusted hazard ratio 0.40 and 0.60, respectively). The respective proportions of appendectomised and non-appendectomised patients who required oral steroids and immunosuppressive therapy were not significantly different (67% vs 70% and 27% vs 19%, respectively). However, during the time period examined, the UC was active for 48% of the time in appendectomised patients and for 62% of the time in non-appendectomised patients. Therefore, previous appendectomy was associated with a less severe course of UC [14].

In a companion paper to the large-scale Danish Cohort published by Hallas *et al.* the authors examined the cases of UC identified through the Danish National Patient Registry during the period from 1981 to 1999. Of all patients with UC, 202 had an appendectomy after their first admission with UC. They compared the incidence rate of hospitalisations for a primary diagnosis of UC during the period between the onset of UC and appendectomy, with the rate of such hospitalisations after appendectomy. To adjust for the clinical course of UC unrelated to appendectomy, they extracted a reference cohort ($n = 808$), matched to the index subjects with respect to age, sex and year of first admission, but with an intact appendix. Their results showed that the rates of admission to hospital due to UC decreased by 47% after appendectomy (RR 0.53). However, the reference cohort showed a similar decline in admission rate (RR 0.51). Thus appendectomy had no apparent beneficial effect on admission rate after adjustment for the clinical course of disease unrelated to appendectomy (adjusted rate ratio 1.05). Their conclusion was that appendectomy had no significant beneficial effect on rates of admission to hospital in patients with UC [15]. Although this study did not support an effect of appendectomies on the rate of hospitalisations for UC, they did not attempt to judge other measures of disease activity such as surgery or the use of immunosuppressive therapy.

In spite of this impressive cumulative evidence supporting a negative association between appendectomies and the development of UC and possibly even an influence on the natural history of the disease, the issue that remains to be resolved is defining the mechanism that might be involved in such an effect.

Pathogenetic hypothesis

In attempting to explain the epidemiological observations pointing to a protective role for appendectomies in preventing UC, we can consider several possibilities. It is possible that appendectomies lead to specific alterations in the mucosal immune response that prevent or counteract those that are involved in the pathogenesis of UC. Alternatively, there may be alterations in the immune system of UC patients that lead to protection against appendicitis and therefore manifest as a lower incidence of appendicitis and a less frequent need for surgical cure thereof. Lastly, we can consider the possibility that UC is driven by an appendiceal-derived immune response either due to abnormal immune cells developing there or due to an infection-driven appendiceal inflammation that spreads to the colon if not excised. Excision of the appendix would then have an immune-modulating effect protecting against UC. The hypotheses presented are difficult to address in humans or animal models of the disease, although some interesting data are available for examination.

The appendix

The appendix was probably first noted during early Egyptian civilization (3000 BC), as the mummification process was one of the earliest practices that allowed for direct observations of the internal human anatomy. The practice was to remove abdominal parts and place them in Coptic jars with inscriptions describing the contents. Some of these jars carried the inscriptions that referred to the 'worm of the intestine.' The jars containing the internal organs often carried depictions of the sons of the God Horus and in one example the jar containing the appendix displayed the falcon head of the God's son, Qebehsenuef.

In the year 30 CE, the Roman physician Aulus Cornelius Celsus probably discovered the appendix because he was allowed to dissect criminals executed by Caesar. Aristotle and Galen did not identify the appendix because they both dissected lower animals, which do not have appendices. Andreas Vesalius survived death sentences under the Inquisition for his dissections when he published *De corporis humani fabrica* (1563), providing the first accurate drawings of human anatomy showing the appendix, although Leonardo da Vinci had depicted the appendix in anatomic drawings in 1492. It was Phillipe Verheyen who coined the term appendix vermiformis in 1710.

In Western countries, approximately 7% of individuals develop appendicitis at some time during their lives. Approximately 200,000 appendectomies are performed annually in the United States. Acute appendicitis is less common in Africa and parts of Asia due in part to the high-residue diets of the inhabitants of those regions. Appendicitis is thought to be related to obstruction of the lumen of the appendix that may occur as a result of lymphoid hyperplasia (60%), a faecalith (35%), a foreign body (4%) or an obstructing tumour (1%).

Function of the appendix

The structural similarities between the appendix and the Peyer's patches found on the anti-mesenteric side of the small intestine raised the possibility that these structures shared immune function, be it recognition of luminal Ag or sampling of enteric bacteria flora. Alternatively, the anatomical location of the appendix at the end of the small intestine conjures up similar speculations of shared function. The mystery of the function of the mammalian appendix has intrigued scientists for centuries.

Another possible function for the appendix is suggested by the finding that the Bursa of Fabricius, an out pouching at the end of the intestine and found only in birds, is responsible for B cell development. Hieronymus Fabricius (1537–1619) was a distinguished Italian anatomist and surgeon, best known as the teacher of William Harvey. His published work on anatomy includes a comparative analysis of the anatomy of the appendix, but he is immortalised in the naming of the out pouching or bursa of the cloacae in birds, in which lymphocytes were identified to undergo mitosis and maturation into B-cells before migrating out into the general body tissues. The Bursa is a blind sac that extends from the dorsal side of the cloacae, wherein one finds a columnar epidermis and connective tissue filled with lymph nodules. Removal of the Bursa of Fabricius, early in life prevents development of B cells and antibody responses [16, 17]. In spite of a considerable effort searching for the mammalian equivalent of the Bursa of Fabricius, none has been found. The possibility that the appendix might serve a similar role in the development of the humoral immune response has not been borne out and, in fact, it is more likely that this role is served by the foetal yolk sac and foetal liver and possibly bone marrow [18–21]. Nonetheless, there have been a few recent studies that showed that neonatal appendectomy in rabbits could alter Ag- specific antibody levels in response to intra-peritoneal and intra-duodenal immunisations with ovalbumin (OVA). More specifically, appendectomy nearly ablated OVA-specific IgA levels in the gut and severely depleted OVA-specific IgG in the gut and serum. These results would support a major role of the rabbit appendix in seeding the intestinal lamina propria with plasma cell precursors, especially those producing IgA [22].

Other studies of the appendix have identified unique subsets of T cells expressing the CD4-CD8-B220+ TCR $\alpha\beta$ phenotype seen in other intra-epithelial sites of the intestine. These cells contained forbidden T cell clones – T cells with the ability to respond to self-Ag. These CD4-CD8-B220+ $\alpha\beta$ T cells seem to originate *in situ* from *c-kit* + stem cells in the appendix, suggesting that the appendix may be a site of primary T cell subset development and may lead to the development of T cells that can develop and express auto-reactivity. The possibility that this might contribute to an auto-immune response or to the initiation of colitis remains speculative [23].

Role of the appendix in the pathogenesis of colitis

A full discussion of the pathogenesis of IBD is beyond the scope of this review. In brief, the focus of much recent work, in particular studies of the animal models of colitis, is that IBD probably represents a genetically determined defect in the interaction of the host immune system and environmental triggers or antigens [24–26]. The defect in the host immune response may involve the innate as well as the cognate immune system. Recent work has focused on the possibility that a defect in regulatory elements of the immune system and in particular regulatory T cells may allow for unopposed immune activation in the intestinal mucosa [27–29]. In addition, studies have begun to identify non-T cells that may function in a regulatory fashion in the intestine, including IEL subsets and B cells [30–34]. It is from these studies that we may have some further insight into how the appendix may influence the development of colitis.

Among the original genetically manipulated mouse models of colitis was the TCR α chain knockout (TCRα −/−) mouse, first published in 1993. These mice developed spontaneous colitis that resembled ulcerative colitis histologically [35]. The inflammation observed in this model is associated with an increase in IL-4 levels (i.e. a Th2 type of inflammatory response). In addition, it appears that although B cells were not required for the development of colitis, B cells can suppress the development of colitis [36]. This model was used to study the potential role of the appendix in the development of spontaneous colitis. Indeed, the authors showed that when TCR-α knockout mice underwent appendectomy at a young age (3–5 weeks) only 3.3% of these mice developed IBD in the 6–7-month period of observation. In contrast, approximately 80% of controls, including the sham-operated TCRα knockout mice developed colitis during this period. They concluded that the lymphoid follicles contained within the appendix are the priming site of cells involved in the induction of development of IBD in TCRα −/− mice [37].

In more recent work CD62L cells were shown to preferentially migrate into the appendix in mice with experimental chronic colitis. The CD62L+CD4+ T cell represent effector T cells and suggest that either the appendix is involved in activating these T cells or represents a second site of T cell-induced inflammation [38].

Few studies have attempted to examine the human appendix in patients with IBD. One such study reported on lymphocyte phenotype and proliferation. Using surgical specimens of the appendix obtained from 5 patients with colon cancer, 5 with acute appendicitis, 12 with UC and 7 with CD, showed that the number of Ki-67(+) proliferating cells, CD19, and CD138 cells was significantly higher in the appendix of patients with UC than in controls, patients with acute appendicitis, and patients with CD. Lamina propria cells in the appendix of patients with UC also showed an increase in proliferation with increased numbers of CD19 and CD138 cells. An increased proportion of Ki-67(+) cells in CD19 and CD138 cells represents proliferation of immature plasma cells in the appendix of patients with UC, and proliferation of such immature plasma cells was seen in both active- and remission-stage UC. Proliferation of immature plasma cells in the appendix of patients with UC suggests a primary role of humeral immune responses in the pathogenesis of UC [39].

Although the exact mechanisms by which appendectomy prevents or delays the onset of colitis in a genetically susceptible host remains to be defined, these results of the animal studies first support the epidemiological evidence of the negative association between appendectomy and ulcerative colitis and suggest that there is a real connection between the appendix and the mechanisms that lead to the colonic inflammation. The question of which immune cells are involved and how this leads to colitis remains unanswered. Nonetheless, the possibility that emerges from this is that appendectomy may serve as a preventive measure in high-risk susceptible individuals or may aid in the treatment of patients with established UC. Confirmation of these speculations will require carefully designed clinical studies.

Clinical studies

The intriguing speculation that appendectomy is of potential benefit to patients with either established UC or who are at risk of developing UC, has already led to a few clinical case reports and small case series. Several case reports have described patients with chronically active UC, usually refractory to medical therapy, who have improved after undergoing an appendectomy. In one report a 21-year-old man was shown to improve and remain in remission for 3 years after an appendectomy. This patient had moderate inflammation that appeared to have been restricted to the rectum. Interestingly, this group showed that increases in tissue interferon γ were reduced after surgery suggesting that appendectomy resulted in altered Th1/Th2 cytokine balance [40]. It is possible that the changes in the cytokine levels were a result of the decrease in inflammation and not necessarily a direct effect of the appendectomy.

A case series of laparoscopic appendectomy in patients with refractory ulcerative colitis was described by Jarnerot et al. In this report appendectomy was performed in six patients with UC refractory to standard treatment and in whom surgery was considered. Unfortunately, five of the six patients failed to respond in a 2–4 year follow-up [41].

In another study histological and immunological characteristics of the appendix in UC were assessed and correlated with the effect of appendectomy on the disease. Nine subjects with mildly active UC were treated by surgical appendectomy. In four subjects, the histological findings of the appendix were compatible with ulcerative appendicitis. CD3+CD4+CD25+, CD3+CD4+CD45RO+ and CD3+CD8+CD45RO+ appendiceal mononuclear cells were significantly higher in UC than in acute appendicitis and in the normal appendix. There was a trend towards higher mRNA transcripts of IFN-γ in the appendix of UC. Clinical activity index decreased significantly 4 weeks after the appendectomy, but the effect did not persist. They concluded that the appendix is a site of involvement in UC [42], but they failed to show a significant beneficial clinical effect. Therefore the significance of the changes in inflammatory cells described remains unknown.

Conclusion

We have explored a significant body of work that shows an intriguing negative association between appendectomies and the development and natural history of UC. This evidence is derived for the most part from a number of large cohort studies. Most intriguingly, these observations were further supported by elegant work in an animal model of spontaneous colitis where appendectomy prevented the development of the colitis, hence recapitulating the epidemiological data. This is the best scenario if we are to define the mechanisms underlying this association and perhaps at the same time increase our understanding of the basic pathogenetic mechanisms underlying the development of UC. It is of some concern that the data in the patients with PSC suggests a possible increased risk of dysplasia or the development of colo-rectal cancer at least in the small subsets of patients with UC associated with PSC. This again raises the intriguing question as to how the removal of that mysterious organ of Qebehsenuef, the appendix, can possibly influence the development of neoplasia. The continued exploration of these and other questions that arise from large-scale epidemiological studies serve to help steer our basic science questions and keep them on a relevant course.

References

1. Gilat T, Hacohen D, Lilos P, Langman MJ. Childhood factors in ulcerative colitis and Crohn's disease: an international cooperative study. *Scand J Gastroenterol* 1987;22:1009–24.
2. Gent AE, Hellier MD, Grace RH, Swarbrick ET, Coggon D. Inflammatory bowel disease and domestic hygiene in infancy. *Lancet* 1994;343:766–7.
3. Rutgeerts P, D'Haens G, Hiele M, Geboes K, Vantrappen G. Appendectomy protects against ulcerative colitis. *Gastroenterology* 1994;106:1251–3.
4. Smithson JE, Radford-Smith G, Jewell DP. Appendectomy and tonsillectomy in patients with inflammatory bowel disease. *J Clin Gastroenterol* 1995;21:283–6.
5. Duggan AE, Usmani I, Neal KR, Logan RF. Appendicectomy, childhood hygiene, *Helicobacter pylori* status, and risk of inflammatory bowel disease: a case control study [see comments]. *Gut* 1998;43:494–8.
6. Koutroubakis IE, Vlachonikolis IG. Appendectomy and the development of ulcerative colitis: results of a metaanalysis of published case-control studies. *Am J Gastroenterol* 2000;95:171–6.
7. Koutroubakis IE, Vlachonikolis IG, Kouroumalis EA. Role of appendicitis and appendectomy in the pathogenesis of ulcerative colitis: a critical review. *Inflamm Bowel Dis* 2002;8:277–86.
8. Hallas J, Gaist D, Sorensen HT. Does appendectomy reduce the risk of ulcerative colitis? *Epidemiology* 2004;15:173–8.
9. Florin TH, Pandeya N, Radford-Smith GL. Epidemiology of appendicectomy in primary sclerosing cholangitis and ulcerative colitis: its influence on the clinical behaviour of these diseases. *Gut* 2004;53:973–9.
10. Blomqvist P, Ljung H, Nyren O, Ekbom A. Appendectomy in Sweden 1989–1993 assessed by the Inpatient Registry. *J Clin Epidemiol* 1998;51:859–65.
11. Andersson RE, Olaison G, Tysk C, Ekbom A. Appendectomy and protection against ulcerative colitis. *N Engl J Med* 2001;344:808–14.
12. Scott IS, Sheaff M, Coumbe A, Feakins RM, Rampton DS. Appendiceal inflammation in ulcerative colitis. *Histopathology* 1998;33:168–73.

13. Radford-Smith GL, Edwards JE, Purdie DM, *et al.* Protective role of appendicectomy on onset and severity of ulcerative colitis and Crohn's disease. *Gut* 2002;51:808–13.
14. Cosnes J, Carbonnel F, Beaugerie L, Blain A, Reijasse D, Gendre JP. Effects of appendicectomy on the course of ulcerative colitis. *Gut* 2002;51:803–7.
15. Hallas J, Gaist D, Vach W, Sorensen HT. Appendicectomy has no beneficial effect on admission rates in patients with ulcerative colitis. *Gut* 2004;53:351–4.
16. Perey DYE, Cooper MD, Good RA. Lymphoepithelial tissues of the intestine and differentiation of antibody production. *Science* 1968;161:265–6.
17. Perey DYE, Bienenstock J. Effects of bursectomy and thymectomy on ontogeny of fowl IgA, IgG and IgM. *J Immunol* 1973;111:633–7.
18. Cooper MD, Perey DY, McKneally MS, Gabrielsen AE, Sutherland DER, Good RA. A mammalian equivalent of the avian bursa of Fabricius. *Lancet* 1966;i:1388–91.
19. Perey DYE, Frommel D, Hong R, Good RA. The mammalian homologue of the avian bursa of Fabricius: II. Extirpation, lethal X-irradiation, and reconstitution in rabbits. Effects on humoral immune responses, immunoglobulins, and lymphoid tissues. *Lab Invest* 1970;22:212–27.
20. Perey DYE. Mammalian analogues of the bursal-thymic systems. In: Cohen S, Cudkowicz G, McCluskey RT, eds. *Second International Convocation on Immunology, Buffalo, 1970. Cellular Interatcitons in the Immune Response*. Basel: Karger; 1971:13–24.
21. Rudzik O, Bienenstock J. Isolation and charcteristics of gut mucosal lymphocytes. *Lab Invest* 1974;30:260–6.
22. Dasso JF, Howell MD. Neonatal appendectomy impairs mucosal immunity in rabbits. *Cell Immunol* 1997;182:29–37.
23. Yamagiwa S, Sugahara S, Shimizu T, *et al.* The primary site of CD4$^-$8$^-$B220$^+$ αβ T cells in *lpr* mice: the appendix in normal mice. *J Immunol* 1998;160:2665–74.
24. Merger M, Croitoru K. Infections in the immunopathogenesis of chronic inflammatory bowel disease. *Semin Immunol* 1998;10:69–78.
25. Elson CO, Konrad A, Cong Y, Weaver CT. Gene disruption and immunity in experimental colitis. *Inflamm Bowel Dis* 2004;10(Suppl 1):S25–8.
26. Bouma G, Strober W. The immunological and genetic basis of inflammatory bowel disease. *Nat Rev Immunol* 2003;3:521–33.
27. Powrie F. Immune regulation in the intestine: a balancing act between effector and regulatory T cell responses. *Ann N Y Acad Sci* 2004;1029:132–41.
28. Powrie F, Maloy KJ. Immunology: regulating the regulators. *Science* 2003;299:1030–1.
29. Nagler-Anderson C, Bhan AK, Podolsky DK, Terhorst C. Control freaks: immune regulatory cells. *Nat Immunol* 2004;5:119–22.
30. Laroux FS, Norris HH, Houghton J, *et al.* Regulation of chronic colitis in athymic nu/nu (nude) mice. *Int Immunol* 2004;16:77–89.
31. Poussier P, Ning T, Banerjee D, Julius M. A unique subset of self-specific intraintestinal T cells maintains gut integrity. *J Exp Med* 2002;195:1491–7.
32. Shevach EM. Regulatory/suppressor T cells in health and disease. *Arthritis Rheum* 2004;50:2721–4.
33. Mizoguchi E, Mizoguchi A, Preffer FI, Bhan AK. Regulatory role of mature B cells in a murine model of inflammatory bowel disease. *Int Immunol* 2000;12:597–605.
34. Wei B, Velazquez P, Turovskaya O, *et al.* Mesenteric B cells centrally inhibit CD4+ T cell colitis through interaction with regulatory T cell subsets. *Proc Natl Acad Sci USA* 2005;102:2010–15.
35. Mombaerts P, Mizoguchi E, Grusby MJ, Glimcher LH, Bhan AK, Tonegawa S. Spontaneous development of inflammatory bowel disease in T cell receptor mutant mice. *Cell* 1993;75:275–82.
36. Mizoguchi A, Mizoguchi E, Smith RN, Preffer FI, Bhan AK. Suppressive role of B cells in chronic colitis of T cell receptor α mutant mice. *J Exp Med* 1997;186:1749–56.
37. Mizoguchi A, Mizoguchi E, Chiba C, Bhan AK. Role of appendix in the development of inflammatory bowel disease in TCR-alpha mutant mice. *J Exp Med* 1996;184:707–15.
38. Farkas SA, Hornung M, Sattler C, *et al.* Preferential migration of CD62L cells into the appendix in mice with experimental chronic colitis. *Eur Surg Res* 2005;37:115–22.
39. Kawachiya T, Oshitani N, Jinno Y, *et al.* Significance of increased proliferation of immature plasma cells in the appendix of patients with ulcerative colitis. *Int J Mol Med* 2005;15:417–23.
40. Okazaki K, Onodera H, Watanabe N, *et al.* A patient with improvement of ulcerative colitis after appendectomy. *Gastroenterology* 2000;119:502–6.
41. Jarnerot G, Andersson M, Franzen L. Laparoscopic appendectomy in patients with refractory ulcerative colitis. *Gastroenterology* 2001;120:1562–3.
42. Jo Y, Matsumoto T, Yada S, *et al.* Histological and immunological features of appendix in patients with ulcerative colitis. *Dig Dis Sci* 2003;48:99–108.

II: Diagnosis and assessment

6: What are the controversies in histopathological diagnosis?

Bryan F. Warren and Neil A. Shepherd

Controversy 1

Can we accurately distinguish acute self-limiting colitis from chronic idiopathic inflammatory bowel disease using routine histological assessment of colorectal biopsies?

The differential diagnosis of an early acute 'colitis' may present considerable difficulties. There are, however, several histological features that may indicate a diagnosis of an acute self-limiting (i.e. infective) colitis or alternatively chronic inflammatory bowel disease (CIBD), even in the absence of well-established diagnostic features of either condition [1]. Crypt architectural distortion takes about 6 weeks to develop in CIBD [2, 3]. Diffuse crypt architectural distortion is a strong pointer towards CIBD, particularly ulcerative colitis (Fig 6.1) as is a villiform surface architecture: these architectural changes are most unusual in infective colitis, being effectively never seen in acute infective colitis and only rarely seen in chronic colitides such as shigellosis and occasionally chronic amoebiasis [4]. The presence of diffuse chronic inflammation is a useful marker of CIBD, although this may occasionally be seen in some infective diseases [5]. Basal lymphoid aggregates are also a good histological pointer to CIBD, in particular ulcerative colitis [4]. Mucin depletion is a variable feature of chronic inflammatory bowel disease: mucin preservation is seen more in Crohn's disease than ulcerative colitis, although this is not an entirely consistent and reliable sign [6, 7].

Acute inflammation is usually diffuse in nature in ulcerative colitis and predominantly involves the epithelium. However, in Crohn's disease and some infections, the polymorph infiltrate may be distinctly patchy and is often more pronounced in the lamina propria than in the epithelium (Fig 6.2) [8, 9]. Occasionally the classical histological features of an acute self-limiting (infective) colitis may be present: these include normal crypt architecture, gross lamina propria oedema and focal collections of neutrophils within the lamina propria with some ingress into the epithelium (Fig 6.3) [4]. Crypt abscesses may also be seen and are often eccentric or demonstrate a classical pattern of crypt beading [4]. However such features are not always seen and some cases of infectious colitis are good mimics of early CIBD. *Campylobacter jejuni* colitis characteristically shows mimicry of CIBD histologically, especially if there is some chronicity to the infection [3]. Amoebic colitis may also be a difficult differential diagnosis. However, if the characteristic haematoxyphilic necrotic slough on the surface of an ulcer is found within the biopsy, it is a good indication for this diagnosis, although one may have to search carefully to see amoebae that have a prominent nuclear karyosome and that have incorporated red blood cells into their cytoplasm (Fig 6.4) [10]. There may be difficulty in differentiating amoebae from macrophages containing red blood cells but here the nuclear detail and size of the cell are useful, as are a periodic acid-Schiff (PAS) stain (which will highlight the amoebae) and an immunohistochemical stain for macrophages (such as CD68).

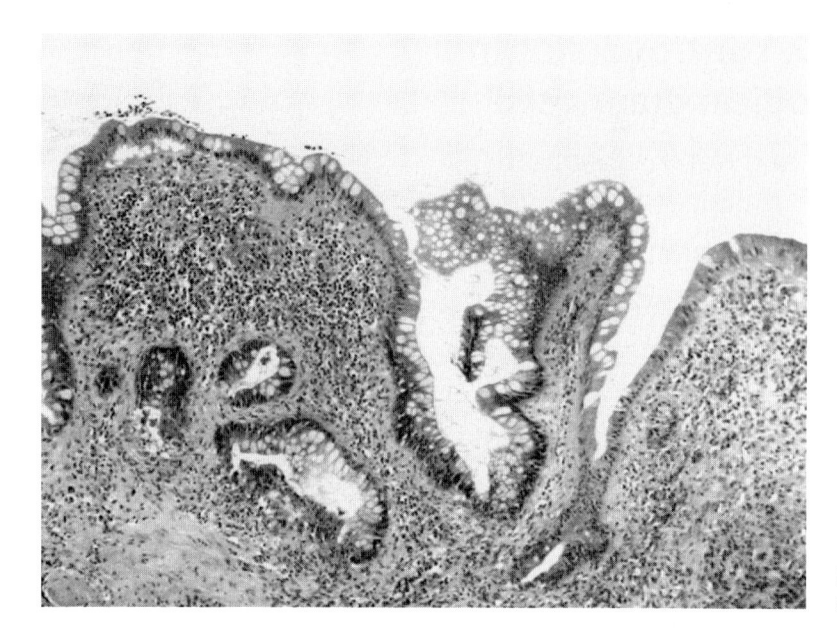

Fig 6.1 Biopsy appearances of ulcerative colitis.

Controversy 2

Do the sequelae of infection include chronic changes in patients who do not develop CIBD?

Most infective colitides resolve without leaving residual histological stigmata. It is notable that the chronic inflammation in *Helicobacter pylori*-associated antral gastritis may persist for up to 1 year after successful eradication of the organism [11]. Occasional patients with pseudomembranous colitis, due to Clostridium difficile toxin [12], will, after resolution, have a degree of crypt architectural distortion and hyperplastic change (personal observations). Perhaps the best example of chronic architectural changes after previous infective colitis, mimicking CIBD, especially chronic ulcerative colitis, is chronic shigellosis [4]. Such pathology is effectively never seen in the Western world but is

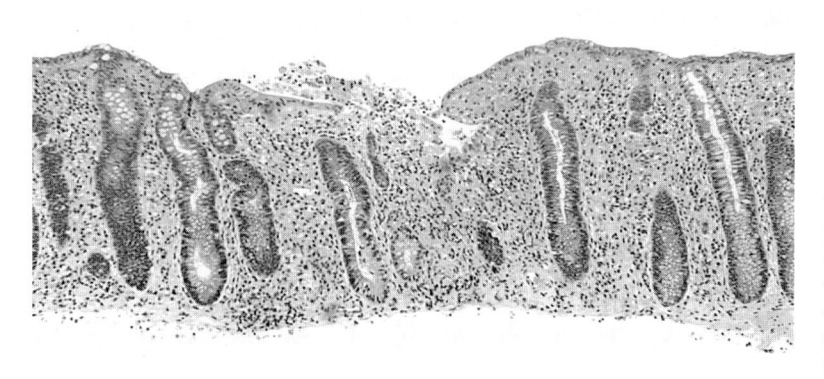

Fig 6.2 Biopsy appearances of Crohn's disease. There is chronic inflammation in the lamina propria with modest crypt architectural disturbance. There is focal active inflammation and ulceration (both seen centrally).

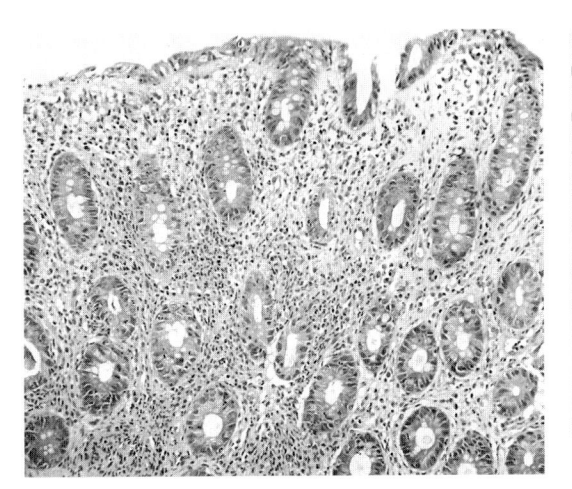

Fig 6.3 Infective colitis. In this biopsy both oedema and polymorph infiltrate are well seen but there is no increase in chronic inflammatory cells.

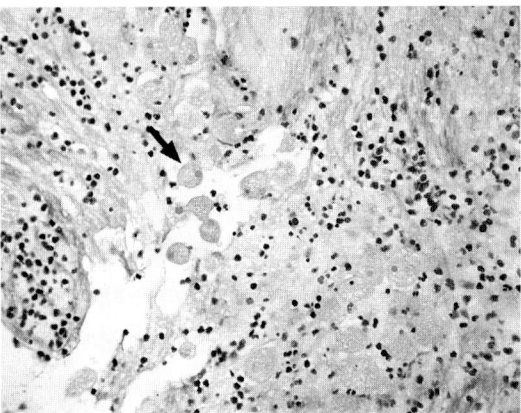

Fig 6.4 Amoebic colitis. In this inflammatory debris from the surface of an ulcerated colonic mucosal biopsy, there are several well-defined amoebae (one arrowed).

relatively common in the tropics: in such a situation even gross crypt architectural distortion should not be taken as evidence for CIBD.

Controversy 3

Are there indeterminate colitides or merely indeterminate pathologists?

Indeterminate colitis was the term originally introduced to describe colectomy specimens in which the macroscopic and microscopic features resembled both Crohn's disease and ulcerative colitis and in which a firm diagnosis of neither was possible [13]. The term has since been sometimes applied to biopsy histopathology in which a diagnosis of CIBD can be confidently made but the features are equivocal for ulcerative colitis and Crohn's disease. We believe this is an inappropriate use of the term indeterminate colitis. We believe that Price's original description of the concept of indeterminate colitis, applied only to resection specimens, is a useful and specific one, which is valuable in the management of CIBD. We believe that the term should not be applied to biopsy material. Cases equivocal for ulcerative colitis and Crohn's disease on biopsy material are best designated as 'CIBD unclassified'. Resections of such cases usually provide definitive evidence of one or other of the two major sub-types of CIBD and do not often show changes characteristic of indeterminate colitis.

So why is there uncertainty in the differential diagnosis of CIBD, even in resection specimens? The main reason is that neither disease displays diagnostic histological features that are universally present in one disease and invariably absent in the other. From a pathological diagnosis point of view, the most difficult colorectal resection specimens are those cases of acute fulminating colitis in which the inflammatory and ulcerative changes are so severe that distinction between the two major sub-types of CIBD becomes very difficult. In most series a diagnosis of indeterminate colitis is made in 10–15% of colectomy specimens performed for fulminant colitis [13]. It is important to note that most cases of indeterminate colitis, when diagnosed (appropriately) at the time of colectomy, behave like ulcerative colitis, and restorative proctocolectomy is generally successful, although patients who undergo such pouch surgery do have a higher incidence of pelvic sepsis but not of, for example, pouchitis [14, 15]. For instance, the prevalence of fistulae may be higher in pouch patients who had indeterminate colitis compared to those with classical ulcerative colitis, although the long-term function may be just as good [16]. In a small proportion, the diagnosis does turn out to be Crohn's disease and these patients have a poorer outcome with pouch failure rates of up to 40% [17].

Those who apply the term indeterminate colitis to biopsy material have suggested that between 3 and 13% of cases of CIBD show such equivocal features [14, 18]. Inevitably this area is confused and complicated because there are so many confounding factors, including the number of biopsies taken, their site and the number of procedures undertaken over varying time periods. Nevertheless there are an appreciable number of cases, and we would agree that the number is about 10%, where standard biopsy protocols, performed during multiple colonoscopic assessments, are unable to positively differentiate between ulcerative colitis and Crohn's disease. It should be emphasised, however, that the pathological assessment must never be performed in isolation, because further clinical, radiological or endoscopic information will often clarify the diagnosis of either Crohn's disease or ulcerative colitis in the absence of definitive differentiating histopathological features on biopsy.

In conclusion, despite the term 'indeterminate colitis' suggesting that pathologists may be less than definitive in their diagnostic opinion, it is in fact a clinically useful, relatively specific, diagnosis that has led to well-defined management strategies and a relatively predictable natural history [19] but only when applied to resection specimens. We believe that much confusion has been caused by applying this term to cases of unclassified or equivocal CIBD and that other terminology should be used in these circumstances.

Controversy 4

Which histopathological features are important in the distinction of ulcerative colitis from Crohn's disease?

Skip lesions

Skip lesions have always been thought to be macroscopic indicators of Crohn's disease. Initially it was thought that they do not occur in ulcerative colitis. It has, however, been recognised recently that macroscopic skip lesions may occur in ulcerative colitis in two distinct circumstances. One is in the appendiceal skip lesion as described and titled by Davison and Dixon [18]. The other is the caecal patch lesion as described by D'Haens et al. [20]. The appendix is involved as an extension of caecal disease in 62% of cases of ulcerative colitis that come to colectomy [21]. This appendiceal involvement may be seen either in association with continuous involvement [21] in total colitis or as a skip lesion [18]. The latter may manifest as appendiceal involvement in the presence of a clearly defined proximal demarcation of active disease, which may be in the ascending colon but may be seen with very distal disease. Such appendiceal involvement, with left-sided ulcerative colitis, is not unusual and it is now recognised that the disease activity in the peri-appendiceal skip lesions of ulcerative colitis will mimic closely the disease activity in the left side of the colonic following treatment [21]. Furthermore, the presence of peri-appendiceal skip lesions may indicate a sub-type of ulcerative colitis, which shows a particularly good response to medical therapy [22].

Patients with both the appendiceal skip lesion and with the caecal patch lesion have, in our experience, a natural history entirely typical of ulcerative colitis, unless there are other features to suggest Crohn's disease, and they have a successful outcome following pouch surgery [23]. Histologically, the caecal patch lesion shows the typical histological changes of ulcerative colitis, as do the appendiceal 'skip lesions' [18, 20, 23]. The latter show quite different histological features from acute appendicitis in that there are chronic changes of crypt architectural distortion and chronic inflammation, in association with acute inflammation. The inflammatory changes are restricted to the mucosa, unlike acute appendicitis, in which there is ulceration and transmural acute inflammation.

Mucin depletion

Mucin depletion has often been quoted as a hallmark of ulcerative colitis when comparing histological appearances with Crohn's disease. However, mucin may be preserved in some cases of ulcerative colitis. This is particularly the case in acute fulminant colitis associated with toxic megacolon in which, mysteriously, the mucin complement seems well preserved in between areas of ulceration. Mucin depletion, in ulcerative colitis without such fulminant change, is usually regarded as proportionate to the amount of acute inflammation and activity [2]. Consequently, in cases of inactive ulcerative colitis there may be little or no mucin depletion. Therefore this is a less valuable discriminator, between Crohn's disease and ulcerative colitis, than has been suggested.

Focality of inflammatory infiltrate

This has been regarded as a hallmark of Crohn's disease rather than ulcerative colitis. It is regularly quoted as an important criterion, although there is little objective evidence for its usage as a discriminator between the two major types of CIBD [2]. It is, admittedly, a parameter with the highest level of intra-observer concordance, of all the regularly used criteria for the diagnosis of CIBD in biopsy material [24]. However, it has been recognised more recently that the evidence for the utility of multiple colonoscopic biopsies in distinguishing ulcerative colitis from Crohn's disease is actually rather scanty [4, 9]. It has also been recognised that some patchiness of inflammation in ulcerative colitis may be apparent in the healing stage, particularly after some modern therapies [9]. This focality of disease in ulcerative colitis may require further evaluation, based on study of cases after treatment.

Mucosal granulomas and microgranulomas

When well-formed granulomas are seen away from crypts within the mucosa, they provide a stronger pointer towards a diagnosis of Crohn's disease [2]. However, it is recognised that granulomas may also be seen in other circumstances, particularly in diversion colitis [25] and in the luminal mucosal inflammatory disease that complicates diverticular disease, usually known as diverticular colitis [26, 27]. The definition of the term microgranuloma has caused some difficulty in the past: it is now accepted that this represents a collection of epithelioid macrophages, greater than five in number [1]. As such, the microgranuloma is characteristic of Crohn's disease but, once again, may be seen in other situations, such as infective colitis [4, 5].

Cryptolytic granulomas are those seen in relation to the rupture or destruction of a colorectal crypt (Fig 6.5) [28]. In one study, a relatively small series, these were shown to be relatively specific for Crohn's disease [28]. Furthermore, the same authors have suggested that this feature is pathognomonic of Crohn's disease [28]. That is not

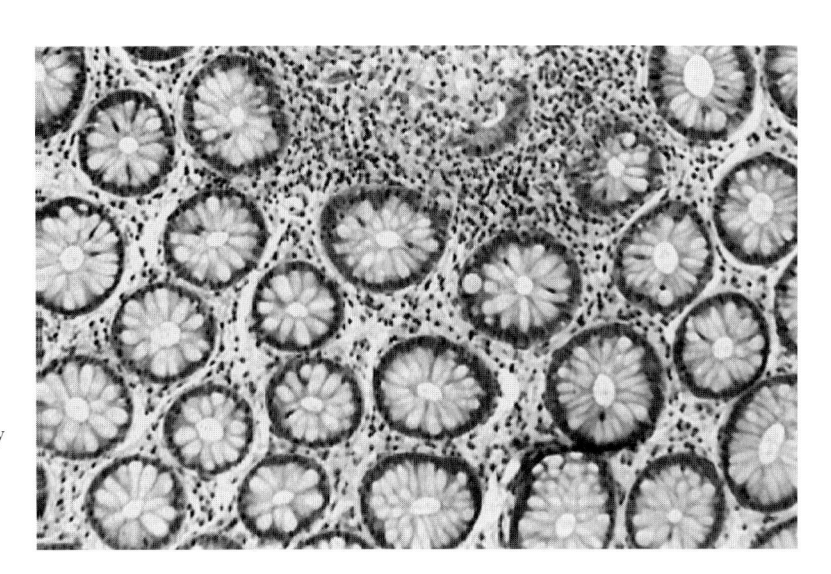

Fig 6.5 Cryptolytic granuloma. Towards the top of this deliberately transversely orientated colonic mucosal biopsy, there is a granulomatous reaction to a disruptive crypt abscess.

our experience and we, and others, have seen such lesions in ulcerative colitis, diverticular colitis, diversion colitis, pouchitis and campylobacter colitis [23, 27, 29]. Granulomas related to crypts might be in response to a disrupted crypt abscess, in which case mucin and neutrophils will be evident within the granuloma. Alternatively the granuloma may be seen in association with a largely intact crypt and appears to be inflicting damage on the epithelium itself [29].

It is important that the pathologist is confident that the structure he or she has identified is truly a granuloma, because, in histological sections, tangential sectioning of crypts may mimic granulomas. In this situation, there appear to be small clusters of epithelioid cells, apparently separate from crypts, with pronounced imitation of a well-formed granuloma. Only by close attention to the multiple levels, which are standard parts of histological assessment of colorectal mucosal biopsies, will these structures be demonstrated to be crypt epithelium and not granulomas.

Inflammatory cell type

Older textbooks, particularly non-pathology textbooks, have often stated that the type of cell in the lamina propria inflammatory infiltrate is important in distinguishing Crohn's disease from ulcerative colitis. In particular, neutrophils have been associated with ulcerative colitis. The truth is that neutrophils are present when inflammatory bowel disease is active and are a reflection of activity rather than disease type. It is a truism that, in Crohn's disease, there will be more aggregates of neutrophils in the lamina propria whereas in ulcerative colitis many more of these will involve the epithelium lining the crypts and surface resulting in crypt abscesses, epithelial destruction and ulceration. However, such inflammatory features are also seen in Crohn's disease, although the involvement of crypts is often patchier [1, 24].

Depth of inflammation

The inflammation in ulcerative colitis is usually stated to be mucosal. However, when there is extensive ulceration, it is inevitable that active inflammation will extend into the submucosa and even deeper into the bowel wall. In fact extension of active inflammation into the muscularis propria, often with myocytolysis and gross telangiectasia, is the characteristic feature of acute fulminant ulcerative colitis and toxic megacolon. Such deep extension, with muscle damage, is the reason for perforation in toxic megacolon. Thus, it can be seen that extension of inflammation, below the level of the mucosa, is inevitable in acute fulminant ulcerative colitis. The context in which deep extension of inflammation is demonstrated in biopsies is therefore critical. If the endoscopic features are relatively mild and there is no evidence of deep ulceration, then the demonstration of extension of inflammation beyond the muscularis mucosae may well be an important sign of Crohn's disease.

Some have suggested that specific histological criteria will reproducibly enable Crohn's colitis to be differentiated from ulcerative colitis. However, in most inter-observer studies of mucosal biopsies, including some using very large datasets, pathologists can accurately differentiate the histological features of inflammatory bowel disease from those of normal mucosa but the distinction of Crohn's disease from ulcerative colitis is poor.

Rupture of crypts into the submucosa

Disruptive crypt abscesses cause much consternation amongst pathologists, when attempting to differentiate Crohn's disease from ulcerative colitis. When crypts rupture downwards, they inevitably involve the muscularis mucosae and the superficial part of the submucosa. This is a further example of extension of active inflammation into the submucosa. Such a feature does not necessarily favour a diagnosis of Crohn's disease. Indeed such crypt rupture is often associated with a histiocytic infiltrate because the inflammatory debris from the crypt, admixed with mucin, is often recognised as 'foreign material' and incites such a reaction. Even in this situation, the appearances may yet represent ulcerative colitis rather than Crohn's disease.

Controversy 5

Is it easy to distinguish backwash ileitis from Crohn's disease histologically?

Backwash ileitis is defined as the extension of the inflammatory process of ulcerative colitis through an incompetent ileocaecal valve to involve the distal few centimetres of the terminal ileum [30]. In resection specimens the differentiation is straightforward because the continuity of disease from the proximal colon into the ileum, with an incompetent ileocaecal valve, can be readily appreciated. In small mucosal biopsies, it can be much more difficult. Backwash ileitis can strongly mimic active Crohn's disease of the ileum. In this situation, accurate information concerning the endoscopic features, notably the extent of disease in the colon and the continuity of disease between colon and ileum, together with information about the ileocaecal valve, should be imparted to the pathologist, to avoid an erroneous diagnosis of Crohn's disease.

Controversy 6

Are there any specific and diagnostic features of Crohn's disease?

Granulomas

Intra-mucosal and cryptolytic granulomas, and microgranulomas, have already been considered above. Granulomas below the level of the mucosa have much more specificity for Crohn's disease but may be seen in several other situations. Complicated diverticular disease is an important mimic of Crohn's disease and this condition is often associated with well-formed granulomas deep in the wall of the bowel [26, 31–33]. The distribution of transmural inflammation in the form of lymphoid aggregates and of transmural granulomas is different in that both will radiate out from around inflamed diverticula and will not be truly transmural in the way that Crohn's granulomas and the associated lymphoid aggregates are. Granulomas in sarcoidosis are, in our experience, indistinguishable from those in Crohn's disease. However, a diagnosis of colorectal sarcoidosis should only be considered if there is good clinical evidence of sarcoidosis elsewhere.

Tuberculosis remains an important differential diagnosis of Crohn's disease, particularly in immigrants from parts of Southern Asia and Africa and in those with poor nutritional status such as alcoholics or vagrants [34]. The granulomas in tuberculosis are usually coalescent (Fig 6.6) and are associated with caseous necrosis. However, only about 40% of ileocolonic tuberculosis will have demonstrable acid and alcohol-fast bacilli [34]. In occasional cases, it can be difficult to positively differentiate tuberculosis from Crohn's disease. In this situation, other

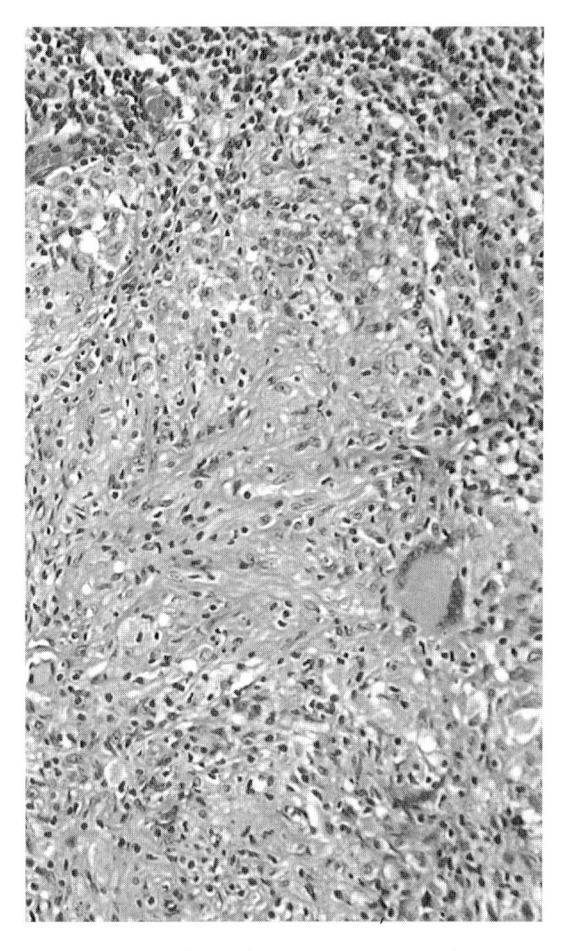

Fig 6.6 The typical granulomatous appearance of tuberculous ileocolitis. There are coalescent granulomas with a very well-defined Langhans-type giant cell.

clinical pointers, such as the results of a Heaf test, the immigration status of the patient and evidence of disease elsewhere, may be required before a diagnosis can be reached.

Granulomatous vasculitis is present when there is destruction of vessel walls by granulomas. It is said to be specific for Crohn's disease [35]. Nevertheless, once again, caution is appropriate. We have seen this in very rare cases of gastrointestinal involvement in Churg-Strauss syndrome, when it is accompanied by an eosinophil infiltrate with peripheral eosinophilia and asthma. Furthermore it has been described in diversion proctitis, in ulcerative colitis [30] and also in diverticulitis [31]. Outside these circumstances, it is an extremely useful histological feature to aid in the distinction of Crohn's disease from ulcerative colitis [36]. It is particularly important to remember that isolated giant cells and well-defined granulomas, away from areas of crypt rupture, do not, as a rule, occur in ulcerative colitis. These do, in a colonoscopic biopsy with features of inflammatory bowel disease, provide a strong indication for a diagnosis of Crohn's disease. However, crypt-related giant cells and granulomas are not reliable discriminatory features to distinguish Crohn's colitis from ulcerative colitis [37].

Fissuring ulcers

Fissuring ulcers may been seen in many forms of colitis. Deep vertical fissuring is certainly characteristic of Crohn's disease. Nevertheless, any acute fulminant colitis, with deep ulceration, may show a degree of lateral fissuring and this is one of the characteristic features of indeterminate colitis [13]. Fissuring ulcers may develop in the diverted rectum in ulcerative colitis where they develop from the basis of ruptured crypts [38] and are also seen in the pelvic ileal reservoir of patients with an unequivocal diagnosis of ulcerative colitis [23].

Fat-wrapping

Crohn's disease is characterised by relatively specific connective tissue changes, which reflect its chronic transmural nature. Thus, fat-wrapping is a highly characteristic and almost pathognomonic feature of Crohn's disease: certainly we have never seen it either in the colon in ulcerative colitis or in the ileum affected by backwash ileitis [39]. It is more difficult to appreciate fat-wrapping in the colon and rectum compared with the small bowel. Its pathogenetic basis is a hyperplasia of the mesenteric and mesocolic fat, with loss of the bowel to mesentery angle and encroachment of fat around the circumference of the bowel in segments of disease-effected bowel. This is useful to the surgeon at laparotomy in identifying areas of Crohn's disease where multiple skip lesions are present. Fat-wrapping correlates well with the transmural inflammation that is such an important part of the pathology of Crohn's disease. However, the exact mechanisms of formation of the connective tissue changes in Crohn's disease, particularly the fat-wrapping, are far from being well understood [39].

Transmural inflammation

Transmural inflammation is a highly characteristic feature of Crohn's disease. However, it should be appreciated that transmural inflammation in the form of lymphoid aggregates, a feature that is such an important and commonplace accompaniment of the plethora of pathological changes of Crohn's disease, may also be seen in other situations. It is commonly seen in complicated diverticular disease [26] but may be seen in any severe colitis, whatever the cause, if there is deep inflammation, particularly when extending into the muscularis propria [23]. Hence it is seen in acute fulminant colitis, whether definitely due to ulcerative colitis or showing the features of indeterminate colitis. If accompanied by some of the other stigmata of Crohn's disease, then it may be impossible to define the type of CIBD in these colectomy specimens. However, the pattern seen in Crohn's disease is quite distinctive, although it may need an overall low-power view to distinguish it from diverticular inflammation. This pattern is the highly distinctive rosary where lymphoid aggregates are sharply defined and often confined to the subserosal tissues immediately beneath the muscularis propria. In only one other condition is this pattern of transmural inflammation so well seen and that is, curiously, colorectal cancer [40]. This 'rosary' is said to impart an excellent prognosis to colorectal cancer suggesting a pronounced host immune response to the carcinoma [40].

Aphthous ulcers

Aphthous ulcers are very common in Crohn's tissue and some believe them to be relatively specific for this type of inflammatory bowel disease, especially when they are demonstrated on the surface of lymphoid follicles in the colorectum and terminal ileum at the time of endoscopy. Nevertheless, they are also seen in other situations: they are a common feature in diverticular disease-associated chronic colitis or diverticular colitis [26, 27]. They are also often seen in diversion colitis, from whatever cause [30, 41].

Connective tissue changes

In Crohn's disease important post-inflammatory components of the disease are the effects on the connective tissues of the bowel wall and the adjacent mesenteric tissues [39]. They characteristically occur in segments of bowel that have been severely diseased or are severely diseased. They affect all layers of the bowel wall. There is thickening and disruption of the muscularis mucosae, resulting in apparent muscularisation of the submucosa. The neural component shows hyperplasia of the nerves of the submucosal and myenteric plexi. There are often marked vascular changes with intimal hyperplasia and duplication of the muscular layer of both arterial and venous components. The muscular propria is often profoundly disordered and there is the distinctive change in adipose tissue, which is both hyperplastic and migratory, leading to the macroscopic feature of fat-wrapping [39, 42]. Some of these changes may be seen in other inflammatory diseases of the small and large bowel, especially pathology from non-steroidal anti-inflammatory drugs (NSAIDs) and diverticular disease [26, 43]. However, of all these changes, fat-wrapping seems to be the one that is most specific to Crohn's disease [39, 42].

Ulcer-associated cell lineage

Ulcer-associated cell lineage (UACL), previously known as pyloric or pseudopyloric metaplasia, has been stated to be pathognomonic of Crohn's disease. However, it is now clear that UACL occurs adjacent to any area of ulceration in the gut: it represents part of the gut healing and repair process [44]. The lineage develops from crypts and undergoes a functional change so that it can secrete epidermal growth factor to help regenerate epithelium over the edges of healing ulcers [42, 44].

Controversy 7

Do the histological appearances of CIBD remain diagnosable irrespective of treatment?

We have already indicated that patchiness, or focality, of inflammation is a weaker discriminator for a diagnosis of Crohn's disease and against a diagnosis of ulcerative colitis than was previously thought. This may be an effect of the effects of more contemporary drug therapy on ulcerative colitis. We are at present profoundly ignorant of the specific effects of such drugs in ulcerative colitis and Crohn's disease. It is, therefore, important that such features are catalogued to enable a revision of the currently accepted diagnostic criteria in differentiating Crohn's disease from ulcerative colitis. Apparent rectal sparing in ulcerative colitis has long been associated with rectal installation of anti-inflammatory drugs [23]. It has to be recognised, however, that a small subset of ulcerative colitis patients has relative rectal sparing in the absence of a history of local instillation of anti-inflammatory agents [45]. Usually in this situation there is evidence of chronic inflammatory and architectural changes of ulcerative colitis in the rectum even though there is little or none of the active inflammation that is present more proximally. A completely normal rectum should always raise suspicions of Crohn's disease [9].

Ciclosporin-induced 'pseudodysplasia'

Villous regeneration and nuclear enlargement in epithelial cells are both seen in regeneration of the mucosa in ulcerative colitis after severe acute inflammation. Both these changes are more pronounced after treatment with ciclosporin and can lead to an erroneous misdiagnosis of dysplasia on biopsy, because they may be very pronounced [46]. In older textbooks, villous architecture has been a valuable pointer towards dysplasia: in our experience villous regeneration is actually more common than villous areas of dysplasia in ulcerative colitis. Such regenerative villous change will be seen even more commonly if the use of ciclosporin therapy becomes more widespread [46].

The effects of diversion: do they modify the criteria for CIBD diagnosis?

It has been recognised for some time that diverting the faecal stream away from Crohn's disease may have therapeutic benefits [47, 48] and that diverting the faecal stream in ulcerative colitis may worsen the inflammation [36, 37]. Curiously, diversion itself may actually be diagnostically useful for the pathologist in some cases of indeterminate colitis as part of the three-stage pouch procedure. A colectomy may be performed for colitis, which has been previously difficult, on the basis of biopsies, to distinguish between ulcerative colitis and Crohn's disease. Even the colectomy specimen may not allow the distinction between the two major forms of CIBD because the changes of acute fulminant colitis may not be specific as previously described. The resultant changes seen in the de-functioned rectum may well provide some insight into the underlying pathology. If the active rectal inflammation ameliorates or resolves, then this is often a pointer towards Crohn's disease, whereas if the rectal inflammation worsens, it will be a strong indicator that this is ulcerative colitis [49]. It must be emphasised that these assessments must be made in the wider context of all other clinical, endoscopic and radiological features. For instance, the presence or absence of perianal disease and/or small-bowel disease will provide further useful information concerning the final diagnosis and suitability for pelvic ileal reservoir surgery. In the past, it has been a source of considerable distress when diversion of the faecal stream from the rectum of an ulcerative colitis patient has led to an erroneous diagnosis of Crohn's disease because of the profound mimicry of Crohn's disease with transmural inflammation in the form of lymphoid aggregates, granulomatous inflammation, fissuring ulceration and granulomatous vasculitis [30, 37]. In a large study of rectal diversion in CIBD, it has been shown that granulomas, in the diverted rectum, are seen more commonly in patients with an initial diagnosis of Crohn's disease, whereas transmural lymphoid aggregates in this study were found in diverted inflammatory bowel disease, whatever its type. Other histological features of diversion in inflammatory bowel disease develop independently of the initial, pre-diversion, diagnosis or of the duration of diversion [50].

Controversy 8

Is there an established evidence base for the value of colonoscopic biopsy series in IBD diagnosis?

There are histological features in current usage that seem to be reliable for the histological distinction between Crohn's disease and ulcerative colitis in colonoscopic biopsy series. Perhaps this is surprising in view of the fact that most of these criteria were developed from the histological analysis of resection specimens and/or single rectal biopsies. In fact, very few of the major publications on this subject have specifically looked at colonoscopic biopsy series. There is clearly much more investigation required on the value of the colonoscopic biopsy series in the differential diagnosis of CIBD, especially with the application of the British Society of Gastroenterology (BSG) Guidelines for reporting the initial biopsies in inflammatory bowel disease [1].

Controversy 9

Does the rectal mucosa ever return to normal in ulcerative colitis?

It has been a long-held view amongst histopathologists that the rectal (and indeed the colonic) mucosa always shows distinctive changes of crypt architectural distortion and/or atrophy after an attack of ulcerative colitis and that this is useful in the confirmation, and the refutation, of a diagnosis of ulcerative colitis. Recent observations suggest that the histological appearances of mucosal biopsies in patients with undoubted evidence of previous ulcerative colitis may return to normal [51]. In this situation, a potential previous infective colitis has to be considered [4] and the reporting pathologist should review all biopsy material. The wording of such a report may present some difficulty and confusion.

Controversy 10

Is histological scoring worthwhile in routine biopsies in ulcerative colitis or Crohn's disease?

Many histological scoring systems for assessing activity in inflammatory bowel disease have been developed [52, 53]. They rarely correlate with clinical activity scoring systems, but they may be extremely useful in animal models where history and examination may be unrevealing. In our experience such scoring systems are also useful in assessing drug therapy in that they provide a numerical score for assessing amelioration and resolution of acute inflammation and/or ulceration with a variety of treatments. Inter-observer reproducibility has not often been assessed, although a more recent scoring system has undergone rigorous evaluation [52]. In routine reporting, we would recommend that activity is best expressed as mild, moderate or severe, as most currently available scoring systems require further evaluation before they can be recommended for routine usage.

In Crohn's disease, histological scoring is much more difficult due to its patchy distribution [54]. The only histological feature, which has evolved from the development of scoring systems that is of any value clinically, is the presence of small groups of neutrophils within the lamina propria [53]. Such a feature may be of value in predicting early relapse in clinically resolved ulcerative colitis following treatment. However, numerical scoring is, in our opinion, of no value in the routine clinical management of inflammatory bowel disease patients. We firmly believe that the only indication for numerical scoring, in routine diagnostic histopathological practice and management of inflammatory bowel disease, is in the assessment of pouchitis (as discussed below).

Controversy 11

Should we be using reporting algorithms, guidelines and/or computer tick boxes? Do they improve reproducibility in the histopathology of inflammatory bowel disease or do they inhibit an investigative mind by limiting the available diagnostic categories?

It seems logical that algorithms would improve reliability and reduce inter-observer and intra-observer variations in the diagnosis of inflammatory bowel disease. The 'tick box' system of the BSG guidelines has attempted to do this in the initial biopsy diagnosis of IBD [1]. There are also other neural networks and computer programs that have been shown to improve diagnostic acumen [55]. Currently there are no widely promulgated recommendations for the routine use of such systems and, for the most part, their use is largely based on personal preference. However, we are aware that the use of proforma reporting has had a markedly beneficial effect on the quality of histopathological reporting of common cancer resection specimens [56]. They particularly ensure that pathological reports document all-important items for patient management. However, it remains uncertain whether their use does anything to improve pathological judgement and assessment of histological features. This is an area ripe for future development and research.

Controversy 12

Is the frozen section of any value in the differential diagnosis of inflammatory bowel disease?

The majority of pathologists would answer strongly in the negative to this question. However, we believe that there is a limited but sometimes important role for frozen section as an inter-operative procedure in cases that have been, up until then, equivocal for the two major types of inflammatory bowel disease, despite the availability of all previous clinical, radiological and pathological data [23]. If there is an apparent skip lesion in what was thought to be ulcerative colitis, other than a caecal patch lesion, frozen sections of the most severely affected piece of colon, of the apparent skip lesion and of any enlarged lymph node can provide useful diagnostic information. The purpose of sampling these three sites is to establish whether any transmural inflammation shows a pattern typical of Crohn's disease in the disease segment [23]. The apparently normal segment is sampled to assess the presence or absence of focality of disease. The largest lymph node is assessed to confirm or refute the presence of well-formed epithelioid cell granulomas, clearly a feature that would strongly suggest Crohn's disease.

Provided the surgeon and the pathologist are both aware of the limitations of this technique, we have found it extremely useful on a small number of occasions. The presence of continuity of disease, the lack of transmural inflammation in the form of lymphoid aggregates, and the absence of granulomas will be quite reassuring. However, it must be emphasised that the pathologist is only examining but a small part of a relatively extensive disease: he or she can only really say there is no evidence of Crohn's disease in the tissues examined. Should there be features that do suggest Crohn's disease, then the surgeon can resort to a three-stage pouch procedure to allow full histopathological examination of the resection specimen. A considerable number of cases have undergone a change of diagnosis after one-stage pouch procedures from ulcerative colitis to Crohn's disease upon full histopathological examination of the colectomy specimen [57]. It is likely that intra-operative frozen section consultation can considerably reduce the number of these unfortunate cases [23].

Controversy 13

How should we grade dysplasia in inflammatory bowel disease?

The time-honoured method for grading dysplasia in the intestines, most notably in adenomas, has been with three categories of mild, moderate and severe dysplasia [58]. More recently it has been recognised that inter-observer variation is marked when using such categories and that the grading system has not been clinically useful [59, 60]. In 1983, Riddell et al. [61] recommended the use of two definitive categories for dysplasia, low grade and high grade: this provides much more useful management guidance and is now universally recommended for routine use [61]. Furthermore, Riddell's classification introduced the concept of 'indefinite for dysplasia' [61]. We believe this category to be an important one. It accepts that the assessment of dysplasia is inevitably subjective and it further implies that not all cases are definitive, especially when there is associated active inflammation. The term does not imply (usually) that the reporting pathologist is indefinite but rather that he or she is being realistic and is fully accepting the often equivocal features seen on routine histological assessment.

Controversy 14

Can we distinguish dysplasia-associated lesion or mass from sporadic adenoma?

A patient with long-term chronic ulcerative colitis is just as likely to develop sporadic adenomas as any other patient. The differentiation of such sporadic adenomas from polypoid dysplasia in ulcerative colitis is fraught with difficulties [62, 63]. Nevertheless, the distinction is of critical importance because the standard treatment of an adenoma is local excision whereas the accepted management of dysplasia-associated lesion or mass (DALM) has been total colectomy. There have been attempts at establishing criteria for distinguishing the histopathological features of sporadic adenoma in ulcerative colitis from polypoid dysplasia or DALM [62, 63]. In fact, the distinction is often relatively straightforward, especially if the adenoma is in a site, usually the right colon, which has not been affected by ulcerative colitis, especially if occurring in the older patient with a higher propensity to adenoma formation [63]. On the other hand, a flat or sessile lesion in a young patient, especially if in the rectum or distal colon, is much more likely to be a DALM. The sessile lesion in an older patient presents more difficulty. If it is clearly outside the area of colitis, then it is likely to be a sessile adenoma.

Despite the confidence that the literature espouses in enabling a differentiation between sporadic adenoma, adenoma-like lesions and DALM on microscopic criteria [62, 63], unfortunately, in some patients, there is often a degree of overlap between these conditions. Undoubtedly the most useful investigation is to biopsy not only the lesion (and extensive biopsy at that) but also to biopsy the adjacent flat mucosa. The presence of dysplasia in flat mucosa adjacent to the polypoid mucosa strongly aids in the substantiation of a diagnosis of DALM. The detection of dysplasia and its treatment by means of colonoscopy are now in question following two recent studies. Firstly, it has been demonstrated that careful colonoscopy renders most dysplastic lesions in ulcerative colitis visible [64]. Furthermore, one study has shown that local excision of dysplastic lesions, in 34 ulcerative colitis patients, whatever the subtype of the lesion, may be adequate treatment with favourable long-term follow up [65].

Controversy 15

Should a specialist pathologist, or a generalist, report dysplasia? Should dysplasia be confirmed by a second observer?

In our view, double reporting is invaluable: the recent adverse publicity surrounding the reporting of histopathology has ensured that many departments have introduced procedures for the double reporting of cancer specimens. This is certainly for the protection of patients and also aids the clinician by enhancing the level of confidence in a diagnosis that might well imply major surgery. Furthermore, we believe that such double reporting provides an invaluable educational and audit tool for pathologists. We would thoroughly recommend that a diagnosis such as high-grade dysplasia in chronic ulcerative colitis that may well obligate major surgery, should be confirmed by a second experienced observer. Such double reporting has not been the subject of any formal assessment, audit or trial, as far as we are aware. Nevertheless, the alarming inter-observer and intra-observer variation in the diagnosis of dysplasia in inflammatory bowel disease [66, 67] clearly indicates, to us at least, that such co-operation has to be regarded as best practice. Currently, in the UK, we do not have the resources to insist that all such diagnoses be made by specialist pathologists. We believe that the reporting of dysplasia in the gastrointestinal tract is best performed by specialist pathologists, but we accept that such a recommendation is not achievable at present.

Controversy 16

How should we diagnose pouchitis? Is histopathology the only criterion?

We firmly believe that the diagnosis of pouchitis should have three phases: clinical, endoscopic and histological [23]. The diagnosis should be based on the presence of clinical symptoms and signs: diarrhoea and/or discharge with associated systemic symptoms [68]. There must be endoscopic evidence of generalised inflammation within the pouch mucosa, appearing similar to the features of CIBD elsewhere in the intestines [68]. Finally, biopsies must reveal evidence of severe acute inflammation and ulceration (Fig 6.7) [69]. We do not believe that a diagnosis of pouchitis could, or should, be based solely on histopathological features. This is because other causes of inflammation within the pouch may cause just as much inflammation and ulceration as pouchitis: we have seen biopsies from patients with reservoir inflammation caused by ischaemia, mucosal prolapse, Crohn's disease and even infective enteritis that have all shown enough histopathological abnormality to justify a diagnosis of pouchitis according to current criteria [70]. Furthermore, the little recognised entity of secondary pouchitis, in which an external mass (usually a pelvic abscess but occasionally desmoid tumour or carcinoma) can cause florid inflammatory changes in the pouch mucosa, may show histopathological changes that strongly mimic pouchitis. In many centres, scoring systems have been used to grade the amount of histopathological abnormality [69, 71]. The amount of ulceration and acute inflammation required to correlate with a clinical and endoscopic diagnosis of pouchitis is usually dictated by the St Mark's scoring system

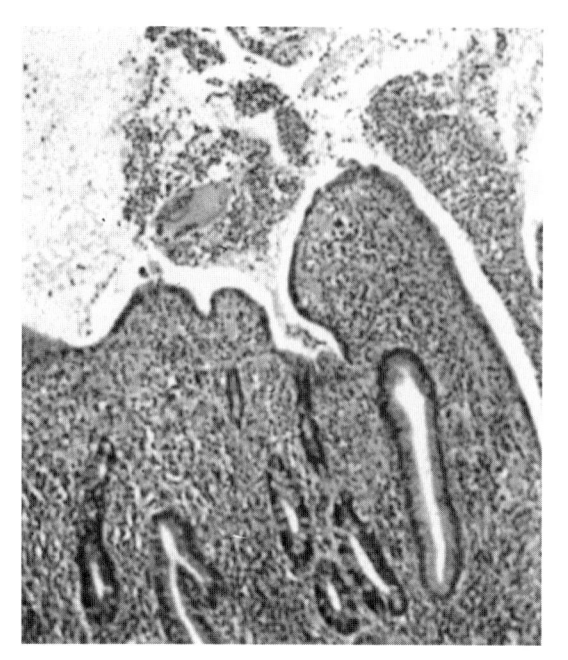

Fig 6.7 Pouchitis. There is surface pus indicating ulceration elsewhere and there is villous atrophy, diffuse chronic inflammation and a large erupting crypt abscess (at right).

[71]: in this system an acute inflammatory score of four or more usually implies pouchitis. It is only the acute inflammatory score that correlates well with the clinical and endoscopic features of pouchitis [72]. A study of the Heidelberg pouchitis activity index has highlighted that, whilst histological and endoscopic scoring is reasonably reproducible, the clinical scoring system is less reliable [73].

Controversy 17

Does dysplasia really occur in pouch mucosa?

We have not seen dysplasia in ileal mucosa of the pelvic ileal reservoir in our own practices, although a few reports do exist in the literature [72–74]. Although there are theoretical reasons why dysplasia could be a considerable problem in an ileal mucosa subject to colonic phenotypic change and to inflammation with associated hyperproliferation [75], we now believe that concerns over potentially high rates of neoplasia in the ileal mucosa itself may have been over-called [23]. The operation has been established for almost 30 years and it would seem unlikely to us that the reservoir will suffer the same levels of neoplastic change that the colon does in ulcerative colitis patients. This is certainly supported by evidence from Kock's continent ileostomy operations, in which there has been no notable increase in neoplastic change and, indeed, it would appear that the mucosa could revert to normality after 20 years [76]. This does not make us complacent and there is considerable concern about any remaining rectal or cuff mucosa at the lower end of the pouch. This cuff mucosa may well have considerable neoplastic potential [23, 77].

Controversy 18

Should we follow up pouch patients?

There are reports of dysplasia and carcinoma in the pouch mucosa but recent data suggest that the neoplastic risk is generally low [78, 79]. Nevertheless, we believe that ileal reservoirs should be subject to some form of surveillance [23, 70]. It has been recommended that patients undergo endoscopic surveillance every year [70]. Protocols recommend that biopsies be taken from several different sites in the pouch, according to standardised methodology, because the histological changes of colonic phenotypic change and inflammation may be patchy in the pouch mucosa [80, 81].

More recently, although not yet published, the International Organisation for IBD has asked a working group to study the whole question of neoplastic risk in and around the pouch and to make recommendations with regard to surveillance. They maintain that all patients do require surveillance but that only those with severe inflammatory changes, those with so-called type C histology, have a high risk of pouchitis and, at the same time, presumably, a somewhat higher risk of developing dysplasia and cancer in the ileal mucosa of the pouch. These patients as well as those with 'cuffitis' and/or a substantial remaining anal transitional zone (ATZ: cuff) should be kept under very close surveillance.

A small subset of patients with an apparently clear diagnosis of ulcerative colitis may have pouch surgery and, at a later date, develop Crohn's disease. In one series, this occurred in 32 patients out of 790 [82]. Crohn's disease should not be diagnosed on the basis of histological findings in the pouch alone. In this study pre-operative clinical, endoscopic or pathological features were not useful predictors of either pouch failure or of patient outcome.

Controversy 19

What is the role and value of upper GI endoscopy in the diagnosis, and differential diagnosis, of chronic inflammatory bowel disease?

There is increasing interest in gastro-duodenal involvement in Crohn's disease, not least because minor abnormalities, easily detectable in mucosal biopsies at the time of upper gastro-intestinal endoscopy, appear to be much more common than previously thought. These abnormalities may provide corroborative evidence for a diagnosis of Crohn's disease, especially when symptoms and signs are caused by more distal occult small intestinal disease, poorly accessible to conventional diagnostic modalities. About 15% of patients with Crohn's disease will have duodenal histological abnormalities, although gross involvement only affects about 2% of patients. On the other hand, focal active gastritis, sometimes known as focally enhanced gastritis, in the absence of *H. pylori* involvement, is said to be characteristic of gastric Crohn's disease. However, we firmly believe that this association has been over-called in the literature and there is support for our views from a recent study that indicates that such focally enhanced gastritis is neither a specific nor sensitive marker for CD [83]. Even if these upper gastrointestinal pathological changes occur in a setting of known CIBD, then some caution is appropriate as some clear-cut cases of ulcerative colitis may also have upper gastrointestinal tract lesions identical to those seen in Crohn's disease [84]. In paediatric disease, some authors have found oesophagogastroduodenoscopy a helpful investigation in cases of CIBD that are difficult to classify [85].

Conclusions

In this revised chapter, for the second edition of this book, we have, once again, deliberately raised more questions than we have provided answers. We believe it is the histopathologist's role to continually question perceived dogma in the diagnosis of inflammatory bowel disease (as exemplified by the change in attitude to the possible treatment of dysplastic lesions in ulcerative colitis). Histopathologists need to be fully aware of changes in disease with time and those introduced by newer drug therapies. There is also a need for continuing reassessment of diagnostic criteria of Crohn's disease- and ulcerative colitis. There is also an ongoing need for inter-observer and intra-observer studies. Likewise we should be required to review and, if necessary, modify our diagnostic criteria for dysplasia on a regular basis. The full potential of the pathologist's role in the management of CIBD is only fully realised, we believe, when the inter-disciplinary management team works together to benefit patient care. Pathologists should not work in isolation and should be kept informed, by being given all relevant clinical details on the pathology request form and by means of regular clinicopathological meetings, in which the pathologist plays a full and active role. We hope this chapter has raised enough items of interest to encourage pathologists and clinicians alike to continue with an active role in research and audit into improved diagnosis and management of CIBD and its complications.

References

1. Jenkins D, Balsitis M, Gallivan S, *et al*. Guidelines for the initial biopsy diagnosis of suspected chronic idiopathic inflammatory bowel disease. The British Society of Gastroenterology initiative. *J Clin Pathol* 1997;50:93–105.
2. Surawicz CM, Belic L. Rectal biopsy helps to distinguish acute self-limited colitis from idiopathic inflammatory bowel disease. *Gastroenterology* 1984;86:104–13.
3. Surawicz CM, Haggitt RC, Husseman M, *et al*. Mucosal biopsy diagnosis of colitis: acute self-limited colitis from ulcerative colitis. *Gastroenterology* 1994;107:755–63.

4 Day DW, Mandal BK, Morson BC. The rectal biopsy in salmonella colitis. *Histopathology* 1978;2:117–31.
5 Nostrant TT, Kumar NB, Appelman HD. Histopathology differentiates acute self-limiting colitis from ulcerative colitis. *Gastroenterology* 1987;92:313–28.
6 Hellstrom HR, Fisher ER. Estimation of mucosal mucin as an aid in the differentiation of Crohn's disease of the colon and chronic ulcerative colitis. *Am J Clin Pathol* 1967;48:259–68.
7 Goldman H. Ulcerative colitis and Crohn's disease. In: Ming SC, Goldman H, eds. *Pathology of the Gastrointestinal Tract*. 2nd ed. New York: Springer; 1998:673–718.
8 Tanaka M, Riddell RH. The pathological diagnosis and differential diagnosis of Crohn's disease. *Hepatogastroenterology* 1990;37:18–31.
9 Kleer CG, Appelman HD. Ulcerative colitis: patterns of involvement in colorectal biopsies and changes with time. *Am J Surg Pathol* 1998;22:983–9.
10 Pittman FE, Hennigar GR. Sigmoidoscopic and colonic mucosal biopsy findings in amoebic colitis. *Arch Pathol Med* 1974;97:155–8.
11 Wyatt J, Rathbone BJ, Sobala GM, et al. Gastric epithelium in the duodenum and its association with *Helicobacter pylori* infection. *J Clin Pathol* 1990;43:981–6.
12 Price AB, Davies DR. Pseudomembranous colitis. *J Clin Pathol* 1977;30:1–12.
13 Price AB. Overlap in the spectrum of non-specific chronic inflammatory bowel disease: colitis indeterminate. *J Clin Pathol* 1978;31:567–77.
14 Pezim ME, Pemberton JH, Beart RW, et al. Outcome of indeterminate colitis following ileal pouch anal anastomosis. *Dis Colon Rectum* 1989;32:653–8.
15 McIntyre PB, Pemberton JH, Wolff BG, Dozois RR, Beart RW. Indeterminate colitis: long-term outcome in patients after ileal pouch-anal anastomosis. *Dis Colon Rectum* 1995;38:51–4.
16 Rudolph WG, Uthoff SM, Mcauliffet L, Goode ET, Petras RE, Galandiuk S. Indeterminate colitis: the real story. *Dis Colon Rectum* 2002;45:1528–34.
17 Lucarotti ME, Freeman BJ, Warren BF, Durdey P. Synchronous proctocolectomy and ileoanal pouch formation and the risk of Crohn's disease. *Br J Surg* 1995;82:755–6.
18 Davison AM, Dixon MF. The appendix as a skip lesion in ulcerative colitis. *Histopathology* 1990;16:93–5.
19 Guindi M, Riddell RH. Indeterminate colitis. *J Clin Pathol* 2004;57:1233–44.
20 D'Haens G, Geboes K, Peeters M, Baert F, Ectors N, Rutgeerts P. Patchy caecal inflammation associated with distal ulcerative colitis: a prospective endoscopic study. *Am J Gastroenterol* 1997;92:1275–9.
21 Yamagishi N, Iizuka B, Nakamura T, Suzuki S, Hayashi N. Clinical and colonoscopic investigation of skipped periappendiceal lesions in ulcerative colitis. *Scand J Gastroenterol* 2002;37:177–82.
22 Goldblum JR, Appelman H. The appendix in ulcerative colitis. *Mod Pathol* 1992;5:607–10.
23 Warren BF, Shepherd NA. Surgical pathology of the intestines: the pelvic ileal reservoir and diversion proctocolitis. In: Lowe DG, Underwood JCE, eds. *Recent Advances in Histopathology*. Vol. 18. Edinburgh: Churchill Livingstone; 1999:63–88.
24 Theodossi A, Spiegelhalter DJ, Jass JR, et al. Observer variation and discriminating value of biopsy features in inflammatory bowel disease. *Gut* 1994;35:961–8.
25 Warren BF, Shepherd NA. The role of pathology in pelvic ileal reservoir surgery. *Int J Colorectal Dis* 1992;7:68–75.
26 Shepherd NA. Diverticular disease and chronic idiopathic inflammatory bowel disease: associations and masquerades. *Gut* 1996;38:801–2.
27 Makapugay LM, Dean PJ. Diverticular disease-associated chronic colitis. *Am J Surg Pathol* 1996;20:94–102.
28 Lee FD, Maguire C, Obeidat W, et al. Importance of cryptolytic lesions and pericryptal granulomas in inflammatory bowel disease. *J Clin Pathol* 1997;50:148–52.
29 Warren BF, Shepherd NA, Price AB, Williams GT. Importance of cryptolytic lesions and pericryptal granulomas in inflammatory bowel disease. *J Clin Pathol* 1997;50:880–1.
30 Rice AJ, Abbott CR, Mapstone NM. Granulomatous vasculitis in diversion proctocolitis. *Histopathology* 1999;34:276–7.
31 Burroughs SH, Bowrey DJ, Morris-Stiff GJ, Williams GT. Granulomatous inflammation in sigmoid diverticulitis: two diseases or one? *Histopathology* 1998;33:349–53.
32 Gledhill A, Dixon MF. Crohn's like reaction in diverticular disease. *Gut* 1998;42:392–5.
33 Shepherd Na. Granulomas in the diagnosis of intestinal Crohn's disease: a myth exploded? *Histopathology* 2002;41:166–8.
34 Shepherd NA. Pathological mimics of chronic inflammatory bowel disease. *J Clin Pathol* 1991;44:726 33.
35 Wakefield AJ, Sankey EA, Dhillon AP, et al. Granulomatous vasculitis in Crohn's disease. *Gastroenterology* 1991;100:1279–87.

36 Edwards CM, George BD, Warren BF. Diversion colitis: new light through old windows. *Histopathology* 1999;35:86–7.
37 Mahadeva U, Martin JP, Patel NK, Price AB. Granulomatous ulcerative colitis: a re-appraisal of the mucosal granuloma in the distinction of Crohn's disease from ulcerative colitis. *Histopathology* 2002;41:50–5.
38 Warren BF, Shepherd NA, Bartolo DCC, Bradfield JWB. Pathology of the defunctioned rectum in ulcerative colitis. *Gut* 1993;34:514–16.
39 Sheehan AL, Warren BF, Gear MWL, Shepherd NA. Fat wrapping in Crohn's disease: pathological basis and relevance to clinical practice. *Br J Surg* 1992;79:955–8.
40 Graham DM, Appelman HD. Crohn's-like lymphoid reaction and colorectal carcinoma: a potential histologic prognosticator. *Mod Pathol* 1990;3:332–5.
41 Lusk LB, Reichen J, Levine JS. Aphthous ulceration in diversion colitis: clinical implications. *Gastroenterology* 1984;87:1171–3.
42 Borley NR, Mortensen NJMcC, Jewell DP, Warren BF. The relationship between inflammation and serosal connective tissue changes in ileal Crohn's disease: evidence for a possible causal link. *J Pathol* 2000;190:196–202.
43 Shepherd NA, Jass JR. Neuromuscular and vascular hamartoma of the small intestine: is it Crohn's disease? *Gut* 1987;28:1663–8.
44 Wright NA, Pike C, Elia G. Ulceration induces a novel epidermal growth factor-secreting cell lineage in human gastrointestinal mucosa. *Digestion* 1990;46:125–31.
45 Spiliadis CA, Spiliadis CA, Lennard-Jones JE. Ulcerative colitis with relative sparing of the rectum: clinical features, histology, and prognosis. *Dis Colon Rectum* 1987;30:334–6.
46 Hyde G, Warren BF, Jewell DP. Histological changes associated with the use of intravenous cyclosporin in the treatment of severe ulcerative colitis may mimic dysplasia. *Colorectal Dis* 2002;4(6):455–8.
47 Harper PH, Lee EC, Kettlewell MGW, Bennett MK, Jewell DP. Role of faecal stream in the maintenance of Crohn's colitis. *Gut* 1985;26:279–84.
48 Edwards CM, George BD, Jewell DP, Warren BF, Mortensen NJ, Kettlewell MGW. Role of a defunctioning stoma in the management of large bowel Crohn's disease. *Br J Surg* 2000;87:1063–6.
49 Warren BF, Shepherd NA. Diversion proctocolitis: a review. *Histopathology* 1992;21:91–3.
50 Asplund S, Gramlich T, Fazio V, Petras R. Histologic changes in defunctioned rectums in patients with inflammatory bowel disease: a clinicopathological study of 82 patients with long term follow up. *Dis Colon Rectum* 2002;45:1206–13.
51 Levine TS, Tzardi M, Mitchell S, Sowter C, Price AB. Diagnostic difficulty arising from rectal recovery in ulcerative colitis. *J Clin Pathol* 1996;49: 319–23.
52 Geboes K, Riddell RH, Ost A, Jensfelt B, Persson T, Lofberg R. A reproducible grading scale for histological assessment of inflammation in ulcerative colitis. *Gut* 2000;47:404–9.
53 Riley SA, Mani V, Goodman MJ, Dutt S, Herd ME. Microscopic activity in ulcerative colitis: what does it mean? *Gut* 1991;32:174–8.
54 Geboes K. Is histology useful for the assessment of the efficacy of immunosuppressive agents in IBD and if so, how should it be applied? *Acta Gastroenterol Belg* 2004;67:285–9.
55 Dube AK, Cross SS, Lobo A. Audit of the histopathological diagnosis of non-neoplastic colorectal biopsies: achievable standards for the diagnosis of inflammatory bowel disease. *J Clin Pathol* 1998;51:37–81.
56 Cross SS, Feeley KM, Angel CA. The effect of four interventions on the informational content of histopathology reports of resected colorectal carcinomas. *J Clin Pathol* 1998;51:481–2.
57 Lucarotti ME, Freeman BJ, Warren BF, Durdey P. Synchronous proctocolectomy and ileoanal pouch formation and the risk of Crohn's disease. *Br J Surg* 1995;82:755–6.
58 Konishi F, Morson BC. Pathology of colorectal adenomas: a colonoscopic survey. *J Clin Pathol* 1982;35:830–41.
59 Brown LJ, Smeeton NC, Dixon MF. Assessment of dysplasia in colorectal adenomas: an observer variation and morphometric study. *J Clin Pathol* 1985;38:174–9.
60 Fenger C, Bak M, Kronborg O, Svanholm H. Observer reproducibility in grading dysplasia in colorectal adenomas: comparison between two different grading systems. *J Clin Pathol* 1990;43:320–4.
61 Riddell RH, Goldman H, Ransohoff DF, et al. Dysplasia in inflammatory bowel disease: standardised classification with provisional clinical applications. *Hum Pathol* 1983;14:931–68.
62 Mueller E, Vieth M, Stolte M, Mueller J. The differentiation of true adenoma from colitis associated dysplasia in ulcerative colitis: a comparative immunohistochemical study. *Hum Pathol* 1999;30:898–905.
63 Torres C, Antonioli D, Odze RD. Polypoid dysplasia and adenomas in inflammatory bowel disease: a clinical, pathologic, and follow-up study of 89 polyps from 59 patients. *Am J Surg Pathol* 1998;22:275–84.

64. Rutter MD, Saunders BP, Wilkinson KH, Kamm MA, Williams CB, Forbes A. Most dysplasia in ulcerative colitis is visible at colonoscopy. *Gastrointest Endosc* 2004;60:334–9.
65. Odze RD, Farraye FA, Hecht JL, Hornick JL. Long term follow–up after polypectomy treatment for adenoma–like dysplastic lesions in ulcerative colitis. *Clin Gastroenterol Hepatol* 2004;2:534–41.
66. Melville DM, Jass JR, Shepherd NA, *et al*. Dysplasia and deoxyribonucleic acid aneuploidy in the assessment of precancerous changes in chronic ulcerative colitis: observer variation and correlations. *Gastroenterology* 1988;95:668–75.
67. Melville DM, Jass JR, Morson BC, *et al*. Observer study of the grading of dysplasia in ulcerative colitis: comparison with clinical outcome. *Hum Pathol* 1989;20:1008–14.
68. Shepherd NA, Hulten L, Tytgat GN, *et al*. Pouchitis. *Int J Colorectal Dis* 1989;4:205–29.
69. Moskowitz RL, Shepherd NA, Nicholls RJ. An assessment of inflammation in the reservoir after restorative proctocolectomy with ileoanal ileal reservoir. *Int J Colorectal Dis* 1986;1:167–74.
70. Warren BF, Shepherd NA. Iatrogenic pathology of the gastrointestinal tract. In: Kirkham N, Hall PA, eds. *Progress in Pathology*. Edinburgh: Churchill Livingstone; 1995:31–54.
71. Shepherd NA, Jass JR, Duval I, Moskowitz RL, Nicholls RJ, Morson BC. Restorative proctocolectomy with ileal reservoir: pathological and histochemical study of mucosal biopsy specimens. *J Clin Pathol* 1987;40:601–7.
72. Gullberg K, Stahlberg D, Liljeqvist L, *et al*. Neoplastic transformation of the pelvic pouch mucosa in patients with ulcerative colitis. *Gastroenterology* 1997;112:1487–92.
73. Heuschen UA, Allemeyer EH, Hinz U, *et al*. Diagnosing pouchitis: comparative validation of two scoring systems in routine follow up. *Dis Colon Rectum* 2002;45:776–86.
74. Stern H, Walfisch S, Mullen B, McLeod R, Cohen Z. Cancer in an ileoanal reservoir: a new late complication? *Gut* 1990;31:473–5.
75. Shepherd NA. The pelvic ileal reservoir: apocalypse later? *Br Med J* 1990;301:886–7.
76. Helander KG, Ahren C, Philipson BM, Samuelsson BM, Ojerskog B. Structure of mucosa in continent ileal reservoirs 15–19 years after construction. *Hum Pathol* 1990;21:1235–8.
77. Sequens R. Cancer in the anal canal (transitional zone) after restorative proctocolectomy with stapled ileal pouch-anal anastomosis. *Int J Colorectal Dis* 1997;12:254–5.
78. Borjesson L, Willen R, Haboubi N, Duff SE, Hulten L. The risk of dysplasia and cancer in the ileal pouch mucosa after restorative proctocolectomy for ulcerative proctocolitis is low: a long term follow-up study. *Colorect Dis* 2004;6:494–8.
79. Hulten L, Willen R, Nilsson O, Safarani N, Haboubi N. Mucosal assessment for dysplasia and cancer in the ileal pouch mucosa in patients operated on for ulcerative colitis – a 30-year follow up study. *Dis Colon Rectum* 2002;45:448–52.
80. Shepherd NA, Healey CJ, Warren BF, Richman PI, Thomson WHF, Wilkinson SP. Distribution of mucosal pathology and an assessment of colonic phenotypic change in the pelvic ileal reservoir. *Gut* 1993;34:101–5.
81. Setti-Carraro P, Talbot IC, Nicholls RJ. Long term appraisal of the histological appearances of the ileal mucosa after restorative proctocolectomy for ulcerative colitis. *Gut* 1994;35:1721–7.
82. Braveman JM, Schoetz DJ Jr, Marcello PW, *et al*. The fate of the ileal pouch in patients developing Crohn's disease. *Dis Colon Rectum* 2004;47:1613–1614.
83. Xin W, Greenson JK. The clinical significance of focally enhanced gastritis. *Am J Surg Pathol* 2004;28:1347–51.
84. Oberhuber G, Hirsch M, Stolte M. High incidence of upper gastrointestinal tract involvement in Crohn's disease. *Virchows Arch* 1998;432(1):49–52.
85. Abdullah BA, Gupta SK, Croffie JM, *et al*. The role of esophagogastroduodenoscopy in the initial evaluation of childhood inflammatory bowel disease: a seven-year study. *J Pediatr Gastroenterol Nutr* 2002;35:636–40.

7: The challenges of using capsule endoscopy in the diagnosis and management of inflammatory bowel disease

Gary C. Chen and Simon K. Lo

Introduction

Inflammatory bowel disease (IBD) is a chronic inflammatory disorder consisting of two main entities: Crohn's disease and ulcerative colitis. Establishing the correct diagnosis in patients with IBD is extremely important because the natural history and outcomes, medical management and surgical management of these two entities are quite different. Despite the advances in modern medical technology, diagnosing IBD in patients with chronic abdominal symptoms and properly differentiating Crohn's from ulcerative colitis can sometimes still present a challenge to gastroenterologists. Approximately 70% of patients with Crohn's disease have involvement of the small intestine, and in 30% the disease is limited to the small intestine [1, 2].The diagnosis of Crohn's disease is usually established with contrast imaging techniques or direct visualisation on endoscopy or at surgery. Laboratory data are only used as adjunctive evidence. Histopathological findings are preferred but not required [3]. Because the disease pattern and behaviour are the only reliable clues for Crohn's disease, identification of active intestinal mucosal disease is the key to the diagnosis.

Traditional modalities in diagnosing small intestinal Crohn's disease

Small bowel radiography

Because the small intestine mucosa is traditionally difficult to visualise, contrast small bowel radiography has been the main diagnostic imaging modality used to evaluate small intestinal Crohn's disease [4]. A single contrast small bowel series is the most commonly ordered luminal radiographic study, although enteroclysis is considered the diagnostic examination of choice because of the ability to distend the intestinal lumen for a detailed double contrast examination [5, 6]. However, because there is not a single pathognomonic radiographic feature that defines Crohn's disease, the radiological diagnosis is based on subjective radiologist interpretations that take into consideration a wide range of possible findings. When the disease is mild and confined to the mucosa, it is possible for small bowel radiography to miss such lesions. This diagnostic modality also exposes patients to significant radiation.

Traditional endoscopy

Most of the small intestine is beyond the reach of standard endoscopes. Oesophagogastrodudenoscopic examination may identify Crohn's lesions if there is disease involvement in the upper gastrointestinal tract of the patient. Although retrograde ileoscopy is perhaps the most useful and definitive way of diagnosing small intestinal Crohn's disease via colonoscopy, some small intestinal Crohn's disease lesions may not involve the terminal ileum or are not possible to examine because of technical difficulty in passing an endoscope through the ileocaecal valve, especially if there is significant degree of inflammation due to Crohn's disease around the ileocaecal valve.

Enteroscopy

Push enteroscopy was designed with the hope that the longer endoscope would enter deeper inside the small intestine. However, in practice, it can rarely be passed 100 cm beyond the ligament of Treitz [7]. Sonde enteroscopy reaches the ileum in approximately 75% of the time, but this procedure typically takes 8 h or longer to complete and is associated with significant patient discomfort [7]. For these reasons, it is seldom performed and only available at a few centres worldwide [8]. Another diagnostic form of enteroscopy is intra-operative push enteroscopy, which is usually reserved for severe cases. Using this approach the endoscope can usually examine the entire small intestine. However, the downsides of this procedure include the drawbacks associated with exploratory surgery, general anaesthesia, prolonged post-operative ileus and costs of hospitalisation. The recently introduced double-balloon enteroscopy (Fujinon Corporation, Saitama, Japan), which can be inserted from either an oral or anal approach, has the capability to perform biopsy and certain therapeutic measures. One series reported that double-balloon enteroscopy achieved total small bowel examination by combining both the oral and anal approaches in 84% of the patients [9]. However, it is also a labour-intensive procedure that may take more than 2 h to perform in each direction. Preliminary results from a multi-centre study on 41 patients who underwent 47 double-balloon enteroscopy procedures showed that the average procedure time was 115 min and the mean distance reached by double-balloon enteroscopy was 389 (40–665) cm (distal jejunum) [10]. In addition, potentially serious complications that are seen with intra-operative push enteroscopy, such as serosal tears, haematoma, perforation, avulsion of mesenteric vasculature and prolonged ileus can probably be encountered in this procedure. Although the prospect of total enteroscopy with the possibility of performing biopsy and therapy is intriguing, it is not certain that double-balloon enteroscopy will become a routine test used for examination of small intestinal Crohn's disease.

Inadequacy of the traditional diagnostic modalities

As stated above, each of these diagnostic modalities has its limitations. In reality, a majority of the bowel is often not thoroughly examined in the work-up of these patients. Delay in therapy, repetitive studies or improper treatment may occur as a result. There are multiple case scenarios in which a more sensitive diagnostic modality is desired. For example, patients who have ulcerative colitis but still experience significant symptoms, such as unexplained haematochezia or melaena, abdominal pain and/or nutritional deficiency, should be screened for small intestinal Crohn's disease. Even in patients with established Crohn's disease, confirming the presence or absence of suspected active disease activity in the small intestine can be critical in determining the best treatment options. Furthermore, patients with chronic abdominal symptoms suggestive of Crohn's disease, but without definite proof of the disease, deserve to be investigated further. From a financial standpoint, the inadequate small bowel examination may lead to excessive utilisation of health care resources, decrease in work productivity and increase in disability. A better diagnostic modality for small intestinal Crohn's disease is clearly needed.

Capsule endoscopy

Recent advances in medical technology have led to the development of capsule endoscopy (Figs 7.1–7.2), which was first described by Iddan and Sturlesi's team from Israel in 1997 [11]. Paul Swain underwent the first capsule endoscopy in August 1999 and stated that the capsule 'was easily swallowed and caused no discomfort' [12]. Capsule endoscopy is a diagnostic procedure developed for the complete examination of the small intestine through video images transmitted from an ingestible video camera. Originally named the M2A capsule, the PillCam™ Capsule Endoscopy and Diagnostic Imaging System (Given Imaging, Inc., Yoqneam, Israel) is a commercially available system consisting of three major components: (1) a PillCam™ capsule (measures 11 mm in diameter and 26 mm in

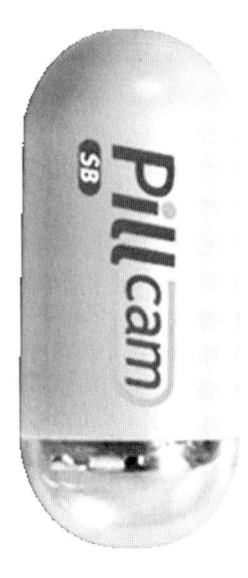

Fig 7.1 The PillCam™ capsule endoscope.

length and weighs 3.7 g) that contains a miniature complementary metal oxide silicon (CMOS) chip video camera, six light-emitting (LED) illumination sources, two silver oxide batteries, an UHF band

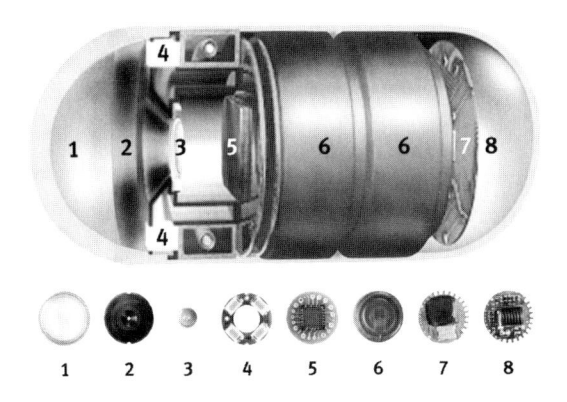

INSIDE THE *PillCam*

1. Optical dome
2. Lens holder
3. Lens
4. Illuminating LEDs (light emitting diode)
5. CMOS (complementary metal oxide semiconductor) imager
6. Battery
7. ASIC (application specific integrated circuit) transmitter
8. Antenna

Fig 7.2 Inside the PillCam™ capsule endoscope.

radio-frequency transmitter and an antenna; (2) sensor array and data recorder that are attached to the patient's body to receive and record data transmitted from the PillCam™ capsule; (3) a RAPID™ workstation that is used to initialise the data recorder and to download and process the raw data from the data recorder [13, 14]. The PillCam™ capsule captures images and transmits digital pictures at the rate of 2 frames/s. The processed information, composed of approximately 50,000 still images collected over an 8-hour period, can be reviewed as a continuous video stream at various speeds using the proprietary Rapid Reader software (Given Imaging, Inc., Yoqneam, Israel). Another form of capsule endoscopy has recently been developed and tested using animal models (Olympus Medical Systems Co., Tokyo, Japan) [15].

A number of studies have now demonstrated the superior sensitivity and specificity of capsule endoscopy over traditional diagnostic studies of the small intestine for the evaluation of gastrointestinal bleeding [16–20]. The major advantages of capsule endoscopy over traditional imaging and endoscopic modalities include: (1) the ability to visualise the entire small bowel; (2) the ability to detect small, flat mucosal lesions; (3) it is a non-invasive procedure; and (4) it is an ambulatory procedure that does not require sedation or hospitalisation and is well accepted by patients. In other words, capsule endoscopy is capable of providing detailed and extensive endoscopic images of the entire small bowel and carries great promise in taking on many of the imaging roles occupied by the existing but inadequate diagnostic modalities. For these reasons, capsule endoscopy has recently been used as a new diagnostic modality for Crohn's disease, after having been primarily used in the evaluation of gastrointestinal bleeding.

Case examples of using capsule endoscopy in IBD patients

Case 1

A middle-aged female patient with a history of Crohn's disease was evaluated for severe abdominal pain despite negative oesophagogastrodudenoscopy (OGD), colonoscopy and small bowel follow through (SBFT). It was previously thought that she had chronic pain syndrome with possible secondary gain. However, her capsule endoscopy study showed extensive Crohn's ulcerations throughout the small intestine. Afterwards, she was treated accordingly for Crohn's disease.

Case 2

The first case of a retained capsule, in our experience, occurred incidentally in a female patient with a long-standing history of right lower quadrant abdominal pain, recurrent nausea and vomiting, as well as abdominal bloating. Multiple endoscopic, CT and small bowel radiography studies were unremarkable. The patient suspected that she had obstructive disease that could not be proven using conventional means. When warned of potential capsule retention in the setting of an obstructive anatomical lesion, she informed the gastroenterology staff that she would be delighted because she would readily accept surgical intervention if required. Indeed, the capsule held up in the distal ileum, but the aetiology could not be identified on capsule images because of a large amount of food debris in the same region. The patient then underwent an ileal resection and the tissue specimen confirmed stenosing Crohn's ileitis. She remained asymptomatic for more than 1 year after her surgery. This case exemplifies the possibility of intestinal obstruction despite multiple negative endoscopic and intestinal imaging studies. Her long-standing symptoms might have eventually led her to surgical resection even if Crohn's disease had been diagnosed and capsule endoscopy examination never been performed. Nonetheless, our current rule of practice is to investigate for possible obstructive symptoms before proceeding with any capsule endoscopy examination. All patients with symptoms suggestive of obstruction are required to have a prior barium small bowel follow through study with presumed non-obstructive results before they can proceed to capsule endoscopy examination.

Current clinical experience in adult patients

Following Fireman *et al.* 's [21] paper published on the utility of capsule endoscopy for Crohn's disease in 2003, a few other studies have also been published in full manuscripts [21–28] and abstracts [29, 30–35] (Table 7.1). In addition, several other studies have included patients with Crohn's disease or with suspected Crohn's disease among larger studies primarily aimed for the evaluation of patients with obscure gastrointestinal bleeding [19, 37–39]. Virtually all the studies designed to detect Crohn's disease have reported on less than 60 patients, but almost all showed evidence that capsule endoscopy could be useful in the diagnosis and management of small intestinal Crohn's disease.

In a prospective study from Israel, Fireman *et al.* performed capsule endoscopy on 17 highly selected patients suspected of having Crohn's disease with symptoms including abdominal pain, diarrhoea, iron deficiency anaemia and/or weight loss [21]. These patients all had negative results on OGD, colonoscopy and barium small bowel radiography. A large proportion of patients (71%) were found to have intestinal lesions compatible with Crohn's disease by capsule endoscopy, with the majority of the lesions found in the distal small bowel. However, only 6 of the 12 patients had their ileum intubated with retrograde ileoscopy and had confirmatory biopsy. These 12 patients were treated with aminosalicylates and corticosteroid therapy and 10 patients had clinical improvement of their symptoms. This small study provided the first insight into the inadequacy of traditional diagnostic modalities in diagnosing Crohn's disease and stimulated more investigations into the usefulness of capsule endoscopy for this condition.

Herrerias *et al.* [22] prospectively studied the utility of capsule endoscopy in 21 patients in Spain with suspected Crohn's disease, after negative workups with OGD, colonoscopy and barium small bowel radiography. Capsule endoscopy was able to identify 9 patients with findings consistent with Crohn's disease. The lesions detected included aphthous lesions, linear or irregular ulcers and fissures.

Table 7.1 Comparison of diagnostic yield for Crohn's disease from selected studies of capsule endoscopy.

Study	n	Comparator	Patients	CE	Small bowel radiography	EGD	Ileoscopy	Push enteroscopy	CT enteroclysis
Fireman [21] (Paper)	17	Small bowel radiography, EGD, ileoscopy	Suspected CD	70.6%	0%	0%	50% (6/12 exams)	ND	ND
Herrerias [22] (Paper)	21	SBFT, EGD, ileoscopy	Suspected CD	43%	0%	0%	35% (6/17 exams)	ND	ND
Ge [23] (Paper)	20	SBFT, EGD, ileoscopy	Suspected CD	65%	0%	0%	NR	ND	ND
Mow [25] (Paper)	50	SBFT, ileoscopy	Known and suspected IBD	40%	NR	ND	NR	ND	ND
Eliakim [24] (Paper)	35	SBFT, CT enterography	Suspected CD	77%	23%	ND	NR	ND	20%
Dubcenco [33] (Abstract)	31	SBFT, ileoscopy	Known and suspected CD	77.4%	16.1%	ND	45.1%	ND	ND
Solem [35] (Abstract)	21	SBFT, ileoscopy, CT enterography	Known CD	87% (21/23 exams)	45% (5/11 exams)	ND	13% (2/15 exams)	ND	29% (2/7 exams)
Bloom [34] (Abstract)	16	SBFT, ileoscopy	Known and suspected CD	56%	19%	ND	50%	ND	ND
Toth [29] (Abstract)	47	Small bowel radiography, ileoscopy, push enteroscopy	Known and suspected CD	88%	24%	ND	68%	16%	ND
Buchman [28] (Paper)	30	SBFT	Known CD	70%	66.7%	ND	ND	ND	ND
Voderholzer [27] (Paper)	30	EGD, CT enteroclysis, ileoscopy	Known and suspected CD	48%	ND	NR	NR	ND	13%
Costamagna [19] (Paper)	3	SBFT	Known and suspected CD	67%	33%	ND	ND	ND	ND
Scapa [36] (Paper)	13	SBFT, EGD, colonoscopy	Suspected CD	46%	0%	0%	NR	ND	ND
Liangpunsakul [37] (Paper)	3	Enteroclysis	Abdominal pain, Iron deficiency anaemia	100%	0%	ND	ND	ND	ND
Chong [26] (Paper)	43	Small bowel enteroclysis, push enteroscopy	Known and suspected CD	44%	9%	ND	ND	7%	ND

CD: Crohn's disease; IBD: inflammatory bowel disease; n: number of patients; CE: capsule endoscopy; SBFT: small bowel-follow through; EGD: esophagogastroduodenoscopy; CT: computed-tomography; ND: not done; NR: not reported.

Retrograde ileoscopy was successfully performed in 17 patients, with 6 patients found to have inflammatory changes on biopsy. The 9 patients with findings of Crohn's disease on capsule endoscopy all went into clinical remission after they were subsequently treated with aminosalicylates and corticosteroid. However, no specific details on the treatment courses of these patients were discussed.

Ge et al. [23] prospectively examined 20 patients with suspected Crohn's disease in China with capsule endoscopy. All the patients had normal barium small bowel radiography, OGD, colonoscopy (16 patients) and abdominal CT (14 patients) prior to undergoing capsule endoscopic examinations. Thirteen patients had findings on capsule endoscopy consistent with small intestinal Crohn's disease. The distribution of the lesions was mainly in the distal part of the small bowel. The findings detected by capsule endoscopy included mucosal erosions, aphthous ulcers, nodularity, large ulcers and ulcerated stenosis. Of these 13 patients, 11 showed 'good clinical' improvement after treatment with aminosalicylates and short-term corticosteroid, while the other two patients showed 'some improvement' in their clinical symptoms only. Once again, the researchers did not elaborate on the description of the treatment courses. More importantly, because only 5 patients had their terminal ileums intubated with ileoscopy and not all of the patients had colonoscopy examination, one must be concerned that the findings on capsule endoscopy were actually backwash ileitis or intestinal tuberculosis rather than Crohn's disease, because ulcerative colitis and tuberculous ileitis are more common than Crohn's disease in China [40–42].

Eliakim et al. [24] compared the diagnostic yields of capsule endoscopy, SBFT and multi-planar spiral entero-computed tomography (CT) in 35 patients suspected of having Crohn's disease. The symptoms of these Israeli patients were chronic diarrhoea, abdominal pain and/or weight loss. Capsule endoscopy detected 77% of the patients with Crohn's disease, which was superior to SBFT (23%) and CT enterography (20%). Furthermore, capsule endoscopy was able to detect all the lesions identified by the other two diagnostic modalities. The findings identified by capsule endoscopy included aphthous ulcers, erosions, ulcerations, erythema, nodular lymphoid hyperplasia and blunted or absent mucosal villi. However, the diagnosis of Crohn's disease may have been inflated by the use of non-specific findings such as erythema and absent mucosal villi as diagnostic criteria, especially because they did not perform confirmatory biopsy.

Mow et al. [25] performed capsule endoscopy in another highly selected group of 50 patients with ongoing IBD symptoms. There were 22 patients with only known colitis, 20 patients with Crohn's disease and uncertain extent of small bowel disease and 8 patients with suspected IBD. Patients with significant obstructive signs or symptoms were excluded from the study. Forty of the 50 patients had undergone barium SBFT within 1 year of the capsule endoscopy examination and 68% of the SBFT were reported as normal. Ileoscopy was performed in 43 patients, with 41 patients having undergone ileoscopy within 1 year of their capsule endoscopy examinations. Overall, ileoscopy was unremarkable in 18 patients, although the rest of the patients had at least some degree of abnormality. In terms of capsule endoscopy examinations, 20 (40%) were felt to be diagnostic of Crohn's disease while 10 patients (20%) were felt to be suspicious for small intestinal Crohn's disease. Capsule endoscopy findings were diagnostic of Crohn's disease in 3 of 8 patients who had suspicious symptoms, but without having a prior established diagnosis of IBD. Eighty per cent of the patients with diagnostic or suspicious findings on the capsule improved clinically with intensified medical treatment for IBD. Twelve patients with a previous history of ulcerative colitis or indeterminate colitis were found to have lesions in the small bowel and resulted in a change in diagnosis to Crohn's disease. Subsequent ileoscopy with biopsies definitely confirmed the diagnosis of small intestinal Crohn's disease in 5 of these patients. In this clinical setting, the findings on capsule endoscopy led to more aggressive medical treatment rather than performing colectomy [25].

Chong et al. prospectively compared the diagnostic yields of capsule endoscopy, small bowel enteroclysis and push enteroscopy in 22 patients with known and 21 patients with suspected small intestinal Crohn's disease [26]. Capsule endoscopy had findings consistent with small intestinal Crohn's disease in 17/22 patients with known Crohn's disease and in 2/21 patients with suspected Crohn's disease. However, small bowel enteroclysis had findings compatible with Crohn's disease in 4/21 patients with established Crohn's disease and none of the patients with suspected Crohn's disease. Lastly, push enteroscopy only demonstrated findings consistent with small intestinal Crohn's disease in 3 of the patients with known Crohn's disease and none of the patients with suspected Crohn's disease. The authors also surveyed their referring physicians and found that the management of the patients in their study was modified in 70% of the patients [26].

A Swedish group compared the diagnostic yields of capsule endoscopy, barium small bowel radiography (89% enteroclysis, 11% SBFT), push enteroscopy and ileocolonoscopy in 47 patients with suspected or active Crohn's disease in a prospective, controlled study published in abstract form [29]. All 47 patients completed all 4 diagnostic examinations within 3 months, except for ileocolonoscopy, in which only 44 patients had successful intubation of the ileum. Lesions compatible with small intestinal Crohn's disease were identified by one or more methods in 25 patients. Capsule endoscopy had the highest diagnostic yield (88%), although the other modalities were less sensitive: ileocolonoscopy (68%), barium small bowel radiography (24%) and push enteroscopy (16%) [29].

Voderholzer et al. prospectively compared the diagnostic yield of capsule endoscopy with CT enteroclysis in 56 patients with Crohn's disease [27]. The 56 patients first underwent CT enteroclysis and 15 were excluded for capsule endoscopy procedure after strictures were detected on CT enteroclysis. Of the remaining 41 patients, 25 were found to have jejunal or ileal lesions by capsule endoscopy compared with 12 by CT enteroclysis ($p = 0.004$). Although these two diagnostic modalities did not differ significantly in the detection of lesions in the terminal ileum (capsule endoscopy detected 24/41, while CT enteroclysis detected 20/41), the capsule was able to detect more lesions proximally. Findings on capsule endoscopy led to changes in treatment in 10 patients, all of whom responded clinically [27]. Likewise, a study comparing the diagnostic yield of capsule endoscopy with MR enteroclysis in 10 patients with Crohn's disease who have terminal ileum involvement also showed capsule endoscopy to be the superior test [30]. However, these abstracts do not mention if confirmatory biopsy was performed. Caution should be used before labelling patients with Crohn's disease on the basis of minor findings such as villous denudation and fibrinous lesions without biopsy or other confirmatory studies.

Legnani et al. [31] published, in abstract form, a longer period of patient follow-up. In 32 patients with either 'abnormal' (detailed definition not provided in the abstract) small bowel radiography or abdominal pain, 30 had negative capsule endoscopy examinations. After a mean follow-up of 19 months, none of these 30 patients developed any evidence of Crohn's disease (criteria not provided in the abstract), yielding a 100% negative predictive value for capsule endoscopy. In another group of 33 patients with either known IBD with normal small bowel radiography findings or patients with known Crohn's disease with persistent obscure bleeding, 18 had positive capsule endoscopy examinations. Overall, treatment decisions based on diagnostic findings from capsule endoscopy examination in 20/21 patients led to clinical improvement [31]. However, this abstract did not provide details of the treatment course, nor was confirmatory biopsy performed on the patients.

A published abstract by these authors reviewed retrospectively 97 capsule endoscopy procedures that were performed on 88 symptomatic patients with documented Crohn's disease over a 2-year period [31]. Forty-eight of 96 (50%) patients had findings diagnostic of active Crohn's disease and 10 (10%) patients had findings suggestive of active Crohn's disease on capsule endoscopy, while 33 (34%) patients had normal findings on the capsule. Twenty-two patients had colonoscopy data within 90 days (mean = 30 days) of their capsule endoscopy examinations for comparison. Although 55% patients had disease findings on capsule endoscopy, only one patient (5%) had a single aphthous ulcer on colonoscopy. Furthermore, SBFT was performed within 90 days of the capsule endoscopy examination (mean = 30 days) in 32 cases, capsule endoscopy was found to be superior to

SBFT in detecting active Crohn's lesions (Fisher's Exact Test $p = 0.05$). This published abstract, based on selected patients, suggested that SBFT and colonoscopy added little value in assessing active disease in symptomatic Crohn's patients. In clinical practice, we feel that capsule endoscopy may be the preferred modality in evaluating established small intestinal Crohn's disease patients who present with active symptoms after the likelihood of stricture is ruled out. Large-scale, well-controlled prospective studies are needed to address this issue definitively.

In spite of the rapidly increasing number of studies on the utility of capsule endoscopy for diagnosing Crohn's disease and the apparent high diagnostic yield of active disease in many of these studies, care must be taken to not assume similar findings in a less selected population. The mere discovery of mucosal ulcers or erosions does not clinch the diagnosis and responses to Crohn's disease treatment have not been reported in sufficient detail. Several questions have also been raised about these studies: (1) the criteria for clinical suspicion of Crohn's disease were not well-described or uniform; (2) diagnostic criteria and terminology for capsule endoscopy findings have not been fully established; (3) patient selection and exclusion were different in these studies; (4) long term follow-up was generally lacking in these studies; and (5) each study lacked detailed description of treatment course. Large-scale, well-controlled prospective studies are needed to confirm these preliminary data.

Comparison of capsule endoscopy with traditional diagnostic modalities

The preliminary results from these studies suggest that capsule endoscopy has the potential to achieve higher diagnostic yield than traditional modalities for the detection of small intestinal Crohn's disease. A meta-analysis of capsule endoscopy compared to other modalities in patients with suspected or known non-stricturing small intestinal Crohn's disease was published in abstract form [43]. This meta-analysis included 10 studies comparing the diagnostic yields of capsule endoscopy and small bowel radiography, which were 62 and 27% ($n = 226$), respectively. The authors also analysed 4 studies that compared diagnostic yields of capsule endoscopy and ileoscopy, which were 57 and 43% ($n = 117$), respectively. They also examined 3 studies that compared the diagnostic yields of capsule endoscopy and CT enterography, which were 73 and 41% ($n = 70$), respectively. Finally, they evaluated 2 studies that compared the diagnostic yields of capsule endoscopy and push enteroscopy, which were 47 and 7% ($n = 75$), respectively [43]. The low sensitivity and general lack of additional information to findings of capsule endoscopy from the preliminary studies have raised substantial scepticism in regards to the value of the small bowel radiography. However, in the published paper by Buchman et al. [28], 30 patients suspected of recurrent Crohn's disease were evaluated with both SBFT and capsule endoscopy within a single week, and the results were quite different from those of all other published studies. Capsule endoscopy found 21/30 patients with active Crohn's disease, while SBFT found 20/30 patients, and complete agreement between these two modalities occurred in 13 patients [32]. In addition, despite the results of these studies, standard practice still routinely uses small bowel radiography as a screening measure for obvious small bowel lesions and to exclude obstructions in patients who have symptoms and signs of possible obstructions. Capsule endoscopy is still reserved for symptomatic patients without obvious obstruction. The shortcoming of both CT enterography and MR enterography appears to be the fact that both of these studies may be normal when Crohn's disease is mild and inflammatory changes are confined to the mucosa. Therefore, these two new diagnostic tools might not add much to the existing small bowel radiography, although more sophisticated technology may yield improved results. Instead, the most appropriate role for these two modalities is the detection of extra-luminal complications of Crohn's disease. CT enterography is quite useful in identifying abscesses, fistulas, bowel wall thickening and extra-intestinal inflammation [5]. In addition, this technique has the advantage of allowing the simultaneous study of the mucosa and bowel wall, which makes it an ideal replacement of barium small bowel studies. Likewise, MR enteroclysis is capable of detecting Crohn's disease lesions, such as thickening and distortion of the small intestinal folds, but the resolution is insufficient for the depiction of more subtle lesions such as aphthous ulcers [44]. Large-scale, well-controlled prospective studies are needed to confirm these preliminary results.

Push enteroscopy has not been in widespread use for the diagnosis of Crohn's disease because Crohn's disease tends to have distal ileum and/or colonic involvement. Results from studies mentioned above have echoed this perception [26, 29]. The yield of positive biopsy results from the upper gastrointestinal tract in symptomatic Crohn's disease patients is also not satisfactory. Hence, push enteroscopy is unlikely to be useful in the diagnosis of Crohn's disease.

Based on the number of studies thus far, it appears that capsule endoscopy is valuable in examining the terminal ileum, although it offers only a slight advantage over retrograde ileoscopy via colonoscopy. Capsule endoscopy seems more helpful for patients in whom it is not technically feasible to perform a retrograde ileoscopy, and when it is clinically necessary to examine the other regions of the small intestine. However, most of these data were presented only in abstract form and specific details on the study designs and descriptive findings of these studies are lacking. Whether the capsule endoscopy findings from these studies truly represent small intestinal Crohn's disease, or lesions due to other aetiologies, is unclear. Therefore, larger-scale, well-controlled prospective studies are required to confirm these preliminary conclusions. Until then, capsule endoscopy should be performed after ileocolonoscopy in the diagnostic work-up for patients with suspected Crohn's disease.

Distribution of Crohn's disease lesions on capsule endoscopy

Traditionally, intestinal Crohn's lesions are believed to localise in the distal ileum. With the development of capsule endoscopy, we are now able to directly visualise the small bowel mucosa to gain insight as to the localistion and distribution of Crohn's disease. Tabizbadeh *et al.* [45] have reported on the distribution of small bowel erosions or ulcerations in patients presenting for capsule endoscopy. The authors have evaluated the distribution of small bowel lesions in 97 capsule endoscopy procedures that were performed on 88 symptomatic patients with documented Crohn's. Forty-four of 96 (46%) procedures showed lesions in more than one region of the small bowel. The distribution of the lesions in the small bowel were: 23% of the lesions were found in the duodenum, 34% of the lesions were found in the jejunum, 42% of the lesions were found in the proximal ileum, and 61% of the lesions were found in the terminal ileum. Only 5 cases showed lesions in the duodenum, jejunum, or proximal ileum without lesions in the distal ileum (Fisher's Exact Test $p < 0.0001$). Although this result confirmed the theory that most of the Crohn's disease lesions are located in the distal ileum, the surprisingly high number of lesions detected in the more proximal regions suggested that perhaps Crohn's disease is more evenly distributed than once thought.

Appearance of Crohn's disease lesions on capsule endoscopy

Using capsule endoscopy to diagnose small intestinal Crohn's disease can be a challenging task simply for the reason that the small bowel mucosal lining has never been visualised in detail before. The natural assumption is that the typical ulcers, erosions and inflammation seen in the terminal ileum and duodenum by conventional endoscopy would appear the same in the other locations of the small bowel on capsule endoscopy. Capsule endoscopy has the ability to identify Crohn's lesions between the two ends of the small intestine. Indeed, the appearance of lesions on capsule endoscopy closely resembles those captured with traditional endoscopy (Fig 7.3).

However, as described in the studies above, numerous terms describing lesions identified by capsule endoscopy have appeared from various studies. A standardised terminology system for capsule endoscopy findings is warranted in order to compare findings, define diagnoses and determine the severity of the disease. This is of particular importance in describing these findings because there is limited ability in gauging the depth of many mucosal lesions [46]. Gastroenterologists from a tertiary medical centre in New York have designed a Crohn's disease

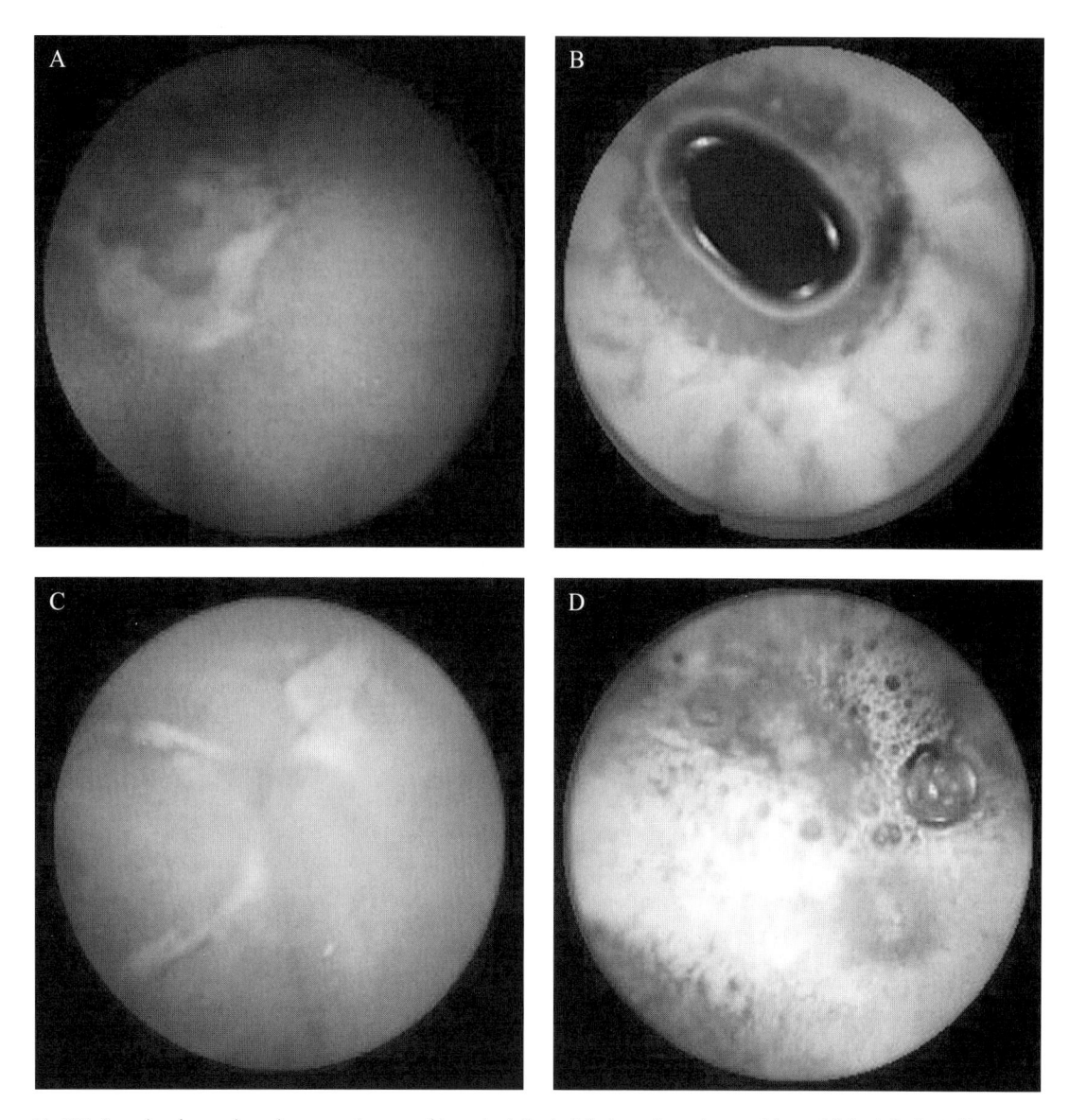

Fig 7.3 Sample of capsule endoscopy pictures of intestinal Crohn's lesions, in patients with established Crohn's disease, captured with the PillCam™ capsule endoscope. (a) Small bowel ulcer with surrounding edema, which is commonly seen but not exclusively in Crohn's disease. (b) Jejunal Crohn's stricture, which was subsequently confirmed in surgical resected specimen. (c) Linear, serpiginous ulcer commonly seen in Crohn's disease. (d) Aphthous lesion.

capsule endoscopic scoring index scale called the 'Lewis scoring system' for the description of small intestinal lesions detected on capsule endoscopy [47]. Whether this scoring index will be applicable and useful is still to be determined. In addition, future studies should address whether lesions in the ileum detected by capsule endoscopy can be scored with Crohn's disease endoscopic index of severity (CDEIS), which measures disease activity on the basis of colonoscopy findings [48].

A major concern with the findings on capsule endoscopy is that patients with advanced Crohn's disease may have typical endoscopic lesions, but many of the less severe lesions can be difficult to differentiate from lesions caused by non-steroidal anti-inflammatory drugs (NSAIDS) [49]. Furthermore, published abstracts suggested that small lesions in the intestine could even occur in asymptomatic control subjects not taking NSAIDS [50, 51]. A few scattered erosions, erythema or mucosal breaks are insufficient to establish the diagnosis of Crohn's disease, although large ulcers located in the small bowel are perhaps more specific for Crohn's disease [46]. Voderholzer *et al.* suggested that the finding of more than 10 apthous ulcers on capsule endoscopy raises high index of suspicion for Crohn's disease [27]. However, Mehdizadeh *et al.* classified symptomatic patients with more than three small bowel ulcers on capsule endoscopy examination as having active Crohn's disease [32]. Therefore, extreme caution is warranted before diagnosing patients with CD, which is a life-long disease, simply based on a few small and scattered small bowel lesions detected on capsule endoscopy. It is the opinion of these authors that practicing physicians should correlate capsule endoscopy findings with clinical findings. Nonetheless, the possibility of 'silent' Crohn's disease must always be kept in mind even in asymptomatic patients.

Use of capsule endoscopy in the pediatric patients with Crohn's disease

Few studies have so far evaluated the utility of capsule endoscopy in paediatric patients with Crohn's disease [52, 53]. Arguelles-Arias *et al.* [52] found capsule endoscopy to be well tolerated and safe in 12 paediatric patients (age 12–16) suspected of having Crohn's disease. Seven of the 12 patients were found to have lesions suggestive of small intestinal Crohn's disease on capsule endoscopy after negative findings with OGD, colonoscopy (5 patients had ileoscopy) and SBFT. The children with findings consistent with Crohn's disease were treated with corticosteroid and oral aminosalicylates, and all went into either clinical remission or analytical remission (term not explained) with at least 3 months of follow-up [52]. The limited data suggest that capsule endoscopy may be safe and well tolerated in paediatric patients and may be effective in diagnosing Crohn's disease. Nonetheless, larger-scale, prospective studies are needed to confirm capsule endoscopy as a routine diagnostic modality in detecting Crohn's disease in the paediatric population. It would be a welcome improvement if capsule endoscopy could replace small bowel radiography and reduce radiation exposure in children. Moreover, permanent trapping of a capsule proximal to a Crohn's lesion may be a more common event in children who have a naturally smaller intestinal calibre than in adults. Furthermore, future studies must determine the smallest size or youngest age of patients who can undergo capsule endoscopy examination, as well as standardised approaches to insert the capsule in paediatric patients who cannot or refuse to swallow the capsule. Nevertheless, capsule endoscopy in carefully chosen young patients may lead to early treatment and restore proper growth and development.

Experience of capsule endoscopy in patients with ulcerative colitis

Studies on the utility of capsule endoscopy in the IBD world have been mostly limited to the diagnosis of Crohn's disease. Its role in patients with established ulcerative colitis is unknown. The authors have retrospectively examined the case records at our centre and identified all patients with moderate to severe ulcerative colitis who underwent capsule endoscopy over a 3-year period. A single experienced endoscopist reviewed all the capsule endoscopy images (Simon K. Lo). The finding of multiple ulcerations (>3) on capsule endoscopy was classified as diagnostic of small intestinal Crohn's disease. Seventy-one patients with known moderate to severe ulcerative colitis underwent 73 capsule endoscopy procedures during the 3-year period. Patients were grouped as follows: Group A, consisting of 61 (86%) patients with moderate to severe ulcerative colitis with either symptoms out of proportion to colitis such as severe abdominal pain, or non-bloody diarrhoea or steroid refractory disease and, Group B, consisting of 10 (14%) patients with previous colectomy who continued to have, or developed new onset of, symptoms including diarrhoea and/or abdominal pain and pouchitis refractory to antibiotic therapy. Eleven of 61 (18%) patients in Group A had findings consistent with Crohn's disease and 3 of 10 (30%) patients with previous colectomy (Group B) had findings consistent with Crohn's disease on capsule endoscopy. Among the 14 patients with positive findings on capsule endoscopy, 9 had a SBFT within 32 days of the capsule, but none showed evidence of Crohn's disease. Most of these 14 patients have been followed-up after their capsule endoscopy examinations, with clinical information that supported their change in diagnosis to Crohn's disease.

From these results, we conclude that a small but significant number of patients with moderate to severe ulcerative colitis have the potential to be reclassified as Crohn's disease when further evaluated by capsule endoscopy. The sensitivity of SBFT was found to be inferior to capsule endoscopy in these patients. These preliminary findings suggest that capsule endoscopy could be useful in evaluating ulcerative colitis patients who have persistent symptoms. It is logical to assume that if capsule endoscopy is proven to be useful in reclassifying a subset of ulcerative colitis patients to Crohn's disease, it may impact upon the choice of medical or surgical therapy and may alter the course of illness in these patients. A negative capsule endoscopy study may be equally valuable as it may exclude Crohn's disease in ulcerative colitis patients who have persistent or extraordinary symptoms.

Experience of capsule endoscopy in patients with indeterminate colitis

Indeterminate colitis is defined here as established isolated colitis in which available endoscopic, pathologic, laboratory and radiological studies are inconclusive for ulcerative colitis or Crohn's disease. Up to 10% of patients with IBD are considered to have indeterminate colitis [4]. The diagnosis of indeterminate colitis in these patients would be changed to Crohn's disease if lesions were identified in the small intestine [54]. Forty-five patients with indeterminate colitis had capsule endoscopy examination at our institution. Twenty-two (49%) had small intestine lesions suggestive of active Crohn's disease and had therapeutic changes [3]. Whitaker et al. [55] examined 7 indeterminate colitis patients (including 3 patients with history of procto-colectomy) with capsule endoscopy. In 2 patients, lesions consistent with small intestinal Crohn's disease were detected by capsule endoscopy, and 3 other patients had subtle changes including isolated erosions and aphthous ulceration in the distal small bowel. In the 4th International Conference on Capsule Endoscopy, Mascarenhas-Saraiva of Portugal presented 27 patients with indeterminate colitis who had chronic colonic inflammation that had capsule endoscopy examinations [56]. In these 27 patients, 22% of the patients had mucosal alterations in the small bowel compatible with Crohn's disease, while 7.4% of the patients had findings suspicious for Crohn's disease. These preliminary data suggest that capsule endoscopy could be a useful modality in patients with indeterminate colitis. However, clinical significance of subtle small bowel lesions is unknown and long-term follow up of these patients is certainly warranted. Furthermore, whether a negative capsule endoscopy study can fully exclude small intestinal Crohn's disease in patients with indeterminate colitis remains to be investigated in future studies.

Challenges and concerns of using capsule endoscopy in IBD patients

Capsule retention

Although a number of the studies on the utilisation of capsule endoscopy for Crohn's disease have been promising, there are still concerns and questions about performing capsule endoscopy in this setting because intestinal obstruction may occur in 35–54% of patients with Crohn's disease [57]. Many physicians and patients are concerned that the capsule may stick proximal to the stricture and lead to intestinal obstruction. Even if a retained capsule does not induce obstructive symptoms, it must be removed before the capsule's contents, come in contact with the intestinal lining and cause injury. Therefore, it is important to address the question of whether capsule endoscopy is safe to perform on patients with known or suspected small intestinal Crohn's disease.

Out of the initial 26,500 patients undergoing capsule endoscopy for various indications, only 28 failed to pass the capsule because of unsuspected obstructive lesions (0.1%) [58]. Furthermore, in all 28 patients with retained capsules, capsule endoscopy identified the cause of capsule retention and led to proper treatment. Another study showed that the capsule was retained in 7 of 272 patients (3.6%) with 5 patients requiring surgical intervention and 2 patients requiring endoscopic removal of the capsule [59]. Given the higher frequency of strictures in patients with Crohn's disease, it is likely that the true incidence of capsule retention in Crohn's disease is significantly higher than the reported 0.1–3.6% for all indications. One of the main reasons that the capsule retention rate has not been as high as expected in Crohn's disease patients is that most of the studies conducted had excluded patients with symptoms suggestive of obstructive disease. Of the first 97 capsule endoscopy cases that we retrospectively reviewed, which were performed on 88 symptomatic patients with documented Crohn's disease, 3 capsules were retained. Two of the 3 patients required surgical removal while the other one passed the capsule spontaneously after 3 weeks.

Another published abstract retrospectively reviewed 38 patients with known Crohn's disease who had undergone capsule endoscopy and found retention of the capsule proximal to a stricture in 5 of 6 patients with retained capsules [60]. Of the 6 patients with retained capsule, 3 patients had strictures that were not detected by prior SBFT while the other 3 patients were suspected of having strictures prior to capsule endoscopy examination. In 5 patients, the obstructing lesions were resected and led to complete resolution of the patients' underlying symptoms. More importantly, acute small bowel obstruction did not occur in any of these 6 patients. As a result, the authors of the study proposed that a retained capsule might be considered a 'therapeutic complication' that can be of value in the evaluation and management in patients with known or suspected Crohn's disease [60]. Whether or not it is clinically advantageous to have a capsule stuck proximal to a Crohn's stricture or not, it is important for gastroenterologists to clearly explain to the patients about the potential risk involved with capsule endoscopy examination as well as the possible consequences that might require surgical intervention. Most experts feel that for patients that had capsule endoscopy examinations but the capsule video recordings do not show images of the colon and the patients fail to notice the capsule endoscope in the stool, an abdominal X-ray is warranted in 7 days to check for capsule retention [61].

Standard practice favours performing SBFT prior to capsule endoscopy to rule out strictures, but this is surprisingly not a reliable way to exclude short or moderate strictures. As a result, Given Imaging (Yoqneam, Israel) is investigating the possibility of screening patients with a potential silent stricture using a dissolvable test capsule before subjecting them to the real capsule studies. This Patency capsule system consists of two components: (1) an ingestible, dissolvable capsule that is has the exact dimension as the PillCam™ capsule (11 × 27 mm) with a tiny radio frequency ID (RFID) tag, and (2) a hand-held scanner used to detect the RFID tag. The Patency capsule can be identified by either the hand-held scanner or fluoroscopy because it contains a small amount of barium. This capsule is designed to disintegrate into small components and pass naturally after 40–100 h. If the capsule passes whole in a timely fashion, then the regular PillCam™ capsule can theoretically be safely administered to the patient.

A multi-centre trial has been conducted to assess the ability of the Patency capsule to verify functional small bowel patency in 85 patients with suspected or confirmed small bowel strictures (80 patients with strictures confirmed by conventional radiology and 61% with Crohn's disease) [62]. The Patency capsule was excreted intact in 39 of 80 patients with radiographically confirmed strictures and non-intact in 41 patients. The Patency capsule was excreted intact in all 5 patients with suspected strictures. Twenty of the 85 patients experienced abdominal pain that either resolved spontaneously or with treatment (treatment method was not discussed in the abstract). Thirty-three patients who had their gastrointestinal tract patency verified then underwent capsule endoscopy and the capsule passed naturally in all cases [62]. The results of these studies raises some questions about adopting Patency capsules as part of clinical practice because it can still lead to severe abdominal pain requiring treatment in a significant number of patients. It has been suggested that abdominal pain in these circumstances could be due to temporary intestinal occlusion induced by the Patency capsule [63]. Furthermore, some Patency capsules disintegrate prematurely and therefore potentially lead to false negative results. Therefore, the exact role of Patency capsule is still to be determined. Till then, the Patency capsule should be used cautiously in patients who are at risk of having strictures.

Incomplete small bowel examination

Another consideration is that capsule endoscopy cannot achieve complete small bowel examination in many patients. Mergener et al. [59] found that the capsule endoscope failed to complete examination of the small bowel in 59/197 patients. Hyun et al. [64] retrospectively reviewed 197 capsule endoscopy cases and found that the capsule successfully examined the entire small bowel in 65% of the cases. Another abstract retrospectively reviewed 282 capsule endoscopy cases in 266 patients and found 64 cases had incomplete examination of the small bowel [65]. In our experience, in 89 patients with established Crohn's disease presenting with symptoms who underwent 96 capsule endoscopy procedures, the capsule was able to reach the caecum in 64 of 96 (67%) procedures.

Many of these patients who had incomplete examination of the small bowel by capsule endoscopy have risk factors that may cause delayed capsule transit time. A series, reported in abstract form, reviewed 463 capsule endoscopy cases and factors such as prior abdominal surgery, Crohn's disease, diabetes, hypothyroidism and space-occupying intraluminal lesions were analysed [66]. The capsule failed to pass the entire length of the small bowel in 145 cases. Prior abdominal surgery and diabetes had the highest risks for delayed transit time [66]. Failure to completely investigate the small bowel may lead to a false negative examination or under-estimate the extent of the patient's disease because the ileum is extremely important to evaluate in Crohn's disease patients. Manufacturing a capsule with longer battery life or smaller size could alleviate this problem. A smaller size capsule could, theoretically, be safer in pediatric patients as well.

Bowel preparations and prokinetic agents have also been investigated to alleviate this problem. Fireman et al. [67] measured the gastric, small bowel and colon transit times by capsule endoscopy, with and without bowel preparation, in 62 patients with small bowel and colon pathologies. The patients were divided into 3 groups: (1) prepared with polyethylene glycol ($n = 9$); (2) prepared with sodium phosphate ($n = 13$); and (3) with no preparation ($n = 40$). The results showed that, compared to both sodium phosphate and no preparation, oral polyethylene glycol significantly shortened the transit time of the capsule through the stomach and small bowel. Likewise, metoclopramide, erythromycin and tegaserod have been found to enhance capsule transit time [68–70]. A published study prospectively evaluated the small bowel transit in 150 patients undergoing capsule endoscopy, in which metoclopramide was not administered to the first 83 patients, but was given orally to the subsequent 67 patients, and found a much higher likelihood that the capsule reached the colon in the latter group of patients [68]. However, pro-kinetic agents should not be administered intentionally when there is a known stricture in the small intestine.

Image quality

Factors such as food debris, air bubble, faecal matter, mucous secretions, inadequate lighting and bile may compromise the quality of video images. Most gastroenterologists employ the standard practice, which is to start the NPO period about 8–12 h prior to capsule endoscopy examination. The extent to which pre-treatment with oral purging solution optimises the quality of the examination is still being debated. Niv et al. [71] retrospectively evaluated 32 patients who underwent capsule endoscopy examination, with the first 10 patients prepared with overnight fasting only, while the next 22 had oral sodium phosphate. An experienced endoscopist and endoscopy nurse, who were blinded to the method used, graded the quality of the video images and found 5 of 10 patients in the overnight fasting group had poor preparation rating in contrast to only 1 of the 22 patients given oral sodium phosphate ($p = 0.01$). Another study also found that bowel preparation improved the visualisation of the small bowel in patients undergoing capsule endoscopy [72].

Mucosal healing

Endoscopic examination is the most widely used modality for the assessment of the extent and the severity of Crohn's disease in the small bowel and the colon [73]. Hence, after confirming the diagnosis of Crohn's disease, one needs to question whether the lesions detected on capsule endoscopy are correlated with clinical symptoms and if mucosal healing represents remission of the disease. If the answer to the question is yes, then capsule endoscopy may become a critically important tool in the management of Crohn's disease. Although earlier studies have clearly shown that mucosal healing is not correlated with response to oral corticosteroids and that mucosal healing does not accompany improvement of disease activity of Crohn's disease [74–76], newer and more potent therapies for Crohn's disease have since been shown to induce mucosal healing [73]. D'Haens et al. [77] observed complete or partial healing of colonic lesions in 95% of their 20 patients in clinical remission treated by azathioprine. Furthermore, treatment with infliximab has also demonstrated mucosal healing as early as 4 weeks after a single infusion [78]. Debinski assessed mucosal healing by infliximab infusion using the Crohn's disease capsule endoscopic scoring index ('the Lewis scoring system') in 13 patients with clinically active small intestinal Crohn's disease documented by capsule endoscopy [79]. In this study, infliximab infusion was administered in these 13 patients at weeks 0 and 6, and then at weeks 8–10 the patients underwent a second capsule endoscopy examination, which showed complete mucosal healing in 46% of the patients. It is conceivable that capsule endoscopy has the potential to be used in the future to document objectively clinical improvement and remission. Therefore, it is important for future studies to investigate this issue further, as well as whether findings on capsule endoscopy can predict response to a specific treatment regimen.

Inability to perform biopsy

The inability to perform mucosal biopsy in order to obtain histological specimens is one shortcoming of capsule endoscopy. The mere detection of small bowel ulcerations does not mean the patient would have Crohn's disease. Furthermore, established diagnostic criteria for IBD, such as those of Lennard-Jones [80], are based on multi-modality work-up and tend to rely on histological findings not obtainable with capsule endoscopy. Due to the inability to obtain tissue specimens, the recently introduced double-balloon enteroscopy (Fujinon Corporation, Saitama, Japan), might be able to complement the limitations of capsule endoscopy.

A recent multi-centre retrospective study in the United States compared the diagnostic yields of double-balloon enteroscopy with capsule endoscopy [10]. In this study, 13 patients with gastrointestinal bleeding had concordant double-balloon enteroscopy and capsule endoscopy test results; only 2 patients had a negative capsule study but a positive double-balloon enteroscopy procedure. All 9 capsule endoscopy studies for non-gastrointestinal bleeding indications showed non-specific findings, including submucosal nodules, thickened edematous folds and blunted villi. On the contrary, only 3 of these patients had positive findings on double-balloon enteroscopy, including a large ileal carcinoid that was confirmed at biopsy. The mean time for the double-balloon enteroscopy procedure was 115 min, whereas historical data on capsule endoscopy reading time is approximately 60 min. This study concluded that these 2 modalities might have complementary roles in the evaluation of unexplained gastrointestinal blood loss. Both endoscopic techniques are reasonably sensitive ($>50\%$) in identifying the source of unexplained gastrointestinal bleeding. A distinct advantage of double-balloon enteroscopy over capsule endoscopy is the ability to deliver therapy and perform biopsy, whereas capsule endoscopy seems to have a much shorter procedure time and is less invasive. Hence, the issue of correlating findings on capsule endoscopy to histology or conventional endoscopy in IBD patients may soon be clarified.

Inter-observer variability of capsule endoscopy image analysis

The process of capsule endoscopy image interpretation has not been standardised with respect to the (1) selection and training of individual readers; (2) determination of the gold standard to which findings are compared to assess sensitivity and false positive rates; and (3) inadequate assessment on inter-observer variability between readers. Survey from the 2003 International Conference of Capsule Endoscopy (ICCE) found that 82% of gastroenterologists reported that they were the first reader to interpret the capsule endoscopy case recordings, although 18% used a resident, physician assistant and/or nurse to interpret the capsule endoscopy case recordings first [81]. Preliminary studies of inter-observer variability have mostly been limited to comparison between 1 and 4 different readers [82, 83]. Although most studies have shown good concordance rates between physicians and non-physicians/gastroenterology fellows, the concordance rates from these studies were simply correlations between identification of major lesions [82, 83]. Chen *et al.* [84] found a sensitivity of 80% in detecting clinically significant lesions on wireless capsule endoscopy, but a moderate rate of inter-observer disagreement on minor findings in a group of untrained capsule readers ($n = 10$). Therefore, whether physician extenders can serve as the initial screeners to help save physicians' time in interpreting capsule images is still waiting to be seen. Because of the inter-observer variations on the minor findings, standardisations of capsule endoscopy image interpretation and proper reader training must be addressed in future studies. Another published abstract assessed the inter-observer agreement between 2 experienced capsule endoscopists (each has performed over 100 capsule endoscopy cases) by using capsule endoscopy recordings from 27 patients [85]. The 2 capsule endoscopists were found to have a high level of agreement with respect to Crohn's lesions in the duodenum and jejunum, but the agreement decreased significantly in the proximal and terminal ileum [85].

Transmural disease

Although capsule endoscopy has revolutionised the examination of small bowel by transmitting high quality images, it is unable to detect transmural disease, which can be important in patients with Crohn's disease. The inability to assess fistulas and abscesses could place capsule endoscopy at a disadvantage in patients with advanced Crohn's disease. New, modified CT and MRI can help the practicing gastroenterologist to assess transmural disease.

Other concerns associated with capsule endoscopy

There are other minor, but important, concerns that need to be addressed as well. First, the safety of capsule endoscopy in pregnant patients has not yet been established [12, 13]. It is unlikely that there is a direct health impact on pregnancy or the foetus. Rather, the clinical circumstance related to capsule retention could lead to an abdominal surgery, radiological capsule localisation and potential obstructive symptoms. Second, the exact safety profile and possibility of interference of data recording in patients with cardiac pacemaker or defibrillator have not been fully established. Recently, a case was reported of a patient with a cardiac pacemaker implanted in the abdominal wall who underwent capsule endoscopy examination [86]. After capsule ingestion, cardiac monitoring showed no modification of the pacemaker compartment, but the capsule recording revealed more than 3 h of image loss. Another study evaluated 5 patients with cardiac pacemaker who underwent capsule endoscopy examination, but did not find any interference or adverse cardiac events [87]. It appears capsule endoscopy is safe in patients with cardiac pacemakers, but, whether the cardiac pacers can lead to loss of endoscopy images is not certain.

Economic decision model

Goldfarb *et al.* developed a decision tree model designed to evaluate the economics of two diagnostic approaches in Crohn's disease – colonoscopy and SBFT or capsule endoscopy [88]. They estimated that capsule endoscopy produces a cost saving of $291 USD for each case presenting for diagnostic work-up for Crohn's disease. Sensitivity analysis was performed using varying diagnostic yields of colonoscopy and SBFT versus capsule endoscopy, based upon data from the available literature. The investigators found that capsule endoscopy is still less costly than colonoscopy, even at the highest reported diagnostic yields of SBFT and colonoscopy, as long as the diagnostic yield of capsule endoscopy is 64.1% or better [88]. Hence, the payers may find capsule endoscopy as the first-line diagnostic procedure to be more cost effective than the traditional approach for diagnosing small intestinal Crohn's disease after obstructive symptoms are excluded. However, data from larger- scale, well-controlled prospective studies are needed in order to design a definitive economic decision model.

Conclusion

IBD is a condition that affects at least the mucosal lining and has remained a diagnostic challenge to gastroenterologists since its initial description more than 70 years ago [89]. After decades of diagnostic refinements, direct visualisation of disease activity within the small intestine remains an important component in disease confirmation. Conventional imaging tests and surgical exploration are insensitive, imprecise or impractical to rely upon for this purpose. Capsule endoscopy may have finally arrived as the diagnostic modality of choice. Preliminary studies have shown evidence that the capsule study could be superior to traditional imaging modalities to inspect the small intestine for active Crohn's disease. Anecdotal experiences mostly based on abstract reports, have already suggested that it is useful in diagnosing new Crohn's disease, monitoring disease activity, better defining indeterminate colitis and re-classifying ulcerative colitis. Capsule endoscopy is also potentially capable of altering disease management and improving clinical outcomes, and perhaps providing physicians with valuable information on the natural history of inflammatory bowel disease. Although histological proof is not necessary to confirm Crohn's disease, it is important for correlation with endoscopic findings in order to establish uniformity in endoscopic nomenclature and interpretation of findings at this early stage of capsule endoscopy. Indeed, a disadvantage of capsule endoscopy compared with conventional endoscopy is its inability to take tissue samples. Large-scale, well-controlled prospective studies with long-term follow-ups are needed to confirm the clinical relevance of this new technology in the field of inflammatory bowel disease. Until then, the most appropriate role for capsule endoscopy in IBD patients appears to be for the evaluation of patients with suspected Crohn's disease, or Crohn's disease patients with atypical symptoms after retrograde ileoscopy evaluation. There is currently no indication for capsule endoscopy in patients with established ulcerative colitis except for differential diagnosis purpose if the diagnosis is in doubt. Our view is that it could become a useful diagnostic standard for diagnosing intestinal Crohn's disease.

References

1. Delaney CP, Fazio VW. Crohn's disease of the small bowel. *Surg Clin North Am* 2001;81:137–58.
2. Mekhian HS, Smith DM, Melnyk CS, *et al*. Clinical features and natural history of Crohn's disease. *Gastroenterology* 1979;68:627–35.
3. Lo SK. Capsule endoscopy in the diagnosis and management of inflammatory bowel disease. *Gastrointest Endosc Clin N Am* 2004;24:179–93.
4. Sands BE. Crohn's disease. In: Feldman M, Friedman LS, Sleisenger MH, eds. *Sleisenger & Fordtran's Gastrointestinal and Liver disease*. 7th ed. Philadelphia: Saunders; 2002:2005–38.
5. Scotiniotis I, Rubesin SE, Ginsberg GG. Imaging modalities in inflammatory bowel disease. *Gastroenterol Clin N Am* 1999;28:391–421.
6. Maglinte DDT, Lappas JC, Heitkamp DE, *et al*. Technical refinements in enteroclysis. *Radiol Clin N Am* 2003;41(2):213–29.
7. Eisen GM, Dominitz JA, Faigel DO, *et al*. Ethnic issues in endoscopy. *Gastrointest Endosc* 2001;53:874–5.
8. Cohen RD, Lee SD. Endoscopy in inflammatory bowel disease. *Gastroenterol Clin N Am* 2002;31:119–32.

9. Yamamoto H, Kita H, Sunada K, et al. Endoscopic diagnosis and treatment of small intestinal diseases using the double-balloon endoscopy [Abstract]. *Gastrointest Endosc* 2004;59(5):AB100.
10. Lo SK, Leighton JA, Ross A, et al. Double balloon push enteroscopy: technical details and early experience in 6 U.S. tertiary care centres. *Gastrointest Endosc* 2005;61(5):AB212.
11. Fritscher-Ravens A, Swain PC. The wireless capsule: new light in the darkness. *Dig Dis* 2002;20:127–33.
12. Swain P. Wireless capsule endoscopy. *Gut* 2003; 52(Suppl 4):iv, 48–50.
13. Buchman AL. Inflammatory bowel diseases of the small intestine. In: Halper M, Jacob H, eds. *Atlas of Capsule Endoscopy*. Yoqneam, Israel: Given Imaging, 2002, 33–47.
14. Yu M. M2A capsule endosocpy: a breakthrough diagnostic tool for small intestine imaging. *Gastroenterol Nurs* 2002;25:24–7.
15. Ogata H, Kumai K, Imaeda H, et al. The development of a new capsule endoscope: function-confirming test using animal model. *Gastrointest Endosc* 2005; 61(5):AB177.
16. Appleyard M, Fireman Z, Glukhovsky A, et al. A randomized trial comparing wireless capsule endoscopy with push enteroscopy for the detection of small-bowel lesions.*Gastroenterology* 2000;119: 1431–8.
17. Appleyard M, Glukhovsky A, Swain P. Wireless capsule diagnostic endoscopy for recurrent small bowel bleeding. *N Eng J Med* 2001;344:232–3.
18. Ell C, Remke S, May A, et al. The first prospective controlled trial comparing wireless capsule endoscopy with push enteroscopy in chronic gastrointestinal bleeding. *Endoscopy* 2002;34:685–90.
19. Costamagna G, Shah SK, Riccioni ME, et al. A prospective trial comparing small bowel radiographs and video capsule endoscopy for suspected small bowel disease.*Gastroenterology* 2002;123: 999–1005.
20. Blue Cross Blue Shield Association Technology Evaluation Center. Wireless capsule endoscopy in obscure digestive tract bleeding. *Technologica MAP Suppl* 2001;6;42–3.
21. Fireman Z, Mahajna E, Broide E, et al. Diagnosing small bowel Crohn's disease with wireless capsule endoscopy. *Gut* 2003;52:390–2.
22. Herrerias JM, Caunedo A, Rodriguez-Tellez M, et al. Capsule endoscopy in patients with suspected Crohn's disease and negative endoscopy. *Endoscopy* 2003;35:564–8.
23. Ge ZZ, Hu YB, Xiao SD. Capsule endoscopy in diagnosis of small bowel Crohn's disease. *World J Gastroenterol* 2004;10(9):1349–52.
24. Eliakim R, Suissa A, Yassin K, et al. Wireless capsule video endoscopy compared to barium follow-through and computerized tomography in patients with suspect Crohn's disease-final rep ort. *Dig Liver Dis* 2004;36(8):519–22.
25. Mow MS, Lo SK, Targan SR, et al. Initial experience with wireless capsule enteroscopy in the diagnosis and management of inflammatory bowel disease. *Clin Gastroenterol Hep* 2004;2:31–40.
26. Chong AK, Taylor A, Miller A, et al. Capsule endoscopy vs. push enteroscopy and enteroclysis in suspected small-bowel Crohn's disease. *Gastrointest Endosc* 2005;61:255–61.
27. Voderholzer WA, Beinhoelzl J, Rogalla P, et al. Small bowel involvement in Crohn's disease: a prospective comparison of wireless capsule endoscopy and computed tomography enteroclysis. *Gut* 2005;54: 369–73.
28. Buchman AL, Miller F, Wallin A, et al. Videocapsule endoscopy versus barium contrast studies for the diagnosis of Crohn's disease recurrence involving the small intestine. *Am J Gastroenterol* 2004;99(11): 2171–7.
29. Toth E, Fork FT, Almqvist P, et al. Wireless capsule entersocopy: a comparison with enterography, push enteroscopy and ileo-colonoscopy in the diagnosis of small bowel Crohn's disease. *Gastrointest Endosc* 2004;57(5):AB173.
30. Tillack C, Herrmann K, Seiderer J, et al. Capsule endoscopy in patients with Crohn's disease and small bowel involvement distal to the terminal ileum, detected by MR enteroclysis [Abstract]. *Gastroenterology* 2004;126(4 Suppl 2):A204.
31. Legnani PE, Kornbluth A, George J, et al. Capsule endoscopy in IBD: findings and effects on clinical outcomes [Abstract]. *Gastroenterology* 2004; 126(4 Suppl 2):A77.
32. Mehdizadeh S, Chen G, Enayati P. Utility of wireless capsule endoscopy in evaluating Crohn's disease patients with abdominal symptoms. *Gastrointest Endosc* 2005;61(5):AB175.
33. Dubcenco E, Jeejeebhoy KN, Petroniene R, et al. Diagnosing Crohn's disease of the small bowel: should capsule endoscopy be used? CE vs. other diagnostic modalities [Abstract]. *Gastrointest Endosc* 2004;57(5):AB174.
34. Bloom PD, Rosenberg MD, Klein SD, et al. Wireless capsule endoscopy is more informative than ileoscopy and SBFT for the evaluation of the small intestine in patients with known or suspected Crohn's disease [Abstract]. *Gastroenterology* 2004;126(4 Suppl 2): A203.
35. Solem CA, Loftus EV, Petersen BT, et al. Retrospective experience with capsule endoscopy in Crohn's disease

[Abstract]. *Am J Gastroenterol* 2004;99(Suppl 10): 830.
36. Scapa E, Jacob H, Lewkowicz S, *et al.* Initial experience of wireless capsule endoscopy for evaluating occult gastrointestinal bleeding and suspected small bowel pathology. *Am J Gastroenterol* 2002;97:2776–9.
37. Liangpunsakul S, Chadalwada V, Rex DK, *et al.* Wireless capsule endoscopy detects small bowel ulcers in patients with normal results from state of the art enteroclysis. *Am J Gastroenterol* 2003;98: 1294–98.
38. Pennazio M, Santucci R, Rondonotti E, *et al.* Outcome of patients with obscure gastrointestinal bleeding after capsule endoscopy: report of 100 consecutive cases. *Gastroenterology* 2004;126:643–53.
39. Maieron A, Hubner D, Blaha B, *et al.* Multicenter retrospective evaluation of capsule endoscopy in clinical routine. *Endoscopy* 2004;36(10):864–8.
40. Jiang XL, Cui HF. An analysis of 10218 ulcerative colitis cases in China. *World J Gastroenterol* 2002;8(1):158–61.
41. Leong RW, Lau JY, Sung JJ. The epidemiology and phenotype of Crohn's disease in the Chinese population. *Inflamm Bowel Dis* 2004;10(5):646–51.
42. Zheng JJ, Shi XH, Chu XQ, *et al.* Clinical features and management of Crohn's disease in Chinese patients. *Chin Med J (Engl)* 2004;117(2): 183–8.
43. Triester SL, Leighton JA, Gurudu SR, *et al.* A meta-analysis of capsule endoscopy compared to other modalities in patients with non-stricturing small bowel Crohn's disease [Abstract]. *Am J Gastroenterol* 2004;99(10 Suppl):834.
44. Umschaden HW, Gaser J. MR enteroclysis. *Radiol Clin N Am* 2003;41(2):231–48.
45. Tabibzadeh S, Kimble J, Zaidel O, *et al.* Distribution of small bowel erosions or ulcerations in patients presenting for wireless capsule enteroscopy [Abstract]. *Gastrointest Endosc* 2003;57(5):AB171.
46. Kornbluth A, Legnani P, Lewis BS. Video capsule endoscopy in inflammatory bowel disease: past, present, and future. *Inflamm Bowel Dis* 2004;10(3):278–85.
47. Lewis BS, Legnani P, Gralnek I, *et al.* The Crohn's disease capsule endoscopic scoring index: a new disease activity scale [Abstract]. *Gastroenterology* 2004;126(4 Suppl 1):880.
48. Mary JY, Modigliani R. Development and validation of an endoscopic index of the severity for Crohn's disease: a prospective multicentre study. *Gut* 1989;30:983–9.
49. Arnott ID, Lo SK. The clinical utility of wireless capsule endoscopy. *Dig Dis Sci* 2004;49(6):893–901.
50. Goldstein J, Eisen G, Lewis BS, *et al.* Abnormal small bowel findings are common in healthy subjects screened for a multicenter, double blind, randomized, placebo controlled trial using capsule endoscopy [Abstract]. *Gastroenterology* 2003;124(4 Suppl 1): A37.
51. Graham DY, Opekun AR, Willingham FF, *et al.* Visible small-intestinal mucosal injury in chronic NSAID users. *Clin Gastroenterol Hepatol* 2005;3(1): 55–9.
52. Arguelles-Arias F, Caunedo A, Romero J, *et al.* The value of capsule endoscopy in pediatric patients with a suspicion of Crohn's Disease. *Endoscopy* 2004;36:869–73.
53. Bizzari B, Fornaroli F, Del Rossi C, *et al.* Ileoscopy with videocapsule in pediatric-juvenile age [Abstract]. *Am J Gastroenterol* 2004;99(10 Suppl):966.
54. Papadakis KA, Tabibzadeh S. Diagnosis and misdiagnosis of inflammatory bowel disease. *Gastrointest Endosc Clin N Am* 2002;12:433–49.
55. Whitaker DA, Hume G, Radford-Smith GL, *et al.* Can capsule endoscopy help differentiate the aetiology of indeterminate colitis [Abstract]. *Gastrointest Endosc* 2004;59(5):AB177.
56. Mascarenhas-Saraiva M. Capsule endoscopy: a valuable help for the differential diagnosis of indeterminate colitis. In: *4th International Conference on Capsule Endoscopy Conference Report*, Miami, 2005.
57. Berg DF. Acute surgical emergencies in inflammatory bowel disease. *Am J Surgery* 2002;184:45–51.
58. Loftus EV. Capsule endoscopy for Crohn's disease: ready for prime time? *Clin Gastroenterol Hep* 2004;2:14–16.
59. Mergener K, Enns R, Brandabur JJ, *et al.* Complications and problems with capsule endoscopy: results from two referral centers [Abstract]. *Gastrointest Endosc* 2003;57(5):AB170.
60. Cheifetz AS, Kornbluth AA, Legnani PE, *et al.* Incidence and outcome of the retained video capsule endoscope in Crohn's disease: is it a 'therapeutic complication' [Abstract]? *Am J Gastroenterol* 2004;99(10 Suppl):807.
61. Swain P. Wireless capsule endoscopy and Crohn's disease. *Gut* 2005;54:323–6.
62. Costamagna G, Spada C, Spera G, *et al.* Given patency system is a new diagnostic tool for verifying functional patency of the small bowel [Abstract]. *Am J Gastroenterol* 2004;99(10 Suppl):188.
63. Gay G, Delvaux M, Laurent V. Temporary intestinal occlusion induced by a 'patency capsule' in a patient with Crohn's disease. *Endoscopy* 2005;37(2):174–7.
64. Hyun JH, Keum BR, Choung RS, *et al.* Analysis of incomplete small bowel investigation in capsule

endoscopy [Abstract]. *Gastrointest Endosc* 2004;59(5):AB177.
65 Sachdev RM, Cave DR. Incomplete small intestinal transit and the retained video-capsule: a cloud with a silver lining [Abstract]. *Am J Gastroenterol* 2004;99(10 Suppl):186.
66 Chan S, Wang J, Daniels JM, *et al.* A retrospective evaluation of wireless capsule endoscopy: determination of factors that influence transit time [Abstract]. *Gastrointest Endosc* 2004; 59(5):AB175.
67 Fireman Z, Kopelman Y, Fish L, *et al.* Effect of oral purgatives on gastric and small bowel transit time in capsule endoscopy. *Isr Med Assoc J* 2004;6(9):521–3.
68 Selby W. Complete small-bowel transit in patients undergoing capsule endoscopy: determining factors and improvement with metoclopramide. *Gastrointest Endosc* 2005;61(1):80–5.
69 Schmelkin IJ. Tegaserod decreases small bowel transit times in patients undergoing capsule endoscopy [Abstract]. *Gastrointest Endosc* 2004;59(5):AB176.
70 Fireman Z, Mahajna E, Fish L, *et al.* Effect of Erythromycin on gastric and small bowel transit time of video capsule endoscopy [Abstract]. *Gastrointest Endosc* 2003;57(5):AB163.
71 Niv Y, Niv G. Capsule endoscopy: role of bowel preparation in successful visualization. *Scand J Gastroenterol* 2004;39(10):1005–9.
72 Dai N, Gubler C, Hengstler P, *et al.* Improved capsule endoscopy after bowel preparation. *Gastrointest Endosc* 2005;61(1):28–31.
73 Daperno M, D'Haens G, Van Assche G, *et al.* Simplified endoscopic activity score for Crohn's disease: the SES-CD. *Gastrointest Endosc* 2004;60(4):505–12.
74 Modigliani R, Mary JY, Simon JF, *et al.* Clinical, biological, and endoscopic picture of attacks of Crohn's disease. Evolution on prednisolone. *Gastroenterology* 1997;98:811–8.
75 Olaisson B, Sjodahl R, Tagesson C. Glucocorticoid treatment in ileal Crohn's disease: relief of symptoms but not of endoscopically viewed inflammation. *Gut* 1990;31:325–8.
76 Cellier C, Sahmoud T, Froguel E, *et al.* Correlations between clinical activity, endoscopic severity, and biological parameters in colonic or ileocolonic Crohn's disease: a prospective multicenter study of 121 cases. *Gut* 1994;35:231–5.

77 D'Haens G, Geboes K, Rutgeerts P. Endoscopic and histologic healing of Crohn's ileo-colitis with azathioprine. *Gastrointest Endosc* 1999;50:667–71.
78 D'Haens G, Van Deventer S, Van Hogezand R, *et al.* Endoscopic and histological healing with infliximab anti-tumor necrosis factor antibodies in Crohn's disease: a European multicentre trial. *Gastroenterology* 1999;116:1029–34.
79 Debinski H. Mucosal healing in small bowel Crohn's disease following therapy with infliximab. Assessment using the Crohn's disease capsule endoscopic index. In: *4th International Conference on Capsule Endoscopy Conference Report*, Miami, 2005.
80 Lennard-Jones JE. Classification of inflammatory bowel disease. *Scand J Gastroenterol* 1989(Suppl);170:2–6.
81 Consensus Statement. *Given International Conference*, Berlin, 2003.
82 Levinthal GN, Burke CA, Santisi JM. The accuracy of an endoscopy nurse in interpreting capsule endoscopy. *Am J Gastroenterol* 2003;98(12):2669–71.
83 Adler DG, Knipschield M, Gostout C. A prospective comparison of capsule endoscopy and push enteroscopy in patients with GI bleeding of obscure origin. *Gastrointest Endosc* 2004;59(4):492–8.
84 Chen G, Enayati P, Tran T, *et al.* Sensitivity and inter-observer variability for capsule endoscopy image analysis in a cohort of novice readers [Abstract]. *Gastrointest Endosc* 2004;59(5):AB165.
85 Boivin ML, Voderholzer W, Ortner MA. Interobserver agreement of wireless capsule endoscopy in patients with Crohn's disease [Abstract]. *Gastroenterology* 2005;128(4 Suppl 2):A647.
86 Guyomar Y, Vandeville L, Heuls S, *et al.* Interference between pacemaker and video capsule endoscopy. *Pacing Clin Electrophysiol* 2004;27(9):1329–30.
87 Leighton JA, Sharma VK, Srivathsan K, *et al.* Safety of capsule endoscopy in patients with pacemakers. *Gastrointest Endosc* 2004;59(4):567–9.
88 Goldfarb NI, Pizzi LT, Fuhr JP, *et al.* Diagnosing Crohn's disease: an economic analysis comparing wireless capsule endoscopy with traditional diagnostic procedures. *Dis Manag* 2004;7(4):292–304.
89 Crohn BB, Ginzburg L, Oppenheimer GD. Regional ileitis, a pathological and clinical entity. *JAMA* 1932;99:1323–7.

8: Cross-sectional imaging of inflammatory bowel disease

Stuart Taylor and Steve Halligan

Introduction

After entering the twenty-first century, it has become clear that imaging will remain pivotal for diagnosis and management of inflammatory bowel disease (IBD). Although modern endoscopic techniques allow unprecedented access to the gastrointestinal tract, many parts remain relatively inaccessible despite technological advances, notably the small bowel and any areas upstream of tight strictures. Furthermore, the bewildering array of extra-luminal complications associated with IBD makes it almost unique in non-neoplastic gastrointestinal disease, and fuels the ongoing demand for imaging.

The modern radiologist has a vast armamentarium of modalities and techniques available, but conventional barium-based studies such as the small bowel follow-through continue to be the workhorses of day-to-day patient management. Fluoroscopic imaging provides both functional and anatomical information, remains the gold standard for radiological detection of mucosal disease, and is well understood by referring physicians and surgeons alike. It is clear, however, that these studies have weaknesses, particularly for detection of extra-luminal complications such as fistula and abscess. Modern cross-sectional modalities such as computed tomography (CT), magnetic resonance imaging (MRI) and ultrasound (USS) allow unprecedented opportunity to characterise disease both in, and particularly outside the bowel lumen. Such techniques provide diagnostic information from the whole bowel wall and not just the mucosal surface, and are increasingly able to guide clinical management decisions by providing an additional assessment of disease activity. This chapter will outline the complementary relationship between cross-sectional techniques and conventional barium radiology, and will also detail some horizon scanning for possible future applications.

CT scanning

CT scanning utilises ionising radiation and produces sequential axial slices through the region of interest. The recent introduction of multi-detector row (multi-slice) technology permits very rapid acquisition of data with improved spatial resolution. For example, the abdomen and pelvis can be scanned in less than 10–15 seconds with individual slice thickness of 1mm or less. CT thus lends itself especially well to imaging ill and/or immobile patients who will not tolerate prolonged examination times.

Standard techniques

Patients routinely drink dilute barium- or iodine-based contrast agents prior to abdomino-pelvic CT. This opacifies and also distends the small bowel lumen, facilitating analysis of the bowel wall and improving detection of extra-luminal complications. Volumes up to 1500 ml are routine, usually administered over the 90 minutes prior to imaging. Poor bowel distension, however, occasionally remains a problem with oral administration, both reducing sensitivity and mimicking wall thickening and stricturing. Some authors, therefore, advocate infusion of contrast medium via a naso-jejunal tube [1, 2] so-called CT-enteroclysis. Careful control of infusion rates can induce small bowel hypotonia and achieve excellent distension. Naso-jejunal tube insertion may, however, be difficult for both the patient and radiologist alike, and the technique essentially negates one of the intrinsic advantages of CT, which is rapid and non-invasive image acquisition. Intravenous contrast is also routinely administered during abdomino-pelvic CT. Normal bowel wall enhances avidly and abnormal enhancement patterns are well described in patients with IBD, providing additional diagnostic information (see CT scanning: disease activity below) CT images are conventionally viewed as 2-D axial slices but acquisition of near isotropic data with thin collimation (slice thickness) multi-detector – row CT protocols allow excellent multi-planar (coronal, sagittal) reconstructions [3].

It should always be borne in mind that CT scanning conveys a significant radiation burden (7–8mSV–13.3mSV [4]) and should always be used judiciously, especially when so many IBD patients are young and may need repetitive examination, over time.

Diagnosis

Normal bowel is easily seen on CT and individual wall thickness should not exceed 2–3 mm in the distended state [5].

Inflammatory bowel disease classically manifest as bowel wall thickening on CT. The mean colonic wall thickness is usually greater in Crohn's disease (11–13 mm) compared to ulcerative colitis (7.8 mm) [6, 7] which may aid differentiation in those with isolated colonic disease, although considerable overlap exists. Eccentric thickening, small bowel involvement and skip lesions favour Crohns's over ulcerative colitis [8]. Experience of CT scanning for primary diagnosis of IBD remains limited at present, probably because subtle mucosal abnormalities such as aphthoid ulceration are invisible with CT [9]. Indeed, recent comparative studies have confirmed the superiority of endoscopy and barium studies over CT for diagnosis of early mucosal lesions in Crohn's disease [2, 9–11].

In patients with established IBD, CT may reveal additional sites of luminal disease missed by conventional contrast studies [12], particularly in the paediatric age group, who may be difficult to examine using fluoroscopic techniques [9, 13]. At present, however, CT remains a second-line investigation for primary diagnosis of IBD, with endoscopy and conventional barium studies preferred.

Extra-luminal complications

CT images the extra-luminal tissues in exquisite detail because of its high contrast and spatial resolution. Fistulae and abscesses are common complications of Crohn's disease and their detection often precipitates more aggressive therapeutic intervention [14]. CT is established as the radiological reference standard for detection of intra-abdominal abscesses complicating IBD (Fig 8.1), although ultrasound may have similar sensitivity in experienced hands (see Ultrasound: extra-luminal complications below). The literature series suggests the sensitivity of CT for abscess detection is between 59–85% [15, 16]. Furthermore, CT allows safe and effective image guidance for percutaneous abscess drainage [17, 18].

The ability of CT to reliably detect internal fistulae is more controversial. Conventional barium techniques are still considered the reference radiological standard, although in reality these may miss up to 50% of fistulae identified at laparotomy [19–21]. A recent report suggests CT may be comparable with conventional enteroclysis for the detection of fistulae (around 70% sensitivity) [16], although smaller older studies have reported inferior performance when using CT [10].

CT scanning also has an important role for the investigation of those IBD patients presenting with acute bowel obstruction, allowing diagnosis of extra-luminal complications such as abscesses, detection of adhesions and providing information about the bowel upstream, which is often inaccessible to an endoscope [22].

Studies suggest that detection of unsuspected extra-luminal complications by CT changes the intended management plan in up to 28% of patients [7, 11], and it is clear that judicious use of CT scanning adds considerable benefit to the diagnostic work-up in those with suspected complications.

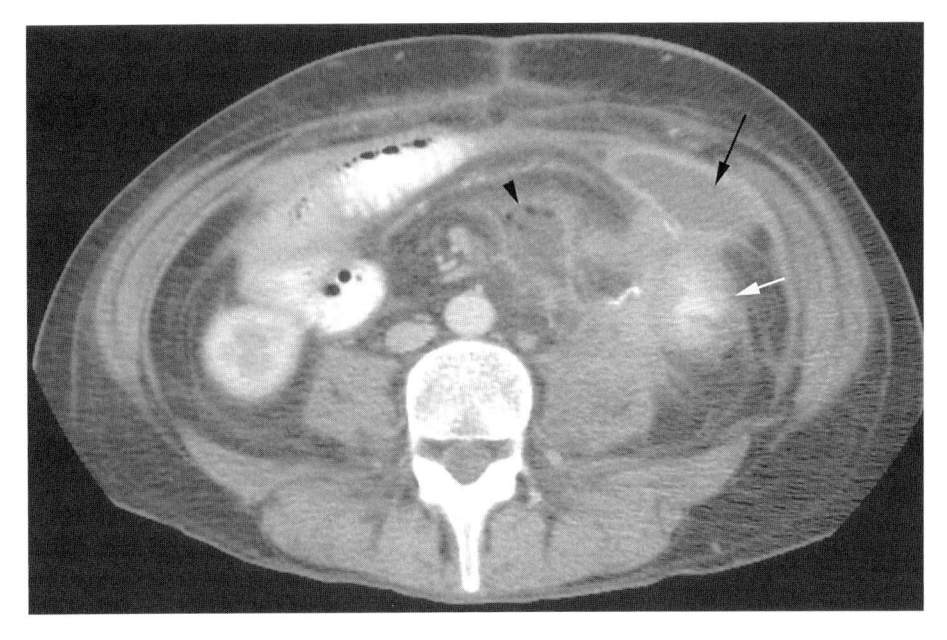

Fig 8.1 Axial CT scan through the upper pelvis in a 20-year-old male with active Crohn's disease. The superficial collection (long black arrow) was identified with ultrasound, but the deeper gas filled abscess (arrow head) was only identified on CT. Note the thickened small bowel loop (white arrow).

Disease activity

CT has conventionally been regarded as relatively poor when predicting disease activity, and probably inferior to other radiological techniques such as 99 mTc-white blood cell scintigraphy [23]. However, it is increasingly clear that patterns of contrast enhancement in affected bowel loops are correlated with disease activity [24]. A recent retrospective analysis reported that homogenous bowel wall enhancement was associated with quiescent disease whereas multi-layered mural stratification or a double layer of mural enhancement separated by low attenuation submucosa was associated with active disease [25]. Such mural enhancement patterns may help classify patients into those with active or inactive disease, but probably lack the required sensitivity and specificity for absolute disease characterisation.

Fibrofatty proliferation, increased vascularity of the vasa recta (comb sign) and mesenteric lymphadenopathy are all well described in IBD and are easily demonstrated with CT [8, 22]. Although adenopathy may be associated with active disease (see MRI: disease activity below), recent data suggests that increased pericolic or perienteric vasculature is seen more commonly [26]. Again, although not absolute, such a finding may be of use in helping to guide patient classification.

Novel CT techniques

Virtual CT colonoscopy is becoming an established method for detecting colonic neoplasia [27, 28], but may potentially also have a role in IBD. Patients undergo full purgation and the colon is distended with air or carbon dioxide before a thin collimation CT scan. The data can then be rendered to create a 3-D endoluminal view – hence the name 'virtual colonoscopy'. Data is relatively sparse, but it is clear that with present technology subtle mucosal changes such as superficial ulceration remain well beyond the resolution of the technique [29]. Recent data suggests virtual colonoscopy is comparable to colonoscopy for detecting elevated lesions of Crohn's colitis and may have a role in patients with impassible strictures [30]. However, the relative insensitivity for flat and ulcerated lesions sounds a strong note of caution for the use of virtual colonoscopy for colonic surveillance in chronic IBD.

Magnetic resonance imaging

As a method of enteric imaging, MRI has many intrinsic advantages. Soft tissue contrast is superior to that of CT and multi-planar imaging is routine and easily achieved. Significantly, there is no radiation burden, which is a very major advantage in the IBD population who are likely to be subjected to repeated imaging due to the chronic nature of their disease. Until relatively recently, enteric MRI was severely hampered by prolonged image acquisition times, with the effect that physiological bowel motion significantly detracted from image quality. However, recent advances in MRI hard- and software, particularly development of ultra-fast image sequences, mean that high quality images of the whole bowel can be acquired in less then 20 seconds and MRI is currently challenging more established imaging techniques in IBD.

Technique

The principles of MRI technique are comparable to those of CT. Oral contrast medium is vital to outline and distend the bowel lumen, and ideally should provide homogeneous opacification with minimal intestinal absorption. Depending on their chemical composition, contrast agents can appear bright (positive), dark (negative) or both bright and dark (biphasic) according to the imaging sequence used [31]. There is no consensus as to the best oral contrast agent, or indeed whether positive or negative agents are superior. Various workers have advocated methylcellulose [1], dilute barium [32], mannitol [33], manganese [34] or even blueberry juice [35], although ultimately the choice will be largely governed by local availability and costs.

Many workers strongly favour infusing the contrast agent through a naso-jejunal tube to optimise bowel distension as it is clear that good luminal distension, maximises detection of mucosal abnormalities [31, 36]. In common with both CT and conventional enteroclysis, insertion of the naso-jejunal tube prior to MRI can be difficult and time-consuming, often requiring fluoroscopic guidance, and essentially negating the benefit of MRI's lack of ionising radiation. Although orally ingested agents in themselves may not always produce reliable bowel distension [37], abnormal bowel is usually easily detected, and this may be sufficient to plan patient management. Furthermore, considerable interest has been generated in various additives to oral preparations that improve luminal distension, notably locust bean gum, which produces excellent bowel distension in normal volunteers [38].

Many sequences have been advocated to maximise diagnostic information from MRI. Both T1- and T2-weighted sequences in axial and coronal planes are mandatory to provide adequate information regarding the bowel lumen and wall, and extra-luminal tissues. Most workers also advocate the use of IV gadolinium to highlight abnormal bowel and perhaps provide some assessment of disease activity (see MRI: disease activity below). Ultimately the choice of sequences will depend on the available hardware and manufacturer of software, but a protocol based around true fast imaging with a steady precession (True FISP), half-Fourier acquired single-shot fast spin-echo (HASTE), T2-weighted turbo spin-echo, and gadolinium-enhanced fat-suppressed spoiled gradient-echo sequences is increasingly popular [31, 36]. Although individual sequences have relatively short acquisition times, the number employed prolongs examination times to several minutes and administration of an anti-spasmolytic is routine to reduce peristaltic artifact.

Diagnosis

In common with CT scanning, IBD usually manifests as bowel wall thickening on MRI. In comparison to CT, however, MRI appears to provide improved depiction of relatively early mucosal disease. Deep ulceration and cobble-stoning are visible, especially on True FISP sequences [31] but early and subtle changes, such as aphthous ulceration, currently remain beyond the resolution of the technique. Recent reports suggest MRI may have a role in the primary diagnosis of terminal ileal Crohn's disease in a paediatric population [39], but again, superficial erosions were not depicted and sensitivity for endoscopically confirmed ulcerative colitis was poor in this series. An earlier, albeit smaller, study reported a relatively poor sensitivity of just 50% for the primary diagnosis of Crohn's disease in this patient population [40].

In those with established IBD, several reports suggest that MRI enteroclysis is comparable and possibly superior to conventional enteroclysis for the detection, localisation and length estimation of involved small bowel segments, with excellent sensitivity for small bowel obstruction [1, 36, 41]. The multi-planar capabilities of MRI often reveal segments of diseased bowel not readily apparent on conventional fluoroscopic images. There have been few studies directly comparing CT with MRI, although Low and colleagues reported improved sensitivity for bowel wall thickening when using MRI compared to single slice CT [42]. However, using state-of-the-art multi-slice technology, Schmidt and colleagues found CT was superior to MRI for detection of abnormal small bowel, with greater interobserver agreement [43]. The authors did however conclude that that further improvements in technology would probably allow MRI to 'catch' up with CT in the near future.

Extra-luminal complications

MRI provides detailed information regarding extra-luminal tissues. Recent reports suggest it may be equivalent to CT for the detection of intra-abdominal abscesses, although comparative studies with a surgical gold standard are lacking. In a series of 84 patients, Reiber reported a sensitivity of 77.8% for the detection of abscesses (none of which were detected by conventional enteroclysis) [41].

Data on sensitivity for enteric fistula is also relatively sparse. A sensitivity of 83% was reported by Reiber [44] compared to a surgical gold standard, although this fell to 70.6% in a larger study from the same group [41]. In a series of 32 patients, Prassopoulos and colleagues found MRI enteroclysis depicted all fistulas shown at conventional enteroclysis, but only half of the sinus tracts were visible on MRI [36]. Although MRI is clearly promising in its ability to detect extra-luminal complications, further data is awaited.

Perianal disease

Over 25% of patients afflicted with Crohn's disease will suffer from perianal fistulae during the course of their disease [45]. Fistulae complicating IBD tend to be more complex compared to cryptoglandular disease, and also are more refractory to treatment [46]. The exquisite soft tissue contrast afforded by MRI makes this the gold standard technique for pre-operative imaging of perianal fistulae, the aim of which is to determine the course of the fistula relative to the anal sphincter while also detecting areas of sepsis that might be missed during examination under anaesthetic (EUA) (Fig 8.2). Sepsis missed at EUA is the major cause of treatment failure [47] and recent work has shown that pre-operative MRI can reduce fistulae recurrence by as much as 75% [48]. Such is the accuracy of MRI that it is doubtful

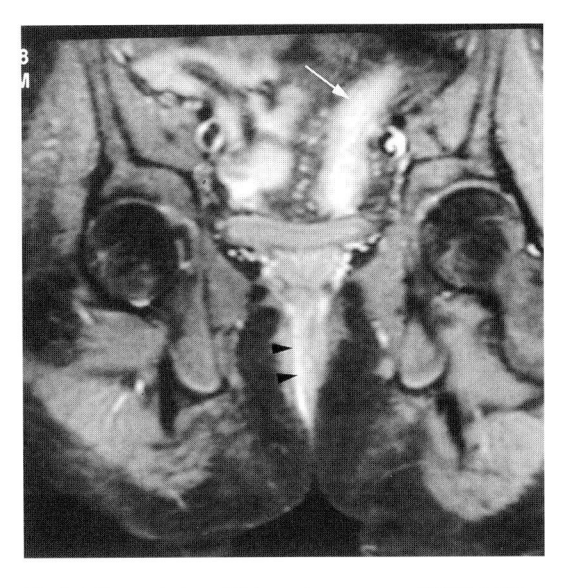

Fig 8.2 Coronal short TI-inversion recovery (STIR) MRI image through the anal canal in an 18-year-old male with perianal Crohn's disease. A fistula (arrow heads) ascends in the inter-sphincteric plane. Note the thickened sigmoid loop (white arrow) in keeping with associated Crohn's colitis.

whether surgery for complex or recurrent disease should be attempted without it, if available. MRI has also proved useful in assessing pharmacological treatments for active perianal Crohn's disease, notably assessing the response of fistulae to Infliximab [49]. In particular, MRI can reveal extensive underlying disease even though the external opening has healed.

Disease activity

Assessment of disease activity using MRI is based both on anatomical observations such as wall thickening and fibrofatty proliferation, and also on patterns of contrast enhancement in an acutely inflamed bowel.

Simple measurement of bowel wall thickness may help indicate the level of disease activity in affected bowel segments. Using a cut-off of 4 mm, Koh *et al.* reported a sensitivity of 54% and a specificity of 98% for active disease [50]. Similarly, Maccioni *et al.* found reasonable correlation between wall thickness and disease activity, but did report overlap with inactive disease [51]. However, both groups observed high signal within bowel wall on T2-weighted images in the most actively inflamed bowel segments. The presence of fibrofatty proliferation is a poor discriminator between inactive and active disease, but increased signal within fat surrounding bowel loops on T2-weighted images is a good indicator of active inflammation (perhaps reflecting oedema) [33, 50, 51].

Several groups have described prominent lymphadenopathy in association with Crohn's disease [52, 53] and there is some evidence that nodes, which enhance avidly after intravenous gadolinium, may reflect regionally active disease [31]. In common with CT, the presence of increased mesenteric vascularity ('comb sign') is a reasonable indicator of active disease [36] with reported sensitivity and specificity of 78% and 57%, respectively [50].

Considerable interest has been generated by patterns of intravenous gadolinium enhancement as indicators of disease activity. As with CT, a layered or stratified appearance to the bowel wall after contrast is very specific for active disease but lacks sensitivity [50]. Using dynamic MRI (i.e. repeated image acquisitions at a single level after an intravenous contrast bolus), a clear association can be demonstrated between disease activity and the degree of mural enhancement [52, 54, 55]. Correlation with the Crohn's disease activity index (CDAI) is often only moderate (perhaps reflecting the inadequacy of this index), but interestingly a much stronger correlation exists with serum-acute inflammatory markers such as C-reactive protein (CRP) [52]. The mechanism for increased mural enhancement in active disease is assumed to be increased capillary permeability secondary to increased local inflammatory mediators [54]. Although dynamic MRI may provide greater quantification of mural enhancement, the technique is technically challenging and not yet suited to routine practice outside a research setting. Simple semi-quantitative assessment of enhancement on routine post-contrast images is presently a more attractive proposition for routine clinical application and such an approach has already proved useful when assessing disease activity [50, 51].

Overall, it is clear that assessment of disease activity using MRI is highly promising and it is likely that a combination of observations will produce the best results. Relatively small series suggest a per patient sensitivity of around 90% for active disease [50, 51], but larger prospective studies are required before more widespread clinical implementation.

Ultrasound

As an imaging modality, ultrasound also has many attractive properties. It is relatively cheap and quick, and requires little patient preparation. There is no radiation burden and it is well tolerated by patients. It does, however, remain highly operator-dependent and may be technically difficult, especially in obese or immobile patients.

Technique

Most enteric ultrasound is performed without oral or intravenous contrast agents, using standard resolution probes (3–5 MHz) supplemented with higher resolution probes (7–12 MHz) for more detailed assessment. The normal bowel wall thickness measures around 3 mm and is composed of multiple layers (classically 5) of alternating echogenicity. The ultra-sonographer uses graded compression [56] to gently compress the underlying bowel and separate loops for interrogation. Systematic analysis is performed of both the small bowel and colon. Blood flow can be readily assessed both in the bowel wall and in the main superior and inferior mesenteric arteries. Intravenous contrast is unnecessary when using standard Doppler functions, which may help document disease activity (see Ultrasound: disease activity below).

Diagnosis

Inflammatory bowel disease produces bowel wall thickening on USS. Depending on the stage of the disease, this ranges from thickening of individual layers (e.g. the submucosa) to thickening of the whole bowel wall with loss of the normal layered stratification. Such findings are however relatively non-specific and are common to a variety of conditions including both infections and neoplasia. Abnormalities in ulcerative colitis are often less marked than Crohn's disease although superficial ulceration with submucosal oedema can be demonstrated using high resolution USS. Extra-luminal changes such as fat hypertrophy are readily appreciated and fistulation can also be detected [57, 58].

Several studies have examined the use of USS as a primary diagnostic tool in suspected IBD. Quoted sensitivities lie between 78–95% with specificity around 90% [59–63]. Performance is operator-dependent and a clear learning curve has been demonstrated [60]. USS often cannot demonstrate subtle mucosal abnormalities and as would be expected, sensitivity is much lower for early disease [56, 64]. There is some evidence that sensitivity is higher for Crohn's disease than ulcerative colitis [65], probably because the superficial nature of the latter. Assessment of the extent of disease is less accurate than that for detection, with accuracy around 80% [64, 66], although good correlation between the length of small bowel involved has been reported when using conventional barium studies for comparison [67, 68]. Sensitivity of USS for detection of bowel stenosis is moderate (58–90%), and USS remains inferior to both conventional enteroclysis and MRI in this respect [56, 69, 70].

Extra-luminal complications

The reported ability of USS to detect extra-luminal complications of IBD is variable, but it is clear that the technique is a very useful tool in the right hands. Maconi and colleagues initially reported an overall sensitivity of 67% and 83% for detection of fistulae and intra-abdominal abscesses, respectively [71]. In a subsequent larger series, including 128 patients undergoing surgery acting as reference standard, the same group showed USS and conventional barium studies to be complimentary for the diagnosis of internal fistulae, with sensitivities of around 70% [16]. The same study suggested USS and CT had comparable sensitivities for the diagnosis of abscesses (around 90%), although CT was a little more specific. Gasche and colleagues reported a sensitivity of 87% for internal fistulae in a small cohort of 30 patients undergoing surgery for IBD [72], although Potthast found USS very poor in a study of 46 patients, with sensitivity of just 31% for fistula detection compared to 87% for MRI [70]. However, despite its inferiority to MRI, USS had a respectable sensitivity of 89% in detecting abscesses in this study [70].

Although the precise role of USS in the primary diagnosis and detection of extra-luminal complications in IBD remains unresolved, the test is safe, quick and relatively cheap and it is clear that in experienced hands it has a significant role to play in day-to-day patient management.

Disease activity

In common with other cross-sectional techniques, assessment of disease activity with USS is dependent on structural findings, including bowel wall thickening, and functional parameters, notably Doppler indices of blood flow.

Bowel wall thickening tends to be greater in active compared to quiescent Crohn's disease [73], but there is considerable overlap, which limits the measurement as a reliable indicator of disease activity [67]. Some workers have suggested mild wall thickening with preservation of mural stratification on USS reflects early disease, while loss of recognisable layers suggests more active disease [56]; again significant overlap exists.

Vessel density within thickened bowel wall as determined by Doppler techniques is however more promising. Both Heyne *et al.* and Spalinger *et al.* reported a good correlation between active disease (based on CDAI) and bowel wall vascularity using a semi-quantitative score of vessel number per square cm [73, 74]. Similar results were obtained by Esteban *et al.* who described obvious increased mural vascularity in 44 patients with active Crohn's disease compared to none of 35 patients with quiescent disease [75]. There are some data suggesting that semi-quantatative assessment of mural vascularity may also be useful in assessing response of active disease to medication such as sulphasalazine [76]. Increased vascularity around intestinal fistulae has also been documented, again correlating with more standard measurements of disease activity [77]. It must be stressed that all these methods are only semi-quantative and are to a large extent reliant on technical parameters and subjective assessment, which may limit widespread implementation, although overall intra-observer agreement appears to be good.

Several workers have concentrated on flow measurement in the main arterial supply to the gut in an attempt to assess disease activity, based on the well documented increase in neo-vascularisation that occurs in IBD. Using Doppler sonography, Van Oostayen *et al.* described increased arterial volume flow in the superior mesenteric artery (SMA) in 10 patients with active Crohn's disease when compared to 10 patients with quiescent disease and 10 healthy controls [78]. Several other workers have since replicated this finding, documenting increased portal vein flow and decreased vascular resistance, over and above the changes in SMA blood flow [79, 80]. Mirk *et al.* also found that similar results could be obtained when applying the technique to the inferior mesenteric artery (IMA) [81]. Changes in Doppler flow parameters have also been shown in response to treatment [82] raising the possibility of non-invasive monitoring of treatment regimens.

Although definite strong associations exist between Doppler blood flow parameters and IBD, the clinical utility of such measurements remain undetermined. Indeed, some workers have suggested that changes in flow parameters merely reflect the extent of disease rather than any actual disease activity [83]. Furthermore, it is clear that there is considerable normal overlap for various Doppler indices, suggesting that absolute levels may not be clinically useful when attempting to separate patients into active or inactive groups [84]. Therefore, Doppler studies, although providing a guide to disease activity, may actually prove more useful for follow-up of individual patients, assessing their response to therapy and perhaps predicting relapse [80].

Other techniques

Recent work suggests that 18F-flurodeoxyglucose positron emission tomography (FDG-PET) may be a useful tool for assessment of disease activity. The technique is expensive, time-consuming and also conveys a significant radiation dose, which ultimately may limit its use. However, recent data suggests it may be more sensitive than either MRI or immunoscintigraphy in detecting active disease [85]. Further studies are awaited.

Conclusions

Cross-sectional techniques will have an increasing role in the management of patients with IBD. Although conventional barium studies remain the radiological reference standard for the diagnosis of early IBD, it is clear that CT, MRI and ultrasound, either alone or in combination, are superior for the detection of many extra-luminal complications and possibly disease extent. Reliable assessment of disease activity is becoming increasingly possible with newer techniques, and will ultimately play a significant role both in individual patient management and assessment of newer experimental treatment regimens. Cross-sectional imaging may be able to provide a 'one-stop' assessment of IBD patients in the not too distant future.

References

1. Umschaden HW, Szolar D, Gasser J, Umschaden M, Haselbach H. Small-bowel disease: comparison of MR enteroclysis images with conventional enteroclysis and surgical findings. Radiology 2000;215(3):717–25.
2. Hassan C, Cerro P, Zullo A, Spina C, Morini S. Computed tomography enteroclysis in comparison with ileoscopy in patients with Crohn's disease. Int J Colorectal Dis 2003;18(2):121–5.
3. Raptopoulos V, Schwartz RK, McNicholas MM, Movson J, Pearlman J, Joffe N. Multiplanar helical CT enterography in patients with Crohn's disease. AJR Am J Roentgenol 1997;169(6):1545–50.
4. Bitterling H, Rock C, Reiser M. Computed tomography in the diagnosis of inflammatory bowel disease – methodology of MSCT and clinical results. Radiologe 2003;43(1):17–25.
5. Desai RK, Tagliabue JR, Wegryn SA, Einstein DM. CT evaluation of wall thickening in the alimentary tract. Radiographics 1991;11(5):771–83.
6. Philpotts LE, Heiken JP, Westcott MA, Gore RM. Colitis: use of CT findings in differential diagnosis. Radiology 1994;190(2):445–9.
7. Fishman EK, Wolf EJ, Jones B, Bayless TM, Siegelman SS. CT evaluation of Crohn's disease: effect on patient management. AJR Am J Roentgenol 1987;148(3):537–40.
8. Horton KM, Corl FM, Fishman EK. CT evaluation of the colon: inflammatory disease. Radiographics 2000;20(2):399–418.
9. Jamieson DH, Shipman PJ, Israel DM, Jacobson K. Comparison of multidetector CT and barium studies of the small bowel: inflammatory bowel disease in children. AJR Am J Roentgenol 2003;180(5):1211–16.
10. Orel SG, Rubesin SE, Jones B, Fishman EK, Bayless TM, Siegelman SS. Computed tomography vs barium studies in the acutely symptomatic patient with Crohn disease. J Comput Assist Tomogr 1987;11(6):1009–16.
11. Mako EK, Mester AR, Tarjan Z, Karlinger K, Toth G. Enteroclysis and spiral CT examination in diagnosis and evaluation of small bowel Crohn's disease. Eur J Radiol 2000;35(3):168–175.
12. Reittner P, Goritschnig T, Petritsch W, et al. Multiplanar spiral CT enterography in patients with Crohn's disease using a negative oral contrast material: initial results of a noninvasive imaging approach. Eur Radiol 2002;12(9):2253–7.
13. Hyer W, Beattie RM, Walker-Smith JA, McLean A. Computed tomography in chronic inflammatory bowel disease. Arch Dis Child 1997;76(5):428–31.
14. Mekhjian HS, Switz DM, Melnyk CS, Rankin GB, Brooks RK. Clinical features and natural history of Crohn's disease. Gastroenterology 1979;77(4, Pt 2):898–906.
15. Gore RM, Cohen MI, Vogelzang RL, Neiman HL, Tsang TK. Value of computed tomography in the detection of complications of Crohn's disease. Dig Dis Sci 1985;30(8):701–9.
16. Maconi G, Sampietro GM, Parente F, et al. Contrast radiology, computed tomography and ultrasonography in detecting internal fistulas and intra-abdominal abscesses in Crohn's disease: a prospective comparative study. Am J Gastroenterol 2003;98(7):1545–55.
17. Strotzer M, Manke C, Lock G, Bregenzer N, Scholmerich J, Feuerbach S. Percutaneous abscess drainage in Crohn disease. Rofo Fortschr Geb Rontgenstr Neuen Bildgeb Verfahr 1998;169(5):510–14.
18. Casola G, vanSonnenberg E, Neff CC, Saba RM, Withers C, Emarine CW. Abscesses in Crohn disease: percutaneous drainage. Radiology 1987;163(1):19–22.
19. Maglinte DD, Chernish SM, Kelvin FM, O'Connor KW, Hage JP. Crohn disease of the small intestine: accuracy and relevance of enteroclysis. Radiology 1992;184(2):541–5.
20. Nolan DJ. The true yield of the small-intestinal barium study. Endoscopy 1997;29(6):447–53.
21. Michelassi F, Stella M, Balestracci T, Giuliante F, Marogna P, Block GE. Incidence, diagnosis, and treatment of enteric and colorectal fistulae in patients with Crohn's disease. Ann Surg 1993;218(5):660–6.
22. Furukawa A, Saotome T, Yamasaki M, et al. Cross-sectional Imaging in Crohn Disease. Radiographics 2004;24(3):689–702.
23. Charron M, Di LC, Kocoshis S. CT and 99mTc-WBC vs colonoscopy in the evaluation of inflammation and complications of inflammatory bowel diseases. J Gastroenterol 2002;37(1):23–28.
24. Gore RM, Balthazar EJ, Ghahremani GG, Miller FH. CT features of ulcerative colitis and Crohn's disease. AJR Am J Roentgenol 1996;167(1):3–15.
25. Choi D, Jin LS, Ah CY, et al. Bowel wall thickening in patients with Crohn's disease: CT patterns and correlation with inflammatory activity. Clin Radiol 2003;58(1):68–74.
26. Lee SS, Ha HK, Yang SK, et al. CT of prominent pericolic or perienteric vasculature in patients with Crohn's disease: correlation with clinical disease activity and findings on barium studies. AJR Am J Roentgenol 2002;179(4):1029–36.

27 Pickhardt PJ, Choi JR, Hwang I, *et al.* Computed tomographic virtual colonoscopy to screen for colorectal neoplasia in asymptomatic adults. *N Engl J Med* 2003;349(23):2191–2200.

28 Yee J, Akerkar GA, Hung RK, Steinauer-Gebauer AM, Wall SD, McQuaid KR. Colorectal neoplasia: performance characteristics of CT colonography for detection in 300 patients. *Radiology* 2001;219(3):685–92.

29 Tarjan Z, Zagoni T, Gyorke T, Mester A, Karlinger K, Mako EK. Spiral CT colonography in inflammatory bowel disease. *Eur J Radiol* 2000;35(3):193–8.

30 Ota Y, Matsui T, Ono H, *et al.* Value of virtual computed tomographic colonography for Crohn's colitis: comparison with endoscopy and barium enema. *Abdom Imaging* 2003;28(6):778–83.

31 Papanikolaou N, Prassopoulos P, Grammatikakis I, Maris T, Gourtsoyiannis NC. Technical challenges and clinical applications of magnetic resonance enteroclysis. *Top Magn Reson Imaging* 2002;13(6):397–408.

32 Low RN, Francis IR. MR imaging of the gastrointestinal tract with i.v. gadolinium and diluted barium oral contrast media compared with unenhanced MR imaging and CT. *AJR Am J Roentgenol* 1997;169(4):1051–9.

33 Schunk K. Small bowel magnetic resonance imaging for inflammatory bowel disease. *Top Magn Reson Imaging* 2002;13(6):409–25.

34 Bernardino ME, Weinreb JC, Mitchell DG, Small WC, Morris M. Safety and optimum concentration of a manganese chloride-based oral MR contrast agent. *J Magn Reson Imaging* 1994;4(6):872–6.

35 Karantanas AH, Papanikolaou N, Kalef-Ezra J, Challa A, Gourtsoyiannis N. Blueberry juice used per os in upper abdominal MR imaging: composition and initial clinical data. *Eur Radiol* 2000;10(6):909–13.

36 Prassopoulos P, Papanikolaou N, Grammatikakis J, Rousomoustakaki M, Maris T, Gourtsoyiannis N. MR enteroclysis imaging of Crohn disease. *Radiographics* 2001;21 Spec No:S161–72.

37 Minowa O, Ozaki Y, Kyogoku S, Shindoh N, Sumi Y, Katayama H. MR imaging of the small bowel using water as a contrast agent in a preliminary study with healthy volunteers. *AJR Am J Roentgenol* 1999;173(3):581–2.

38 Lauenstein TC, Schneemann H, Vogt FM, Herborn CU, Ruhm SG, Debatin JF. Optimization of oral contrast agents for MR imaging of the small bowel. *Radiology* 2003;228(1):279–83.

39 Laghi A, Borrelli O, Paolantonio P, *et al.* Contrast enhanced magnetic resonance imaging of the terminal ileum in children with Crohn's disease. *Gut* 2003;52(3):393–7.

40 Durno CA, Sherman P, Williams T, Shuckett B, Dupuis A, Griffiths AM. Magnetic resonance imaging to distinguish the type and severity of pediatric inflammatory bowel diseases. *J Pediatr Gastroenterol Nutr* 2000;30(2):170–4.

41 Rieber A, Wruk D, Potthast S, *et al.* Diagnostic imaging in Crohn's disease: comparison of magnetic resonance imaging and conventional imaging methods. *Int J Colorectal Dis* 2000;15(3):176–181.

42 Low RN, Francis IR, Politoske D, Bennett M. Crohn's disease evaluation: comparison of contrast-enhanced MR imaging and single-phase helical CT scanning. *J Magn Reson Imaging* 2000;11(2):127–35.

43 Schmidt S, Lepori D, Meuwly JY, *et al.* Prospective comparison of MR enteroclysis with multidetector spiral-CT enteroclysis: interobserver agreement and sensitivity by means of 'sign-by-sign' correlation. *Eur Radiol* 2003;13(6):1303–11.

44 Rieber A, Aschoff A, Nussle K, *et al.* MRI in the diagnosis of small bowel disease: use of positive and negative oral contrast media in combination with enteroclysis. *Eur Radiol* 2000;10(9):1377–82.

45 Schwartz DA, Loftus EV Jr, Tremaine WJ, *et al.* The natural history of fistulizing Crohn's disease in Olmsted County, Minnesota. *Gastroenterology* 2002;122(4):875–80.

46 Williams DR, Coller JA, Corman ML, Nugent FW, Veidenheimer MC. Anal complications in Crohn's disease. *Dis Colon Rectum* 1981;24(1):22–4.

47 Halligan S, Buchanan G. MR imaging of fistula-in-ano. *Eur J Radiol* 2003;47(2):98–107.

48 Buchanan G, Halligan S, Williams A, *et al.* Effect of MRI on clinical outcome of recurrent fistula-in-ano. *Lancet* 2002;360(9346):1661–2.

49 Van Assche G, Vanbeckevoort D, Bielen D, *et al.* Magnetic resonance imaging of the effects of infliximab on perianal fistulizing Crohn's disease. *Am J Gastroenterol* 2003;98(2):332–9.

50 Koh DM, Miao Y, Chinn RJ, *et al.* MR imaging evaluation of the activity of Crohn's disease. *AJR Am J Roentgenol* 2001;177(6):1325–32.

51 Maccioni F, Viscido A, Broglia L, *et al.* Evaluation of Crohn disease activity with magnetic resonance imaging. *Abdom Imaging* 2000;25(3):219–28.

52 Schunk K, Kern A, Oberholzer K, *et al.* Hydro-MRI in Crohn's disease: appraisal of disease activity. *Invest Radiol* 2000;35(7):431–7.

53 Rieber A, Wruk D, Nussle K, *et al.* MRI of the abdomen combined with enteroclysis in Crohn disease using oral and intravenous Gd-DTPA. *Radiologe* 1998;38(1):23–8.

54. Shoenut JP, Semelka RC, Magro CM, Silverman R, Yaffe CS, Micflikier AB. Comparison of magnetic resonance imaging and endoscopy in distinguishing the type and severity of inflammatory bowel disease. *J Clin Gastroenterol* 1994;19(1):31–5.
55. Pauls S, Kratzer W, Rieber A, et al. Quantifying the inflammatory activity in Crohn's disease using CE dynamic MRI. *Rofo Fortschr Geb Rontgenstr Neuen Bildgeb Verfahr* 2003;175(8):1093–9.
56. Tarjan Z, Toth G, Gyorke T, Mester A, Karlinger K, Mako EK. Ultrasound in Crohn's disease of the small bowel. *Eur J Radiol* 2000;35(3):176–82.
57. Sarrazin J, Wilson SR. Manifestations of Crohn disease at US. *Radiographics* 1996;16(3):499–520.
58. O'Malley ME, Wilson SR. US of gastrointestinal tract abnormalities with CT correlation. *Radiographics* 2003;23(1):59–72.
59. Bozkurt T, Richter F, Lux G. Ultrasonography as a primary diagnostic tool in patients with inflammatory disease and tumors of the small intestine and large bowel. *J Clin Ultrasound* 1994;22(2):85–91.
60. Sheridan MB, Nicholson DA, Martin DF. Transabdominal ultrasonography as the primary investigation in patients with suspected Crohn's disease or recurrence: a prospective study. *Clin Radiol* 1993;48(6):402–4.
61. Lim JH, Ko YT, Lee DH, Lim JW, Kim TH. Sonography of inflammatory bowel disease: findings and value in differential diagnosis. *AJR Am J Roentgenol* 1994;163(2):343–7.
62. Solvig J, Ekberg O, Lindgren S, Floren CH, Nilsson P. Ultrasound examination of the small bowel: comparison with enteroclysis in patients with Crohn disease. *Abdom Imaging* 1995;20(4):323–6.
63. Hollerbach S, Geissler A, Schiegl H, et al. The accuracy of abdominal ultrasound in the assessment of bowel disorders. *Scand J Gastroenterol* 1998;33(11):1201–8.
64. Pradel JA, David XR, Taourel P, Djafari M, Veyrac M, Bruel JM. Sonographic assessment of the normal and abnormal bowel wall in nondiverticular ileitis and colitis. *Abdom Imaging* 1997;22(2):167–72.
65. Sonnenberg A, Erckenbrecht J, Peter P, Niederau C. Detection of Crohn's disease by ultrasound. *Gastroenterology* 1982;83(2):430–4.
66. Reimund JM, Jung-Chaigneau E, Chamouard P, Wittersheim C, Duclos B, Baumann R. Diagnostic value of high resolution sonography in Crohn's disease and ulcerative colitis. *Gastroenterol Clin Biol* 1999;23(6-7):740–6.
67. Maconi G, Parente F, Bollani S, Cesana B, Bianchi PG. Abdominal ultrasound in the assessment of extent and activity of Crohn's disease: clinical significance and implication of bowel wall thickening. *Am J Gastroenterol* 1996;91(8):1604–9.
68. Parente F, Greco S, Molteni M, et al. Role of early ultrasound in detecting inflammatory intestinal disorders and identifying their anatomical location within the bowel. *Aliment Pharmacol Ther* 2003;18(10):1009–16.
69. Parente F, Maconi G, Bollani S, et al. Bowel ultrasound in assessment of Crohn's disease and detection of related small bowel strictures: a prospective comparative study versus x ray and intraoperative findings. *Gut* 2002;50(4):490–5.
70. Potthast S, Rieber A, Von Tirpitz C, Wruk D, Adler G, Brambs HJ. Ultrasound and magnetic resonance imaging in Crohn's disease: a comparison. *Eur Radiol* 2002;12(6):1416–22.
71. Maconi G, Bollani S, Bianchi PG. Ultrasonographic detection of intestinal complications in Crohn's disease. *Dig Dis Sci* 1996;41(8):1643–8.
72. Gasche C, Moser G, Turetschek K, Schober E, Moeschl P, Oberhuber G. Transabdominal bowel sonography for the detection of intestinal complications in Crohn's disease. *Gut* 1999;44(1):112–7.
73. Heyne R, Rickes S, Bock P, Schreiber S, Wermke W, Lochs H. Non-invasive evaluation of activity in inflammatory bowel disease by power Doppler sonography. *Z Gastroenterol* 2002;40(3):171–5.
74. Spalinger J, Patriquin H, Miron MC, et al. Doppler US in patients with crohn disease: vessel density in the diseased bowel reflects disease activity. *Radiology* 2000;217(3):787–91.
75. Esteban JM, Maldonado L, Sanchiz V, Minguez M, Benages A. Activity of Crohn's disease assessed by colour Doppler ultrasound analysis of the affected loops. *Eur Radiol* 2001;11(8):1423–8.
76. Rogoveanu I, Saftoiu A, Cazacu S, Ciurea T. Color Doppler transabdominal ultrasonography for the assessment of the patients with inflammatory bowel disease during treatment. *Rom J Gastroenterol* 2003;12(4):277–81.
77. Maconi G, Sampietro GM, Russo A, et al. The vascularity of internal fistulae in Crohn's disease: an *in vivo* power Doppler ultrasonography assessment. *Gut* 2002;50(4):496–500.
78. van Oostayen JA, Wasser MN, van Hogezand RA, Griffioen G, de Roos A. Activity of Crohn disease assessed by measurement of superior mesenteric artery flow with Doppler US. *Radiology* 1994;193(2):551–4.
79. Bolondi L, Gaiani S, Brignola C, et al. Changes in splanchnic hemodynamics in inflammatory bowel disease. Non-invasive assessment by Doppler

ultrasound flowmetry. *Scand J Gastroenterol* 1992;27(6):501–7.
80 Ludwig D, Wiener S, Bruning A, Schwarting K, Jantschek G, Stange EF. Mesenteric blood flow is related to disease activity and risk of relapse in Crohn's disease: a prospective follow-up study. *Am J Gastroenterol* 1999;94(10):2942–50.
81 Mirk P, Palazzoni G, Gimondo P. Doppler sonography of hemodynamic changes of the inferior mesenteric artery in inflammatory bowel disease: preliminary data. *AJR Am J Roentgenol* 1999;173(2):381–7.
82 Britton I, Maguire C, Adams C, Russell RI, Leen E. Assessment of the role and reliability of sonographic post-prandial flow response in grading Crohn's disease activity. *Clin Radiol* 1998;53(8):599–603.
83 Maconi G, Parente F, Bollani S, *et al*. Factors affecting splanchnic haemodynamics in Crohn's disease: a prospective controlled study using Doppler ultrasound. *Gut* 1998;43(5):645–50.
84 Byrne MF, Farrell MA, Abass S, *et al*. Assessment of Crohn's disease activity by Doppler sonography of the superior mesenteric artery, clinical evaluation and the Crohn's disease activity index: a prospective study. *Clin Radiol* 2001;56(12):973–8.
85 Neurath MF, Vehling D, Schunk K, *et al*. Noninvasive assessment of Crohn's disease activity: a comparison of 18F-fluorodeoxyglucose positron emission tomography, hydromagnetic resonance imaging, and granulocyte scintigraphy with labeled antibodies. *Am J Gastroenterol* 2002;97(8):1978–85.

III: Management of ulcerative colitis

9: Mesalazine for maintenance therapy in ulcerative colitis – how much, how long?

Miles P. Sparrow, Wee-Chian Lim and Stephen B. Hanauer

Mesalazine for maintenance therapy in ulcerative colitis – how much, how long?

Crohn's disease (CD) and ulcerative colitis (UC), which together comprise the idiopathic inflammatory bowel diseases (IBD), are chronic, relapsing and remitting conditions that require biphasic pharmacologic therapy: first with induction agents and then with maintenance agents. Aminosalicylates or 5-aminosalicylic acid (5-ASA, mesalazine, mesalamine) remain the mainstay of therapy for both the induction and maintenance of remission in UC, and with these agents annual relapse rates can be reduced to 30–50%, as compared to 80% if no maintenance agent is added [1].

Sulphasalazine, the prototype aminosalicylate that combines sulphapyridine (an antibiotic) with the anti-inflammatory 5-ASA was found to be efficacious for UC in the 1940s. It was not until the 1970s that 5-ASA was recognised as the active moiety, with the sulphapyridine component acting as an inert carrier molecule that delivers the 5-ASA to the site of active mucosal inflammation in the colon [2]. This discovery and the recognition that the 'sulpha' component was responsible for most of the allergic and dose-dependent side effects of sulphasalazine, led to the development of various sulpha-free mesalazine formulations that carry 5-ASA to the inflamed small bowel and colonic mucosa.

Broadly speaking, the newer 5-ASA formulations can be categorised as either sulpha-free azo-bonded pro-drugs or sulpha-free coated 5-ASAs. Pro-drugs (sulphasalazine, balsalazide and olsalazine) contain azo-bonds that conjugate different carrier molecules to the 5-ASA moiety, which are then released when the azo-bond is cleaved by colonic bacterial azo-reductases. In balsalazide, the inert carrier molecule is 4-aminobenzoyl-β alanine; olsalazine consists of two 5-ASA molecules joined by an azo-bond. The sulpha-free coated 5-ASA preparations include pH-dependent delayed-release (Asacol®) and time-dependent controlled-release (Pentasa®) formulations. Delayed-release Asacol® is a 5-ASA coated with Eudragit-S, an acrylic-based resin, which dissolves at pH 7 or higher, beginning in the terminal ileum or caecum. Controlled-release Pentasa® incorporates 5-ASA into microgranules of ethylcellulose, a semi-permeable membrane that dissolves when hydrated, releasing mesalamine in a time-dependent fashion throughout the small bowel and colon. At the molecular level, aminosalicylates are known to possess a wide array of anti-inflammatory and immunomodulatory actions, but the exact mechanism of action of 5-ASAs in IBD is unknown; it is theorised that the 5-ASAs exert a topical effect on the intestinal mucosa rather than a systemic effect [3]. In the background of this brief introduction to aminosalicylate formulations and their delivery, the evidence regarding their use in UC, with emphasis on their role as maintenance agents, will now be reviewed. Mesalazine maintenance therapy of UC: how much should be given? As an induction agent in mild-moderate UC, mesalazine induces remission in 40–74% of patients at doses of 1.5–4.8 g daily [4], with a dose-response demonstrated for doses up to 3 g (olsalazine) [5], 4.8 g (Asacol®) [6] and 6.75 g (balsalazide) [7]. Despite this knowledge, the optimal 5-ASA dose for the treatment of active disease is yet to be determined; however, based on trials with Asacol®, the current recommendation is for dose-titration up to 4.8 g/day [6].

Once complete remission of UC has been induced, maintenance therapy should be instituted; but again, the optimal dose of 5-ASA therapy needed to prevent relapse is unknown. Sulphasalazine maintains remission in 71–88% of patients when given at doses of 1–4 g/day, with a dose response demonstrated up to 4 g/day. However, at these higher doses adverse effects attributable to the sulphapyridine component become problematic in 30–40% of patients; maintenance doses of 2 g/day are more commonly employed [8]. In the only maintenance dose-ranging studies for mesalazine, there was no dose-response between 800 mg and 1.6 g daily of Asacol® [9]. In another study comparing 1.5 g daily and 3 g daily Pentasa®, there was a trend favouring the higher dose that nearly reached statistical significance ($p = 0.057$) [10]. However, neither of these trials looked at the dose response in patients who required higher doses of mesalazine to achieve remission, and it is probable that a dose response exists up to 4.8 g daily [11].

A recent Cochrane systematic review showed that mesalazine at doses of 0.8–4 g daily was superior to placebo at maintaining remission in UC, with a pooled odds ratio (OR) for relapse of 0.47 (CI 0.36–0.62) and a number needed to treat (NNT) of 6; however a dose-dependent trend was not seen ($p = 0.489$). This same meta-analysis compared the efficacy of sulphasalazine and mesalazine formulations as maintenance agents, and the odds ratio for maintenance of remission favoured sulphasalazine over mesalazine (OR 1.20; CI 1.05–1.57), unlike for induction therapy where the odds ratio favoured mesalazine (OR 0.87; CI 0.63–1.21) [12].

Whereas it used to be common to reduce the aminosalicylate dosage once remission had been attained, the current standard of care is to maintain the same dose of mesalazine for induction and maintenance therapy [13]. There is evidence to demonstrate the long-term safety of mesalazine at doses of up to 5 g daily [14]. Numerous gaps in the data remain, such as confirmation of the dose response for maintenance therapy, and dose-ranging studies are needed to clarify whether oral mesalazine can maintain corticosteroid-induced remissions.

With respect to choosing which formulation of mesalazine should be used for maintaining remission in UC, there is currently insufficient evidence to suggest that one formulation is superior to another, and a recent systematic review found no difference in the pharmacokinetic profile of the various oral 5-ASA formulations [15]. Hence, the selection of oral 5-ASA formulation or 5-ASA pro-drug as a maintenance agent should be based on a combination of efficacy data, the potential for adverse effects and practical issues such as compliance and cost [16].

Patients with left-sided UC should be treated with topical (rectal) 5-ASA for both the induction and maintenance of remission. Given that 80% of incident cases of UC have endoscopic disease distal to the splenic flexure, and 95% of incident cases are mild or moderate in severity, the majority of patients with UC could benefit from rectal 5-ASA therapy over the course of their disease. In practice, oral aminosalicylates are used more commonly in this setting due to patient preferences [17]. The delivery formulations available as topical 5-ASA therapies include suppositories, foams and liquid enemas; the appropriate form for each patient depends on the proximal extent of mucosal disease. Suppositories reach the upper rectum, foams typically reach the proximal sigmoid and enemas typically reach the splenic flexure. As induction agents in left-sided disease, meta-analyses have shown topical mesalazine to be superior to placebo, oral mesalazine and topical corticosteroids, although a dose response has not been demonstrated for doses greater than 1 g/day [18, 19]. In patients not responding to either topical mesalazine or topical corticosteroid, the combination of the two is superior to using either agent alone [20], and similarly, the combination of oral and topical mesalazine therapy is more efficacious than using either agent alone [21].

As maintenance agents in left-sided UC, topical mesalazine in doses as low as 1 g/day have been shown to be as efficacious as oral mesalazine [22], and efficacy can be maintained even if the dosing interval is reduced to every other day or every third day [19]. A combination of oral and topical mesalazine may prove to be the most effective way to maintain remission. In a 1-year double-blind study of 72 patients who had experienced two or more relapses in the previous year, but were currently in remission, relapse occurred in 64% of patients taking oral therapy alone, but in only 36% of patients receiving the combination of oral mesalazine 1.6 g/day and twice weekly mesalamine enemas 4 g/100 mL [23]. In patients with proctitis, suppositories of 5-ASA are effective in maintaining remission. In a double-blind study comparing 5-ASA suppositories 500 mg twice daily with placebo, cumulative 1-year relapse rates were 47% in the placebo group versus 10% in the treatment group [24].

Mesalazine for maintenance therapy in UC: how long should it be used?

Although aminosalicylates are effective maintenance agents in quiescent UC [12], the duration of therapy remains controversial. It is not clear if all patients should be treated indefinitely or whether there exists a subgroup of patients whose treatment can be discontinued. Foundational 5-ASA maintenance trials had follow-up durations of less than 2 years, and 'longer term' maintenance efficacy rates compared with placebo remain unexplored. Although a recent prospective cohort study revealed that all patients with newly diagnosed UC relapsed within 10 years despite long-term 5-ASA maintenance therapy, in particular those with extensive disease, with the majority of patients doing so in the first 2–3 years, the oral maintenance dose of 1.6 g daily may not have been optimal [25]. Several randomised trials that have attempted to answer these questions also produced conflicting results. An early withdrawal trial did not find a difference in relapse rates at 6 months, in patients who had been in remission for at least 1 year with sulphasalazine, after randomisation to either continuing maintenance treatment with sulphasalazine or placebo, suggesting that perhaps maintenance treatment may be discontinued in this group of patients [26]. This finding was disputed by a subsequent study that recommended indefinite maintenance therapy. Sixty-four patients with prolonged clinical, endoscopic and histological remission while taking sulphasalazine were randomised to continue treatment or placebo in a double-blind, double-dummy trial; at 6 months, placebo-treated patients had more than four times the relapse rate of those receiving sulphasalazine [27]. However, these early studies do suffer from methodological flaws and failed to clearly define the baseline characteristics of enrolled patients (duration and extent of disease, length of remission and previous treatment received). Therefore, these studies did not allow identification of patient subgroups with higher relapse risks that would benefit from continuing therapy.

In the latest placebo-controlled trial with a longer duration of follow-up (12 months), mesalazine maintenance therapy significantly reduced the relapse rates in UC patients who had been in clinical, endoscopic and histological remission for 1–2 years with aminosalicylate therapy. This was true in a subset of older patients who had been in remission for more than 2 years, had a longer duration of disease and a lower mean risk of relapse per year [28]. However, the statistical power of this study was compromised due to insufficient recruitment and should be interpreted with caution. Until more convincing data emerges, aminosalicylate maintenance therapy should be continued on a long-term basis to prevent disease relapse.

The recent flurry of data demonstrating the potential for aminosalicylates to reduce cancer risk provides yet another compelling reason to continue long-term maintenance therapy. Although one study did not find a significant difference in 5-ASA use between colorectal cancer cases and controls, the duration of 5-ASA therapy was less than 2 years [29]. In contrast, data from retrospective case control and cohort studies supports a protective effect for sulphasalazine in compliant patients [30] who had taken doses of more than 2 g/day [31] for at least 3 months [32]. Similarly, regular mesalazine (in patients on it for less than 1 year, and without medications in a 5–10-year period) also conferred a protective effect, decreasing the risk of cancer by 81% at doses of more than 1.2 g/day [31]. These findings were corroborated in a similar study that demonstrated a 76% cancer risk reduction for patients taking more than 1.2 g/day of mesalazine [33].

Finally, patient adherence is crucial to the success of long-term pharmacological maintenance therapy. Single men, multiple concomitant medications [34] and frequent dosing [35] are associated with non-adherence and increasing the risk of relapse among patients with quiescent ulcerative colitis [36]. Patient education, self-directed management strategies [37] and single-dosing schedules [38] will help improve patient compliance and eventual outcome.

References

1. Klotz U. The role of aminosalicylates at the beginning of the new millennium in the treatment of chronic inflammatory bowel disease. *Eur J Clin Pharmacol* 2000;56(5):353–62.
2. Azad Khan AK, Piris J, Truelove SC. An experiment to determine the active therapeutic moiety of sulphasalazine. *Lancet* 1977;2(8044):892–5.
3. MacDermott RP. Progress in understanding the mechanisms of action of 5-aminosalicylic acid. *Am J Gastroenterol* 2000;95(12):3343–5.
4. Sutherland L, MacDonald JK. Oral 5-aminosalicylic acid for induction of remission in ulcerative colitis. *Cochrane Database Syst Rev* 2003;(3):CD000543.
5. Meyers S, Sachar DB, Present DH, Janowitz HD. Olsalazine sodium in the treatment of ulcerative colitis among patients intolerant of sulphasalazine: a prospective, randomized, placebo-controlled, double-blind, dose-ranging clinical trial. *Gastroenterology* 1987;93(6):1255–62.
6. Schroeder KW, Tremaine WJ, Ilstrup DM. Coated oral 5-aminosalicylic acid therapy for mildly to moderately active ulcerative colitis: a randomized study. *N Engl J Med* 1987;317(26):1625–9.
7. Levine DS, Riff DS, Pruitt R, Wruble L, Koval G, Sales D, Bell JK, Johnson LK. A randomized, double blind, dose-response comparison of balsalazide (6.75 g), balsalazide (2.25 g), and mesalamine (2.4 g) in the treatment of active, mild-to-moderate ulcerative colitis. *Am J Gastroenterol* 2002;97(6):1398–407.
8. Azad Khan AK, Howes DT, Piris J, Truelove SC. AQ Optimum dose of sulphasalazine for maintenance treatment in ulcerative colitis. *Gut* 1980;21(3):232–40.
9. Hanaller SB, Sninsky CA, Robinson M, Powers BJ, McHattie JO, Mayle JE, Elson CO, DeMicco MP, Butt JH, Pruitt RE, Bozdech JM, Safdi MA. An oral preparation of mesalamine as long-term maintenance therapy for ulcerative colitis: a randomized, placebo-controlled trial. The mesalamine study group. *Ann Intern Med* 1996;124(2):204–11.
10. Fockens P, Mulder CJ, Tytgat, GN, Blok P, Ferwerda J, Meuwissen SG, Tuynman HA, Dekker W, Gasthuis K, Van Hee PA. Comparison of the efficacy and safety of 1.5 compared with 3.0 g oral slow-release mesalazine (pentasa) in the maintenance treatment of ulcerative colitis. Dutch Pentasa study group. *Eur J Gastroenterol Hepatol* 1995;7(11):1025–30.
11. Kornbluth A, Sachar DB. Ulcerative colitis practice guidelines in adults. American College of Gastroenterology, Practice Parameters Committee. *Am J Gastroenterol* 1997;92(2):204–11.
12. Sutherland L, Roth D, Beck P, MayG, Makiyama K. Oral 5-aminosalicylic acid for maintenance of remission in ulcerative colitis. *Cochrane Database Syst Rev* 2002;(4):CD000544.
13. Hanauer SB, Present DH. The state of the art in the management of inflammatory bowel disease. *Rev Gastroenterol Disord* 2003;3(2):81–92.
14. Cunliffe RN, Scott BB. Review article: monitoring for drug side-effects in inflammatory bowel disease. *Aliment Pharmacol Ther* 2002;16(4):647–62.
15. Sandborn WJ, Hanauer SB. Systematic review: the pharmacokinetic profiles of oral mesalazine formulations and mesalazine pro-drugs used in the management of ulcerative colitis. *Aliment Pharmacol Ther* 2003;17(1):29–42.
16. Sandborn WJ. Rational selection of oral 5-aminosalicylate formulations and prodrugs for the treatment of ulcerative colitis. *Am J Gastroenterol* 2002;97(12):2939–41.
17. Marshall JK, Irvine EJ. Putting rectal 5-aminosalicylic acid in its place: the role in distal ulcerative colitis. *Am J Gastroenterol* 2000;95(7):1628–36.
18. Marshall JK, Irvine EJ. Rectal aminosalicylate therapy for distal ulcerative colitis: a meta-analysis. *Aliment Pharmacol Ther* 1995;9(3):293–300.
19. Cohen RD, Woseth DM, Thisted RA, Hanauer SB. A meta-analysis and overview of the literature on treatment options for left-sided ulcerative colitis and ulcerative proctitis. *Am J Gastroenterol* 2000;95(5):1263–76.
20. Mulder CJ, Focken P, Meijier JW, Van der Heide H, Wiltink EH, Tytgat GN. Beclomethasone dipropionate (3 mg) versus 5-aminosalicylic acid (2 g) versus the combination of both (3 mg/2 g) as retention enemas in active ulcerative proctitis. *Eur J Gastroenterol Hepatol* 1996;8(6):549–53.
21. Safdi M, DeMicco M, Sninsky C, Bank P, Wruble L, Deren J, Koval G, Nichols T, Targan S, Fleishman C, Wiita B. A double-blind comparison of oral versus rectal mesalamine versus combination therapy in the

22. Trallori G, Messori A, Scuffi C, Bardazzi G, Silvano R, d'Albario G, Pacini F. 5-Aminosalicylic acid enemas to maintain remission in left-sided ulcerative colitis: a meta- and economic analysis. *J Clin Gastroenterol* 1995;20(3):257–9.

23. d'Albasio G, Pacini F, Camarri E, Messori A, Trallori G, Bonanomi AG, Bardazzi G, Milla M, Ferrero S, Biagini M, Quaranta S, Amorosi A. Combined therapy with 5-aminosalicylic acid tablets and enemas for maintaining remission in ulcerative colitis: a randomized double-blind study. *Am J Gastroenterol* 1997;92(7):1143–7.

24. d'Albasio G, Paoluzi P, Campieri M, Porro GB, Pera A, Prantera C, Sturniolo GE, Miglioli, M. Maintenance treatment of ulcerative proctitis with mesalazine suppositories: a double-blind placebo-controlled trial. The Italian IBD study group. *Am J Gastroenterol* 1998;93(5):799–803.

25. Bresci G, Parisi G, Bertoni M, Capria A. Long-term maintenance treatment in ulcerative colitis: a 10-year follow-up. *Dig Liver Dis* 2002;34(6):419–23.

26. Riis P, Anthonisen P, Wulff HR, Folkenburg O, Bonnevie O, Binder V. The prophylactic effect of salazosulphapyridine in ulcerative colitis during long-term treatment: a double-blind trial on patients asymptomatic for one year. *Scand J Gastroenterol* 1973;8(1):71–4.

27. Dissanayake A S, Truelove SC. A controlled therapeutic trial of long-term maintenance treatment of ulcerative colitis with sulphazalazine (salazopyrin). *Gut* 1973;14(12):923–6.

28. Ardizzone S, Petrillo M, Imbesi V, Cerutti R, Bollani S, Bianchi S, Bianch Porro G. Is maintenance therapy always necessary for patients with ulcerative colitis in remission? *Aliment Pharmacol Ther* 1999;13(3):373–9.

29. Bernstein CN, Blanchard JF, Metge C, Yogendran M. Does the use of 5-aminosalicylates in inflammatory bowel disease prevent the development of colorectal cancer? *Am J Gastroenterol* 2003;98(12):2784–8.

30. Moody GA, Jayanthi V, Probert CS, Mackey H, Mayberry JF. Long-term therapy with sulphasalazine protects against colorectal cancer in ulcerative colitis: a retrospective study of colorectal cancer risk and compliance with treatment in Leicestershire. *Eur J Gastroenterol Hepatol* 1996;8(12):1179–83.

31. Eaden J, Arams K, Ekbom A, Jackson E, Mayberry J. Colorectal cancer prevention in ulcerative colitis: a case-control study. *Aliment Pharmacol Ther* 2000;14(2):145–53.

32. Pinczowski D, Ekbom A, Baron J, Yuen J, Adami HO. Risk factors for colorectal cancer in patients with ulcerative colitis: a case-control study. *Gastroenterology* 1994;107(1):117–20.

33. Rubin D. Use of 5-ASA is associated with decreased risk of dysplasia and colon cancer in ulcerative colitis. *Gastroenterology* 2003;124:A279.

34. Kane SV, Cohen RD, Aikens JE, Hanauer SB. Prevalence of nonadherence with maintenance mesalamine in quiescent ulcerative colitis. *Am J Gastroenterol* 2001;96(10):2929–33.

35. Shale MJ, Riley SA. Studies of compliance with delayed-release mesalazine therapy in patients with inflammatory bowel disease. *Aliment Pharmacol Ther* 2003;18(2):191–8.

36. Kane S, Huo D, Aikens J, Hanauer S. Medication nonadherence and the outcomes of patients with quiescent ulcerative colitis. *Am J Med* 2003;114(1):39–43.

37. Robinson A, Thompson DG, Wilkin D, Roberts C. Guided self-management and patient-directed follow-up of ulcerative colitis: a randomised trial. *Lancet* 2001;358(9286):976–81.

38. Kane S, Huo D, Magnanti K. A pilot feasibility study of once daily versus conventional dosing mesalamine for maintenance of ulcerative colitis. *Clin Gastroenterol Hepatol* 2003;1(3):170–3.

10: Refractory distal colitis
Simon Travis

Refractory distal colitis

Refractory distal colitis remains a common clinical dilemma. The reasons for refractoriness and optimum management are debated and the very definition of refractoriness is controversial. This reflects the paucity of data. Consequently, the management approach presented in this chapter is based as much on opinion as on scientific evidence. Nevertheless, it is essential to have a strategy for such patients, because there is otherwise a tendency for a haphazard series of therapeutic trials during which both the patient and doctor become demoralised by persistent symptoms.

Definition

What is meant by refractoriness?

Refractoriness implies an inadequate response to conventional treatment. Both response and treatment need to be specified. An adequate response must mean a return to the patient's normal bowel function, which, for the sake of an objective criterion, implies three or fewer stools/day without visible bleeding or urgency. All too frequently, clinical improvement is considered an acceptable response, leaving patients to put up with persistent symptoms from inadequately treated disease. This is as true of clinical trials as it is in practice, making therapeutic comparisons difficult [1]. The three criteria for evaluating response to treatment in therapeutic trials must be clinical, endoscopic and histological remission. Of these, clinical remission is the most important, because this is what matters to the patient.

What constitutes conventional treatment is more debatable. For some this means treatment with oral aminosalicylates and topical steroids, with refractoriness defined as an inadequate response after 6–8 weeks [2]. Others identify different components of refractoriness, including inability to withdraw steroids without a flare-up of activity, relapse unresponsive to re-treatment, limited duration of remission after steroid withdrawal or proximal extension of disease on therapy [3]. Trials indicate that oral salicylates and topical steroids are inadequate in comparison to systemic steroids (see below). For the purposes of this chapter, refractory distal colitis is defined as persistent symptoms due to colonic inflammation confined to the rectum or recto-sigmoid colon despite treatment with oral and topical steroids for 6–8 weeks.

What is the prevalence of refractoriness?

The prevalence of refractory distal colitis is around 20%, but is uncertain just because the management of active distal colitis is so variable. When 40 consecutive patients with active distal colitis (24 proctitis, 16 proctosigmoiditis), median age 48 (23–86) years were treated by a staged management protocol (Fig 10.1), 22/40 (55%) achieved remission with topical therapy [4]. Of the remaining, 8/40 (20%) had active disease after oral steroids and met the criteria of refractoriness. Of these 8, 3 responded to further oral steroids and mesalazine enemas,

Relapse in a patient with distal colitis
Oral aminosalicylates ≥4 g/day
with hydrocortisone foam enemas or mesalazine enemas

Remission

2–4 weeks

Symptoms continue: evaluate severity and pattern of disease
Prednisolone 40 mg/day, tapering over 8 week (moderate)
20 mg, tapering over 6 week (mild), with steroid enema

6–8 weeks

Remission

Olsalazine 2 g/day maintenance

Symptoms continue
Refractory distal colitis

Consider differential diagnosis (Table 10.1)
Sigmoidoscopy, biopsy and stool culture
Start mesalazine foam enemas 1 g at night (distal colitis)
or mesalazine 1 g suppositories (proctitis)

4 weeks

Remission

Olsalazine 2 g/day maintenance
or
rectal mesalazine 1 g/day

Symptoms continue
Plain abdominal X-ray: treat proximal constipation
Repeat sigmoidoscopy
Prednisolone 40 mg daily
Azathioprine 2 mg/kg/day
Use steroid enema in the morning, mesalazine enema at night
Change mesalazine enemas to suppositories if not tolerated

2–4 weeks

Improvement

Continue

No change in symptoms
Admit for intensive treatment
Flexible sigmoidoscopy to re-evaluate disease extent
Discuss views on surgery; see stomatherapist

1 week

Remission

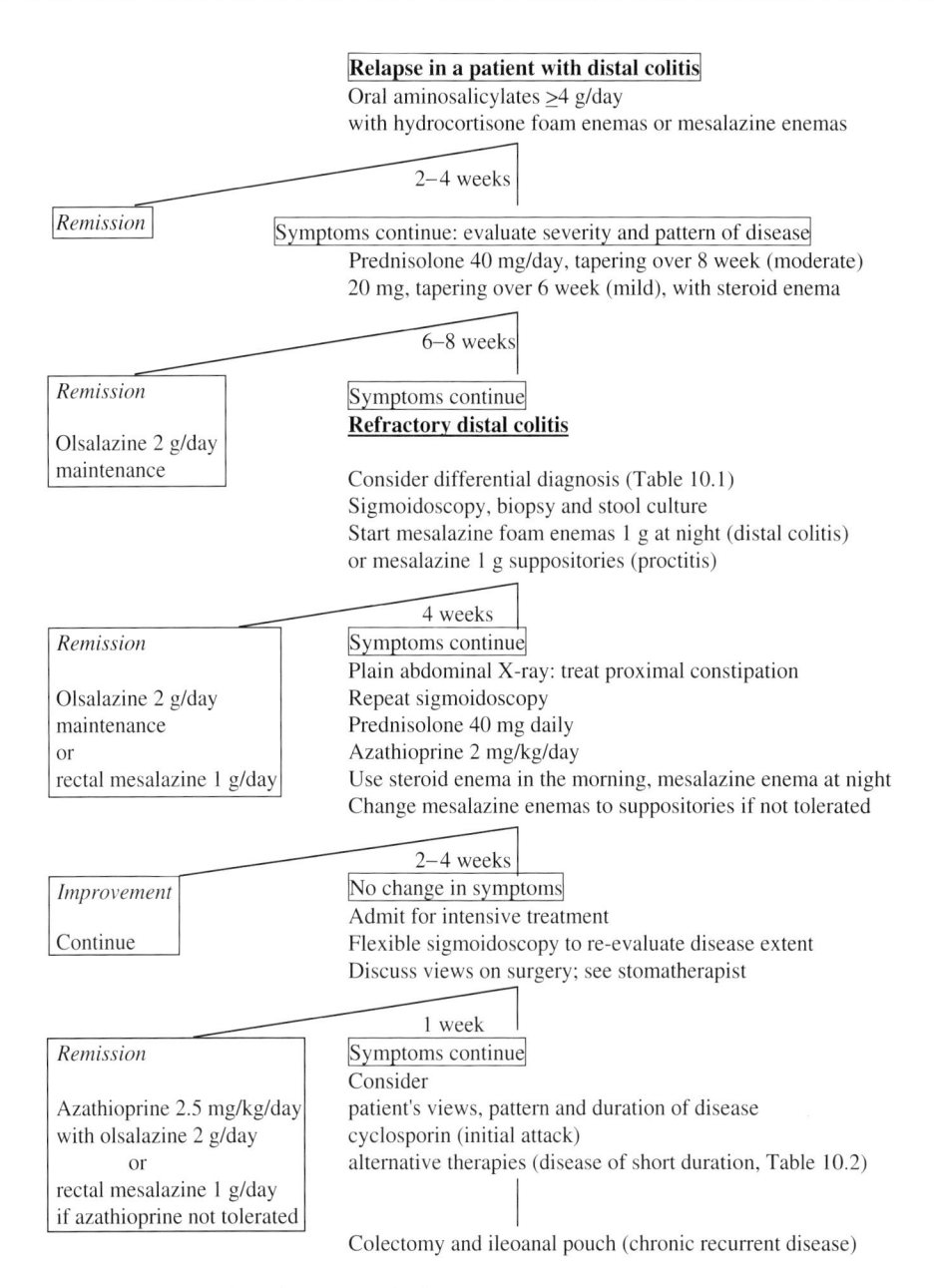

Azathioprine 2.5 mg/kg/day
with olsalazine 2 g/day
or
rectal mesalazine 1 g/day
if azathioprine not tolerated

Symptoms continue
Consider
patient's views, pattern and duration of disease
cyclosporin (initial attack)
alternative therapies (disease of short duration, Table 10.2)

Colectomy and ileoanal pouch (chronic recurrent disease)

Fig 10.1 Management algorithm for refractory distal colitis.

1 entered remission after treatment of proximal constipation and 3 after intensive intravenous treatment. One came to colectomy. Numbers are small, but they represent clinical practice and such patients are over-represented in outpatient clinics because of frequent attendance.

Pathophysiology

What defines distal disease?

The extent of disease reflects differences between one part of the colon and another. There are physiological differences between the proximal and distal colon, including energy substrate, epithelial permeability and electrolyte transport [5]. Toll-like receptor [6] and Paneth cell distribution [7], cytokine profiles [8] and stromal influences on cell function [9]. The proximal colonic epithelium, for instance, uses glutamine and glucose as well as short-chain fatty acids for oxidative metabolism, whereas the distal colonic epithelium is primarily dependent on butyrate [10]. This influences mucosal integrity, leucocyte recruitment [11] and resistance to injury, although it is a paradox that colitis starts in the less permeable epithelium of the distal colon. Mucosal blood flow [12], neuronal distribution [13] and motility [14] also differ between proximal and distal colon during inflammation, thereby influencing colonic epithelial function. A fuller discussion of colonic heterogeneity and how host-bacterial interactions might provoke pro-inflammatory responses that lead to colitis is discussed in Chapter 4 [15].

The endoscopic limit of inflammation in distal colitis can be very striking and none of the differences between proximal and distal colon (other, perhaps, than neuronal distribution) appear abrupt enough to account for the sharp demarcation between inflamed and normal mucosa that is often observed within a centimetre or two. Furthermore, the extent of colonic involvement is clearly dynamic, as illustrated by the proximal extension of proctitis or regression of more extensive disease over time [16, 17]. This argues against the micro-vascular supply determining the proximal extent of disease [18], so other explanations have to be sought. One is a threshold phenomenon. Epithelial and mucosal changes from normal to inflamed colon may indeed be gradual, but there may be a threshold above which destructive inflammation is triggered. A threshold phenomenon would explain the abrupt line of demarcation, as well as the variable extent of disease, and still be consistent with other biological concepts, including that of controlled inflammation as a physiological process in the colon [15]. Another explanation is neuroimmune. The limit of inflammation may be controlled by interactions between enteric neurones, stromal myoepithelial cells and fibroblasts, other constituents of the mucosal matrix and immune cell apoptosis that have yet to be fully defined [19]. Peripheral evidence to support this view is provided by the increased cell density and total cellularity in distal colitis compared to the mucosa of patients with extensive disease [20], as well as the increased numbers of mast cells at the line of demarcation [21]. The leading edge of inflammation in distal colitis needs further attention.

Why does distal colitis become refractory?

The reasons that distal disease becomes refractory can be divided into the environmental and physiological. Environmental factors include patient adherence with therapy, inadequate concentrations of the active drug, the wrong drug, or co-existent infection. Apart from adherence and the delivery system, the choice of drug is clearly relevant. Topical corticosteroids, for instance, are less effective than topical salicylates (below) and the possibility that co-existing therapy (such as non-steroidal anti-inflammatory drugs) or infection might be causing refractory disease should always be considered.

Adherence

The issue of adherence (or compliance) with therapy is shockingly simple. Note that adherence implies choice, with the onus on the doctor to inform and the patient to decide about taking treatment, although compliance implies expectation and fault. In a follow-up study of 99 patients, all those who relapsed within 6 months took less than 80% of the prescribed dose and at 12 months, 68% (13/19 who relapsed) were non-adherent, compared to 26% who took more than 80% of the prescribed dose [22]. The risk of relapse in poorly adherent patients was increased five-fold (OR 5.5, CI 2.3–13.2). The prevalence of non-adherence with maintenance therapy is high. Out of 98 Sheffield patients with UC, 42% reported taking less than 80% of the prescribed dose, but urine analysis of 5-ASA and N-acetyl 5-ASA showed that self-reporting identified only 66% of those with poor adherence [23]. This is similar to the Chicago experience, where the median dispensed dose of 5-ASA was 71% of that prescribed (range 8–130%) [24]. Factors associated with poor adherence include being male (OR 2.1, CI 1.2–4.9), four or more prescriptions (OR 2.5, CI 1.4–5.7), full time employment (OR 2.7, CI 1.1–6.9) and three times daily dosing (OR

3.1, CI 1.8–8.4). Being married helped (OR for poor adherence 0.46, CI 0.39–0.57). Adherence of patients with refractory disease needing thiopurines may be slightly better, but 4/82 patients (5%) on azathioprine or mercaptopurine had no detectable serum thioguanine, indicating that they were taking none of the medication [25]. Although adherence or compliance is typically more problematic in maintenance therapy for asymptomatic individuals, these studies underscore the relatively high rate of non-adherence in this patient population. Explanation and patient education regarding the principles of disease management and techniques of drug administration are required if outcome is to improve.

Tissue concentration of 5ASA

Inadequate drug concentrations also affect relapse and reflect the delivery system. The mucosal concentration of 5-ASA is inversely proportional to endoscopic and histological activity in ulcerative colitis ($r = 0.712$, $p < 0.001$) [26]. For oral salicylates, azo-bonded compounds (such as sulphasalazine, olsalazine, or balsalazide) deliver a higher concentration of 5-aminosalicylic acid to the distal colon at equivalent doses than controlled-release Pentasa or Asacol [27]. The mucosal concentration of 5-ASA has been reported to be higher with sulphasalazine than mesalazine in one study [28], but not another [29, 30]. What is clear, however, is that topical 5-ASA massively increases the concentration of mucosal 5-ASA [28, 29]. Frieri and colleagues have shown that increasing the tissue concentration of 5-ASA by up to 100-fold by doubling the dose of oral and topical 5-ASA reduced the relapse rate 10-fold in patients with refractory disease over a 2-year period [31]. The aim should also be to achieve a high concentration of 5-ASA in the rectal mucosa of those with refractory distal colitis.

Pharmacokinetics of rectal therapy

A suppository, once dissolved, has greater viscosity and mucosal adherence than liquid or foam enemas, but only coats the rectum and recto-sigmoid junction [32]. The distribution of a foam or liquid enema, however, depends on the volume and rectal response to installation. In healthy volunteers, a 100 mL enema reached the splenic flexure in 7 out of 8 subjects, whilst a 40 mL foam enema remained in the sigmoid colon in 50% [33]. Reflex rectal contraction aids proximal distribution, but the greater the contraction, the less medication contact time there is in the rectum. In 31 patients with active disease, less than 10% of 30, 60 or 100 mL enemas remained in the rectum as measured by scintigraphy, with most (66–99%) in the sigmoid colon [34]. When gels were examined by scintigraphy, a low volume (20 mL) had a similar distribution to 80 mL (up to the descending colon), but the study rather missed the point that length is not everything and efficacy may depend on the amount remaining in the rectum [35]. Gels are a logical formulation for topical therapy and more variety (5-ASA, ropivacaine) should become available. Given the anorectal instability associated with active distal inflammation, the pressure generated by rectal contraction after instillation of an enema can overcome anal sphincter tone and lead to immediate evacuation. This means that suppositories may be better tolerated, achieve a higher concentration of drug at the site of inflammation and be effective where enemas have failed. Suppositories may be a useful adjunct to treatment with enemas for distal disease.

Physiological factors that may contribute to refractory disease include cellular steroid receptor expression and poor rectal compliance. Steroid receptors express either an active α chain, or a β chain that is an intra-cellular antagonist of glucocorticoid activity. β chain mRNA was detectable in 10 of 12 poor responders to corticosteroids, but in only 1 of 11 responders and 2 of 20 healthy subjects. All expressed the α chain [36]. Steroid receptor sensitivity has been examined by using the concentration of dexamethasone necessary to inhibit T cell proliferation stimulated by phytohaemaglutinin. In severe colitis treated with intravenous steroids, all 11 complete responders had T cells sensitive (>60% inhibition of proliferation) to less than 150 nM dexamethasone, compared to 2 of 7 poor responders [37]. Such trials have not addressed response in distal colitis, but offer an intriguing insight into the mechanisms of refractoriness. Poor rectal compliance as a consequence of chronic inflammation, however, can cause persistent symptoms even in the absence of inflammation and, as indicated above, may diminish mucosal contact time for topical therapies. With diminished rectal compliance urgency and stool frequency increase, because the desire to defecate is triggered by low stool volume.

Management approach

Strategy

The importance of a management strategy to avoid haphazard therapeutic trials of treatment in refractory distal colitis cannot be over emphasised. The stages should be discussed with the patient, who usually appreciates the sense of direction, even if the response remains poor. My own approach when symptoms persist after initial treatment is first to review the diagnosis followed by a trial of mesalazine enemas. Proximal constipation is then treated, before introducing azathioprine with further corticosteroids. If colitis remains active after this, the patient is admitted for intensive treatment and the extent of disease reassessed at colonoscopy. The opportunity is taken during admission to discuss progress, the impact of continuing symptoms on lifestyle, the patient's own wishes and the possibility of surgery. As a final stage, alternative therapies may be given a trial, largely based on anecdotal evidence, before surgery (Fig 10.1).

Conventional treatment of active distal colitis

Therapeutic trials in ulcerative colitis suffer from many problems that make comparison difficult [1, 38]. Lack of controlled data, insufficient statistical power, clinical heterogeneity, incomplete reporting of follow-up and ill-defined endpoints, are the main problems. Meta-analyses have attempted to resolve these issues, although in one analysis of rectal corticosteroids [39], 50 of 83 trials were rejected because of lack of randomisation, inclusion of patients with extensive colitis or Crohn's disease or duplicate reporting of data. In one key area (that of comparing oral salicylates with oral steroids) there are almost no comparative data. This matters when considering the speed of response to treatment, which is as much of concern to patients suffering miserable symptoms, as potential side effects. For each patient it is fundamental to assess both the severity of relapse (mild, moderate or severe) and the clinical pattern of disease (intermittent, frequently relapsing or chronic continuous), according to well-established criteria [1, 40, 41].

Oral aminosalicylates and rectal steroids

Oral aminosalicylates and rectal corticosteroids are commonly used as initial treatment for active ulcerative colitis, but in controlled trials around half of mild to moderate attacks of colitis do not respond within 6 weeks. For example, in 158 patients given Asacol 2.4 g, 1.6 g or placebo daily with rectal steroids, the response (not remission) rate after 6 weeks was 49, 43 and 23%, respectively [42]. Clinical response characteristically occurs at twice the remission rate. In a meta-analysis of oral 5-ASA compounds for active disease [38], the outcome of interest on an intention to treat principle was the failure to induce remission. A pooled odds ratio of less than 1.0 indicated one treatment to be more effective than another. Mesalazine was about twice as effective as placebo (OR 0.51, CI 0.35–0.76), but not significantly better than sulphasalazine (OR 0.87, CI 0.63–1.21). Meta-analyses, however, have not addressed the speed of response. It is often the speed of response that matters most to patients, who want rapid resolution of symptoms that are interfering with their life. Because aminosalicylates are well tolerated, there is a vogue (especially in the United States) for using very high doses (>4 g/day) to treat active colitis. The most recent trial examined oral Asacol 4.8 g versus 2.4 g daily in 268 patients with moderate UC, 50% of who had distal disease [43]. The treatment response at 6 weeks was 72% in the 4.8 g group and 59% in the 2.4 g group ($p = 0.036$), regardless of the extent of disease, although complete remission was achieved in only 20 and 17%, respectively. When the time to relief of specific symptoms was examined, 80% given 4.8 g and 70% given 2.4 g had cessation of rectal bleeding within 1 month.

Combination treatment with oral and rectal steroids

The modest response to oral aminosalicylates is in contrast to two early studies on combination therapy with oral and rectal corticosteroids. Oral prednisolone (starting at 40 mg daily) with steroid enemas induced remission in 77% of 118 patients with mild to moderate disease within 2 weeks, compared to 48% treated with 8 g/day sulphasalazine and steroid enemas [44]. Similar findings were reported by Lennard-Jones [45], who found the combination of oral and rectal steroids to be better than either alone. An appropriate regimen for moderately active disease (bloody stool frequency 5–6 times daily with no systemic features) is prednisolone 40 mg/day for 1 week, 30 mg/day for 1 week, then 20 mg/day for 1 month before decreasing by 5 mg/day/week. Topical steroids can be given twice daily whilst there is visible bleeding, then once at night until oral steroids cease. Shorter courses are associated with early relapse and doses of prednisolone less than or equal to 15 mg day are ineffective for active disease [46]. Oral steroids with low systemic bioavailability (prednisolone metasulphobenzoate) and a colonic release mechanism are at a preliminary stage of development [47].

Although it may seem odd to base therapeutic recommendations on trials performed 40 years ago, the evidence they provide on clinical efficacy and speed of response has not been superseded. Side effects to systemic steroids remain a real concern, but when the data on speed of remission are explained to the patient, decisive treatment is usually appreciated when there has been no response to oral salicylates and topical therapy within a fortnight. Persisting with treatment that is ineffective in 50% beyond this period puts a considerable burden on patients when symptoms are interfering with work and lifestyle. Distal disease may respond rapidly to topical salicylates (for example, 64% clinical and 52% endoscopic remission after just 2 weeks on mesalazine suppositories 1 g daily [48]), but distal colitis can be as debilitating as more extensive disease. When symptoms are debilitating, limited disease is better treated as if it was more extensive. There is a clinical suspicion, but as yet no objective evidence, that refractory colitis is less common if a relapse is effectively treated at an early stage.

Differential diagnosis

If symptoms persist after oral and topical steroids, the disease can appropriately be called refractory and the diagnosis needs to be reviewed (Table 10.1). Commonly, a co-existent irritable bowel accounts

Table 10.1 Differential diagnosis of refractory distal colitis.

Condition
Irritable bowel syndrome with anal canal bleeding
Aminosalicylate-induced colitis
Solitary rectal ulcer (mucosal prolapse) syndrome
Crohn's proctitis
Neoplasia (carcinoma, lymphoma)
Infection (*Cytomegalovirus* sp., *Chlamydia* spp., *Herpes simplex*, opportunistic)
Quiescent colitis with poor rectal compliance
Radiation proctitis

for more symptoms than active disease. This should be suspected if abdominal pain and bloating are prominent, with only a granular mucosa visible on sigmoidoscopy. If symptoms are disproportionate to the objective evidence of disease, then they may respond to additional fibre, antispasmodics or other treatment for an irritable bowel. Care should, however, be taken to ensure that topical therapy has not induced relative rectal sparing, leaving active inflammation beyond the reach of a rigid sigmoidoscope. Symptoms of pain and bloating can also be a feature of proximal constipation. The possibility of dietary intolerance or hypolactasia should be excluded.

Other conditions should be evident from a careful review of the history and histology. Rectal mucosal prolapse (solitary rectal ulcer syndrome) classically mimics the symptoms of proctitis, but erythema on the rectal wall is focal and the biopsy shows characteristic interdigitating muscle fibres. Crohn's proctitis usually responds to similar treatment to ulcerative proctitis, but when refractory may indicate local infection that responds to metronidazole. In the absence of granulomas, histological features of discontinuous crypt distortion, focal inflammation and limited goblet cell depletion favour Crohn's [49]. The possibility of secondary colitis (from sepsis in the pelvis) should be considered. An elevated C-reactive protein (CRP), platelet count, or weight loss in distal colitis or proctitis justifies pelvic magnetic resonance imaging and small bowel radiology. Radiation proctitis should be identified by the history. Infective proctitis is rarely chronic, but exceptions are amoebic colitis, Cytomegalovirus in the immunocompromised, or sexually transmitted infection (*Chlamydia* spp.,

Herpes simplex). Very occasionally, salicylate therapy may itself provoke colitis [50]. Patients usually improve within 72 h of stopping treatment and experience a rapid (<24 h) symptomatic and endoscopic relapse if rechallenged with rectal mesalazine [3]. Assuming none of these conditions apply and inflammation remains active, then further treatment of the distal colitis is appropriate, starting with a change in topical therapy.

Topical salicylates

Topical mesalazine (5-ASA) induced remission in active distal colitis in 31–80% (median 67%) compared to 7–11% given placebo in a meta-analysis of 11 trials in 778 patients [51]. The properties and distribution of topical preparations (suppository, foam, liquid enema or gel) need to be taken into account to ensure the maximum concentration of 5-ASA at the site of disease activity (see above).

Advantages over rectal corticosteroids

There is clear evidence that topical mesalazine is more effective than topical steroids. The pooled odds ratio comparing the two in seven trials showed rectal 5-ASA to be superior for disease remission, whether for symptoms (OR 2.42, CI 1.72–3.41), endoscopy (OR 1.89, CI 1.29–2.76), or histology (OR 2.03, CI 1.28–3.20) [39]. In the largest trial of 295 patients treated for 4 weeks, 52% on Asacol foam enemas entered remission compared to 31% on Predfoam ($p < 0.001$, intention to treat) [52]. The combination of high-dose oral and topical mesalazine has also been compared with oral therapy alone in the treatment of active *extensive* colitis [53]. In 127 patients, 90% improved after combination treatment (Pentasa 4 g, Pentasa enema 1 g) for 4 weeks, compared to 62% on Pentasa alone ($p = 0.0008$) and 64% were in remission by 8 weeks compared to 43% ($p = 0.03$) respectively. It begins to approach the efficacy of oral steroids, although the speed of response is slower. It is also consistent with a much-quoted earlier study [54] and clearly indicates that combination oral and topical 5-ASA therapy is preferable to monotherapy.

Topical salicylates compared with steroids of low systemic bioavailability

Two further advantages of topical salicylates over conventional steroid enemas are the absence of adrenal suppression during long-term use and the ability to maintain remission. The potential systemic effects of rectal hydrocortisone or prednisolone may be clinically detectable after 8 weeks [55], but can be exaggerated. Biochemical adrenal suppression is detectable before 8 weeks, but is clinically unimportant. Nevertheless, steroids with low systemic bioavailability have been developed (budesonide, beclomethasone dipropionate, prednisolone metasulphobenzoate, tixocortol pivalate) for topical use. Such 'newer' steroids are still less effective than topical salicylates. Clinical remission after 4 weeks on budesonide enemas was 38% compared with 60% on mesalazine foam enemas ($p = 0.03$) [56]. A dose-ranging study of budesonide enemas in 233 patients with left-sided colitis reported 19% clinical remission on 2.0 mg and 27% remission on 8.0 mg, compared to 4% on placebo after 6 weeks [57]. This is unimpressive, although clearly better than placebo. Of greater interest is a study showing that the combination of beclomethasone dipropionate (3 mg) and mesalazine (2 g) enemas produced significantly better clinical, endoscopic and histological improvement than either agent alone [58]. Consequently, a combination of corticosteroid enemas in the morning and mesalazine enemas in the evening is a useful practical approach for refractory distal disease.

Dose and delivery

All trials in active distal colitis have used at least 1 g rectal 5-ASA daily, but there is no dose-response relationship. In a study of 113 patients with active distal colitis, remission rates after 30 days on 1, 2 and 4g enemas were 63, 67 and 72%, respectively [51, 59]. Disease activity does not influence the distribution of enemas, but less than 10% of an aminosalicylate enema remains in the rectum over 4 h [34]. On the other hand, the type of suppository and delivery system may matter. In 50 patients with active proctitis, a single high-dose suppository (Pentasa 1 g) was more rapidly effective than 500 mg (Claversal) suppositories twice daily [48]. Clinical (and endoscopic) remission occurred in 64% (52%) within 2 weeks on Pentasa, compared with 28% (24%) on Claversal suppositories ($p < 0.01$). Not surprisingly, once daily therapy was more popular with patients. Suppositories or foam salicylate enemas are better tolerated than liquid enemas. In 233 patients with active distal colitis, 81% reported a good acceptance of mesalazine foam enemas compared to 49% given liquid enemas of the same dose [60]. This is likely to affect adherence with therapy.

It will be apparent that most data relate to uncomplicated proctitis or distal colitis rather than refractory disease. For patients with refractory left-sided ulcerative colitis (unresponsive to, or intolerant of, rectal or oral corticosteroids, or oral salicylates), salicylate enemas have been shown to be effective [61]. Remission was achieved in 54% after 12 weeks and 80% after 34 weeks, allowing patients to reduce or discontinue corticosteroids. A novel approach to improving outcome has been to add topical butyrate to 5-ASA enemas. When 51 patients with refractory disease received topical 5-ASA 2 g and butyrate twice daily, remission occurred in 6/24 compared to 1/27 on 5-ASA and saline enemas ($p < 0.05$) [62]. When considered with the results of the Italian study on refractory disease [31], topical salicylates should be started at an early stage. The type of application (enema, foam or suppository) should be changed if one formulation cannot be tolerated and combinations (suppository and enema) considered. There may, however, be other reasons for a poor response, including proximal constipation.

Proximal constipation

Proximal colonic stasis is induced by abnormal intestinal motility in patients with distal ulcerative colitis. The motility disorder is characterised by delayed mouth to caecum transit time, prolonged transit through uninvolved colon and rapid transit through inflamed distal colon [63]. This implies physiological changes in the small bowel and uninvolved colon, presumably through neuroendocrine or neuroimmune pathways. This may influence drug delivery to the distal colon. Scintigraphy has demonstrated that labelled, Eudragit-coated resin remained in the healthy proximal colon (91%,

CI 85–96) in 12 patients with active left-sided disease, so that only 9% (CI 4–15) was in the distal colon compared to 31% (CI 24–37) in 22 healthy controls ($p < 0.001$) [64]. This is a convincing explanation to account for the common clinical experience that relief of proximal constipation leads to resolution of refractory distal colitis. Consequently, if sigmoidoscopic inflammation persists after treatment with topical salicylates and oral steroids, a plain abdominal radiograph is appropriate. If there is visible faecal loading in the descending colon, a vigorous laxative (1–2 sachets of Picolax™) is appropriate, after explaining the paradox of proximal constipation despite distal diarrhoea. Topical salicylates should be continued, but if symptoms do not resolve within another 2–4 weeks, then intensive treatment is usually the best option.

Intensive treatment

Although more commonly a feature of extensive colitis, distal disease can present with a severe relapse (bloody stool frequency >6 daily, with either a pulse rate >90, temperature >37.8°C, haemoglobin <10.5 g/dL, or ESR >30 mm/h). This should be treated promptly by direct admission and intravenous steroids. In one study of 51 episodes of severe colitis, 16% had distal disease and in a further 18% disease was left-sided [65]. The standard treatment regime involves intravenous steroids (e.g. hydrocortisone 400 mg daily), rectal hydrocortisone and correction of electrolyte imbalance, anaemia or nutritional deficiency over 5 days. Antibiotics confer no additional benefit.

Intravenous steroids and ciclosporin

The real dilemma, however, is how best to manage patients with distal disease and continuing mild to moderate activity in spite of a course of oral steroids, topical salicylates and treatment of proximal constipation. Some gastroenterologists opt for further trials of topical therapy, often with alternative agents (see below). Distal colitis in these circumstances is best treated as if it was more extensive or severe. In 39 patients with distal disease refractory to outpatient treatment with oral steroids and salicylates, remission was achieved by intensive treatment within a week in 90% [66]. This is an impressive and rapid response in otherwise refractory disease and is better than that reported with alternative topical therapies. Should the response be poor, the role of ciclosporin is debatable. It certainly has a place in severe distal colitis not responding to intravenous steroids, because colectomy may be avoided in a patient with limited disease, which is especially valuable during an initial attack [67]. The pattern of disease must, however, be taken into account. Ciclosporin should only be used for refractory distal colitis if there is the potential to change the pattern of distal disease by using immunomodulators such as azathioprine.

Reassessing the extent of disease

During admission for intensive treatment of refractory distal colitis, it is appropriate to perform a colonoscopy (or flexible sigmoidoscopy if disease is severe) to re-evaluate the extent of disease. The risk of proximal extension of distal disease has been debated. In a population-based study of 1161 patients with ulcerative colitis, 48% had proctitis or distal disease, 32% left-sided, 18% total colitis and 2% undefined at presentation [68]. Subsequent proximal extension has conventionally been estimated at around 15%, but appears to be higher. In a retrospective study of 145 patients with distal colitis at presentation, disease extension proximal to the sigmoid was recorded in 36% at a median of 6 years, becoming extensive in 29% [16]. Using actuarial analysis, disease extension was predicted for 16% (CI 11–24%) at 5 years and 31% (CI 23–40%) 10 years after diagnosis. A similar proportion (27%) had disease extension in a larger study of 273 patients with distal UC, but only a minority extended beyond the splenic flexure (4 and 10% at 5 and 10 years, respectively) [69]. Interestingly, smoking appeared protective against disease extension. In contrast, in 399 patients with UC, the extent regressed in 22%, with 30% having a normal colonoscopy 14 months after diagnosis [17]. A 'caecal patch' lesion has been recognised in patients with typical clinical, endoscopic and histological features of limited distal ulcerative colitis, who have an isolated area of erythema and inflammation in the caecum [70]. Whether disease extension or refractoriness is more common in the presence of a caecal patch is unknown, but it should not trap the unwary into a diagnosis of Crohn's colitis. Finally, colonoscopy is helpful in excluding malignancy as a cause of refractoriness. Although the risk of colorectal cancer is not increased in distal colitis, sporadic cases may still occur.

Maintaining remission

Assuming that intensive treatment has succeeded in achieving remission, the next issue is how to maintain remission. It has long been established that neither topical nor systemic steroids are effective [71]. In spite of advocating systemic steroids at an early stage to induce effective remission, the effect of long-term (>10 weeks) or recurrent courses (>2/year) on skin, soft tissues and bone should be considered clinically unacceptable. The options are an appropriate type and dose of oral salicylate, continued topical salicylates, or immunosuppression.

Oral aminosalicylates

The main role for oral aminosalicylates is to maintain remission rather than treat active disease, but pharmacokinetic considerations influence the choice (see above, Fig 10.2). Azo-bonded drugs are theoretically preferable in distal colitis, because luminal concentrations of 5-ASA, probably reflecting concentrations in the colonic epithelium, are higher than with slow-release mesalazine [27]. This has been confirmed by measurement of tissue 5-ASA concentrations in some [28] but not all [30] studies and is supported by some clinical trials.

The most recent meta-analysis of maintenance therapy [72] analysed 16 trials on 2341 patients. Mesalazine was more effective than placebo (odds ratio for failure to maintain remission 0.47, CI 0.36–0.62) with an NNT of 6, but sulphasalazine had a small (but statistically significant OR 1.29, CI 1.05–1.57) benefit over mesalazine. In spite of this, there was no difference between the trials using low daily dosages (<2 g) and those using high dosages of mesalazine. This is a little surprising, but may be explained by differences in disease distribution among the patient populations, variable duration of follow-up (4–12 months) and definitions of relapse or remission. Dose is likely to be most relevant in

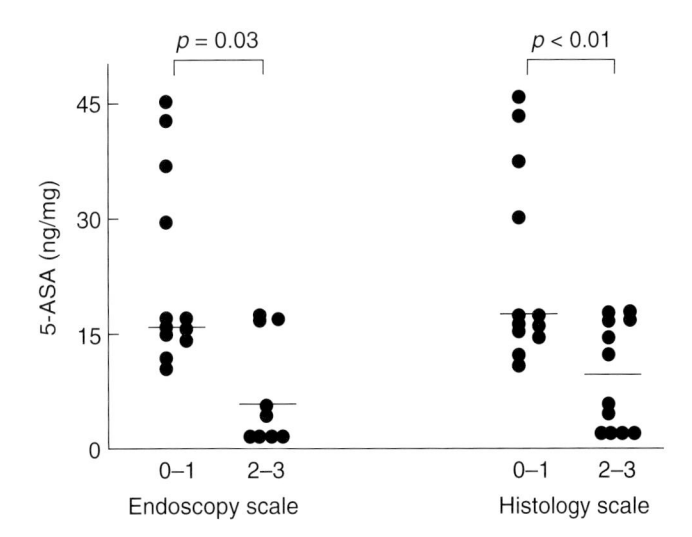

Fig 10.2 Endoscopic and histological activity in relation to mucosal 5-ASA concentrations. The higher the concentration of 5-ASA, the lower the disease activity (from Frieri et al. [26] with permission).

distal disease. When 198 patients were treated with 0.5, 1.0 or 2.0 g olsalazine for 12 months, the highest dose was most effective in proctitis (90% remission, $p = 0.03$) [73]. It was also most effective in those who had recently relapsed (<12 months) prior to the start of the trial. The tendency of olsalazine to induce small intestinal secretion and cause diarrhoea might be used to therapeutic advantage in the proximal constipation associated with refractory distal colitis. Why the choice and dose of salicylate does not appear to matter for more extensive colitis is an interesting question, but is likely to have something to do with the pathobiology of events at the leading edge of inflammation. Prevention of inflammation may be a threshold phenomenon, dependent on the concentration of 5-ASA at the proximal limit of inflammation and thus be largely independent of dose, if 5-ASA is effectively delivered.

Otherwise there are very few comparative trials between the new salicylates. Olsalazine appears to be more effective than Asacol™ [74], consistent with the relatively enhanced delivery to the distal colon by olsalazine. Care must be taken in interpreting this study of 100 patients with left-sided colitis, because it finished early and had an unexpectedly high relapse rate (46% on Asacol™ at 12 months vs 34% on olsalazine). In another maintenance study of 99 patients, balsalazide 3 g/day was more effective than Asacol™ for controlling nocturnal symptoms in remission (90% vs 77% asymptomatic, $p = 0.0011$), but the remission rate (58%) was identical at 12 months [75]. The difference is marginal and there was an exceptionally high withdrawal rate (57%), largely due to relapse. Caution is necessary in interpreting the results of comparative trials between 5-ASA compounds and differences between aminosalicylates other than sulfasalazine appear too small to be detected [76]. In practical terms, if olsalazine 2 g daily does not maintain remission in refractory distal colitis once it has been achieved, then topical maintenance therapy or immunosuppression is appropriate.

Topical salicylates

Topical 5-ASA as a liquid, foam, or suppository is undoubtedly effective at maintaining remission, but is less popular with patients. In 5 trials involving 182 patients given mesalazine suppositories or enemas (0.8–2 g daily, or 4 g intermittently) for 6–24 months, remission was maintained in 54–80% compared to 15–20% on placebo [51]. In two of the trials (98 patients), rectal salicylates were more effective than oral therapy over 2 years (OR 2.41, CI 1.05–5.54). Compliance may be improved with intermittent therapy and mesalazine 1 g (Pentasa) suppositories three times a week maintained remission in 52% over 1 year, compared to 38% on placebo ($p = 0.018$) [77]. Increasing the dose to 1 g daily in those who relapsed induced remission in 61% within 30 days compared to 8% given placebo. Consequently when oral salicylates alone fail,

Pentasa™ 1 g suppositories daily are appropriate for maintaining remission in refractory proctitis, or salicylate (Asacol™) foam enemas for distal colitis. The combination of oral and topical therapy in relatively refractory colitis is better than either alone. This was shown in 72 patients (63 with distal colitis) who had relapsed recently (<3 months) or frequently (>1 relapse/year) [122]. Patients were randomised to mesalazine 1.6 g daily, with placebo or mesalazine enemas twice weekly for 12 months. On combination therapy, 71% remained in remission, compared to 31% on oral therapy alone ($p = 0.036$). If aminosalicylates are ineffective or cannot be tolerated, however, immunosuppression is necessary, which is often the case after intensive treatment for refractory distal colitis.

Immunomodulators

Azathioprine and its metabolite 6-mercaptopurine are effective for patients who have frequent relapses, as well as those with chronically active disease that flares up when oral corticosteroids are reduced [78]. The standard dose for azathioprine is 2 mg/kg/day (1 mg/kg/day for 6-mercaptopurine) and several months of treatment is necessary for maximum effect. Much of the information about azathioprine has been transferred from trials on Crohn's disease, but it is effective as a steroid-sparing agent (NNT = 3) and should be considered for those who relapse rapidly (<6 weeks) after oral steroids, or who relapse at doses less than 15 mg/day. This is as true for distal colitis as for those with more extensive disease, although anecdotal experience from St Mark's on 52 patients who received immunomodulators out of a total of 228 with distal UC, suggested that efficacy may be lower in distal disease. Thiopurines had a clinically useful effect in 43%, were ineffective in 16% and caused toxicity in 34% [79]. This does not, however, reflect our experience.

For the majority who tolerate azathioprine, the question is how long it should be continued. In 67 patients in remission on azathioprine randomised to continue the drug or to placebo, 64% remained in remission on azathioprine at 1 year, compared to 41% on placebo ($p = 0.04$) [80]. A beneficial effect was detected for at least 2 years and if the effect in Crohn's disease can be extrapolated, the benefit may persist for 4–5 years or more [81]. It is customary to continue oral salicylates with azathioprine. There is, however, no evidence that the combination is better than azathioprine alone.

Methotrexate has been disappointing in controlled trials of refractory ulcerative colitis, unlike Crohn's disease, but doses have been low. A weekly dose of 12.5 mg (half of that used in Crohn's disease) was no better than placebo in induction or maintenance of remission in steroid-dependent ulcerative colitis [82]. The potential advantage is that patients who cannot tolerate azathioprine can often tolerate methotrexate (and vice versa). A review of the Oxford experience showed that oral methotrexate at a mean dose of 20 mg/week achieved a good response (steroid withdrawal) in 50% with refractory ulcerative colitis and a sustained remission off steroids in 15/42 patients over a period of 72 weeks [83]. Hence methotrexate can be considered for thiopurine intolerant patients with refractory distal colitis, although the lack of controlled evidence supporting its use should be recognised.

Alternative therapies

The choice of alternative therapies is large, but whilst this reflects the potential refractoriness of distal colitis and proctitis, it also indicates the reluctance of gastroenterologists to treat limited disease systemically. Using the approach outlined above, including intensive treatment, very few patients remain refractory. Some may consider this approach unnecessarily aggressive but it is, after all, much easier for the gastroenterologist to put up with a poor response to therapy than it is for the patient. Nevertheless, there are some patients with limited and troublesome disease rather than disabling symptoms, for whom colectomy might be avoided by patiently persisting with topical therapy. The problem with these alternatives is that most are based on open studies, or trials with insufficient power to detect a difference. The options do, however, illustrate innovative approaches to treatment, with an insight into proposed mechanisms of disease. Table 10.2 summarises the evidence. The choice really depends on local availability and personal preference, because many have to be made up individually by pharmacy. Some novel approaches, such as

Table 10.2 Summary of alternative therapies for distal colitis.

Agent	Proposed mechanism	Dose and duration	Design	n	Outcome	Reference
Anaesthetic gel	Neuroimmune modulation	lignocaine (800 mg) daily. 6–34 weeks	Open	100	Remission 10% proctitis, 83% distal colitis. Most had refractory disease; response in 6 patients with pancolitis	84
		lignocaine (600 mg) daily. 6 weeks	Open	22	12/22 'excellent', 4/22 'very good' response (refractory UC)	85
		ropivacaine (400 mg) daily. 2 weeks	Open	12	Clinical and endoscopic improvement ($p < 0.05$)	86
		ropivacaine (200 mg) single dose	Random	33	Rectal eicosanoid and neuropeptide concentrations similar after ropivacaine in 19 distal UC compared to 14 controls	87
Arsenic	Uncertain	Acetarsol (500 mg) vs prednisolone (5 mg) suppositories. 2 weeks	Random	20	9/10 clinical/endoscopic improvement (refractory distal colitis). Potential toxicity in 6/10 (1 week) 2/10 (4 weeks)	88
Bismuth compounds	Enhanced mucosal barrier? Reduced bacterial adhesion	Bismuth carbomer (450 mg) enema vs 5-ASA (2 g) enema. 4 weeks	Random	63	Bismuth 39% remission, 56% 5-ASA (trend in favour of 5-ASA, $p = 0.16$)	89
Bovine colostrum	Source of growth factors for epithelial restitution	Colostrum 10% (100 mL enema) vs placebo (albumin). 4 weeks	Random	14	Activity index −2.9 (−0.3 to −5.4) in colostrum group, vs +0.5 (−2.4 to +3.4) in placebo	90
Ciclosporin enemas	T cell immunosuppression	Ciclosporin 350 mg vs placebo. 4 weeks	Random	40	Ciclosporin 40% improvement vs placebo 45%. Open trials in refractory distal UC more favourable	91
Epidermal growth factor enemas	Epithelial restitution/repair	EGF 5 mcg (100 mL enema) vs placebo. 12 weeks	Random	24	83% remission at 4 weeks vs 8% on placebo. Rapid and promising; needs repeating. Concern about malignancy	92
Ecabet sodium enema	Mucosal protection	Ecabet sodium 1g in 20–50 mL. 2 weeks	Open	8	Clinical activity index decreased (5.3 ± 1.4–0.5 ± 0.8, $p < 0.05$)	93

(*Continued*)

Table 10.2 (Continued).

Agent	Proposed mechanism	Dose and duration	Design	n	Outcome	Reference
Immunoglobulin G enemas	Immune response promoter	IgG enema	Open	7	Ineffective. 1/7 improved.	94
Interleukin-10 enemas	? IL-10 deficiency in UC	IL-10 100 mcg enema for 10 day	Open	3	Endoscopic response in refractory left-sided colitis	95
Nicotine	Protective influence of smoking; ? neuroimmune	Transdermal nicotine (15–25 mg) vs placebo. 6 weeks	Random	72	Nicotine 48% remission, placebo 24% ($p = 0.03$)	96
		Transdermal nicotine vs placebo. 6 m	Random	80	No difference between groups for maintenance therapy	97
		Transdermal nicotine (15–25 mg) vs prednisolone (5–15 mg). 6 weeks	Random	61	Nicotine 21% remission vs 47% prednisolone ($p = 0.035$), intention to treat; 11/31 nicotine withdrawals (side-effects)	98
		Transdermal nicotine vs placebo. 4 weeks	Random	64	Nicotine 39% clinical response, placebo 9% ($p = 0.007$)	99
		Transdermal nicotine (15 mg) with 5-ASA enema vs enema + mesalazine 2.4 g. 4 weeks	Random	30	Remission 12/15 on nicotine + 5-ASA enema, 5/15 on oral 5-ASA + enema ($p = 0.027$)	100
		Nicotine tartrate enemas (3–6 mg). 4 weeks	Open	10	5/7 improved (previously unresponsive UC); 3 withdrawals	101
		Nicotine carbomer enemas (6 mg). 4 weeks	Open	22	16/17 improved (previously unresponsive. 6 withdrawals	102
Propionyl-L-carnitine (PLC) enemas	Epithelial (SCFA) nutrition	PLC 6 g (200 mL) twice daily.	Open	10	8/10 'improved significantly'	103
Ridogrel	see T × A2 inhibitor					
Short-chain fatty acids (variable composition)	Epithelial nutrition	SCFA mixture vs 5-ASA or steroid enema. 6 weeks	Random	45	Most improved in all three groups	104
		SCFA mixture vs placebo; 6 weeks	Random	40	70% SCFA clinical response, 20% placebo No change in endoscopic or histology scores	105
		SCFA mixture; 6 weeks	Open	10	5/10 responded well (refractory distal colitis)	106
		SCFA mixture vs placebo; 6 weeks	Random	103	No difference in clinical or histological response	107
		SCFA vs butyrate or placebo; 6 weeks	Random	47	No difference between three groups	108
		Butyrate vs placebo; 6 weeks	Random	38	No difference	109

Sucralfate	Enhanced mucosal barrier	Sucralfate 4 g vs prednisolone meta-sulphobenzoate 20 mg enemas; 4 weeks	Random	44	Predenema 71% cessation of bleeding, sucralfate 28%	110
		Sucralfate 10 g vs 5-ASA 2 g vs placebo 4 weeks	Random	50	5-ASA superior. Sucralfate no different from placebo	111
		Sucralfate 10 g vs hydrocortisone 100 mg enemas. 4 weeks	Random	40	Hydrocortisone 42% remission, sucralfate 15%, ($p < 0.05$)	112
		Sucralfate 20 g vs methylprednisolone 20 mg (100 mL) twice daily; 4 weeks.	Random	60	No difference between groups	113
Thromboxane A2 inhibitor	Inhibition of inflammatory mediator	Ridrogel 300 mg vs prednisolone 30 mg enemas; 4 weeks	Random	40	Ridrogel 65% endoscopic remission vs prednisolone 75% (no difference)	114
		Ridogrel 300 mg (40 mL)	Open	11	Decrease in mucosal T × B2, but not other PGs	115
Wheat grass juice	Prebiotic and antioxidant *Triticum aestivum*	WGJ (100 mL) vs placebo	Random	21	Decrease in activity index ($p = 0.031$) and rectal bleeding ($p = 0.025$) comapred to controls	116

antibiotics against *Fusobacterium varium* [117] or leucocytapheresis [118] are appealing, not least because they differ so appreciably from previous therapy. However, it is all the more important that such approaches (and technology-dependent leucocytapheresis in particular) are subjected to randomised controlled trials.

Surgery

Patients with chronically active disease affecting the quality of life or employment, who have not responded to intensive treatment or cannot tolerate immunosuppression, are candidates for surgery. Such a decision should never be precipitate, because refractory distal colitis is a chronic condition that rarely causes the systemic disturbance of more extensive colitis. The decision is quite appropriately deferred until all medical options have been vigorously applied, but a surgical option should be raised when a patient is admitted for intensive treatment, if only to gauge their response. The opportunity to discuss stomas and pouches with an experienced stomatherapist is often appreciated by the patient and relatives, because it provides information, even if this is subsequently unnecessary. Much depends on the individual patient's perception of disability caused by the disease and their attitude to surgery, but it also depends on the working relationship between gastroenterologist and colorectal surgeon. A total colectomy has to be performed, usually with ileoanal pouch formation, because segmental resection leaves that part of the colon most affected and is almost invariably followed by relapse affecting previously normal bowel.

Operation rates for refractory colitis vary widely, whatever the extent of disease. The practice in Copenhagen has a higher proportion of patients coming to surgery than in many centres, but represents the best population-based data available. Out of 498 patients with ulcerative colitis who had distal disease at presentation, 9% came to colectomy in the first year of diagnosis, followed by 1% in subsequent years [68]. This includes those patients whose disease became extensive rather than remaining distal, but at St Mark's Hospital (United Kingdom), 8/52 patients with refractory distal colitis

treated with immunomodulators came to colectomy [79]. This is a specialist practice, but for a general population of 250,000, around 1 colectomy every 1–2 years would be performed for distal disease.

Another surgical approach that has been suggested for the management of refractory ulcerative colitis is appendicectomy. A negative association between appendicectomy and the onset of UC is well recognised: about 2% of patients with UC have had an appendicectomy, compared to 11% of the general population. What is less well recognised is that prior appendicectomy influences the phenotype, with later onset and less severe disease (OR 0.15, CI 0.02–1.15, $p = 0.04$) [119]. The idea that elective appendicectomy may influence that pattern of refractory UC is challenging, but may be sustainable [120].

The outcome of colectomy and pouch formation for distal colitis is usually good. In 263 patients who had a restorative proctocolectomy at one French centre (1986–96), 27 had surgery for distal disease [121]. After surgery there was a significant decrease in mean (SD) diurnal stool frequency 8.2 (4) vs 4.7 (2) stools/day, nocturnal stool frequency and urgency in 26/27 vs 1/27 patients ($p < 0.001$). Previously unknown severe dysplasia was identified in 2 patients. All but one patient were satisfied with the results and 25/27 wished that they had had surgery sooner.

Conclusions

There is a pressing need for data to allow objective decision-making in the management of refractory distal colitis. On the current evidence, the algorithm (Fig 10.1) is a practical approach that should help because it is staged. Combining oral and topical therapy, using salicylate suppositories as an adjunct to enemas, admission for intensive treatment and maintaining remission with immunosuppression should be effective in the vast majority, without resorting to alternative therapies or surgery.

References

1 Irvine EJ. Assessing outcome in randomized clinical trials: inflammatory bowel disease.In: Satsangi J, Sutherland LR, eds.*Inflammatory Bowel Diseases*. London: Churchill Livingstone; 2003:319–33.

2. Jarnerot G, Lennard-Jones JE, Bianchi-Porro G, et al. Medical treatment of refractory distal ulcerative colitis. *Gastroenterol Int* 1991;4:93–8.

3. Griffin MG, Miner PB. Refractory distal colitis – explanations and options. *Aliment Pharmacol Ther* 1996;10:39–48.

4. Travis SPL, Dannatt E, McGovern DPB, Beale A, Jagadeesan S. Managed care for distal ulcerative colitis. *Gut* 2001;48(suppl 2):A87.

5. Amasheh S, Barmeyer C, Koch CS, et al. Cytokine-dependent transcriptional down-regulation of epithelial sodium channels in ulcerative colitis. *Gastroenterology* 2004;126:1711–20.

6. Ortega-Cava CF, Ishihara S, Rumi MA, et al. Strategic compartmentalization of toll-like receptor 4 in the mouse gut. *J Immunol* 2003;170:3977–85.

7. Tanaka M, Saito H, Kusumi T, et al. Spatial distribution and histogenesis of colorectal paneth cell metaplasia in idiopathic inflammatory bowel disease. *J Gastroenterol Hepatol* 2001;16:1353–9.

8. Sangfelt P, Carlson M, Thorn M, et al. Local release of human neutrophil lipocalin (HNL), IL-8 and TNF alpha is decreased as response to topical prednisolone treatment in distal ulcerative colitis and proctitis. *Dig Dis Sci* 2002;47:2064–9.

9. Medina C, Videla S, Radomski A, et al. Increased activity and expression of matrix metalloproteinase-9 ina rat model of distal colitis. *Am J Physiol* 2003;284: G116–22.

10. Velazquez OC, Lederer HM, Rombeau JL. Butyrate and the colonocyte. Production, absorption, metabolism, and therapeutic implications. *Adv Exp Med Biol* 1997;427:123–34.

11. Menzel T, Luhrs H, Zirlik S, et al. Butyrate inhibits leucocyte adhesion to endothelial cells via modulation of VCAM-1. *Inflamm Bowel Dis* 2004;10:122–8.

12. McLaren WJ, Anikijenko P, Thomas SG, et al. In vivo detection of morphological and microvascular changes of the colon in association with colitis using fiberoptic confocal imaging (FOCI). *Dig Dis Sci* 2002;47:2424–33.

13. Beyak MJ, Ramji N, Krol KM, et al. Two TTX-resistant sodium currents in mouse colonic dorsal root ganglia neurones and their role in colitis induced hyperexcitability. *Am J Physiol* 2004;287: G845–55.

14. Linden DR, Sharkey KA, Mawe GM. Enhanced excitability of myenteric AH neurones in the inflamed guinea-pig distal colon. *J Physiol* 2003;547(Pt 2): 589–601.

15. Mahida YR, Rolfe V. Host-bacterial interactions in inflammatory bowel disease. *Clin Sci* 2004;107: 331–41.

16. Ayres RC, Gillen CD, Walmsley RS, Allan RN. Progression of ulcerative proctosigmoiditis: incidence and factors influencing progression. *Eur J Gastroenterol & Hepatol* 1996;8:555–8.

17. Moum B, Ekbom A, Vatn MH, Elgjo K. Change in the extent of colonoscopic and histological involvement in ulcerative colitis over time. *Am J Gastrenterol* 1999; 94:1564–9.

18. Hamilton M, Dick R, Crawford L, et al. Is the proximal demarcation of ulcerative colitis determined by the territory of the inferior mesenteric artery? *Lancet* 1995;345:688–90.

19. Green DR, Kroemer G. The pathophysiology of mitochondrial cell death. *Science* 2004;305:626–9.

20. Jenkins D, Goodall A, Scott BB. Ulcerative colitis: one disease or two (quantitative histological differences between distal and extensive disease). *Gut* 1990;31: 426–30.

21. King TM, Biddle WL, Bhatia P, Moore J, Miner PB. Colonic mucosal mast cell distribution at the line of demarcation of active ulcerative colitis. *Dig Dis Sci* 1992;37:490–5.

22. Kane S, Huo D, Aikens J, Hanauer S. Medication nonadherence and the outcomes of patients with quiescent ulcerative colitis. *Am J Med* 2003;114: 39–43.

23. Shale MJ, Riley SA. Studies of compliance with delayed-release mesalazine therapy in patients with inflammatory bowel disease. *Aliment Pharmacol Ther* 2003;18:191–8.

24. Kane SV, Cohen RD, Aikens JE, Hanauer SB. Prevalence of nonadherence with maintenance mesalamine in quiescent ulcerative colitis. *Am J Gastroenterol* 2001;96:2929–33.

25. Cuffari C, Hunt S, Bayless T. Utilisation of erythrocyte 6-thioguanine metabolite levels to optimise azathioprine therapy in patients with inflammatory bowel disease. *Gut* 2001;48:642–8.

26. Frieri G, Giacomelli R, Pimpo M, et al. Mucosal 5-aminosalicylic acid concentration inversely correlates with severity of colonic inflammation in patients with ulcerative colitis. *Gut* 2000;47: 410–6.

27. Christensen LA, Fallingborg J, Jacobsen BA, et al. Comparative bioavailability of 5-aminosalicylic acid from controlled release preparation and an azo-bond preparation. *Aliment Pharmacol Ther* 1994;8: 289–94.

28. Naganuma M, Iwao Y, Ogata H, et al. Measurement of colonic mucosal concentrations of 5-aminosalicylic acid is useful for estimating its therapeutic efficacy in distal ulcerative colitis: comparison of orally administered mesalamine and sulfasalazine. *Inflamm Bowel Dis* 2001;7:221–5.

29 Hussain FN, Ajjan RA, Kapur K, Moustafa M, Riley SA. Once versus divided daily dosing with delayed-release mesalazine: a study of tissue drug concentrations and standard pharmacokinetic parameters. *Aliment Pharmacol Ther* 2001;15:53–62.

30 Hussain FN, Ajjan RA, Riley SA. Dose loading with delayed-release mesalazine: a study of tissue drug concentrations and standard pharmacokinetic parameters. *Br J Clin Pharmacol* 2000;49: 323–30.

31 Frieri G, Mariateresa P, Brigida G, et al. Long-term oral plus topical mesalazine in frequently relapsing ulcerative colitis. *Dig Liver Dis* 2005;37:92–96.

32 Williams CN, Haber G, Aquino JA. Double-blind, placebo-controlled evaluation of 5-ASA suppositories in active distal proctitis and measurement of extent of spread using 99mTc-labelled 5-ASA suppositories. *Dis Sci* 1987;32:71S–5S.

33 Brown J, Haines S, Wilding IR. Colonic spread of three rectally administered mesalazine (Pentasa) dosage forms in healthy volunteers as assessed by gamma scintigraphy. *Aliment Pharmacol Ther* 1997;11:685–91.

34 Van Bodegraven AA, Boer RO, Lourens J, Tuynman HARE, Sindram JW. Distribution of mesalazine enemas in active and quiescent ulcerative colitis. *Aliment Pharmacol Ther* 1996;10:327–32.

35 Arlander E, Cederlund T, Mare K. No volume effect on retrograde colonic spread of rectally-administered ropivacaine gel. *Aliment Pharmacol Ther* 2003;15: 655–60.

36 Honda M, Orii F, Ayabe T, et al. Expression of glucocorticoid receptor β in lymphocytes of patients with glucocorticoid-resistant ulcerative colitis. *Gastroenterology* 2000;118:819–66.

37 Hearing SD, Norman M, Probert CSJ, et al. Predicting therapeutic outcome in severe ulcerative colitis by measuring *in vitro* steroid sensitivity of proliferating peripheral blood lymphocytes. *Gut* 1999;45:382–8.

38 Sutherland L, MacDonald JK. Oral 5-aminosalicylic acid for induction of remission in ulcerative colitis. *Cochrane Database Syst Rev* 2003;3:CD000543.

39 Marshall JK, Irvine EJ. Rectal corticosteroids versus alternative treatment in ulcerative colitis: a meta-analysis. *Gut* 1997;40:775–81.

40 Truelove SC, Witts LJ. Cortisone in ulcerative colitis: a final report on a therapeutic trial. *Br Med J* 1955;2: 1041–8.

41 Edwards FC, Truelove SC. The course and prognosis of ulcerative colitis. Part I: short-term prognosis. Part II: long-term prognosis. *Gut* 1963;4:299–315.

42 Sninsky CA, Cort DH, Shanahan F, et al. Oral mesalamine (Asacol) for mildly to moderately active ulcerative colitis: a multicentre study. *Ann Intern Med* 1990;115:350–5.

43 Sandborn WJ, Hanauer SB, Katz S, et al. Efficacy and safety of Asacol 4.8 g/day (800 mg tablet) compared to 2.4 g/day (400 mg tablet) in treating moderately active ulcerative colitis. *Am J Gastroenterol* 2005; 100:2478–85.

44 Truelove SC, Watkinson G, Draper G. Comparison of corticosteroid and SASP therapy in ulcerative colitis. *Br Med J* 1962;2:1708-11.

45 Lennard-Jones JE, Longmore AJ, Newell AC, Wilson CWE, Avery Jones F. An assessment of prednisone, Salazopyrin and topical hydrocortisone hemisuccinate used as outpatient treatment for ulcerative colitis. *Gut* 1960;1:217–22.

46 Baron JH, Connell AM, Kanaghinis TG, et al. Outpatient treatment of ulcerative colitis: comparison between three doses of oral prednisone. *Br Med J* 1962;2:441–3.

47 Cameron EA, Binnie JA, Balan K, et al. Oral prednisolone metasulphobenzoate in the treatment of active ulcerative colitis. *Scand J Gastroenterol* 2003;38:535–7.

48 Gionchetti P, Rissole F, Ventura A, et al. Comparison of mesalazine suppositories in proctitis and distal proctosigmoiditis. *Aliment Pharmacol Ther* 1997;11: 1053–7.

49 Jenkins D, Balsitis M, Gallivan S, et al. Guidelines for the initial biopsy diagnosis of suspected chronic idiopathic inflammatory bowel disease. *BSG Guidelines in Gastroenterology*, BSG London 1997, or website http://www.bsg.org.uk/clinical/data/gmpcd.htm.

50 Loftus EV, Kane SV, Bjorkman D. Systematic review: short-term adverse effects of 5-aminosalicylic acid agents in the treatment of ulcerative colitis. *Aliment Pharmacol Ther* 2004;19:179–89.

51 Marshall JK, Irvine EJ. Rectal aminosalicylate therapy for distal ulcerative colitis: a meta-analysis. *Aliment Pharmacol Ther* 1995;9:293–300.

52 Lee FI, Jewell DP, Mani V, et al. A randomised trial comparing mesalazine and prednisolone foam enemas in patients with acute distal ulcerative colitis. *Gut* 1996;38:229–33.

53 Marteau P, Probert C, Lindgren S, et al. Comparison of the efficacy and tolerability of oral 4 g Pentasa (mesalazine) for 8 weeks combined during the initial 4 weeks with either Pentasa 1 g/100 mL enema or placebo enema in extensive mild/moderate active colitis: a randomised, parallel, double-blind trial. *Gut* 2005;54:960–5.

54 Safdi M, DeMicco M, Sninsky C, et al. A double-blind comparison of oral versus rectal mesalamine versus combination therapy in the treatment of distal ulcerative colitis. *Am J Gastroenterol* 1997;92:1867–71.

55 Richter F, Scheppach W. Innovations in topical therapy. *Bailliere's Clin Gastroenterol* 1997;11:97–109.

56 Lemann M, Galian A, Rutgeerts P, et al. Comparison of budesonide and 5-aminosalicylic acid enemas in active distal ulcerative colitis. *Aliment Pharmacol Ther* 1995;9:557–62.

57 Hanauer SB, Robinson M, Pruitt R, et al. Budesonide enema for the treatment of active distal ulcerative colitis and proctitis: a dose-ranging study. *Gastroenterology* 1998;115:525–32.

58 Mulder CJJ, Fockens P, Meijer JWR, et al. Beclomethasone dipropionate (3mg) versus 5-aminosalicylic acid (2 g) versus the combination of both (3 mg/2 g) as retention enemas in active ulcerative proctitis. *Eur J Gastroenterol Hepatol* 1996;8:549–53.

59 Campieri M, Gionchetti P, Belluzzi A, et al. Optimum dosage of 5-aminosalicylic acid as rectal enemas in patients with active ulcerative colitis. *Gut* 1991;32:929–31.

60 Campieri M, Paoluzi P, D'Albaiso G, et al. Better quality of therapy with 5-ASA colonic foam in active ulcerative colitis: a multicenter comparative trial with 5-ASA enemas. *Dig Dis Sci* 1993;38:1843–50.

61 Biddle WL, Miner PB. Long-term use of mesalamine enemas to induce remission in ulcerative colitis. *Gastroenterol* 1990;99:113–8.

62 Vernia P, Annese V, Bresci G, et al. Topical butyrate improves efficacy of 5-ASA in refractory distal ulcerative colitis: results of a multicentre trial. *Eur J Clin Invest* 2003;33:244–8.

63 Rao SSC, Read NW, Brown C, Bruce C, Holdsworth CD. Studies on the mechanism of bowel disturbance in ulcerative colitis. *Gastroenterology* 1987;93:934–40.

64 Hebden JM, Blackshaw PE, Perkins AC, Wilson CG, Spiller RC. Limited exposure of the distal colon to orally-dosed formulation is further exaggerated in active left-sided ulcerative colitis. *Aliment Pharmacol Ther* 2000;14:155–61.

65 Travis SPL, Farrant JM, Ricketts C, et al. Predicting outcome in severe ulcerative colitis. *Gut* 1996;38:905–10.

66 Jarnerot G, Rolny P, Sandberg-Gertzen H. Intensive intravenous treatment of ulcerative colitis. *Gastroenterology* 1985;89:1005–13.

67 Hawthorne AB. Ciclosporin and refractory colitis. *Eur J Gastroenterol Hepatol* 2003;15:239–44.

68 Langholz E, Munkholm P, Davidsen M, Binder V. Course of ulcerative colitis: analysis of changes in disease activity over years. *Gastroenterology* 1994;107:3–11.

69 Meucci G, Vecchi M, Astegiano M, et al. The natural history of ulcerative proctitis: a multicenter, retrospective study. *Am J Gastroenterol* 2000;95:469–73.

70 D'Haens G, Gebboes K, Peeters M, et al. Patchy caecal inflammation associated with distal ulcerative colitis: a prospective endoscopic study. *Am J Gastroenterol* 1997;92:1275–9.

71 Lennard-Jones JE, Misiewicz JJ, Connell AM, et al. Prednisolone as maintenance treatment for ulcerative colitis in remission. *Lancet* 1965;1:188–9.

72 Sutherland L, Roth D, Beck P, May G, Makiyama K. Oral 5-aminosalicylic acid for maintenance of remission in ulcerative colitis. *Cochrane Database Syst Rev* 2002;4:CD000544.

73 Travis SPL, Tysk C, de Silva HJ, et al. Optimum dose of olsalazine for maintaining remission in ulcerative colitis. *Gut* 1994;35:1282–6.

74 Courtney M, Nunes D, Bergin C, et al. Randomised comparison of olsalazine and mesalazine in prevention of relapses in ulcerative colitis. *Lancet* 1992;339:1279–81.

75 Green JRB, Gibson JA, Kerr GD, et al. Maintenance of remission of ulcerative colitis: a comparison between balsalazide 3 g daily and mesalazine 1.2 g daily over 12 months: ABACUS investigator group. *Aliment Pharmacol Ther* 1998;12:1207–16.

76 Hanauer SB. Caution in the interpretation of safety and efficacy differences in clinical trials comparing aminosalicylates for ulcerative colitis. *Am J Gastroenterol* 2003;98:215–6.

77 Marteau P, Crand J, Foucault M, Rambaud J-C. Use of mesalazine slow-release suppositories 1g three times per weeks to maintain remission of ulcerative proctitis: a randomised double blind placebo controlled multicentre study. *Gut* 1998,42:195–9.

78 McGovern DPB, Travis SPL. Thiopurine therapy: when to start and when to stop. *Eur J Gastroenterol Hepatol* 2003;15:219–24.

79 Falasco G, Zinicola R, Forbes A. Review article: immunosuppressants in distal ulcerative colitis. *Aliment Pharmacol Ther* 2002;16:181–7.

80 Hawthorne AB, Logan RFA, Hawkey CJ, et al. Randomised controlled trial of azathioprine withdrawal in ulcerative colitis. *Br Med J* 1992;305:20–2.

81 Lemann M, Bouhnik Y, Colombel J, et al. Randomized, double-blind, placebo-controlled, multicentre, azathioprine withdrawal trial in Crohn's disease. *Gastroenterology* 2002;122:A23.
82 Oren R, Arber N, Odes S, et al. Methotrexate in chronic active ulcerative colitis: a double-blind, randomized, Israeli multicenter trial. *Gastroenterology* 1996;110:1416–21.
83 Cummings JRF, Gorard DA, McIntyre AS, Travis SPL, Jewell DP. Oral methotrexate in ulcerative colitis. *Aliment Pharmacol Ther* 2005;21:385–9.
84 Bjorck S, Dahlstrom A, Ahlman H. Treatment of distal colitis with local anaesthetic agents. *Pharmacol Toxicol* 2002;90:173–80.
85 Saibil FG. Lidocaine enemas for intractable distal ulcerative colitis: efficacy and safety [Abstract]. *Gastroenterology* 1998;114:A1073.
86 Arlander E, Ost A, Stahlberg D, Lofberg R. Ropivacaine gel in active distal ulcerative colitis and proctitis – a pharmacokinetic and exploratory clinical study. *Aliment Pharmacol Ther* 1996;10:73–81.
87 Hillingso JG, Kjeldsen J, Scmidt PT, et al. Effects of topical ropivacaine on eicosanoids and neurotransmitters in the rectum of patients with distal colitis. *Scand J Gastroenterol* 2002;37:325–9.
88 Forbes A, Britton TC, House IM, et al. Safety and efficacy of acetarsol suppositories in unresponsive proctitis. *Aliment Pharmacol Ther* 1989;3:553–6.
89 Pullan RD, Ganesh S, Mani V, et al. Comparison of bismuth citrate and 5-aminosalicylic acid enemas in active distal ulcerative colitis: a controlled trial. *Gut* 1993;34:676–9.
90 Khan Z, Macdonald C, Wicks AC, et al. Use of the 'nutriceutical' bovine colostrum for the treatment of distal colitis: results from an initial study. *Aliment Pharmacol Ther* 2002;16:1917–22.
91 Sandborn WJ, Tremaine WJ, Schroeder KW, et al. A placebo-controlled trial of cyclosporine enemas for mildly to moderately active left-sided ulcerative colitis. *Gastroenterology* 1994;106:1429–35.
92 Sinha A, Nightingale JMD, West KP, Berlanga-Acosta J, Playford RJ. Epidermal growth factor enemas with oral mesalamine for mild-to-moderate left-sided ulcerative colitis or proctitis. *N Engl J Med* 2003;349:350–7.
93 Kono T, Nomura M, Kasai S, Kogho Y. Effect of ecabet sodium enema on mildly to moderately active ulcerative proctosigmoiditis: an open-label study. *Am J Gastroenterol* 2001;96:793–7.
94 Jarlov AE, Munkholm P, Schmidt PN, et al. Treatment of active distal ulcerative colitis with immunoglobulin G enemas. *Aliment Pharmacol Ther* 1993;7:561–5.
95 Schreiber S, Heinig T, Thiele HG, Raedler A. Immunoregulatory role of interleukin-10 in patients with inflammatory bowel disease. *Gastroenterology* 1995;108:1434–44.
96 Pullan RD, Rhodes J, Ganesh S, et al. Transdermal nicotine for active ulcerative colitis. *N Engl J Med* 1994;330:811–95.
97 Thomas GAO, Rhodes J, Mani V, et al. Transdermal nicotine as maintenance therapy for ulcerative colitis. *N Engl J Med* 1995;332:988–92.
98 Thomas GAO, Rhodes J, Ragunath K, et al. Transdermal nicotine compared with oral prednisolone therapy for active ulcerative colitis. *Eur J Gastroenterol Hepatol* 1996;8:769–76.
99 Sandborn WJ, Tremaine W, Offord KP, et al. A randomized, double-blind, placebo controlled trial of transdermal nicotine for mildly to moderately active ulcerative colitis. *Ann Intern Med* 1997;126:364–71.
100 Guslandi M, Frego R, Vitale E, Testoni PA. Distal ulcerative colitis refractory to rectal mesalamine: role of transdermal nicotine versus oral mesalamine. *Can J Gastroenterol* 2002;16:293–6.
101 Sandborn WJ, Tremaine WJ, Leighton JAS, et al. Nicotine tartrate liquid enemas for mildly to moderately active left-sided ulcerative colitis unresponsive to first-line therapy: a pilot study. *Aliment Pharmacol Ther* 1997;11:663–71.
102 Green JT, Thomas GAO, Rhodes J, et al. Nicotine enemas for active ulcerative colitis – a pilot study. *Aliment Pharmacol Ther* 1997;11:859–63.
103 Gasbarrini G, Mingrone G, Giancaterini A, et al. Effects of propionyl-L-carnitine topical irrigation in distal ulcerative colitis: a preliminary report. *Hepatogastroenterolgy* 2003;50:1385–9.
104 Senagore AJ, MacKeigan JM, Scheider M, Ebrom JS. Short-chain fatty acid enemas: a cost-effective alternative in the treatment of non-specific proctosigmoiditis. *Dis Colon Rectum* 1992;35:923–7.
105 Vernia P, Marcheggiano A, Caprilli R, et al. Short-chain fatty acid topical treatment in distal ulcerative colitis. *Aliment Pharmacol Ther* 1995;9:309–13.
106 Patz J, Jacobsohn WZ, Gottschalk-Sabag S, Zeides S, Braverman DZ. Treatment of refractory distal colitis with short-chain fatty acid enemas. *Am J Gastroenterol* 1996;91:731–4.
107 Breuer RI, Soergel KH, Lashner BA, et al. Short-chain fatty acid rectal irrigation for left-sided ulcerative colitis: a randomized, placebo-controlled trial. *Gut* 1997;40:485–91.

108 Scheppach W, Group G-A. Treatment of distal ulcerative colitis with short-chain fatty acid enemas: a placebo-controlled trial. *Dig Dis Sci* 1996;41:2254–9.

109 Steinhart AH, Hiruki T, Brezezinski A, Baker JP. Treatment of left-sided ulcerative colitis with butyrate enemas: a controlled trial. *Aliment Pharmacol Ther* 1996;10:729–36.

110 Riley SA, Gupta I, Mani V. A comparison of sucralfate and prednisolone enemas in the treatment of active distal ulcerative colitis. *Scand J Gastroenterol* 1989;24:1014–18.

111 Campieri M, Gionchetti P, Belluzzi A, et al. Sucralfate, 5-aminosalicylic acid and placebo enemas in the treatment of distal ulcerative colitis. *Eur J Gastroenterol & Hepatol* 1991;3:41–4.

112 Ardizzone S, Petrillo M, Antonacci CM, Bianchi Porro G. Sucralfate and hydrocortisone enemas in the treatment of active ulcerative proctitis – a randomised single-blind comparative study. *Aliment Pharmacol Ther* 1996;10:957–60.

113 Wright JP, Winter TA, Candy S, Marks IS. Sucralfate and methylprednisolone enemas in active ulcerative colitis: a prospective, single-blind study. *Dig Dis Sci* 1999;44:1899–901.

114 van Outryve M, Huble F, van Eeghem P, et al. Comparison of Ridrogel versus prednisolone, both administered rectally, for the treatment of active ulcerative colitis [Abstract]. *Gastroenterology* 1996;110:A1035.

115 Auwerda JJ, Zijlstra FJ, Tak CJ, et al. Ridogrel enemas in distal ulcerative colitis. *Eur J Gastroenterol Hepatol* 2001;13:397–400.

116 Ben-Ayre E, Goldi E, Wengrower D, et al. Wheat grass juice in the treatment of active distal ulcerative colitis: a randomised double-blind placebo controlled trial. *Scand J Gastroenterol* 2002;37:444–9.

117 Ohkusa T, Okayasu I, Ogihara T, et al. Induction of experimental ulcerative colitis by *Fusobacterium varium* isolated from colonic mucosa of patients with ulcerative colitis. *Gut* 2003;52:79–83.

118 Carty E, Rampton DS. Evaluation of new therapies for inflammatory bowel disease. *Br J Clin Pharmacol* 2003;56:351–61.

119 Radford-Smith GS, Edwards JE, Purdie DM, et al. Protective role of appendicectomy on onset and severity of ulcerative colitis and Crohn's disease. *Gut* 2002;51:808–13.

120 Okazaki K, Onodera H, Watanabe N, et al. A patient with improvement of ulcerative colitis after appendectomy. *Gastroenterology* 2000;119:502–6.

121 Brunel M, Penne C, Tiret E, Balladur P, Parc R. Restorative proctocolectomy for distal ulcerative colitis. *Gut* 1999;45:542–5.

122 D'Albasio G, Pacini F, Camarri E, et al. Combined therapy with 5-aminosalicylic acid tablets and enemas for maintaining remission in ulcerative colitis: a randomized double-blind study. *Am J Gastroenterol* 1997;92:1143–7.

11: Pharmabiotics and inflammatory bowel disease – on the verge of evidence-based medicine

Fergus Shanahan, Jude Ryan and Shomik Sibartie

Introduction

Therapeutic manipulation of the enteric flora is emerging as a plausible and realistic option for the management of a diversity of clinical problems. This has contributed to a resurgence of interest in the role of the flora in the development and function of the gastrointestinal tract. Such is the contribution of the flora to mucosal homeostasis that it is no longer acceptable to study intestinal pathophysiology outside the context of the activities of the indigenous bacteria. Indigenous bacteria within the gastrointestinal tract are primarily an asset, conferring protection against pathogenic infections, priming mucosal immunity and producing vitamins, nutrients and other biologically active metabolites. Occasionally, depending on host susceptibility, the bacterial flora may become a liability and contribute to disorders such as Crohn's disease and ulcerative colitis. It follows that any strategy that promotes microbial assets and/or offsets liabilities represents a therapeutic option. Therein lies the rationale for pro-biotic/pre-biotics and other forms of therapeutic manipulation of gut flora [1–3]. Although this is often discussed in simplistic terms as replacing 'bad' bacteria with 'good' bacteria, the interaction between the host and the enteric bacterial flora is a dynamic one, underpinned by continual signalling and engagement of pattern recognition receptors, which maintains mucosal homeostasis. The impact of pro-biotics or pre-biotics is not simply ecologic ('good' for 'bad' bacteria) and almost certainly reflects a change in prokaryotic-eukaryotic signalling [2, 4].

Although the efficacy of pro-biotics in enteric infections and post-antibiotic syndromes appears to be established [5–7], and there is impressive support for pro-biotic therapy in pouchitis [8, 9], convincing evidence for efficacy in other forms of inflammatory bowel disease is less compelling. More importantly, there are several problems and pitfalls that need to be resolved before guidelines for routine clinical use of pro-biotics in Crohn's disease or colitis can be formulated. The clinical implications of host-flora interactions in inflammatory bowel disease, with particular reference to the promise of pro-biotics, is the subject of this overview; other aspects of the gut flora and the scope and promise of pro-biotics have been reviewed elsewhere [1–3, 10–12].

Notes on definition and terminology

The definition of pro-biotics is continually under review [13, 14]; they may be operationally and most simply defined as commensal organisms that can be harnessed for therapeutic benefit. The emphasis has generally been on live micro-organisms, but with clarification of mechanisms of action and identification of therapeutic pro-biotic metabolites; a programme of 'bugs to drugs' discovery may yield a new generation of biologic control agents that will challenge current definitions. For this reason, the more inclusive term *pharmabiotics* may be more appropriate.

The most commonly used pro-biotics are lactobacilli and bifidobacteria, although other bacteria, such as non-pathogenic *E. coli* and even non-bacterial organisms, such as *Saccharomyces boulardii* have been used for pro-biotic effect. In contrast, *pre-biotics* are non-digestible food ingredients that beneficially affect the host by selectively stimulating the growth of bacterial species already established in the colon and thus improve host health. These are usually of a poly- or oligosaccharide nature. The combination of pro-biotics and pre-biotics is referred to as *synbiotics* [15]. It is also noteworthy that the scope for harnessing microbes for therapeutic effect in inflammatory bowel disease is not limited to targeting host-bacterial interactions; helminths and helminthic antigens are currently being investigated with encouraging results in animal models of inflammation and promising early results in humans [16, 17].

Pro-biotics represent one aspect of an emerging class of functional foods at the interface of the food and pharmaceutical industries. Although there is no universally accepted definition of functional foods, there is a consensus that some foods and/or food additives have a distinct health benefit beyond their nutritional content. Although the concept of functional foods is not new, the application of rigorous scientific scrutiny to the area is at an early stage. Clinicians and scientists are beginning to embrace the concept with increasing enthusiasm, and the commercial promise of functional foods is greater than ever. It has been suggested by some economists that future consumers will expect that *all* foods be functional. Realising this promise will require careful scientific underpinning of functional food claims in addition to effective communication across industry, science and society, and clarification of current and future regulatory constraints. The process for the assessment of scientific support for claims on foods (PASSCLAIM) for these problems has recently been addressed [18].

Host-flora interactions in health and disease

The normal enteric flora exerts positive and negative regulatory effects on the development and function of the intestine. This is evident from comparative studies of germ-free and conventionally colonised animals. In the absence of bacteria, there is reduced mucosal cell turnover, digestive enzyme activity, cytokine production, lymphoid tissue, lamina propria cellularity, vascularity, muscle wall thickness and motility. In contrast, there is an increase in enterochromaffin cell area [19]. Modern techniques, such as laser capture micro-dissection and gene array analysis, are now being deployed to probe the molecular events underpinning the regulatory signalling from the lumen and promise to reveal new molecular targets for the design of future therapeutics [20, 21]. When applied to animals colonised with only a single bacterial strain, *Bacteroides thetaiotaomicron*, these experimental techniques have demonstrated the impact of bacterial-derived signalling on the expression of host genes controlling mucosal barrier function, nutrient absorption, angiogenesis and development of the enteric nervous system.

Incoming bacterial signals include secreted chemo-attractants, such as the formylated peptide f-met-leu-phe, cellular constituents such as lipopolysaccharide (LPS) and peptidoglycans, flagellin and bacterial nucleic acids (CpG DNA). Discrimination of pathogens from commensals by the host is mediated, in part, by pattern recognition receptors such as Toll-like receptors (TLRs) that are present on epithelial and immune (dendritic) cells. Engagement of TLRs by ligands from the commensal flora appears to be required for mucosal homeostasis in health. Thus, not only are bacterial signals required for optimal mucosal and immune development, they are actually required to maintain and condition the mucosa for responses to injury [22, 23].

The immune system mediates the sense of microbial danger and responses to injury. Like all senses, immunosensory acuity requires continual education and fine-tuning by environmental experiences such as microbial colonisation and exposure to sporadic mucosal infections. Without the flora, mucosal lymphoid tissue is rudimentary and induction of mucosal immune responses and tolerance are suboptimal [2, 24]. The challenge for host immunosensory performance within the gastrointestinal tract is to maintain tolerance to commensal flora whilst retaining the capacity for rapid responses to episodic challenge with pathogens. Immunologic sampling of the microbial environment across the epithelium is mediated by M cells, which deliver particulate and microbial antigens to underlying immune cells and by mucosal dendritic cells, which appear to extend processes into the lumen between the surface enterocytes without disrupting tight junctions [25]. Intestinal dendritic cells can ingest and retain intact live bacteria, and transit to the mesenteric lymph node where immune responses to commensals are induced locally [26]. Thus, the mesenteric lymph node acts as a gatekeeper, preventing access of commensal bacteria to the internal milieu and protecting the host from harmful systemic immune reactivity. The immunosensory function of dendritic cells is reflected by their remarkable plasticity and versatility of responses [27], depending on the type of organism they encounter. In addition to specific immune responses to enteric bacteria, the surface epithelial cells serve a sensory function for microbial danger by production of chemokines that activate and recruit the host immune response if there is a breach in the mucosal barrier pathogenic infection [28].

Bacterial signals from the lumen are transduced into host immune responses after engagement of TLRs and may trigger more than one molecular cascade. The transcription factor nuclear factor-κB (NF-κB) is the pivotal regulator of epithelial and immune responses to invasive pathogens, but non-pathogenic bacteria can attenuate inflammatory responses by delaying the degradation of IkB, which is counter-regulatory to NF-κB [29]. Other signal transduction pathways probably account for the anti-inflammatory effects pro-biotics and other commensal organisms, such as the anaerobe *Bacteroides thetaiotaomicron*. This can antagonise the pro-inflammatory effects of NF-κB within the epithelial cell by enhancing the nuclear export of its transcriptionally active subunit (RelA), in a peroxisome proliferator activated receptor-α-(PPAR-α)-dependent manner [30].

There is compelling evidence implicating the flora as a contributory factor in the pathogenesis of inflammatory bowel disease (reviewed in [12]). Indeed, many observations of immunological disturbances in these conditions may reflect immune reactivity against components of the flora and this has been exploited to identify the microbes contributing to the pathogenesis of disease. Marker antibodies generated by hybridoma or phage display technology have been used as reagents to identify microbial antigens. For example, anti-neutrophil cytoplasmic antibody (pANCA) associated with ulcerative colitis has been used to identify colonic bacteria expressing a pANCA-related epitope [31]. More recently, serological expression cloning was used to identify bacterial flagellin as a dominant antigen in Crohn's disease [32].

The multiplicity of different defects that may lead to a similar chronic inflammatory outcome in animal models probably also reflects the heterogeneity of these syndromes in humans. Indeed, genetic studies of human inflammatory bowel disease (reviewed elsewhere in this text) underscore the likelihood of distinct subsets of disease. The subset of Crohn's disease linked with the NOD2 (CARD15) polymorphism has highlighted the importance of proteins involved in the regulation of host responses to bacteria within the intestine [33, 34]. It seems likely that additional subsets of disease may be due to other defects at the level of pattern recognition receptor polymorphisms or along the cascade of events following engagement of TLRs by commensal an pathogenic bacteria. Whether non-pathogenic organisms including pro-biotics can be harnessed to offset these defects remains to be seen.

Strain selection: not all pro-biotics are the same

Discussion of pro-biotics in generic terms for clinical medicine is no longer acceptable and far too superficial. Clear distinctions between different bacterial strains are evident and these may translate into variability in efficacy in different clinical conditions. Guidelines for pro-biotic strain identification and functional characterisation have been generated by the Joint Food and Agricultural Organisation (FAO) of the United Nations and the World Health Organisation (WHO) [35]. At present, there is no biomarker from *in vitro* studies that reliably predicts function *in vivo* for putative pro-biotics in any clinical condition. Furthermore, it is unlikely that a single microbial agent or microbial product will be effective in each of the diverse clinical conditions for which pro-biotic efficacy has been claimed.

Comprehensive comparisons of pro-biotic performance using different strains need to be completed in specific disease states. There is emerging evidence in both inflammatory bowel diseases and irritable bowel syndrome that pro-biotic efficacy is not uniform [12, 36]. Furthermore, in light of increasing understanding of pharmacogenomics and nutrigenomics, individual variability in composition of the enteric flora might have to be considered as a determining factor for optimal pro-biotic strain selection. Without resolution of these pivotal issues, pro-biotic therapy will struggle to become established in the arena of evidence-based medicine. The consumer would also benefit from greater regulation of unsubstantiated or exaggerated health claims for some commercially available pro-biotic preparations.

Dosimetry: how much and how often?

There is currently no internationally recognised standardised system for verification of pro-biotic product quality in terms of stability and shelf life. In addition, the dose range, frequency of administration and optimal vehicle of delivery have received limited research attention and may vary for different pro-biotics. Like other biologic agents, pro-biotics may not exhibit a clear dose-response profile like that seen with conventional small molecule drugs. Furthermore, the effective dose of pro-biotics will be influenced by survival during gastric transit, exposure to bile and possibly by the potential for colonisation and multiplication within the colon.

In humans, the optimal dose for pro-biotics may differ in different disease indications. It is, therefore, desirable that studies of pro-biotics include some strategy for quantifying transit and survival of ingested organisms either by conventional culture-dependent methods on faeces or by using molecular probes. In the case of *Lactobacillus salivarius* UCC118, a consistent profile of faecal excreted levels of the pro-biotic after a 3-week feeding period has been demonstrated [37, 38]. The profile of faecal excretion of this lactobacillus and *Bifidobacterium infantis* has also been examined in a murine model of inflammatory bowel disease [39]. In addition, the kinetics of arrival of the pro-biotic at the terminal ileum and, therefore, the ability of the organism to survive gastric acid and bile and small bowel transit has been demonstrated [37].

Monitoring pro-biotic impact on the intestinal ecosystem

One of the great technological limitations to the study of the intestinal flora and the impact of pro-biotics is the inadequacy of traditional culture-dependent methods. Only about 50% of the indigenous gastrointestinal bacteria can be cultured at present. Therefore, little is known of their metabolic activity or variations in composition after ingestion of pro-biotics. This has led to increasing use of culture-independent, molecular methods of examining the enteric flora, including 16S DNA amplification and denaturing gradient gel electrophoresis (DGGE), which have been used to examine the diversity and stability of human intestinal bacteria. Strain-specific primers and probes have refined the technique and have been deployed in other techniques such as fluorescence *in situ* hybridisation (FISH) flow cytometry (FLOW-FISH) [40–43].

Another level of complexity in the gut is the variability in the composition of the flora, both quantitatively and qualitatively, over the long axis and cross-sectional axis of the gastrointestinal tract. Therefore, faecal samples may have limited value in monitoring the enteric ecosystem. Evidence from culture-independent methods suggests that mucosa-associated bacteria differ from those recovered from faeces and supports the idea that host-related factors have a role in determining the enteric flora [44].

The variability in the composition of the flora throughout the alimentary tract also undermines the naïve assumption that any given strategy for therapeutic manipulation of the enteric flora will be equally effective for diseases that variably affect different parts of either the small or large bowel. It follows that depending on the topographic distribution of the lesions in Crohn's disease, a single pro-biotic may not be equally suited to different subsets of patients.

Single strains or combinations

One strategy to accommodate different clinical indications and individual variations in composition of enteric flora is the use of combinations of pro-biotic strains. However, as with all combinations of therapies, the activities of the individual components require definition and optimisation before the combination can be routinely recommended. It is also difficult to see how pro-biotic mechanisms of action will be defined if combinations of different strains are used. In this respect, proponents of pro-biotic therapy should not abandon traditional principles of therapeutics and need to retain the same scientific rigour that is applied to drug therapy. In addition, the use of cocktails of bacteria assumes that the constituents are not mutually antagonistic. It appears that this is not a valid assumption [45 and unpublished].

From theory to practice – the evidence for efficacy

Meta-analyses and a favourable Cochrane review have confirmed the efficacy of pro-biotics in the setting of enteric infections [5–7]. In patients with inflammatory bowel disease, pouchitis appears to be the subset well suited to pro-biotic therapy [8, 9]. Whether other forms of the disease are equally responsive is much less certain. The outcome of the PROGID-controlled trial of maintenance of remission with pro-biotics funded by the European commission is pending. Results from completed small studies to date are inconclusive, but there appear to be subsets of patients who might benefit from this from of therapy (Tables 11.1–11.3) [46–48, 50–60].

From bugs to drugs

The potential to substitute molecules for microbes will become a reality once the mechanism of action of pro-biotics is clarified. As alluded to earlier, current knowledge of the molecular basis of host-flora interactions and pro-biotic-host dialogue has shown the need to move discussions of pro-biotic mechanisms beyond simplistic concepts of replacing 'bad bugs' with 'good bugs'. Pro-biotic therapy is more complex than manipulating the host flora. Rather, it is a question of influencing host-flora signalling. In this context, bacterial metabolites such as anti-microbial peptides (bacteriocins), anti-inflammatory or anti-cancer factors such as conjugated linoleic acid (CLA) and nucleic acids (bacterial CpG DNA), may underpin certain pro-biotic actions in different circumstances [12].

Table 11.1 Summary of human trials of pro-biotic therapy in ulcerative colitis. (N = number of subjects in trial).

Study type	Organism used	Trial outcome	Reference
Randomised controlled trial	E. coli strain (Nissle 1917) $N = 120$	Patients with active colitis demonstrated similar relapse rates compared to patients on mesalazine	Kruis et al., 1997 [46]
Randomised, controlled trial	E. coli strain (Nissle 1917) $N = 116$	Confirmed result from Kruis et al., 1997	Rembacken et al., 1999 [47]
Open labelled trial	VSL# 3 $N = 20$	Maintenance of remission in patients	Venturi et al., 1999 [48]
Randomised controlled trial	E. coli strain (Nissle 1917) $N = 327$	Remission maintained in patients receiving pro-biotic	Kruis et al., 2004 [49]
Open labelled trial	S. boulardii $N = 25$	Treatment given in combination with mesalamine for relapse of ulcerative colitis. Remission achieved in 17 patients	Guslandi et al., 2003 [50]

Table 11.2 Summary of human trials of pro-biotic therapy in pouchitis.

Study type	Organism used	Trial outcome	Reference
Open labelled trial	Pre-biotic fructooligosaccharide and pro-biotic $N = 10$	Effective in inducing remission in combination with antibiotic	Friedman and George, 2000 [51]
Randomised controlled trial	VSL#3 $N = 40$	Maintenance of remission in chronic pouchitis after antibiotic-induced remission 15% relapse rate compared with 100% in control group	Gionchetti et al., 2000 [52]
Randomised controlled trial	VSL#3 $N = 40$	Prevention of acute pouchitis in patients after ileo-anal pouch surgery 10% pouchitis rate in pro-biotic group compared with 40% in control group	Gionchetti et al., 2003 [8]
Randomised controlled trial	VSL#3 (6 g) $N = 36$	Maintenance of remission in recurrent or refractory pouchitis after antibiotic induced remission 85% remained in remission at 1 year, compared with 6% in placebo group	Mimura et al., 2004 [9]

N = number of subjects in trial.

Table 11.3 Summary of human trials of pro-biotic therapy in Crohn's disease.

Study type	Organism used	Trial outcome	Reference
Randomised controlled trial	S. boulardii $N = 20$	Decrease in CDAI in pro-biotic group	Plein and Holz, 1993 [53]
Open labelled trial	Lactobacillus GG $N = 14$	Increase in gut IgA response	Malin et al., 1996 [54]
Randomised controlled trial	E. coli strain Nissle 1917 $N = 28$	Remission achieved in patients on pro-biotics and steroids greater than with steroids alone	Malchow, 1997 [55]
Open labelled trial	Lactobacillus GG in children $N = 4$	Improved intestinal permeability and CDAI	Gupta et al., 2000 [56]
Randomised controlled trial	VSL#3 with antibiotic $N = 40$	Patients with CD had 20% remission when given antibiotic and VSL#3 compared to 40% in mesalamine-treated group	Campieri et al., 2000 [57]
Randomised controlled trial	S. boulardii $N = 32$	Maintenance of remission in treatment group superior as relapse observed in 6.25% of patients receiving pro-biotic plus mesalasine compared to 37.5% on mesalamine alone	Guslandi et al., 2000 [58]
Open labelled trial	L. salivarius 118 $N = 25$	Reduction of mean CDAI and induction of IgA in patients with relapse	McCarthy et al., 2001 [59]
Randomised controlled trial	L. rhamnosus GG $N = 45$	No difference seen in rate of recurrence 1 year after surgery between group given pro-biotic or control	Prantrera et al., 2002 [60]

N = number of subjects in trial, CDAI = Crohn's disease activity index.

Turbo pro-biotics

Even if naturally occurring organisms have insufficient efficacy in inflammatory bowel disease, the use of engineered pro-biotics or food-grade bacteria to deliver anti-inflammatory molecules to the site of intestinal lesions is a realistic proposition [61]. Advantages of this strategy include avoidance of systemic toxicity, lower production costs, convenience, wider scope of indications and perhaps more consistent efficacy. Proof of principle has been demonstrated with a genetically modified (GM) strain of *Lactococcus lactis* engineered to produce the anti-inflammatory cytokine, interleukin-10 (IL-10) [62]. Remarkably, the GM organism was as effective as corticosteroids in a murine model of inflammatory bowel disease. Although the best choice of transgene for treatment of inflammatory bowel disease in humans is uncertain, the delivery of trefoil factors by this method is conceptually appealing because it focuses more on the healing phase of the disease rather than the inflammatory phase [63].

The primary safety concern surrounding GM organisms relates to the public health risk when such organisms are excreted into the environment. A clever strategy to address this has been to insert the therapeutic transgene into the thymidylate synthase (*thy A*) gene locus. Without this enzyme, the organism is dependent on thymine or thymidine in the local micro-environment, but these are not readily available within the external environment, thereby limiting the viability of the excreted GMO. In addition, the transgene would be eliminated from the bacterial genome if the engineered organism re-acquires the *thy A* gene from the wild-type strain [64].

Conclusion

Pro-biotics promise much for clinical medicine. Although they have a sound rationale in inflammatory bowel disease, this therapeutic strategy is still developmental. There are substantial gaps in our understanding of host-bacterial interactions within the gut and several potential pitfalls to the effective use of pro-biotics. Resolution of these problems requires better characterisation of individual strains, clarification of mechanisms of action in different settings and carefully controlled clinical trials. Responsiveness to different pro-biotics is likely to be as variable as that with drug therapy. However, even if naturally occurring pro-biotics lack sufficient efficacy for the more aggressive forms of inflammatory disease, genetically modified organisms may be used in the future for delivery of anti-inflammatory drugs.

Acknowledgements

The author is supported in part by the Science Foundation, Ireland, in the form of a centre grant (Alimentary Pharmabiotic Centre), by the Health Research Board (HRB) of Ireland, the Higher Education Authority (HEA) of Ireland and the European Union (PROGID QLK-2000-00563). The author has been affiliated with a multi-departmental university campus company (Alimentary Health Ltd), which investigates host-flora interactions and the therapeutic manipulation of these interactions in various human and animal disorders. The content of this article was neither influenced nor constrained by this fact.

References

1 Shanahan F. Inflammatory bowel disease: immunodiagnostics, immunotherapeutics and ecotherapeutics. *Gastroenterology* 2001;120:622–35.
2 Shanahan F. Pathophysiological basis and prospects for probiotic therapy in inflammatory bowel disease. *Am J Physiol Gastrointest Liver Physiol* 2005;288(3):G417–21.
3 Shanahan F. Probiotics in inflammatory bowel disease: is there a scientific rationale? *Inflamm Bowel Dis* 2000;6:107–1115.
4 Ghosh S, van Heel D, Playford RJ. Probiotics in inflammatory bowel disease: is it all gut flora modulation? *Gut* 2004;53:620–2.
5 Dunne C, Shanahan F. Role of probiotics in the treatment of intestinal infections and inflammation. *Curr Opin Gastroenterol* 2002;18:40–5.
6 Allen SJ, Okoko B, Martinez E, Gregorio G, Dans LF. Probiotics for treating infectious diarrhoea. *Cochrane Database Syst Rev* 2004;(2):CD003048.
7 D'Souza AL, Rajkumar C, Cooke J, Bulpitt CJ. Probiotics in prevention of antibiotic associated diarrhoea: meta-analysis. *BMJ* 2002;324:1361.

8. Gionchetti P, Rizzello F, Helwig U, et al. Prophylaxis of pouchitis onset with probiotic therapy: a double-blind, placebo-controlled trial. *Gastroenterology* 2003;124(5):1202–9.
9. Mimura T, Rizzello F, Helwig U, et al. Once daily high dose probiotic therapy (VSL#3) for maintaining remission in recurrent or refractory pouchitis. *Gut* 2004;53:108–14.
10. Dunne C, O'Mahony L, Murphy L, et al. In vitro selection criteria for probiotic bacteria of human origin: correlation with *in vivo* findings. *Am J Clin Nutrition* 2001;73(Suppl)(2, Pt 2):386S–92S.
11. Bengmark S. Ecological control of the gastrointestinal tract: the role of probiotic flora. *Gut* 1998;42:2–7.
12. Shanahan F. Host-flora interactions in inflammatory bowel disease. *Inflamm Bowel Dis* 200410(Suppl 1):S16–24.
13. Report of a Joint FAO/WHO Expert Consultation. Health and nutritional properties of probiotics in food including powder milk and live lactic acid bacteria, 2001. http://www.fao.org/es/ESN/Probio/report.Pdf
14. Shanahan F. Probiotics in inflammatory bowel disease: therapeutic rationale and role. *Adv Drug Delivery Rev* 2004;56:809–18.
15. Furrie E, Macfarlane S, Kennedy A, et al. Synbiotic therapy (*Bifidobacterium longum*/Synergy 1) initiates resolution of inflammation in patients with active ulcerative colitis: a randomised controlled pilot trial. *Gut* 2005;54:242–9.
16. Elliott DE, Summers RW, Weinstock JV. Helminths and the modulation of mucosal inflammation. *Curr Opin Gastroenterol* 2005;21:51–8.
17. Summers RW, Elliott DE, Urban JF Jr, Thompson R, Weinstock JV. Trichuris suis therapy in Crohn's disease. *Gut* 2005;54:87–90.
18. Cummings JH, Antoine J-M, Azpiroz F, et al. Passclaim – gut health and immunity. *Eur J Nutr* 2004;43(Suppl 2):II/118–173.
19. Midtvedt T. Microbial functional activities. In: Hanson LA, Yolken RH, eds. *Intestinal Microflora*, Nestle Nutrition Workshop Series. Philadelphia: Lippincott-Raven; 1999;42:79–96.
20. Hooper IV, Wong MH, Thelin A, Hansson L, Falk PG, Gordon JI. Molecular analysis of commensal host-microbial relationships in the intestine. *Science* 2001;291:881–4.
21. Hooper LV, Midvedt T, Gordon JI. How host-microbial interactions shape the nutrient environment of the mammalian intestine. *Annu Rev Nutr* 2002;22:283–307.
22. Rakoff-Nahoum S, Paglino J, Eslami-Varzaneh F, Edberg S, Medzhitov R. Recognition of commensal microflora by toll-like receptors is required for intestinal homeostasis. *Cell* 2004;118:229–41.
23. Madara J. Building an intestine–architectural contributions of commensal bacteria. *N Engl J Med* 2004;351:1685–6.
24. Shanahan F. Nutrient tasting and signaling mechanisms in the gut V. Mechanisms of immunologic sensation of intestinal contents. *Am J Physiol Gastrointest Liver Physiol* 2000;278:G191–6.
25. Rescigno M, Urbano M, Valzasina B, et al. Dendritic cells express tight junction proteins and penetrate gut epithelial monolayers to sample bacteria. *Nat Immunology* 2001;2:361–7.
26. Macpherson AJ, Uhr T. Induction of protective IgA by intestinal dendritic cells carrying commensal bacteria. *Science* 2004;303;1662–5.
27. Huang Q, Liu D, Majewski P, et al. The plasticity of dendritic cell responses to pathogens nd their components. *Science* 2001;294:870–5.
28. Kagnoff MF, Eckmann L. Epithelial cells as sensors for microbial infection. *J Clin Invest* 1997;100: 6–10.
29. Neish AS, Gewirtz AT, Zeng H, et al. Prokaryotic regulation of epithelial responses by inhibition of IκB-αubiquitination. *Science* 2000;289:1560–3.
30. Kelly D, Campbell JI, King TP, et al. Commensal anaerobic gut bacteria attenuate inflammation by regulating nuclear-cytoplasmic shuttling of PPAR-gamma and RelA. *Nat Immunol* 2004;5: 104–12.
31. Dalwadi H, Wei B, Braun J. Defining new pathogens and non-culturable infectious agents. *Curr Opin Gastroenterol* 2000;16:56–59.
32. Lodes MJ, Cong Y, Elson CO, et al. Bacterial flagellin is a dominant antigen in Crohn disease. *J Clin Invest* 2004;113:1296–306.
33. Kobayashi KS, Chamaillard M, Ogura Y, et al. Nod2-dependent regulation of innate and adaptive immunity in the intestinal tract. *Science* 2005;307: 731–4.
34. Maeda S, Hsu LC, Liu H, et al. Nod2 mutation in Crohn's disease potentiates NF-κB activity and IL-1beta processing. *Science* 2005;307:734–8.
35. Working Group Report. Guidelines for the evaluation of probiotics in food. Joint Food and Agriculture Organisation of the United Nations and The World Health Organisation. http://www.fao.org/es/ESN/Probio/probio.htm
36. O'Mahony L, McCarthy J, Kelly P, et al. A randomized, placebo-controlled, double blind comparison of the probiotic bacteria *Lactobacillus* and *Bifidobacterium* in irritable bowel syndrome. *Gastroenterology* 2005; in press.

37 Collins JK, Murphy L, Morrissey D, et al. A randomised controlled trial of a probiotic *Lactobacillus* strain in healthy adults: assessment of its delivery, transit, and influence on microbial flora and enteric immunity. *Microb Ecol Health Dis* 2002;14:81–9.

38 Murphy L, Dunne C, Kiely B, Shanahan F, O'Sullivan GC, Collins JK. *In vivo* assessment of potential probiotic lactobacillus salivarius strains: evaluation of their establishment, persistence and localisation in the murine gastrointestinal tract. *Microb Ecol Health Dis* 1999;11:149–57.

39 McCarthy J, O'Mahony L, O'Callaghan L, et al. Double blind, placebo controlled trial of two probiotic strains in interleukin 10 knockout mice and mechanistic link with cytokine balance. *Gut* 2003;52:975–80.

40 Vaughan EE, Schut F, Heilig HGHJ, Zoetendal EG, de Vos WM, Akkermans ADL. A molecular view of the intestinal ecosystem. *Curr Issues Intest Microbiol* 2000;1:1–12.

41 Akkermans ADL, Zoetendal EG, Favier CF, Heilig HGHJ, Akkermans-van Vliet WM, de Vos WM. Temperature and denaturing gradient gel electrophoresis analysis of 16S rRNA from human faecal samples. *Biosci Microflora* 2000;19:93–8.

42 Qiu X, Wu L, Huang L, et al. Evaluation of PCR-generated chimeras, mutations, and heteroduplexes with 16S rRNA gene based cloning. *Appl Environ Microbiol* 2001;67:880–7.

43 Dalwadi H, Wei B, Braun J. Defining new pathogens and non-culturable infectious agents. *Curr Opin Gastroenterol* 2000;16:56–9.

44 Zoetendal EG, Von Wright A, Vilpponen-Salmela T, Ben-Amor K, Akkermans ADL, de Vos WM. Mucosa-associated bacteria in the human gastrointestinal tract are uniformly distributed along the colon and differ from the community recovered from the feces. *Appl Environ Microbiol* 2000;68:3401–7.

45 Murphy LM, Byrne FR, Collins JK, Shanahan F, O'Sullivan GC. Evaluation and characterisation of probiotic therapy in the CD45RH hi transfer model of colitis. DDW/AGA Orlando Fl. *Gastroenterology* 1999;116:A780.

46 Kruis W, Schutz E, Fric P, Fixa B, Judmaier G, Stolte M. Double blind comparison of an oral *Escherichia coli* preparation and mesalazine in maintaining remission of ulcerative colitis. *Aliment Pharmacol Ther* 1997;11:853–8.

47 Rembacken BJ, Snelling AM, Hawkey PM, Axon ATR. Non-pathogenic *Escherichia coli* versus mesalazine for the treatment of ulcerative colitis: a randomised trial. *Lancet* 1999;354:635–9.

48 Venturi A, Gionchetti P, Rizzello F, et al. Impact on the composition of the faecal flora by a new probiotic preparation: preliminary data on maintenance treatment of patients with ulcerative colitis. *Aliment Pharmacol Ther* 1999;13:1103–8.

49 Kruis W, Fric P, Pokrotnieks J, LuKas M, Fixa B, Kascak M, Kamm MA, Weismueller J, Beglinger C, Stolte M, Wolff C, Schulze J. Maintaining remission of ulcerative colitis with the probiotic Escherichia coli Nissle 1917 is as effective as with standard mesalazine. *Gut* 2004;53:1617–23.

50 Guslandi M, Giollo P, Testoni PA. A pilot trial of *Saccharomyces boulardii* in ulcerative colitis. *Eur J Gastroenterol Hepatol* 2003;15:697–8.

51 Friedman G, George J. Treatment of refractory 'pouchitis' with probiotic and probiotic therapy. *Gastroenterology* 2000;118:A4167.

52 Gionchetti P, Rizzello F, Venturi A, et al. Oral bacteriotherapy as maintenance treatment in patients with chronic pouchitis: a double-blind, placebo-controlled trial. *Gastroenterology* 2000;119:305–9.

53 Plein K, Holz J. Therapeutic effects of *Saccharomyces boulardii* on mild residual symptoms in a stable phase of Crohn's disease with special respect to chronic diarrhoea – a pilot study. *Z Gastroenterol* 1993;31:129–34.

54 Malin M, Suomalainen H, Saxelin M, et al. Promotion of IgA immune response in patients with Crohn's disease by oral bacteriotherapy with *Lactobacillus GG*. *Ann Nutr Metab* 1996;40:137–45.

55 Malchow HA. Crohn's disease and *Escherichia coli*: a new approach in therapy to maintain remission of colonic Crohn's disease? *J Clin Gastroenterol* 1997;25:653–8.

56 Gupta P, Andrew H, Kirschner BS, et al. Is *Lactobacillus GG* helpful in children with Crohn's disease? Results of a preliminary open-label study. *J Pediat Gastroenterol Nutr* 2000;31:453–7.

57 Campieri M, Rizzello F, Venturi A, et al. Combination of antibiotic probiotic treatment is efficacious in prophylaxis of post-operative recurrence of Crohn's disease: a randomised controlled study vs mesalamine [Abstract]. *Gastroenterology* 2000;118:A4179.

58 Guslandi M, Mezzi G, Sorghi M, Testoni PA. *Saccharomyces boulardii* in the maintenance of Crohn's disease. *Dig Dis Sci* 2000;45:1462–4.

59 McCarthy J, O'Mahony L, Dunne C, et al. An open trial of a novel probiotic as an alternative to steroids

60 Prantrera C, Scribano ML, Falasco G, Andreoli A, Luzi C. Ineffectiveness of probiotics in preventing recurrence after curative resection for Crohn's disease: a randomised controlled trial with *Lactobacillus GG*. *Gut* 2002;51:405–9.
61 Shanahan F. Making microbes work for mankind-clever trick or a glimpse of the future for IBD treatment? *Gastroenterology* 2004;127:667–8.
62 Steidler L, Hans W, Schotte L, *et al*. Treatment of murine colitis by *Lactococcus lactis* secreting interleukin-10. *Science* 2000;289:1352–5.
63 Vandenbroucke K, Hans W, Van Huysse J, *et al*. Active delivery of trefoil factors by genetically modified *Lactococcus lactis* prevents and heals acute colitis in mice. *Gastroenterology* 2004;127: 502–13.
64 Steidler L, Neirynck S, Huyghebaert N, *et al*. Biological containment of genetically modified *Lactococcus lactis* for intestinal delivery of human interleukin 10. *Nat Biotechnol* 2003;21:785–9.

in mild/moderately active Crohn's disease [Abstract]. *Gut* 2001; 49(Suppl 3):2447.

12: Current controversies in the surgical management of ulcerative colitis

R. John Nicholls and Mark J. Cheetham

Introduction

Proctocolectomy with permanent ileostomy is curative for ulcerative colitis. Since its introduction 50 years ago [1–3] subsequent surgical developments have been aimed at avoiding a permanent ileostomy. Colectomy with ileorectal anastomosis and restorative proctocolectomy is well accepted but controversies remain on the relative indications for these procedures. In addition, there is some controversy on the indications for surgery against continued medical treatment and questions relating to technical aspects of the procedures.

Emergency surgery

Fulminant colitis

There is no disagreement that surgery is indicated in cases with perforation or megacolon. Most patients in this clinical category have acute severe colitis. Here new agents such as ciclosporin may induce remissions resulting in fewer operations. Patients may not, however, be better served by postponing surgery given the low operative mortality of colectomy with ileostomy resulting in return to normal health without medication. There is evidence that patients having a response to ciclosporin have a high incidence of early relapse [4]. While the results of surgery are submitted to audit, there is no analagous assessment of patients with extensive colitis being maintained on medical treatment. The indications for referral for surgery are at the moment dependent on clinical judgement based upon experience, but they are not entirely objective owing to variation in the approach of gastroenterologists. A new method of quality of life assessment taking into consideration the patient's life end points would be beneficial in assessing outcomes of those still under medical care. For the patient, loss of employment with its financial consequences, the disintegration of social life such as loss of partner or psychosocial dysfunction of the children are important end points. A system to identify these features during medical management would be a clinical advance.

Colectomy with ileostomy

There is general agreement that colectomy with ileostomy and preservation of the rectal stump is the procedure of choice. It has a low mortality and is effective in most cases. Rarely, persisting disease in the rectum is so severe that improvement does not occur, and subsequent rectal excision may be necessary.

In cases with massive bleeding the operation should be modified if bleeding is from ulceration in the rectum. In this case it will be necessary to remove the rectum leaving the anal canal to give the patient the chance of a subsequent restorative procedure.

Mucous fistula

Some debate exists as to whether the rectosigmoid stump should be exteriorised as a mucous fistula or whether it should be closed and returned to the abdomen. There are no prospective clinical trials comparing these options. Retrospective reviews have indicated that closure of the rectal stump is safe [5]. These authors reported 147 consecutive acute colectomies for ulcerative colitis with a mortality of 3%; none related to the rectal stump and only 2% of the total had a pelvic abscess related to leakage of the stump.

A mucous fistula is often troublesome to the patient and can be more of a problem than the ileostomy itself. On the other hand, it is safe especially in an ill patient with malnutrition on high-dose steroid medication in whom the rectal wall may be oedematous and fragile.

Although the matter remains a question of clinical judgement with the emphasis on safety, a compromise has been proposed whereby the stump is closed but brought to a position just under the abdominal wound. If leakage occurs then this should discharge through the wound [6].

Length of rectosigmoid stump

Some surgeons aim to remove as much of the rectum as possible, dividing the stump at the level of pelvic peritoneum. This should be avoided unless it has been necessary to remove the rectum to stop bleeding. It will prejudice the functional result of a subsequent ileorectal anastomosis, and where a rectal excision with or without ileoanal anastomosis is to be undertaken, it can be difficult to find the rectal stump. A long rectosigmoid stump whether exteriorised as a mucous fistula or not should be aimed for routinely. On subsequent re-operation, the rectum is easy to locate.

Elective surgery

The indications for surgery include failed medical treatment, retardation of growth in children and neoplastic transformation. Failed medical treatment is difficult to define but the general indications can be grouped as follows: chronic ill health, recurrent acute exacerbations, severe symptoms, steroid dependence and extra-intestinal manifestations. In many cases these overlap and, furthermore, there is varying opinion as to when medical treatment should be stopped and surgery undertaken.

There are no generally accepted guidelines but the frequency of hospital admissions, loss of time from work, family stresses, other social factors, severity of symptoms, anaemia, poor energy level and evidence of malnutrition must all be taken into account. Bone densitometry allows an objective assessment of the degree of osteoporosis. The recommendation for surgery is also heavily influenced by the patient's wishes.

Most studies have shown an increasing cancer incidence with time in patients with extensive ulcerative colitis. Colonoscopic cancer surveillance with multiple biopsies to identify patients before invasion has occurred can sometimes fail. Carcinoma developed in 13 (7%) of 186 patients with extensive ulcerative colitis followed for over 10 years. Of the 16 carcinomas in the 13 patients, 11 were Dukes' stage A, 3 stage B, 1 stage C, and 1 was inoperable [7]. The presence of low-grade dysplasia is almost as likely as high-grade dysplasia (54% vs 67%) to be associated with the presence of an already established malignancy [8]. There are difficulties in defining dysplasia [9], but based on the application of colectomy for low-grade dysplasia a cost-effective surveillance programme can be devised [10].

Choice of operation

The operations available for elective surgery include proctocolectomy, colectomy with ileorectal anastomosis, and restorative proctocolectomy with ileoanal anastomosis. Each includes a total colectomy, as it has been found that partial colectomy results in a high incidence of recurrent colitis in the remaining colon.

The introduction of restorative proctocolectomy (RPC) has reduced the use of conventional proctocolectomy. Of 422 patients with ulcerative colitis operated on at one hospital between 1976 and 1990, 316 underwent elective surgery. During this period conventional proctocolectomy fell from 60 to 21% and restorative proctocolectomy rose from 7 to 52%. The proportion of patients undergoing colectomy with ileorectal anastomosis fell from 28% in the first 5 years to 11% in the last 5-year period. In 70 patients who had elective surgery after an initial emergency colectomy, only 10 (14%) had a colectomy with ileorectal anastomosis with the majority undergoing restorative proctocolectomy [11].

Colectomy with ileorectal anastomosis

Colectomy with ileorectal anastomosis is a compromise whereby persisting disease in the rectum is accepted in order to avoid a stoma. Poor function owing to continuing inflammation or the occurrence of neoplastic transformation has resulted in a significant failure rate ranging from 10% to more than 30% [12–14].

Suitability for ileorectal anastomosis depends upon the rectum maintaining its function as a capacitance organ. Thus, there should be only minimal or moderate disease and it should be expansile. Contrast radiology and balloon volumetry may be helpful in assessing capacitance. The anal sphincter must be adequate and there must be no evidence of dysplasia or carcinoma within the large bowel unless the patient already has established distant metastases in which case the operation may be the best option provided adequate local clearance of the carcinoma is possible. Colectomy with ileorectal anastomosis has the great advantage of being a low-morbidity procedure from which the patient is likely to make a rapid recovery. In elective cases it is not usual to defunction the anastomosis.

Suitable patients must, however, accept the need for regular indefinite follow-up by endoscopy and biopsy at least yearly. The long-term risk of cancer developing in the rectum has been shown to be around 6% in 20 years and 15% in 30 years [15].

Except for patients with disseminated disease, few patients now are suitable for this operation following the introduction of restorative proctocolectomy (RPC). There is, however, a case for considering it in patients with indeterminate colitis in whom it is not possible to distinguish between Crohn's disease and ulcerative colitis where the rectum is not grossly inflamed. These will be candidates for ileorectal anastomosis provided no anal disease is present and the rectum has adequate capacitance.

Conventional or restorative proctocolectomy?

Restorative proctocolectomy is an alternative to conventional proctocolectomy and not to colectomy with ileorectal anastomosis. It has a higher complication rate. Failure in the first year ranges from 5 to 10% [16–18] with an increasing failure rate with time of around 10–15% at 10–15 years [19, 20]. In contrast, conventional proctocolectomy is less liable to complications and is curative with no pouchitis and no activity-related extra-intestinal manifestations. Its disadvantages, however, include the permanent ileostomy and the cumulative incidence of ileostomy complications requiring subsequent surgery. Furthermore, perineal wound healing may be delayed in as many as 25% of cases at 6 months.

Avoidance of a permanent ileostomy is the only indication for restorative proctocolectomy. Quality of life comparisons of patients with a permanent ileostomy and those after restorative proctocolectomy are not strictly valid because different clinical groups are being compared [21, 22], although they give useful information on general satisfaction levels. These and other assessments [23] demonstrate that the over-riding view of patients is positive. Even those who have experienced failure may feel that the attempt was worthwhile, enabling them to accept a permanent ileostomy more easily.

Age. It has been suggested that older patients should not have a restorative proctocolectomy because of a perception of poor functional results and changes seen in anal physiology [24]. Of 392 patients with ulcerative colitis undergoing restorative proctocolectomy with mucosectomy and hand-sewn ileoanal, 326 were aged 5–49 years and 66 were aged 50–74 years. There was no difference in complications, duration of hospital stay or function. Continence rates were 81.6 and 80% and the mean frequency of defaecation per 24 h was 6.3 ± 0.2 and 7.4 ± 0.5 [25]. Similar findings were recorded by Lewis *et al.* [26] and Takao *et al.* [27]. Others, however, have found the functional outcome poorer and some complications higher in patients older than 55 years [28] but these authors concluded nevertheless that restorative proctocolectomy can be safely performed in the older age group with acceptable results. Age-related changes are not inevitable and the rate of deterioration of anorectal function varies between individuals. It would seem that with careful consideration of the whole patient (including such factors as mobility) it is reasonable to perform restorative proctocolectomy in selected patients over 50 years.

Contraindications to restorative proctocolectomy

Crohn's disease. Approximately 2–5% of patients in reported surgical series of RPC have subsequently been catergorised as having Crohn's disease in the mistaken belief that ulcerative colitis was the diagnosis. Their outcome has been poor with failure rates ranging from 30 to 100% [29, 30]. Panis et al. [31], however, have reported a series of 31 selected patients with Crohn's disease deliberately treated by restorative proctocolectomy. Over a follow-up period of 9–72 months; only two required removal of the pouch, three developed a pouch fistula and two developed recurrent Crohn's disease. The intermediate-term outcome in the 29 patients with an intact pouch at the time of assessment was satisfactory. At 5-year follow-up there were no significant functional differences between patients with Crohn's disease and ulcerative colitis. These results have been updated by Regimbeau et al. [32] in a larger series of 113 patients with a failure rate of 7%.

In the series of Panis et al. and Regimbeau et al., the patients had small bowel and anal sparing with rectal involvement [31, 32]. This distribution is infrequent in clinical practice and it is possible that some of these cases had indeterminate colitis. It has been argued that RPC and colectomy and ileorectal anastomosis for Crohn's disease are analogous [33], but given the high failure rate after the former with the resulting need to remove at least 40 cm of small bowel, most surgeons would regard Crohn's disease as a contraindication.

Indeterminate colitis. The term indeterminate colitis was introduced by Price to describe operation specimens from patients with inflammatory bowel disease in which the histological appearances were typical neither of ulcerative colitis nor Crohn's disease [34]. Ten to fifteen per cent of resection specimens fall into this category, and the dilemma usually arises where the colon has been removed as an emergency during an acute phase of the disease. Thus, of the 30 operative specimens in Price's series, 27 were from patients with severe acute colitis often with megacolon. In another study, histology alone made the final diagnosis of Crohn's disease or ulcerative colitis in 58 (87%) of 67 acute cases [35].

Of 25 patients with indeterminate colitis undergoing restorative proctocolectomy, 8% failed at a mean follow-up of 35 months following closure of the ileostomy. The pelvic sepsis rate was 8%, and occurrence of pouchitis 8% [36]. These rates did not differ from the outcome in the 489 patients with undisputed ulcerative colitis treated during the same period. Thus, it appeared that in the short-term at least indeterminate colitis did not confer a worse prognosis than ulcerative colitis. More recently, however, in a series of 175 patients including 158 with ulcerative colitis and 16 with indeterminate colitis the respective failure rates, 5 and 19% [37] and these rates are very similar to those reported from the Mayo Clinic [38] and St Mark's Hospital [39] of 10 and 16.5%. Indeterminate colitis should not therefore be a contraindication to the procedure but it is clearly important to identify those cases inclining towards ulcerative colitis rather than Crohn's disease. Thus the consideration of clinical and radiological features should be taken into account along with histopathology to assess anal and small bowel involvement that may enable some patients to be categorised confidently as Crohn's disease or inclining towards that diagnosis [40]. Patients with indeterminant colitis should be offered RPC if they so wish with the understanding that the failure rate is marginally but significantly greater than for patients with unequivocal ulcerative colitis.

Cancer. Patients with disseminated disease are not candidates for restorative proctocolectomy owing to the duration of the treatment and the possible complications that are increased in the palliative case. For those with non-disseminated carcinoma the indication should be based on the same criteria used for non-colitis-associated carcinoma particularly of the rectum. In 27 patients there were 3 cancer deaths over a mean follow-up of 4.3 ± 2.6 years indicating that the operation was justified if performed with curative intent and adequate resection margins [41].

Sclerosing cholangitis. Penna *et al.* [42] followed patients with and without sclerosing cholangitis after restorative proctocolectomy. Over a 5-year period the respective incidences of pouchitis were 61 and 36%. Although pouchitis in this study was not confirmed histologically in all cases, the same diagnostic criteria were applied to both groups and it is reasonable to conclude that patients with sclerosing cholangitis should be discouraged from having the operation. There is some evidence that these patients may be at a higher risk of developing dysplasia in the pouch [43].

Female fertility

Olsen *et al.* [44] followed a cohort of female patients with ulcerative colitis of child-bearing age from before the onset of the disease through to the development of colitis and finally after surgery. They studied fecundability, which is an index of fertility combined with the individual's desire or intention to have a child. When compared to the normal population, fecundibility in the cohort was no different before and after the development of ulcerative colitis, but it fell by over 50% after RPC. There was conversely an increased rate of pregnancy resulting from *in vitro* fertilisation in the pouch patients. Subsequent comparison with patients with familial adenomatous polyposis (FAP) having colectomy with ileo-rectal anastomosis and RPC [45] demonstrated that there was no reduction in fecundability after colectomy alone and also that the fall after RPC was greater in the ulcerative colitis than in the FAP patients. There appear therefore to be at least two factors reducing fertility including pelvic dissection and the disease itself. Others have also shown a similar effect on female fertility after pouch surgery [46, 47].

This has important consequences not only for the patient wishing to have children, but also potentially for the health care provider for medicolegal reasons. It is essential that all female patients of child-bearing age are counselled about fertility and that the consultation is recorded in the case notes. The discussion should lead to two broad management options for the patient to decide upon because surgery is necessary owing to the severity of the disease. A colectomy with ileostomy and preservation of the rectal stump will restore the patient to health enabling her to have children with no diminution in fertility. A restorative operation can then be deferred indefinitely to a convenient time for the patient. Alternatively, the patient may prefer to proceed directly to RPC (via an initial colectomy if the disease is severe) accepting the lowered fertility.

Technical aspects of surgery

Rectal dissection

This applies to patients having both conventional and restorative proctocolectomy. There are two technical options including a formal mobilisation of the rectum in the anatomical plane between the presacral fascia and the fascia propria of the rectum and a perimuscular or close rectal dissection. In the former case, the mesorectum is removed, in the latter it is left behind. The important difference between the two techniques lies in the relative potential for damaging pelvic nerves. A perimuscular dissection avoids this.

In patients with dysplasia or an already established carcinoma in any part of the large bowel, a mesorectal dissection should be carried out. The actual state of the rectal mucosa is only known on histopathological examination of the resected specimen. Thus, a patient with dysplasia in the colon as identified by endoscopic biopsy pre-operatively may well have dysplasia or even invasive carcinoma in the rectum when the histopathologist comes to examine the specimen.

Most patients undergoing surgery for ulcerative colitis do not have dysplasia. There are no prospective randomised trials in these cases comparing mesorectal dissection with perimuscular dissection. Mesorectal dissection is easier but there is an incidence of sexual dysfunction, although this is low, for example below 2% [48]. Perimuscular dissection technically is less easy because it does not follow an anatomical plane posteriorly. The mesorectum is left within the patient and thus the dead space in the pelvis after rectal excision is minimised. Very low rates of sexual dysfunction from zero to a few per cent have been reported [49, 50].

Whatever technique is adopted, there is little controversy that the dissection should be kept close to the rectal wall in the region of the lateral ligaments where the autonomic pelvic nerve plexus is most at risk. Identification and preservation of the presacral nerves should be made as they enter the pelvis and Denonvilliers' fascia should be divided in its upper part to reduce the chance of damage to the prostatic nerve plexus.

During conventional proctectomy there is general agreement that removal of the anal canal should be performed through the inter-sphincteric plane whether or not a perimuscular or mesorectal dissection has been carried out.

Pouch design

The triplicated loop S-pouch described by Parks *et al.* [51] resulted in a short distal ileal segment that was joined to the anal canal. Early reports [51] indicated that around 50% of patients could not evacuate spontaneously needing to use a catheter to do so although others reported lower rates [52]. Loss of spontaneous evacuation was therefore a significant disadvantage of the S-reservoir. Using evacuation proctography, Pescatori *et al.* [53] showed this was due to the distal ileal segment causing impedance to evacuation. Using a distal ileal segment of 2 cm or less, catheterisation rates fell to about 10% [52, 54, 55]. Revision of the pouch with removal of the distal ileal segment restored spontaneous evacuation in six out of eight patients [56].

The two-loop J-reservoir directly anastomosed to the anal canal [57] resulted in spontaneous evacuation in almost all cases as does the four loop W-reservoir [58]. The only present indication for employing an 'S' reservoir is in the uncommon situation where mobility of the reservoir to descend to the anal canal is only possible with this design.

Pouch volume is an important determinant of frequency of defaecation. Heppell *et al.* [59] had shown that there was an inverse relationship between frequency and capacitance of the neorectum in patients having a straight ileoanal reconstruction. The same relationship was subsequently described for the ileoanal reservoir [60] and also for the coloanal reservoir [61]. A comparison of three reservoir designs showed that frequency of defaecation was not significantly different for 'S' and 'W' reservoirs but was greater in patients having a J-reservoir. Spontaneous evacuation was much more likely with a J and W than with an S design and the need for anti-diarrhoeal medication was significantly higher for J (58%) than for S or W (20%) [60]. The volume of pouch distension at which large amplitude propulsive waves appeared correlated closely with stool frequency [62]. In a randomised study a larger J pouch (limb length 20 cm) had a similar frequency to the S reservoir again indicating the importance of capacitance [63].

Capacitance increases with time [60, 64]. A randomised comparison between J and a modified Kock (K) pouch showed that the latter attained a greater volume during the first year with a lower frequency of defaecation [64, 65]. A manovolumetric study of the J, K and S pouches at 1 year showed that the S and K designs had greater capacitance [66].

The data indicate that a larger pouch should be constructed for optimal long-term frequency. The ease with which the J reservoir can be constructed using linear stapling devices makes it the most popular design but the W reservoir has the greater capacitance. This and the J share the advantage over the S of not having a distal ileal segment with the disadvantage of non-spontaneous evacuation in some cases.

Mucosectomy

The original operation was based on the concept that all disease-prone mucosa should be removed including not only the colon and rectum but also the columnar epithelium of the anal canal. This required a manual ileoanal anastomosis after mucosectomy. Subsequently stapling at the anorectal junction was claimed to result in improved function [67] possibly due to preservation of sensory receptors within the anal canal. It was equally possible, however, that this was due to internal sphincter damage during manual anastomosis resulting from the anal dilatation.

Randomised prospective trials have shown, however, no difference in functional outcome after stapled or manual ileoanal anastomosis with mucosectomy [68, 69]. Complications were not significantly different, and frequency, urgency and continence were similar. In another trial there was a significant diminution in anal sensation after manual anastomosis, although this was not reflected in worse function [70]. Although resting anal tone was reduced in most cases after manual anastomosis, it was also reduced following stapled anastomosis in about 50% of cases [68].

The disadvantage of stapled anastomosis is the possibility of leaving diseased mucosa in the upper anal canal and in some cases the rectum. This can result in persisting symptoms of proctitis [71] as well as a continuing risk of carcinoma [72, 73]. The anal transitional zone is the area between the squamous epithelium at the dentate line and the columnar epithelium of the proximal large bowel [74]. Thompson-Fawcett and Mortensen [75] have shown that its longitudinal length is variable and it may even be absent. It is difficult therefore to predict the correct level of the anastomosis in the individual case. In patients having a stapled anastomosis subsequent development of dysplasia in the anal mucosa was reported to occur in 3% of patients over an average of 16 months of follow up [48], a rate which, if continued, would be considerable over 20 years.

Unresected inflamed anorectal mucosa may result in persisting symptoms including bleeding, burning and urgency. This occurred in 15–20% of patients undergoing stapled anastomosis [71, 76]. Furthermore, some of these patients suffer from inadequate emptying with the frequent passage of small volumes of stool. Symptoms may be so severe that major surgical revision is necessary involving removal of the rectal stump with ileoanal anastomosis after mucosectomy. Successful outcome of such salvage surgery is about 70%, being lower than if an adequate operation had been performed on the first occasion [77, 78].

Adequate mobility of the pouch to descend to the anus without tension is essential. If despite using manoeuvres to maximise the length of the mesentery there is still the possibility of tension, a stapled anastomosis is preferable. Equally, there are cases where a manual anastomosis is obligatory, for example when the stapler fails or where the anorectal stump is too short for stapling owing to previous surgery.

The surgeon must be capable of using either technique but where stapling is used the anastomosis should be at the correct level to avoid leaving inflamed mucosa behind. Mucosectomy with manual anastomosis should be used in cases with carcinoma or dysplasia elsewhere in the large bowel. There is no evidence that function is different after either method as judged from prospective randomised trials [65, 68, 79].

The number of stages

Some patients will have had an initial colectomy and others a restorative proctocolectomy as the first procedure. Because clinical factors in the individual patient determine the choice (see above), a prospective trial to determine which of these approaches is better is not possible. In a retrospective comparison of patients after either approach there was no difference in the complication rate or function [80].

The need for a defunctioning ileostomy has been questioned since the 1980s. Of 60 patients reported by Everett and Pollard [81], 20 had no ileostomy, of which a defunctioning ileostomy was required in the immediate post-operative period in two cases. In a similar experience, 3 out of 16 patients required a subsequent ileostomy, which was permanent in one [82]. In a randomised trial of 45 patients with ($n = 23$) and without ($n = 22$) an ileostomy there was no difference in leak rate (one in each group) nor any other complication. Overall hospital stay was greater in patients with (23 days (range 13–75)) than without (13 days (range 7–119)) [83]. In contrast in 71 patients having a one-stage and 87 a two-stage operation, respective anastomotic leak rates were 7 and 18% [54]. Patients having a temporary defunctioning ileostomy are at risk of complications due to the stoma amounting to around 25% of cases.

As restorative proctocolectomy is an alternative to conventional proctocolectomy with permanent ileostomy and not to the normal state, it is very useful for the patient to have experienced an ileostomy at some stage during treatment. The surgeon has to balance the advantage of a one-stage procedure resulting in shorter recovery in 80–85% of patients against the disadvantage of faecal peritonitis and re-operation in the minority. A two-stage procedure has the disadvantage of longer treatment time with complications due to the stoma set against the advantage of avoidance of severe faecal sepsis.

Laparoscopic surgery

In expert hands both laparoscopic colectomy and restorative proctocolectomy are feasible [84–87]. Most published series have reported a laparoscopic-assisted approach, with a small Pfannensteil incision used for pevic dissection, transection of the anorectal junction and specimen retrieval. An alternative approach is performing both the colectomy and the pelvic dissection laparoscopically with a small midline incision used for specimen retrieval and pouch construction. The midline incision is closed and stapled pouch-anal anastomosis performed following reintroduction of pneumoperitoneum [87]. These procedures are technically demanding, requiring laparoscopic access to all quadrants of the abdomen and there is a significant learning curve. For these reasons surgeons have been slower to take up laparoscopic surgery for colitis than segmental colectomy for other indications. Operating times of up to seven and three-quarter hours have been reported [87]. There are technical difficulties with cross-stapling the anorectal junction due to difficult access. There are also some concerns that laparoscopic rectal dissection may result in a higher rate of pelvic nerve injury than its open equivalent [88]. The only published randomised-controlled trial to date compared hand-assisted laparoscopic restorative proctocolectomy with open surgery in 60 patients. In this study there was no significant difference in length of stay (median stay of 10 and 11 days respectively) or morbidity between the two groups [89].

Salvage surgery for the failing pouch

Pouch failure (defined as pouch excision or indefinite proximal diversion) continues progressively with time. At 10 years, approximately 10% of patients will have either had the pouch excised or indefinitely defunctioned by an ileostomy [38, 39]. Quantification of the risk of failure based on preoperative and intra-operative variables is already sufficiently refined to be useful in clinical practice as a predictor of failure [90].

The causes of failure include sepsis accounting for more than 50% of cases, poor function in 30% and pouchitis in 10% [39]. In some patients failure when imminent may be avoided by salvage surgery. This can be either abdominal when remodelling or advancement of the pouch is required or perineal when trying to close a low pouch-vaginal fistula.

There is controversy on the effectiveness of abdominal salvage for sepsis due to chronic abscess formation in the pelvis. Fazio et al. [91] reported success defined as avoidance of a permanent ileostomy in 22 of 24 patients undergoing abdominal salvage for sepsis after RPC for ulcerative colitis. Although some patients had poor function, the majority felt the procedure to have been worthwhile. Cohen et al. [92] had had a similar good experience but others in contrast reported disappointing results with success in between 40 and 50% [30, 78, 93, 94]. One factor for this difference is the length of follow-up from the salvage procedure, because failure continues at a rate of about 30% over 5 years [30, 78, 94]. Furthermore the results of salvage surgery for a septic indication are worse than for a non-septic indication by about 20–30% [78, 94, 95]. Thus the evidence to date suggests that abdominal salvage for sepsis should be used with caution and applied to specific clinico-pathological situations such as leakage from the stapled end of a J-pouch or where pouch advancement to a level well below the sepsis or fistula is possible in cases, for example, with a long retained rectal stump. There is less chance of success when the sepsis is low in the pelvis such that it will be adjacent to the new ileo-anal anastomosis. In these circumstances, salvage has a prospect of success of around 70%. Preoperative counselling should be carried out with care and the patient should know that complications are likely and that there is a 30–40% chance of failure over a 5-year period.

Perineal salvage procedures are almost always used to attempt closure of a pouch-vaginal fistula. There is controversy whether an endo-anal or trans-vaginal approach should be employed. Surgeon preference is clearly a major factor, because in the United States the former is most commonly used, while the latter has been favoured in Europe. There appears, however, to be little difference in outcome with successful closure reported in about 60% of patients using either approach [96, 97]. There have been no randomised controlled trials owing to surgeon preference and low patient accrual rates. Nor has there been any comparison of function following either approach. This could be important, however, because the endo-anal approach will result in some degree of dilatation of the anal sphincter.

Follow-up after restorative proctocolectomy

There is general acceptance that patients should be followed-up after RPC. The aims and protocols of this are controversial, however. Aims include the need for the surgeon to know the long-term outcome, the necessity for the patient to remain in contact with the medical team in the event of late complications and functional difficulties, the surveillance for possible haematological and metabolic disturbance and surveillance for possible neoplastic transformation. This last has assumed importance in recent years owing to reports of carcinoma of the ileal pouch itself and of the anorectal mucosa below the ileal pouch anastomosis [98]. These authors reviewed 15 reports from the literature, although at least one [99] may not have been a true development of carcinoma after pouch construction as the tumour almost certainly was present in the rectal stump before the original RPC.

Although the number of cancers is small considering the large number of patients operated on world wide, it will certainly increase in the future. The risk of cancer in the ileal pouch is low. Of 468 patients followed for periods ranging from 1 to more than 21 years with a median of about 10 years, there were four cases of dysplasia and one of carcinoma [100–102]. Hulten *et al.* [103] reported a group of patients followed for a median of 30 years after a Kock ileostomy of who only three developed dysplasia and none carcinoma. With regard to the risk in the residual anorectal stump, follow-up of 178 patients beyond 10 years from RPC identified 8 with dysplasia and none with carcinoma [104] and Coull *et al.* [105] observed no case of dysplasia or carcinoma in 135 patients followed for 1–12 years.

Dysplasia is associated with persisting chronic inflammation (chronic unremitting pouchitis) in the pouch [106] and also in patients with sclerosing cholangitis [43]. The presence of these conditions is therefore an indication of the need for cancer follow-up. Of the patients reviewed by Borjesson *et al.* [98], all had had either dysplasia or an established carcinoma in the original specimen obtained by colectomy or RPC. Thus these patients should be followed. Although carcinoma has been reported at as little as 2 years from RPC, the median interval for the few cases of dysplasia to develop has been of the order of 10–15 years. A regime for cancer follow-up should therefore involve infrequent examination in the early years in the high risk groups identified above, becoming annual from 10 years onwards. Endoscopy with multiple biopsies from the ileal reservoir and the anorectal zone below the distal ileal anastomosis is required. The most practical protocol has not yet been agreed upon.

References

1 Miller GG, Gardner CM, Ripstein CB. Primary resection of the colon in ulcerative colitis. *Can Med Assoc* 1956;60:584.
2 Kartheuser AH, Dozois RR, LaRusso NF, Wiesner RH, Ilstrup DM, Schleck CD. Comparison of surgical treatment of ulcerative colitis associated with primary sclerosing cholangitis: ileal pouch-anal anastomosis versus Brooke ileostomy. *Mayo Clin Proc* 1996;71(8):748–56.
3 Brooke BN. The management of ileostomy. *Lancet* 1952;ii:102–4.
4 Kornbluth A, Present DH, Lichtiger S, Hanauer S. Cyclosporin for severe ulcerative colitis: a user's guide. *Am J Gastroenterol* 1997;92(9):1424–8.
5 Wojdemann M, Wettergren A, Hartvigsen A, Myrhoj T, Svendsen LB, Bulow S. Closure of rectal stump after colectomy for acute colitis. *Int J Colorectal Dis* 1995;10(4):197–9.
6 Ng RL, Davies AH, Grace RH, Mortensen NJ. Subcutaneous rectal stump closure after emergency subtotal colectomy. *Br J Surg* 1992;79(7):701–3.
7 Lennard-Jones JE, Morson BC, Ritchie JK, Williams CB. Cancer surveillance in ulcerative colitis. Experience over 15 years. *Lancet* 1983;2(8342):149–52.
8 Connell WR, Lennard-Jones JE, Williams CB, Talbot IC, Price AB, Wilkinson KH. Factors affecting the

outcome of endoscopic surveillance for cancer in ulcerative colitis. *Gastroenterology* 1994;107(4): 934–44.
9. Riddell RH, Goldman H, Ransohoff DF, et al. Dysplasia in inflammatory bowel disease: standardized classification with provisional clinical applications. *Hum Pathol* 1983;14(11): 931–68.
10. Provenzale D, Wong JB, Onken JE, Lipscomb J. Performing a cost-effectiveness analysis: surveillance of patients with ulcerative colitis. *Am J Gastroenterol* 1998;93(6):872–80.
11. Melville DM, Ritchie JK, Nicholls RJ, Hawley PR. Surgery for ulcerative colitis in the era of the pouch: the St Mark's Hospital experience. *Gut* 1994;35(8): 1076–80.
12. Watts JM, Hughes ES. Ulcerative colitis and Crohn's disease: results after colectomy and ileorectal anastomosis. *Br J Surg* 1977;64(2):77–83.
13. Baker WN. The results of ileorectal anastomosis at St Mark's Hospital from 1953 to 1968. *Gut* 1970;11(3):235–9.
14. Hawley PR. Ileorectal anastomosis. *Br J Surg* 1985;72(Suppl):S75–6.
15. Baker WN, Glass RE, Ritchie JK, Aylett SO. Cancer of the rectum following colectomy and ileorectal anastomosis for ulcerative colitis. *Br J Surg* 1978;65 (12):862–8.
16. Belliveau P, Trudel J, Vasilevsky CA, Stein B, Gordon PH. Ileoanal anastomosis with reservoirs: complications and long-term results. *Can J Surg* 1999;42(5):345–52.
17. Gemlo BT, Wong WD, Rothenberger DA, Goldberg SM. Ileal pouch-anal anastomosis: patterns of failure. *Arch Surg* 1992;127(7):784–6.
18. Jarvinen HJ, Luukkonen P. Experience with restorative proctocolectomy in 201 patients. *Ann Chir Gynaecol* 1993;82(3):159–64.
19. Setti-Carraro P, Ritchie JK, Wilkinson KH, Nicholls RJ, Hawley PR. The first 10 years' experience of restorative proctocolectomy for ulcerative colitis. *Gut* 1994;35(8):1070–5.
20. Korsgen S, Keighley MR. Causes of failure and life expectancy of the ileoanal pouch. *Int J Colorectal Dis* 1997;12(1):4–8.
21. Kohler L, Troidl H. The ileoanal pouch: a risk-benefit analysis. *Br J Surg* 1995;82(4):443–7.
22. McLeod RS, Baxter NN. Quality of life of patients with inflammatory bowel disease after surgery. *World J Surg* 1998;22(4):375–81.
23. Pezim ME, Nicholls RJ. Quality of life after restorative proctocolectomy with pelvic ileal reservoir. *Br J Surg* 1985;72(1):31–3.
24. Stryker SJ, Kelly KA, Phillips SF, Dozois RR, Beart RW Jr. Anal and neorectal function after ileal pouch-anal anastomosis. *Ann Surg* 1986;203(1): 55–61.
25. Bauer JJ, Gorfine SR, Gelernt IM, Harris MT, Kreel I. Restorative proctocolectomy in patients older than fifty years. *Dis Colon Rectum* 1997;40(5):562–5.
26. Lewis WG, Sagar PM, Holdsworth PJ, Axon AT, Johnston D. Restorative proctocolectomy with end to end pouch-anal anastomosis in patients over the age of fifty. *Gut* 1993;34(7):948–52.
27. Takao Y, Gilliland R, Nogueras JJ, Weiss EG, Wexner SD. Is age relevant to functional outcome after restorative proctocolectomy for ulcerative colitis: prospective assessment of 122 cases. *Ann Surg* 1998;227(2):187–94.
28. Dayton MT, Larsen KR. Should older patients undergo ileal pouch-anal anastomosis? *Am J Surg* 1996;172(5):444–7.
29. Nicholls RJ. Restorative proctocolectomy with various types of reservoir. *World J Surg* 1987;11(6):751–62.
30. Galandiuk S, Scott NA, Dozois RR, et al. Ileal pouch-anal anastomosis: reoperation for pouch-related complications. *Ann Surg* 1990;212(4): 446–52.
31. Panis Y, Poupard B, Nemeth J, Lavergne A, Hautefeuille P, Valleur P. Ileal pouch/anal anastomosis for Crohn's disease. *Lancet* 1996;347(9005):854–7.
32. Regimbeau JM, Panis Y, Pocard M, et al. Long-term results of ileal pouch-anal anastomosis for colorectal Crohn's disease. *Dis Colon Rectum* 2001;44(6): 769–78.
33. Phillips RKS. Ileal pouch-anal anastomosis for Crohn's disease. *Gut* 1998;43(3):303–4.
34. Price AB. Overlap in the spectrum of non-specific inflammatory bowel disease – 'colitis indeterminate'. *J Clin Pathol* 1978;31(6):567–77.
35. Swan NC, Geoghegan JG, O'Donoghue DP, Hyland JM, Sheahan K. Fulminant colitis in inflammatory bowel disease: detailed pathologic and clinical analysis. *Dis Colon Rectum* 1998;41(12):1511–15.
36. Pezim ME, Pemberton JH, Beart RW Jr, et al. Outcome of 'indeterminant' colitis following ileal pouch-anal anastomosis. *Dis Colon Rectum* 1989;32(8):653–8.
37. Atkinson KG, Owen DA, Wankling G. Restorative proctocolectomy and indeterminate colitis. *Am J Surg* 1994;167(5):516–18.
38. Yu CS, Pemberton JH, Larson D. Ileal pouch-anal anastomosis in patients with indeterminate colitis: long-term results. *Dis Colon Rectum* 2000;43(11): 1487–96.
39. Tulchinsky H, Hawley PR, Nicholls J. Long-term failure after restorative proctocolectomy for

40 Wells AD, McMillan I, Price AB, Ritchie JK, Nicholls RJ. Natural history of indeterminate colitis. *Br J Surg* 1991;78(2):179–81.

41 Ziv Y, Fazio VW, Strong SA, Oakley JR, Milsom JW, Lavery IC. Ulcerative colitis and coexisting colorectal cancer: recurrence rate after restorative proctocolectomy. *Ann Surg Oncol* 1994;1(6):512–5.

42 Penna C, Dozois R, Tremaine W, et al. Pouchitis after ileal pouch-anal anastomosis for ulcerative colitis occurs with increased frequency in patients with associated primary sclerosing cholangitis. *Gut* 1996;38(2):234–9.

43 Stahlberg D, Veress B, Tribukait B, Broome U. Atrophy and neoplastic transformation of the ileal pouch mucosa in patients with ulcerative colitis and primary sclerosing cholangitis: a case control study. *Dis Colon Rectum* 2003;46(6):770–8.

44 Olsen KO, Joelsson M, Laurberg S, Oresland T. Fertility after ileal pouch-anal anastomosis in women with ulcerative colitis. *Br J Surg* 1999;86(4):493–5.

45 Olsen KO, Juul S, Bulow S, et al. Female fecundity before and after operation for familial adenomatous polyposis. *Br J Surg* 2003;90(2):227–31.

46 Johnson P, Richard C, Ravid A, et al. Female infertility after ileal pouch-anal anastomosis for ulcerative colitis. *Dis Colon Rectum* 2004;47(7):1119–26.

47 Gorgun E, Remzi FH, Goldberg JM, et al. Fertility is reduced after restorative proctocolectomy with ileal pouch anal anastomosis: a study of 300 patients. *Surgery* 2004;136(4):795–803.

48 Ziv Y, Fazio VW, Sirimarco MT, Lavery IC, Goldblum JR, Petras RE. Incidence, risk factors, and treatment of dysplasia in the anal transitional zone after ileal pouch-anal anastomosis. *Dis Colon Rectum* 1994;37(12):1281–5.

49 Lyttle JA, Parks AG. Intersphincteric excision of the rectum. *Br J Surg* 1977;64(6):413–16.

50 Berry AR, de CR, Lee EC. Perineal and pelvic morbidity following perimuscular excision of the rectum for inflammatory bowel disease. *Br J Surg* 1986;73(8):675–7.

51 Parks AG, Nicholls RJ, Belliveau P. Proctocolectomy with ileal reservoir and anal anastomosis. *Br J Surg* 1980;67(8):533–8.

52 Rothenberger DA, Vermeulen FD, Christenson CE, et al. Restorative proctocolectomy with ileal reservoir and ileoanal anastomosis. *Am J Surg* 1983;145(1):82–8.

53 Pescatori M, Manhire A, Bartram CI. Evacuation pouchography in the evaluation of ileoanal reservoir function. *Dis Colon Rectum* 1983;26(6):365–8.

54 Cohen Z, McLeod RS, Stern H, Grant D, Nordgren S. The pelvic pouch and ileoanal anastomosis procedure: surgical technique and initial results. *Am J Surg* 1985;150(5):601–7.

55 Vasilevsky CA, Rothenberger DA, Goldberg SM. The S ileal pouch-anal anastomosis. *World J Surg* 1987;11(6):742–50.

56 Nicholls RJ, Gilbert JM. Surgical correction of the efferent ileal limb for disordered defaecation following restorative proctocolectomy with the S ileal reservoir. *Br J Surg* 1990;77(2):152–4.

57 Utsunomiya J, Iwama T, Imajo M, et al. Total colectomy, mucosal proctectomy, and ileoanal anastomosis. *Dis Colon Rectum* 1980;23(7):459–66.

58 Nicholls RJ, Lubowski DZ. Restorative proctocolectomy: the four loop (W) reservoir. *Br J Surg* 1987;74(7):564–6.

59 Heppell J, Kelly KA, Phillips SF, Beart RW Jr, Telander RL, Perrault J. Physiologic aspects of continence after colectomy, mucosal proctectomy, and endorectal ileo-anal anastomosis. *Ann Surg* 1982;195(4):435–43.

60 Nicholls RJ, Pezim ME. Restorative proctocolectomy with ileal reservoir for ulcerative colitis and familial adenomatous polyposis: a comparison of three reservoir designs. *Br J Surg* 1985;72(6):470–4.

61 Lazorthes F, Gamagami R, Chiotasso P, Istvan G, Muhammad S. Prospective, randomized study comparing clinical results between small and large colonic J-pouch following coloanal anastomosis. *Dis Colon Rectum* 1997;40(12):1409–13.

62 O'Connell PR, Pemberton JH, Brown ML, Kelly KA. Determinants of stool frequency after ileal pouch-anal anastomosis. *Am J Surg* 1987;153(2):157–64.

63 Keighley MR, Yoshioka K, Kmiot W. Prospective randomized trial to compare the stapled double lumen pouch and the sutured quadruple pouch for restorative proctocolectomy. *Br J Surg* 1988;75(10):1008–11.

64 Oresland T, Fasth S, Nordgren S, Hallgren T, Hulten L. A prospective randomized comparison of two different pelvic pouch designs. *Scand J Gastroenterol* 1990;25(10):986–96.

65 Hallgren T, Fasth S, Nordgren S, Oresland T, Hulten L. The stapled ileal pouch–anal anastomosis. A randomized study comparing two different pouch designs. *Scand J Gastroenterol* 1990;25(11):1161–8.

66 Hallgren T, Fasth S, Nordgren S, Oresland T, Hallsberg L, Hulten L. Manovolumetric characteristics and functional results in three different pelvic pouch designs. *Int J Colorectal Dis* 1989;4(3):156–60.

67 Johnston D, Holdsworth PJ, Nasmyth DG, et al. Preservation of the entire anal canal in conservative proctocolectomy for ulcerative colitis: a pilot study comparing end-to-end ileo-anal anastomosis without mucosal resection with mucosal proctectomy and endo-anal anastomosis. Br J Surg 1987;74(10): 940–4.

68 Seow Choen F, Tsunoda A, Nicholls RJ. Prospective randomized trial comparing anal function after hand sewn ileoanal anastomosis with mucosectomy versus stapled ileoanal anastomosis without mucosectomy in restorative proctocolectomy. Br J Surg 1991;78(4): 430–4.

69 Hallgren TA, Fasth SB, Oresland TO, Hulten LA. Ileal pouch anal function after endoanal mucosectomy and handsewn ileoanal anastomosis compared with stapled anastomosis without mucosectomy. Eur J Surg 1995;161(12):915–21.

70 Keighley MR, Winslet MC, Yoshioka K, Lightwood R. Discrimination is not impaired by excision of the anal transition zone after restorative proctocolectomy. Br J Surg 1987;74(12):1118–21.

71 Lavery IC, Sirimarco MT, Ziv Y, Fazio VW. Anal canal inflammation after ileal pouch-anal anastomosis. The need for treatment. Dis Colon Rectum 1995;38(8):803–6.

72 Tsunoda A, Talbot IC, Nicholls RJ. Incidence of dysplasia in the anorectal mucosa in patients having restorative proctocolectomy. Br J Surg 1990;77(5): 506–8.

73 King DW, Lubowski DZ, Cook TA. Anal canal mucosa in restorative proctocolectomy for ulcerative colitis. Br J Surg 1989;76(9):970–2.

74 Fenger C. The anal transitional zone. Location and extent. Acta Pathol Microbiol Scand [A] 1979;87A(5):379–86.

75 Thompson-Fawcett MW, Warren BF, Mortensen NJ. A new look at the anal transitional zone with reference to restorative proctocolectomy and the columnar cuff. Br J Surg 1998;85(11): 1517–21.

76 Schmitt SL, Wexner SD, Lucas FV, James K, Nogueras JJ, Jagelman DG. Retained mucosa after double-stapled ileal reservoir and ileoanal anastomosis. Dis Colon Rectum 1992;35(11): 1051–6.

77 Tulchinsky H, McCourtney JS, Rao KV, et al. Salvage abdominal surgery in patients with a retained rectal stump after restorative proctocolectomy and stapled anastomosis. Br J Surg 2001;88(12):1602–6.

78 Tekkis PP, Heriot AG, Smith JJ, Das P, Canero A, Nicholls RJ. Long-term results of abdominal salvage surgery following restorative proctocolectomy. Br J Surg 2005: in press.

79 McIntyre PB, Pemberton JH, Beart RW Jr, Devine RM, Nivatvongs S. Double-stapled vs. handsewn ileal pouch-anal anastomosis in patients with chronic ulcerative colitis. Dis Colon Rectum 1994;37(5): 430–3.

80 Nicholls RJ, Holt SD, Lubowski DZ. Restorative proctocolectomy with ileal reservoir. Comparison of two-stage vs. three-stage procedures and analysis of factors that might affect outcome. Dis Colon Rectum 1989;32(4):323–6.

81 Everett WG, Pollard SG. Restorative proctocolectomy without temporary ileostomy. Br J Surg 1990;77(6):621–2.

82 Kmiot WA, Keighley MR. Totally stapled abdominal restorative proctocolectomy. Br J Surg 1989;76(9): 961–4.

83 Grobler SP, Hosie KB, Keighley MR. Randomized trial of loop ileostomy in restorative proctocolectomy. Br J Surg 1992;79(9):903–6.

84 Marcello PW, Milsom JW, Wong SK, et al. Laparoscopic restorative proctocolectomy: case-matched comparative study with open restorative proctocolectomy. Dis Colon Rectum 2000;43(5):604–8.

85 Ky AJ, Sonoda T, Milsom JW. One-stage laparoscopic restorative proctocolectomy: an alternative to the conventional approach? Dis Colon Rectum 2002;45(2):207–10.

86 Kienle P, Weitz J, Benner A, Herfarth C, Schmidt J. Laparoscopically assisted colectomy and ileoanal pouch procedure with and without protective ileostomy. Surg Endosc 2003;17(5):716–20.

87 Kienle P, Z'graggen K, Schmidt J, Benner A, Weitz J, Buchler MW. Laparoscopic restorative proctocolectomy. Br J Surg 2005;92(1):88–93.

88 Bemelman WA, D'Hoore A. Laparoscopic restorative proctocolectomy (Br J Surg 2005;92:88–93). Br J Surg 2005;92(4):493.

89 Maartense S, Dunker MS, Slors JF, et al. Hand-assisted laparoscopic versus open restorative proctocolectomy with ileal pouch anal anastomosis: a randomized trial. Ann Surg 2004;240(6):984–91.

90 Fazio VW, Tekkis PP, Remzi F, et al. Quantification of risk for pouch failure after ileal pouch anal anastomosis surgery. Ann Surg 2003;238(4):605–14.

91 Fazio VW, Wu JS, Lavery IC. Repeat ileal pouch-anal anastomosis to salvage septic complications of pelvic pouches: clinical outcome and quality of life assessment. Ann Surg 1998;228(4):588–97.

92 Cohen Z, Smith D, McLeod R. Reconstructive surgery for pelvic pouches. World J Surg 1998;22(4): 342–6.

93 Paye F, Penna C, Chiche L, Tiret E, Frileux P, Parc R. Pouch-related fistula following restorative

proctocolectomy. *Br J Surg* 1996;83(11): 1574–7.
94 Heuschen UA, Allemeyer EH, Hinz U, Lucas M, Herfarth C, Heuschen G. Outcome after septic complications in J pouch procedures. *Br J Surg* 2002;89(2):194–200.
95 Tulchinsky H, Cohen CR, Nicholls RJ. Salvage surgery after restorative proctocolectomy. *Br J Surg* 2003;90(8):909–21.
96 Shah NS, Remzi F, Massmann A, Baixauli J, Fazio VW. Management and treatment outcome of pouch-vaginal fistulas following restorative proctocolectomy. *Dis Colon Rectum* 2003;46(7): 911–7.
97 Heriot AG, Tekkis PP, Smith JJ, Bona R, Cohen RG, Nicholls RJ. Management and outcome of pouch-vaginal fistulas following restorative proctocolectomy. *Dis Colon Rectum* 2005;48(3): 451–8.
98 Borjesson L, Willen R, Haboubi N, Duff SE, Hulten L. The risk of dysplasia and cancer in the ileal pouch mucosa after restorative proctocolectomy for ulcerative proctocolitis is low: a long-term term follow-up study. *Colorectal Dis* 2004;6(6):494–8.
99 Stern H, Walfisch S, Mullen B, McLeod R, Cohen Z. Cancer in an ileoanal reservoir: a new late complication? *Gut* 1990;31(4):473–5.
100 Veress B, Reinholt FP, Lindquist K, Lofberg R, Liljeqvist L. Long-term histomorphological surveillance of the pelvic ileal pouch: dysplasia develops in a subgroup of patients. *Gastroenterology* 1995;109(4):1090–7.
101 Thompson-Fawcett MW, Marcus V, Redston M, Cohen Z, McLeod RS. Risk of dysplasia in long-term ileal pouches and pouches with chronic pouchitis. *Gastroenterology* 2001;121(2):275–81.
102 Heuschen UA, Heuschen G, Autschbach F, Allemeyer EH, Herfarth C. Adenocarcinoma in the ileal pouch: late risk of cancer after restorative proctocolectomy. *Int J Colorectal Dis* 2001;16(2):126–30.
103 Hulten L, Willen R, Nilsson O, Safarani N, Haboubi N. Mucosal assessment for dysplasia and cancer in the ileal pouch mucosa in patients operated on for ulcerative colitis – a 30-year follow-up study. *Dis Colon Rectum* 2002;45(4):448–52.
104 Remzi FH, Fazio VW, Delaney CP, *et al*. Dysplasia of the anal transitional zone after ileal pouch-anal anastomosis: results of prospective evaluation after a minimum of ten years. *Dis Colon Rectum* 2003;46(1):6–13.
105 Coull DB, Lee FD, Henderson AP, Anderson JH, McKee RF, Finlay IG. Risk of dysplasia in the columnar cuff after stapled restorative proctocolectomy. *Br J Surg* 2003;90(1):72–5.
106 Gullberg K, Stahlberg D, Liljeqvist L, *et al*. Neoplastic transformation of the pelvic pouch mucosa in patients with ulcerative colitis. *Gastroenterology* 1997;112(5):1487–92.

13: What are the causes and treatment of ileoanal pouch dysfunction?

Alan F. Horgan, William J. Sandborn and John H. Pemberton

Introduction

From the time Donald Peck and Alan Parks described the original operation of restorative proctocolectomy, ileal pouch anal anastomosis has become a standard approach for patients requiring proctocolectomy for chronic ulcerative colitis. Importantly, long-term outcomes are good [1], and the quality of life improved compared to the previous standard operation of Brooke ileostomy [2]. Variations in pouch design have been described but actual functional differences between pouch designs remain unproven. The ideal outcome following ileal pouch-anal anastomosis (IPAA) consists of four to six semi-formed bowel motions occurring during daytime hours with no nocturnal stools, no incontinence and no necessity for long-term medications. Unfortunately, many patients fall short of this ideal, and pouch dysfunction remains a major cause of morbidity in a subset of patients following ileoanal pouch construction. In this chapter we discuss the aetiology and treatment of ileoanal pouch dysfunction and provide algorithms for approaching the evaluation of pouch dysfunction based on presenting symptoms.

Pouch function is most commonly determined by four major factors, i.e. stool frequency, continence, ability to defaecate spontaneously and ability to defer defaecation. Pouch dysfunction may result from increased stool frequency, incontinence and fistula formation. Importantly, however, outcomes often depend upon patients' expectations and what is perceived to be an excellent result for some may be less than satisfactory for others. There are limited techniques available for objective assessment of pouch function but valuable quantifiable information can be gained in some instances by the use of anal canal manometry, pouch capacity and compliance, static contrast pouchography and videopouchography, scintigraphy, pouch endoscopy with mucosal biopsy and pelvic MRI.

Pouch dysfunction caused by increased stool frequency

Wide variations in stool frequency are seen between patients following restorative proctocolectomy. Although some of these represent variations in normal motility and evacuation, others represent disorders of pouch construction, design or a pouch-specific complication. The majority of patients will respond to hypomotility agents, such as opioid analogues, which have been shown to reduce bowel frequency by reducing total stool weight [3]. However, it must be kept in mind that there are a number of specific pouch-related complications that present with increased stool frequency, and a careful search must be made for an underlying cause in patients who are refractory to first-line therapy.

Stool frequency as a function of pouch construction

It has long been debated if larger pouches are associated with lower stool frequency. Hallgren et al. [4] compared stool frequency between S and J pouches and found the mean stool frequency of the J pouch group to be six motions per 24 h, compared with eight stools per day in patients with S pouches. In contrast, however, Tuckson and Fazio [5] found that mean stool frequency per 24 h was six in patients who had a J pouch, compared with four in patients who had an S pouch. Similarly, the four-limbed W pouch has been shown in some studies to be associated with significantly lower stool frequency compared with S pouches [6]. Similarly, night evacuation has been shown to be higher in patients with J pouches (mean nocturnal frequency 1.2) compared with patients with W pouches whose average nocturnal frequency appears to be significantly less [7, 8]. Whichever pouch design is used, it appears certain that frequency decreases with time as the pouch capacity increases.

Varying claims have been made comparing hand-sewn and stapled pouch-anal anastomoses with regard to stool frequency. However, in the four prospective randomised studies that have been published to date [9–12] there has been no significant difference between hand-sewn and stapled pouch-anal anastomoses with regard to either daytime or nocturnal frequency of pouch evacuation.

Small-bowel motility disorders

Some patients with increased stool frequency, in the absence of any other definable cause, are labelled as suffering from a variant of irritable bowel syndrome (IBS). A final consideration in patients with ileal pouch dysfunction is IBS, recently dubbed the irritable pouch syndrome [13]. This protean affliction may become unmasked after colectomy. Indeed, patients may experience exactly the same symptoms of IBS, as do their unoperated counterparts. These symptoms include bloating, alternating watery and formed stools, abdominal pain, urgency, frequency and a sense of incomplete evacuation. Medications found to be helpful in patients with IBS but without an IPAA, such as amitriptyline (low dose) anticholinergics, and stool-bulking agents will likewise be helpful to the IPAA patient as well. In some patients who have dilated pouches and IBS, daily catheter drainage is quite helpful.

A study of small-bowel motility in patients with good pouch function, i.e. median bowel frequency four per day, compared with patients with poor pouch function, i.e. median bowel frequency of 12 per day, measured small-bowel motility over a 24-h period [14]. It was found that patients with increased stool frequency had a significantly greater number of migrating motor complexes in the small bowel proximal to the pouch compared to those patients with good pouch function. Twenty-four-hour stool output appeared similar in both groups but the median maximum tolerated volume on reservoir distension was significantly lower for patients with poor function compared with those with good function. Soper et al. [15] documented further that compared to controls, proctocolectomy slowed small-bowel transit, but not gastric emptying. Moreover, compared to patients with Brooke ileostomy, patients with an IPAA experienced even slower small-bowel transit.

Specific infections

Specific infections such as bacterial infections with *Salmonella*, *Shigella*, *Escherichia coli* or *Campylobacter* are rare. Stool culture for these bacteria, in addition to viral titres for specific viruses such as cytomegalovirus and the search for *Clostridium difficile* toxins should be performed in the appropriate clinical setting.

Crohn's disease

Despite certain studies that advocate IPAA as an alternative to Brooke ileostomy in selected patients with Crohn's disease (without anoperineal or small-bowel manifestations) [16], Crohn's disease remains a contraindication to IPAA. However, as the distinction between ulcerative colitis and Crohn's disease of the colon continues to be difficult, some patients with Crohn's disease will undergo IPAA inadvertently. Increased stool frequency may be accompanied in these patients by the development of complex fistulae, perianal infection or extra-intestinal manifestations. Direct visualisation of the pouch with biopsy or contrast radiography of the proximal small bowel may show features suggestive of Crohn's disease in these patients. Inadvertent IPAA for Crohn's disease in these patients is historically associated with a high failure rate (45%) [17] but an acceptable long-term functional result can be achieved through the use of immunosuppressive therapy for Crohn's disease if the pouch can be kept *in situ* [18].

Pelvic sepsis

Pelvic sepsis following IPAA will commonly result in decreased pouch compliance with a consequent increase in stool frequency. The incidence of pelvic sepsis in various series has been quoted to be between 10 and 30% [19]. However, rates of pelvic sepsis have declined steadily, such that currently 5% of patients can be expected to have pelvic sepsis post-operatively [20]. This may be due to either an infected pelvic haematoma or a defect in the pouch or pouch-anal anastomotic suture or staple line. Such an event will lead to pouch excision in approximately 5–10% of patients. Moreover, in those pouches that survive, the ensuing fibrosis often leads to unacceptable functional results. The maximum tolerated volume of such pouches, reflected by pouch size, sensitivity, compliance or a combination of these, appears to be the major determinant of pouch function [21]. A retrospective analysis looked at the usefulness of pouchography prior to closure of a defunctioning ileostomy in 25 consecutive patients following IPAA [22]. This group found that the predictive value of a negative test is high (89%) and found that leak of contrast from the anastomosis is a specific (81%), but not sensitive (56%), indicator of pelvic sepsis. The use of prophylactic antibiotics or pre-operative corticosteroids does not appear to influence the incidence of pelvic sepsis, the rate of which appears to decrease with increasing experience of the operating surgeon.

Pouchitis

Pouchitis is defined as an idiopathic inflammation of the ileal pouch mucosa. It is the most frequent long-term complication following IPAA. The Mayo Clinic experience reported the cumulative probability of developing at least one episode of pouchitis during follow-up as 32% [23]. Stahlberg *et al.* [24] found the incidence of pouchitis was highest (23.1%) in the first 6 months after IPAA. The incidence during the next 6-month period fell to 11.4% and was 3.1% thereafter. Nevertheless, the cumulative risk of developing a first episode of pouchitis increases over time. Recent studies from the Mayo Clinic reported that the cumulative risk for the first episode of pouchitis at 1, 5 and 10 years following IPAA is 15, 36 and 46%, respectively [23]. Symptoms of pouchitis include increased stool frequency, rectal bleeding, abdominal cramping, rectal urgency and tenesmus, incontinence, fever, malaise and occasionally reactivation of extra-intestinal manifestations. The definition, however, should include endoscopic and histological confirmation of acute inflammatory changes. Endoscopic examination may show inflammatory changes including mucosal oedema, granularity, contact bleeding, loss of vascular pattern, haemorrhage and ulceration. Histological examination shows acute inflammatory changes including neutrophil infiltration and mucosal ulceration, superimposed on a background of chronic inflammation including villous atrophy, crypt hyperplasia and chronic inflammatory cell infiltration [25]. It must be stressed that it is acute rather than chronic inflammatory changes that are diagnostic of pouchitis. In a series from St Mark's Hospital [26] 80% of pouches examined showed some degree of chronic inflammatory changes but only 30% showed acute changes, and symptoms of pouchitis correlated only with those showing acute inflammation. The pouchitis disease activity index (PDAI) is a quantitative 18-point index of pouchitis including both clinical symptoms and endoscopic and histological findings [27]. Active pouchitis using this scoring system is defined as a PDAI score greater than or equal to 7 points and remission is defined as a PDAI score of less than 7 points in a patient with a history of pouchitis.

The implications of pouchitis based on long-term functional results after restorative proctocolectomy have been studied by Hurst *et al.* [28]. They found that patients with a history of pouchitis had significantly more bowel movements per day and were more likely to have minor or major incontinence. Even in the absence of clinically active pouchitis, patients who had suffered at least one episode of pouchitis had a poor long-term functional result following IPAA. Our experience, however, and that of others [29] does not support this conclusion. In a study of 291 patients following IPAA, 65 patients (22%) were found to have suffered at least one episode of pouchitis. These patients were matched with a similar number of patients without pouchitis and no difference in long-term stool frequency or incontinence was found, thus leading to the conclusion that episodic pouchitis causes minimal functional consequences in the long term.

Risk factors and aetiology of pouchitis

The development of pouchitis appears to occur exclusively in patients who have an underlying diagnosis of ulcerative colitis with a much lower (if any) incidence in patients with familial polyposis. In addition, it appears that patients who had total colitis rather than distal colitis appear to be more at risk of developing pouchitis [30], although other studies have not confirmed this association. The theory that pre-operative backwash ileitis was responsible for the subsequent development of pouchitis was studied by Gustavsson et al. [31] who looked at 131 patients, 20 of whom had developed pouchitis following IPAA. This correlated with only 2 out of the 15 patients who had been found to have backwash ileitis pre-operatively.

Strong links have been documented between patients with extra-intestinal manifestations of inflammatory bowel disease [32] including primary sclerosing cholangitis (PSC) and pouchitis, suggesting a common link in their pathogenesis. PSC is present in 5% of patients with CUC and pouchitis has been shown to occur in 63% of these patients post-operatively compared with 32% of those without PSC [23]. Cumulative risk of developing pouchitis in patients with PSC at 1, 2, 5 and 10 years post-IPAA was 22, 43, 61 and 79%, respectively, compared with 15.5, 22.5, 26 and 45.5%, respectively, in those without PSC.

The prevalence of antineutrophil cytoplasmic antibodies with perinuclear staining pattern appears to be increased in patients with pouchitis compared with patients without pouchitis.

Pouchitis has been shown to respond favourably to antibiotic therapy in the majority of cases, and bacterial overgrowth in the ileal pouch is therefore postulated as a possible cause for pouchitis. Patients with IPAA have been shown to have a total stool anaerobe and *Bacteroides* concentrations that are higher than ileostomy controls and similar to that of the colon. However, there is no evidence that the concentration or composition of bacteria flora in the pouch differs in patients with and without pouchitis.

Alterations in the luminal concentration of short-chain fatty acids (which are the preferred source of energy for colonic enterocytes) have also been suggested as a cause for pouchitis. However, studies, comparing luminal concentrations of short-chain fatty acids within ileal reservoirs have been inconsistent. Likewise, ileal pouch short chain fatty acid concentrations correlate poorly with the development of pouchitis [33].

Faecal stasis and inefficient pouch evacuation have also been implicated in pouchitis. Emptying efficiency, however, does not appear to correlate with the occurrence of pouchitis and no differences have been found in the frequency of pouchitis among patients with J-, S- or W-shaped pouches (which differ in volume, compliance and emptying efficiency) [19, 34]. O'Connell et al. [35] studied reservoir stasis in 20 patients following IPAA. They found that the enteric bacterial count and the efficiency of ileal pouch evacuation were no different in patients with recurrent pouchitis compared to those with good clinical outcome. The fact that pouchitis is only seen following restoration of intestinal continuity when the defunctioning ileostomy is closed would appear to support the argument that pouchitis occurs only in the presence of bacteria. Chronic (but not acute) histological changes in the pouch mucosa significantly increase at 3, 6 and 12 months after ileostomy closure [36]. These histological changes do not, however, appear to correlate with efficiency of pouch emptying, which suggests that these findings result from exposure to the faecal stream rather than faecal stasis.

Columnar cuff disorders

Histological examination of the columnar mucosa of the anal transitional zone (ATZ: a better, more accurate term for which is residual epithelial cuff) has shown inflammatory changes similar to those seen in the rectal mucosa in patients with ulcerative colitis [37]. This area has the potential for dysplasia, neoplasia and continuing inflammation following IPAA even when mucosectomy has been performed.

Inflammation of the epithelial cuff following pouch construction can lead to symptoms similar to, and sometimes indistinguishable from, pouchitis or a flare of colitis. Lavery et al. [38] followed 217 patients after restorative proctocolectomy, finding endoscopic and histological evidence of inflammation in 22.1%. Symptoms of urgency, pain and bleeding were present in 14.7% and 13.8% had associated inflammatory changes in the pouch.

The incidence of dysplasia in the retained rectal mucosa following restorative proctocolectomy is difficult to quantify, depending largely on the frequency and aggressiveness of follow-up. Examination of 109 rectal 'doughnuts' following double-stapled pouch-anal anastomosis for chronic ulcerative colitis showed dysplasia in 0.9% [39]. Examination of mucosectomy specimens following IPAA have shown dysplasia in 7.9% in those who had ulcerative colitis for more than 10 years, decreasing to zero in those who had the disease for less than 10 years. The risk of dysplasia appears to be higher in patients who had dysplasia or cancer (10 and 25%) in the original proctocolectomy specimen.

The question of follow-up of the cuff has been addressed by a number of groups. The Cleveland Clinic reported their experience with 254 patients who had double-stapled IPAA and who were followed by annual post-operative ATZ biopsies [40]. During a mean follow-up of 2.3 years, low-grade dysplasia was found in eight patients (3.1%). Repeat biopsies confirmed dysplasia in only two of these eight patients. Significant correlation was seen between dysplasia in the cuff and concurrent dysplasia or cancer of the large bowel *pre-operatively*. There was no association with age, sex, duration of disease, anastomotic technique or length of rectal cuff.

Controversy persists as to whether or not these patients should be regularly subjected to endoscopic and histological surveillance. Reports of a cancer detected histologically in a mucosectomy specimen [41] and in the cuff post-operatively [42] has strengthened the case of those who advocate this technique in all patients.

Evacuation disorders

Disorders of pouch evacuation can be functional or mechanical. Functional evacuation disorders are poorly understood and may involve alterations in pouch motility with or without disorganisation of pelvic floor defaecatory mechanisms. Mechanical causes of outlet obstruction can be due to a long efferent limb of the pouch, a long rectal stump below the pouch-anal anastomosis, stricture of the pouch, or more commonly stricture of the pouch-anal anastomosis.

Long efferent limbs are seen only with the S-shaped pouch design. Early S pouches were associated with kinking of the efferent limb, which has essentially eliminated the use of this pouch design [43]. Secondly, the use of double stapling techniques in inexperienced hands can leave, *in situ*, a long rectal stump below the anastomosis. Consequently, inefficient emptying of the pouch may necessitate self-catheterisation. A study comparing 'high' and 'low' stapled anastomoses followed two groups of patients after IPAA [44]. Patients with a short rectal cuff had a significantly lower resting anal pressure and absent recto-anal inhibitory reflex. Despite this, these patients had significantly better function than those with a long rectal cuff, in terms of nocturnal continence and daytime frequency [44]. In addition, the potential for dysplastic or neoplastic change in the residual rectal mucosa would, theoretically, be directly proportional to the length of the rectal stump.

The most commonly encountered form of mechanical outlet obstruction is stricture. Strictures, which form early following pouch construction, are usually at the pouch-anal anastomosis and take the form of a very short web-like stricture reducing the anastomotic lumen. This is readily dilated at closure of the ileostomy and rarely, if ever, recurs. It is essential therefore that digital rectal examination be performed on all patients at the time of closure of defunctioning loop ileostomy following restorative proctocolectomy. Late stricture formation is a more difficult problem. Risk factors include technical difficulty at the time of surgery such as tension on the anastomosis or post-operative leak or may be due to underlying Crohn's disease. Strictures above the pouch-anal anastomosis are more likely to be associated with an underlying diagnosis of Crohn's disease and carry much poorer prognoses. The incidence of anastomotic stricturing following IPAA is reported between 1 and 8% [45, 46]. Biopsies should be taken from recurrent strictures or whenever Crohn's disease is suspected.

Therefore, the full assessment of a patient who presents with pouch evacuation difficulties includes digital rectal examination, pouch endoscopy, pouchography to delineate the anatomy of the pouch, and functional studies such as defaecating pouchography or nuclear scintigraphy emptying studies.

Pouch dysfunction due to fistula formation

Fistula formation following restorative proctocolectomy occurs uncommonly but may have devastating consequences and is difficult to treat successfully [47]. Rates of fistula formation are significantly higher in those patients with an underlying diagnosis of Crohn's disease or indeterminate colitis. However, an overall incidence of 6.8% was found in one multi-centre North American study [48]. Thirty per cent of these presented before ileostomy closure and only 12% were found to suffer from Crohn's disease. In a review of 25 cases of pouch-vaginal fistula from the Cleveland Clinic [49], the majority had a tendency to occur in the early post-operative period (0.5 months) in patients without Crohn's disease compared with 16.5 months in those patients with a final diagnosis of Crohn's disease. Fistulae occurred in this study following both stapled (1.9%) and hand-sewn (7.4%) anastomosis. Sepsis appears to be the most common aetiological factor and prognosis is poor in those patients with a delayed diagnosis of Crohn's disease, where pouch excision rates of up to 50% are reported.

Pouch dysfunction due to incontinence

The reported rates of incontinence following IPAA vary but minor incontinence rates as high as 40% have been reported [50, 51]. Loss of anal sensitivity, anal manipulation and surgical trauma have all been implicated as contributing factors. However, similar rates of incontinence have been reported with hand-sewn and stapled pouch-anal anastomoses, and persistence of incontinence despite return of resting anal sphincter pressure to normal suggests an aetiology other than the surgical technique. Interestingly, the level of pouch-anal anastomosis *does* appear to influence continence. As described above in one study, patients with a low-stapled anastomosis with a short rectal cuff had significantly better function than those with a long rectal cuff in terms of nocturnal continence and daytime frequency [44].

There is now some information available concerning the long-term functional outcome of patients following pouch surgery. The Mayo Clinic followed a group of 75 patients after IPAA and compared functional results at 1 year with the same patients after 10 years [52]. Seventy-eight per cent of those patients who had excellent continence at 1 year post-operative remained unchanged at 10 years, 20% developed minor incontinence and one patient developed poor control. Forty per cent of those with initial minor incontinence remained unchanged, 40% improved and 20% worsened. Nocturnal faecal spotting increased over the 10-year period but not significantly (38% increased to 52%). Stool frequency remained unchanged throughout the study period.

Treatment of pouch dysfunction

Disorders of pouch function must be dealt with using a systematic approach. By doing so the patient can be easily placed into one of the categories outlined above and a specific line of investigation and treatment can be undertaken. Non-surgical intervention including modifications in diet and lifestyle, with or without the addition of medications, will solve the majority of problems. In a minority, however, surgical intervention is necessary. When surgery becomes necessary it should be performed only by a surgeon experienced in such matters. Local procedures will often be sufficient to solve the problem and thankfully it is only rarely necessary to proceed to pouch excision with or without reconstruction.

Infection

Rarely, specific infections of the ileoanal pouch may be identified that require treatment with antimicrobial agents. *Campylobacter* is treated with oral erythromycin or ciprofloxacin for 7 days. *Shigella* is treated with oral ciprofloxacin or trimethoprim/sulfamathoxazole for 5 days. *Salmonella* infection is generally self-limited and treatment is usually not recommended. If treatment is necessary the regimen is the same as for *Shigella*. Enteroinvasive *E. coli* is also a self-limiting infection and treatment is usually not recommended. *C. difficile* may be treated with oral vancomycin or metronidazole for 10 days but it is debatable whether it causes disease in the pouch because ileal epithelial cells lack the receptor for the bacterial toxin. Cytomegalovirus is treated with intravenous ganciclovir as a 14–21-day course.

Pouch capacity and compliance

Inadequate pouch capacity or compliance can result in less than satisfactory stool frequency or continence. Treatment of this condition depends on the underlying cause. Idiopathic decreases in pouch compliance can be treated symptomatically with frequent small-volume meals and anti-diarrhoeal medications. Lack of pouch compliance when secondary to pelvic sepsis should be treated with the appropriate antibiotic, with or without surgical or radiological drainage of any associated abscesses. Defunctioning of the pouch by means of a loop ileostomy is often necessary in these patients. When these measures fail then a poorly functioning ileal J pouch reservoir secondary to limited capacity or compliance can sometimes be successfully managed with conversion to a W IPAA. The resultant increase in pouch capacity has been shown to be associated with improvements in compliance and widening of the pouch to anal pressure gradients, providing significantly better functional results with a decrease in 24-h and nocturnal stool frequency, increase in mean pouch evacuation volume and improvement in the daytime and nocturnal continence despite no significant change between pre-operative and post-operative anal manometric pressures [53].

Treatment of pouchitis

Antibiotics

The use of metronidazole and ciprofloxacin for the treatment of pouchitis appears to be successful in approximately 80% of patients [54–56].

Symptomatic improvement usually occurs within 1–2 days, although patients with relapsing pouchitis may require chronic maintenance metronidazole therapy. The success of metronidazole may be based on its anti-anaerobic function. It also has been shown to inhibit superoxide production and therefore reduces oxygen-derived free radical-induced mucosal damage [57]. The dose of metronidazole used is 250 mg t.i.d. for 10 days. The dose of ciprofloxacin is 500 mg b.i.d. for 10 days. Relapse following response to metronidazole or ciprofloxacin is usually treated with a second course. A third occurrence is usually an indication for maintenance therapy with metronidazole or ciprofloxacin. Side effects associated with the use of metronidazole can occur in up to 55% of patients during treatment. These include neuropathies, nausea, vomiting, abdominal discomfort, headache and skin rash. For those patients who do develop side effects, or fail to respond to metronidazole ciprofloxacin can be used as second-line therapy. Ciprofloxacin is generally better tolerated and for this reason is the first-line antibiotic of choice for some clinicians. The use of probiotics has been demonstrated to be effective for primary prevention of pouchitis and for maintenance of remission in patients with chronic pouchitis following induction therapy with antibiotics [58–60]. In patients who appear to develop bacterial resistance after prolonged suppressive antibiotic treatment, cycling of three or four antibiotics in 1-week intervals may be useful.

Anti-inflammatory agents

There have been some uncontrolled studies that suggest that topical 5-aminosalicylic acid (5-ASA) enemas may be beneficial for patients with active pouchitis [61, 62]. Similar uncontrolled reports have suggested that oral and topical corticosteroids may be of benefit in patients with active pouchitis [61, 63]. Budesonide suppositories (0.5 mg t.i.d) resulted in clinical and endoscopic improvement or remission in 10 out of 10 patients with active acute pouchitis [64]. Budesonide enemas (2 mg) were as effective as oral metronidazole in treating active pouchitis [65]. 5-ASA suppositories also appear to be effective for the treatment of cuffitis [66].

Nutritional agents

Therapy with short-chain fatty acid enemas and glutamine suppositories may be useful in treating pouchitis [67]. The data, however, are uncontrolled and the low overall clinical response rate suggests that short-chain fatty acid enemas or suppositories are not beneficial for active pouchitis.

Other agents

The theory that pouchitis may be secondary to oxygen-derived free radical-induced mucosal damage led to the suggestion that treatment with allopurinol may be beneficial to these patients [68]. This, as a xanthine oxidase inhibitor, has been shown in an uncontrolled study to induce clinical improvement in four out of eight patients with acute pouchitis. However, a subsequent placebo-controlled trial failed to confirm these results [69].

Other agents that have been tried include bismuth and endotoxin-binding resins. Controlled data supporting their efficacy, however, are not available.

Surgical treatment of pouchitis

Approximately 3% of patients will be refractory to medical therapy and will require an operative approach with use of an ileostomy and either exclusion or excision of the pouch. Formation of a temporary loop ileostomy obviously eliminates incontinence, but the intensity of the inflammatory changes are not influenced. Closure of the temporary defunctioning loop ileostomy is therefore unlikely to lead to the resolution of symptoms.

Natural history of pouchitis

At the Mayo Clinic, in patients with IPAA for ulcerative colitis, the cumulative risk of developing at least one episode of pouchitis is 50–60%. Of those patients who develop pouchitis, 36% have one to two acute pouchitis episodes, which respond to treatment with antibiotics. Forty-nine per cent relapse more frequently (at least three acute episodes) but respond to antibiotics, and 15% require maintenance suppressive therapy and have been labelled chronic pouchitis. Of this group with chronic pouchitis, up to 50% (or 3% of *all* patients after IPAA) may require surgical exclusion or excision of the pouch [70]. Other studies confirm the incidence of pouch excision as being around 1%.

Treatment of outlet obstruction

Evacuation difficulties secondary to outlet obstruction can be due to a long efferent limb in the case of S-shaped pouches, a long rectal stump or stricture formation, usually at the level of the pouch-anal anastomosis.

Strictures

Most strictures will respond to simple digital dilatation of the pouch-anal anastomosis at the time of closure of loop ileostomy. The majority of patients will need no further dilatations. Occasionally, however, strictures caused by anastomotic dehiscence and fibrosis will require repeated digital dilatation or use of bougies. Having attempted the above measures, if a stricture persists then scar excision may occasionally be successful. If severe, however, pouch excision may be necessary with construction of a new pouch, provided that Crohn's disease has been excluded.

Efferent limb obstruction

This is seen almost exclusively in patients who have undergone construction in an S-shaped pouch. Surgical correction has been shown to result in good functional results. One study of salvage surgery for ileal pouch outlet obstruction showed significant improvement in function following abdominal mobilisation of the pouch with excision of the long efferent limb and hand-sewn ileoanal anastomosis to the dentate line [43].

Long rectal stump

This complication is exclusive to the use of the double-stapled anastomotic technique. Surgical correction involves mobilisation of the pouch from above, including the rectal stump, as far as the pelvic floor. A hand-sewn pouch-anal anastomosis can then be constructed following excision of the rectal stump.

Treatment of fistulae

Treatment of pouch-vaginal fistulae usually involves diversion of the faecal stream together with local measures initially, such as an endoanal advancement flap. If this fails then excision of the pouch with or without reconstruction may be the only alternative. Treatment of pouch-perineal fistulae is usually initially attempted by means of fistulotomy or seton placement, depending on the distance from the anal verge, the degree of anal sphincter involvement and the anal sphincter function pre-operatively. Concomitant diversion of the faecal stream by means of loop ileostomy may be necessary. Reconstruction of the pouch can be attempted if local measures fail, but a significant number will ultimately lose their pouch.

Natural history of pouch dysfunction

The consequences of ileoanal pouch dysfunction, however, can be devastating with protracted medical therapy and numerous hospital admissions. Re-operations for complications is difficult and associated with a high number of further complications. In one series of 114 patients who required re-operation following pouch surgery [71], 70 patients required subsequent operations. After a mean follow-up of 3 years, 22 patients had had their pouch excised, 15 had ileostomies with intact pouches and 77 had functioning pouches. Of these, 77 patients, 70% had a satisfactory functional result. Sixty-nine per cent of patients requiring more than one operation for pouch-related complications had their pouch excised compared to 14% who had only one operation for pouch-related complications.

Conclusion

Diagnostic evaluation of any patient with pouch dysfunction should be based on the patient's symptoms at presentation and a systematic, logical stepwise approach undertaken, and specific treatments instituted. This will be successful in restoring most patients to an acceptable pouch function.

References

1 Farouk R, Pemberton JH, Wolff BG, Browning S, Larson D. Functional outcomes after ileal pouch-anal anastomosis for chronic ulcerative colitis. *Ann Surg* 2000;231:919–26.
2 Pemberton JH, Phillips SF, Ready RR, Zinmeister AR, Beahrs OH. Quality of life after Brooke ileostomy and ileal pouch-anal anastomosis. *Ann Surg* 1989;209: 620–8.
3 Herbst F, Kamm MA, Nicholls RJ. Effects of loperamide on ileoanal pouch function. *Br J Surg* 1998;85:1428–32.
4 Hallgren TA, Fasth SB, Nordgren S, Oresland T, Hallberg L, Hulten L. Manovolumetric characteristics and functional results in three different pelvic pouch designs. *Int J Colorectal Dis* 1989;4:156–60.
5 Tuckson WB, Fazio VW. Functional comparison between double and triple ileal loop pouches. *Dis Colon Rectum* 1991;34:17–21.
6 Sagar PM, Holdsworth PJ, Godwin GR, Quirke P, Smith AN, Johnson D. Comparison of triplicated (S) and quadruplicated (W) pelvic ileal reservoirs: studies on manuvolume try, fecal bacteriology, fecal volatile fatty acids, mucosal morphology, and functional results. *Gastroenterology* 1992;102:520–8.
7 Dozois RR, Goldberg SM, Rothenberger DA, *et al*. Symposium on restorative proctocolectomy with ileal reservoir. *Int J Colorectal Dis* 1986;1:2–19.

8 Nicholls RJ, Lubowski DZ. Restorative proctocolectomy: the four loop (W) reservoir. *Br J Surg* 1987;74:564–6.
9 Seow-Choen Tsunoda A, Nicholls RJ. Prospective randomized trial comparing anal function after hand-sewn ileoanal anastomosis with mucosectomy versus stapled ileoanal anastomosis without mucosectomy in restorative proctocolectomy. *Br J Surg* 1991;78:430–4.
10 Luukkonen P, Jarvinen H. Stapled vs hand-sutured ileoanal anastomosis in restorative proctocolectomy: a prospective randomized study. *Arch Surg* 1993;128:437–40.
11 Hallgren TA, Fasth SB, Oresland TO, Hulten LA. Ileal pouch anal function after endoanal mucosectomy and handsewn ileoanal anastomosis compared with stapled anastomosis without mucosectomy. *Eur J Surg* 1995;161:915–21.
12 Reilly WT, Pemberton JH, Wolff BG, *et al*. Randomized prospective trial comparing ileal pouch-anal anastomosis performed by excising the anal mucosa to ileal pouch-anal anastomosis performed by preserving the anal mucosa. *Ann Surg* 1997;225:666–77.
13 Shen B, Achkar JP, Lashner BA, *et al*. Irritable pouch syndrome: a new category of diagnosis for symptomatic patients with ileal pouch-anal anastomosis. *Am J Gastroenterol* 2002;97:972–7.
14 Groom JS, Kamm MA, Nicholls RJ. Relationship of small bowel motility to ileoanal reservoir function. *Gut* 1994;35:523–9.
15 Soper NJ, Orkin BA, Kelly KA, Brown ML. Gastrointestinal transit after proctocolectomy with ileal pouch-anal anastomosis or ileostomy. *J Surg Res* 1989;46:300–5.
16 Panis Y, Poupard B, Nemeth J, Lavergne A, Hautefeuille P, Valleur P. Ileal pouch/anal anastomosis for Crohn's disease. *Lancet* 1996;347:854–7.
17 Sagar PM, Dozois RR, Wolff BG, Kelly KA. Disconnection pouch revision and reconnection of the ileal pouch-anal anastomosis. *Br J Surg* 1996;83:1401–4.
18 Colombel JF, Ricart E, Loftus EV Jr, *et al*. Management of Crohn's disease of the ileoanal pouch with infliximab. *Am J Gastroenterol* 2003;98(10):2239–44.
19 Nicholls RJ. Restorative proctocolectomy with various types of reservoir. *World J Surg* 1987;11:751–62.
20 Farouk R, Dozois RR, Pemberton JH, Larson D. Incidence and subsequent impact of pelvic abscess after ileal pouch-anal anastomosis for chronic ulcerative colitis. *Dis Colon Rectum* 1998;41:1239–43.
21 Goldberg PA, Kamm MA, Nicholls RJ, Morris G, Britton KE. Contribution of gastrointestinal transit and pouch characteristics in determining pouch function. *Gut* 1997;40:790–3.
22 Malcolm PN, Bhagat KK, Chapman MA, Davies SG, Williams NS, Murfitt JB. Complications of the ileal pouch: is the pouchogram a useful predictor? *Clin Radiol* 1995;50:613–17.
23 Penna C, Dozois R, Tremaine W, *et al*. Pouchitis after ileal pouch-anal anastomosis for ulcerative colitis occurs with increased frequency in patients with associated primary sclerosing cholangitis. *Gut* 1996;38:234–9.
24 Stahlberg D, Gullberg K, Liljeqvist L, Hellers G, Lofberg R. Pouchitis following pelvic pouch operation for ulcerative colitis. Incidence, cumulative risk, and risk factors. *Dis Colon Rectum* 1996;39:1012–18.
25 Moskowitz RL, Shepherd NA, Nicholls RJ. An assessment of inflammation in the reservoir after restorative proctocolectomy with ileoanal reservoir. *Int J Colorectal Dis* 1986;1:167–74.
26 Nicholls RJ, Holt SDH, Lubowski DZ. Restorative proctocolectomy with ileal reservoir: comparison of two-stage vs three-stage procedures and analysis of factors that might affect outcome. *Dis Colon Rectum* 1989;32:323–6.
27 Sandborn WJ, Tremaine WJ, Batts KP, Pemberton JH, Phillips SF. Pouchitis after ileal pouch-anal anastomosis: a pouchitis disease activity index. *Mayo Clin Proc* 1994;69:409–15.
28 Hurst RD, Chung TP, Rubin M, Michelassi F. The implications of acute pouchitis on the long-term functional results after restorative proctocolectomy. *Inflamm Bowel Dis* 1998;4:280–4.
29 Keranen U, Luukkonen P, Jarvinen H. Functional results after restorative proctocolectomy complicated by pouchitis. *Dis Colon Rectum* 1997;40:746–9.
30 Madden MV, Farthing MJG, Nicholls RJ. Inflammation in ileal reservoirs: 'pouchitis'. *Gut* 1990;31:247–9.
31 Gustavsson S, Weiland LH, Kelly KA. Relationship of backwash ileitis to ileal pouchitis after ileal pouch-anal anastomosis. *Dis Colon Rectum* 1987;30:25–8.
32 Lohmuller JL, Pemberton JH, Dozois RR, Ilstrup D, van Heerden J. Pouchitis and extraintestinal manifestations of inflammatory bowel disease after pouch-anal anastomosis. *Ann Surg* 1990;211:622–8.
33 Ambrose WL, Pemberton JH, Phillips SF, Bell AM, Haddad AC. Fecal short-chain fatty acid concentrations and effect on ileal pouch function. *Dis Colon Rectum* 1993;36:235–9.

34. Sagar PM, Dozois RR, Wolff BG. Long-term results of ileal pouch-anal anastomosis in patients with Crohn's disease. *Dis Colon Rectum* 1996;39:893–8.
35. O'Connell PR, Rankin DR, Weiland LH, Kelly KA. Enteric bacteriology, absorption morphology and emptying after pouch-anal anastomosis. *Br J Surg* 1986;73:909–14.
36. De Silva HJ, Millard PR, Kettlewell M, et al. Mucosal characteristic of pelvic ileal pouches. *Gut* 1991;32:61–5.
37. Ambrose WL, Pemberton JH, Dozois RR, Carpenter HA, O'Rourke JS, Ilstrup DM. The histological pattern and pathological involvement of anal transition zone in patients with ulcerative colitis. *Gastroenterology* 1993;104:514–18.
38. Lavery IC, Sirimarco MT, Ziv Y, Fazio VW. Anal canal inflammation after ileal pouch-anal anastomosis. *Dis Colon Rectum* 1995;38:803–6.
39. Haray PN, Amarnath B, Weiss EG, Nogueras JJ, Wexner SD. Short note: low malignant potential of the double-stapled ileal pouch-anal anastomosis. *Br J Surg* 1996;83:1406–8.
40. Ziv Y, Fazio VW, Sirimarco MT, Lavery IC, Goldblum JR, Petras RE. Incidence risk factors, and treatment of dysplasia in the anal transition zone after ileal pouch-anal anastomosis. *Dis Colon Rectum* 1994;37:1281–5.
41. King DW, Lubowski DZ, Cook TA. Anal canal mucosa in restorative proctocolectomy for ulcerative colitis. *Br J Surg* 1989;76:970–2.
42. Sequens R. Cancer in the anal canal (transitional zone) after restorative proctocolectomy with stapled ileal pouch-anal anastomosis. *Int J Colorectal Dis* 1997;12:254–5.
43. Herbst F, Sielezneff I, Nicholls RJ. Salvage surgery for ileal pouch outlet obstruction. *Br J Surg* 1996;83:368–71.
44. Annibali R, Oresland T, Hulten L. Does the level of stapled ileoanal anastomosis influence physiologic and functional outcome? *Dis Colon Rectum* 1994;37:321–9.
45. Skarsgard ED, Atkinson KG, Bell GA, et al. Function and quality of life after ileal pouch surgery for ulcerative colitis and familial polyposis. *Am J Surg* 1989;157:467–71.
46. Wexner SD, Wong WD, Rothenberger DA, Goldberg SM. The ileoanal reservoir. *Am J Surg* 1990;159:178–88.
47. Keighley MR, Grother SP. Fistula complicating restorative proctocolectomy. *Br J Surg* 1993;80:1065–7.
48. Wexner SD, Rothenberger DA, Jensen L, et al. Ileal pouch-vaginal fistulas: incidence, etiology and management. *Dis Colon Rectum* 1989;32:460–5.
49. Lee PY, Fazio VW, Church JM, Hull TL, Eu KW, Lavery IC. Vaginal fistula following restorative proctocolectomy. *Dis Colon Rectum* 1997;40(7):752–9.
50. Goldberg SM. Proctocolectomy and ileoanal anastomosis with an S pouch: functional results. *Can J Surg* 1987;30:359–60.
51. McIntyre PB, Pemberton JH, Beart RW, Devine RM, Nivatvongs S. Double stapled vs handsewn ileal pouch-anal anastomosis in patients with chronic ulcerative colitis. *Dis Colon Rectum* 1994;37:430–3.
52. McIntyre PB, Pemberton JH, Wolff BG, Beart RW, Dozois RR. Comparing functional results one year and ten years after ileal pouch-anal anastomosis for chronic ulcerative colitis. *Dis Colon Rectum* 1994;37:303–7.
53. Klas J, Myers GA, Starling JR, Harms BA. Physiologic evaluation and surgical management of failed ileoanal pouch. *Dis Colon Rectum* 1998;41:854–61.
54. Madden MV, McIntyre AS, Nicholls RJ. Double-blind crossover trial of metronidazole versus placebo in chronic unremitting pouchitis. *Dig Dis Sci* 1994;39:93–6.
55. Shen B, Achkar JP, Lashner BA, et al. A randomised clinical trial of ciprofloxacin and metronidazole to treat acute pouchitis. *Inflamm Bowel Dis* 2001;7:1–5.
56. Sambuelli A, Boerr L, Negreira S, Gil A, Camartino G, Huernos S, Kogan Z, Cabanne A, Graziano A, Peredo H, Doldan I, Gonzalez O, Sugai E, Lumi M, Bai JC. Budesonide enema in pouchitis–a double-blind, double-dummy, controlled trial. *Aliment Pharmacol Ther* 2002;16:27–34.
57. Rauh SM, Schoetz DJ, Roberts PL, Murray JJ, Collar JA, Veidenheimer MC. Pouchitis: Is it a wastebasket diagnosis? *Dis Colon Rectum* 1991;34:685–8.
58. Gionchetti P, Rizzello F, Helwig U, et al. Prophylaxis of pouchitis onset with probiotic therapy: a double-blind, placebo-controlled trial. *Gastroenterology* 2003;124:2–9.
59. Gionchetti P, Rizzello F, Venturi A, et al. Oral bacteriotherapy as maintenance treatment in patients with chronic pouchitis: a double-blind, placebo-controlled trial. *Gastroenterology* 2000;119:5–9.
60. Mimura T, Rizzello F, Helwig U, et al. Once daily high dose probiotic therapy (VSL#3) for maintaining remission in recurrent or refractory pouchitis. *Gut* 2004;53:8–14.
61. Shepherd NA, Hulten L, Tytgat GNJ, et al. Workshop: pouchitis. *Int J Colorectal Dis* 1989;4:205–29.
62. Di Febo G, Miglioli M, Lauri A, et al. Endoscopic assessment of acute inflammation of the reservoir after restorative ileoanal anastomosis. *Gastrointest Endosc* 1990;36:6–9.

63 Tytgat GNJ, van Deventer SJH. Pouchitis. *Int J Colorectal Dis* 1988;3:226–8.
64 Beluzzi A, Campeiri M, Miglioli M, *et al*. Evaluation of flogistic pattern in 'pouchitis' before and after the treatment with budesonide suppositories. *Gastroenterology* 1992;102:A5933.
65 Sambuelli A, Boerr L, Negreira S, *et al*. Budesonide enema in pouchitis – a double-blind, double-dummy, controlled trial. *Aliment Pharmacol Ther* 2002;16: 27–34.
66 Shen B, Lashner BA, Bennett AE, *et al*. Treatment of rectal cuff inflammation (cuffitis) in patients with ulcerative colitis following restorative proctocolectomy and ileal pouch-anal anastomosis. *Am J of Gastroenterol* 2004;99:1527–31.
67 Wischmeyer P, Pemberton JH, Phillips SF. Chronic pouchitis after ileal pouch-anal anastomosis: a pouch disease activity index. *Mayo Clin Proc* 1993;68: 978–81.
68 Levin KE, Pemberton JH, Phillips SF, Zinsmeister AR, Pezim ME. Role of oxygen free radicals in the etiology of pouchitis. *Dis Colon Rectum* 1992;35:452–6.
69 Joelsson M, Andersson M, Bark T, *et al*. Allopurinol as prophylaxis against pouchitis following ileal pouch-anal anastomosis for ulcerative colitis: a randomized placebo-controlled double-blind study. *Scand J Gastroenterol* 2001;36(11):1179–84.
70 Sandborn WJ. Pouchitis following ileal pouch-anal anastomosis: definition, pathogenesis, and treatment. *Gastroenterology* 1994;107:1856–60.
71 Galandiuk S, Scott NA, Dozois RR, *et al*. Ileal pouch-anal anastomosis: reoperation for pouch-related complications. *Ann Surg* 1990;212: 446–52.

IV: Management of Crohn's disease

14: Is mesalazine useful in Crohn's disease?

A. Hillary Steinhart

Introduction

After the landmark discovery of Azad Kahn *et al.* [1] in which mesalazine (5-aminosalicylic acid) was demonstrated to be the active moiety in sulphasalazine, it has been hoped that the use of mesalazine without the sulpha moiety would result in improved efficacy and reduced side-effects and toxicity in patients with inflammatory bowel disease. In addition, the ability to incorporate mesalazine in various controlled-release formats that target different segments of the gastrointestinal tract has raised the possibility that mesalazine could be used for both the short- and long-term treatment of Crohn's disease. It has now been over 20 years since that first study and, since that time, there have been several mesalazine-based formulations developed and marketed for the treatment of inflammatory bowel disease. In this chapter, the role of mesalazine in the treatment of Crohn's disease will be examined in light of the existing data, the development of new therapeutic agents and the current understanding of the pathophysiology of Crohn's disease.

Treatment of active disease

Prior to the development of controlled-release preparations of mesalazine, sulphasalazine was commonly used in the treatment of patients with symptoms of active Crohn's disease. The use of sulphasalazine, which consists of mesalazine bound to sulphapyridine by a diazo bond, was examined in a controlled manner in several studies [2–8]. In the National Co-operative Crohn's Disease Study (NCCDS), patient outcome rankings were superior after 17 weeks of treatment with sulphasalazine (1 g/15 kg body wt/day; max dose = 5 g/day) as compared to those patients who were randomised to receive placebo [6]. The observed benefit was limited primarily to patients with colonic disease (with or without small-intestinal involvement) and to those not receiving corticosteroids prior to the study. However, sulphasalazine did not appear to be as effective as prednisone, particularly in inducing remission by the end of the study period. Although the proportion of patients in remission was approximately 30% in the placebo arm and 43% in those receiving sulphasalazine, this difference did not quite reach statistical significance ($p = 0.08$) whereas the difference between placebo and prednisone (approx 30–60%) was statistically and clinically significant. In the European Co-operative Crohn's Disease Study (ECCDS) patients with active Crohn's disease were randomised to receive methylprednisolone 48 mg/day followed by tapering to 8 mg/day, sulphasalazine 3 g/day, combination methylprednisolone and sulphasalazine or placebo [3]. Clinical response was seen by the end of the 16-week study period in 50% of patients receiving sulphasalazine alone as compared with 34% of those receiving placebo. Methylprednisolone was the most effective treatment (83% response) particularly in patients with small intestinal disease. Although the combination of methylprednisolone and sulphasalazine was no better than methylprednisolone alone, it did seem to be more effective in patients who had colonic disease or those who

Table 14.1 Oral controlled-release preparations of mesalazine.

Brand name	Description	Release mechanism	Site of delivery
Asacol	Eudragit-S coated tablet	pH > 7	Colon +/− terminal ileum
Salofalk	Eudragit-L coated tablet	pH > 6	Colon + ileum
Mesasal	Eudragit-L coated tablet	pH > 6	Colon + ileum
Pentasa	Ethylcellulose coated tablet	Time-dependent	Colon + ileum + jejunum

had previously not been treated. In two other small controlled trials sulphasalazine was shown to be superior to placebo, at least in certain subsets of CD patients [2, 8]. In a 4-week cross-over trial of sulphasalazine given at a dose of 1.5 g/day for 3 days followed by 3 g/day, sulphasalazine produced clinical improvement in patients who had not previously undergone intestinal resection [2]. In a 26-week trial of 26 patients, treatment with sulphasalazine was associated with a greater than 25% reduction in the inflammatory activity index in 62% of patients [8]. Similar reductions in activity were observed in only 8% of placebo-treated patients.

In the Co-operative Crohn's Disease Study in Sweden, sulphasalazine 1.5 g b.i.d was compared to metronidazole 400 mg b.i.d for 4 months followed by a further 4 months cross-over period [7]. There was no placebo arm in the study. In the initial 4-month period significant reductions were noted in the Crohn's disease activity index (CDAI) scores in both treatment arms, but the reductions were not different between the two. In both treatment arms it was noted that patients with colonic disease, with or without small intestinal involvement, experienced more favourable outcomes on average. The results of these studies support the notion that sulphasalazine has modest efficacy in treating the symptoms of active Crohn's disease, particularly when there is colonic involvement, but perhaps not as effective as corticosteroids. Following the demonstration by Azad Khan *et al.* [1] that mesalazine is the principal active component of the sulphasalazine molecule, it was hoped that by formulating mesalazine in a controlled-release preparation it would be possible to improve efficacy by allowing higher doses of mesalazine to be used with fewer adverse effects than would be associated with the use of sulphasalazine (Tables 14.1 and 14.2). It was also hoped that the use of controlled-release preparations would facilitate targeting of drug release in the ileocolonic areas most commonly affected by Crohn's disease. Since then there have been many studies attempting to define the role of the

Table 14.2 Other preparations of mesalazine.

Brand name	Description	Release mechanism	Site of delivery
Salazopyrine (sulphasalazine)	Sulphapyridine and mesalazine joined by diazo bond	Bacterial azoreductase cleavage	Colon
Dipentum (olsalazine)	Two mesalazine molecules joined by diazo bond	Bacterial azoreductase cleavage	Colon
Colazide (balsalazide)	4-aminobenzoyl β alanine and mesalazine joined by diazo bond	Bactcrial azoreductase cleavage	Colon

controlled-release preparations of mesalazine in the treatment of active Crohn's disease and in the maintenance of remission.

The first reported use of mesalazine for the treatment of symptoms of acute Crohn's disease was published by Rasmussen et al. [9]. In that open study 18 patients with small-intestinal Crohn's disease were treated with Pentasa 500 mg t.i.d for 6 weeks. Pentasa, which consists of mesalazine coated in ethylcellulose granules, releases the mesalazine in a time- and pH-dependent fashion throughout the small and large intestine of normal volunteers. It is important to note that no data regarding the release kinetics of Pentasa (or any of the other mesalazine-containing preparations) are available in patients with active Crohn's disease. However, in Rasmussen's initial pilot study, Pentasa was noted to be safe, and 13 out of the 18 patients were rated as being improved on treatment. The same group later published a small, randomised, placebo-controlled trial of Pentasa 1500 mg/day for 16 weeks and found no difference in outcomes between the 30 patients randomised to Pentasa as compared with the 37 randomised to placebo [10]. Improvement was reported in 40 and 30% of the patients in the two arms, respectively. Given the relatively small sample size, this difference was not statistically significant. The modest effect of mesalazine observed in that study may have been, in part, due to the low dose used. However, the 33% improvement in response rate is not entirely out of keeping with the results of subsequent studies using higher doses of mesalazine. The lack of a statistically significant difference in this study may have been due to the fact that the study did not have sufficient power to detect such a difference [11]. Mahida and Jewell reported a 40-patient randomised controlled trial of mesalazine (Pentasa) in patients with active Crohn's disease [11]. They found no difference in response rates over the 6-week study period in the 40 study subjects.

The majority of the evidence supporting the presence of a biological effect of mesalazine, in the form of Pentasa, comes from a single large placebo-controlled dose-finding study carried out in the United States. [12]. In that study, 310 patients with Crohn's disease of the terminal ileum alone or terminal ileum and colon were randomly assigned to receive placebo, 1, 2 or 4 g of Pentasa daily. After 8 weeks of treatment, the patients in the 4 g arm experienced a mean 72-point reduction in the CDAI as compared with a 21-point reduction in patients receiving placebo. Although this was shown to be statistically significantly different and does appear to suggest that mesalazine has some effect on symptomatic status in Crohn's disease, the clinical significance of a 50-point differential is debatable. When the proportion of patients in remission (as defined by a CDAI < 150) at the end of treatment was examined, the 4 g/day group was found to have fared better than those receiving placebo (43% in remission on Pentasa 4 g/day vs 18% on placebo). There were no statistically or clinically significant differences between the placebo, 1 g/day or 2 g/day arms with respect to CDAI scores or proportion of patients in remission at the end of the treatment. The authors subsequently reported quality of life scores that confirmed the superiority of mesalazine at the 4 g/day dose [13]. A second similar study that omitted the 1 g dose was carried out in 232 patients but did not demonstrate superiority of Pentasa over placebo [14]. However, the second study was reported only as a brief correspondence, and no details of the trial methodology were available for review. The author suggested that a pooled analysis of the two trials demonstrated a statistically significant superiority of the 4-g dose over placebo and a statistically significant dose-response trend. A third randomised controlled trial of Pentasa was performed but the results, which showed no difference in CDAI reduction between mesalazine and placebo, were not presented in an independent report. The data from that study were combined with the data from the first two Pentasa trials and the aggregate results were presented within a meta-analysis of the three similarly designed Pentasa-active CD trials [15]. For the meta-analysis, the results from the 4-g/day groups in the three studies were combined ($n = 154$) and compared to the aggregate results of the placebo groups ($n = 156$). The mean Crohn's disease activity index (CDAI) reduction observed in placebo-treated patients was 45 and was 63 in the mesalazine-treated patients. Although this difference was statistically significant ($p < 0.04$) the clinical significance of this difference is questionable.

In a smaller study, Tremaine et al. [16] randomised 38 patients with Crohn's disease of the colon or terminal ileum and colon to receive mesalazine, in the form of Asacol 800 mg q.i.d, or placebo for 16 weeks. Asacol tablets consist of mesalazine in a coating (Eudragit S), which releases the active medication at a pH above 7. It is designed to release mesalazine primarily in the colon with some release in the terminal ileum. In this study, patients receiving Asacol experienced a 60% rate of complete or partial 'success' as compared with 22% in the placebo-treated arm. Complete success was defined as a final CDAI score of less than 150 and at least 70 points lower than baseline. Partial success was a final CDAI score at least 70 points lower than baseline but greater than 150. The results bordered on statistical significance depending on the method of analysis used, but appeared to show a reasonably important clinical difference between the two treatment arms. When only complete success, as defined by attainment of remission, was examined, 45% of the patients in the Asacol group achieved that threshold as compared with 22% of the placebo-treated patients. The validity of the results of this study is supported by the observed placebo remission rate, which is in keeping with that observed in the placebo groups of several other clinical trials in Crohn's disease. In addition, the remission rate in the Asacol arm is in the same range as that seen in other trials of mesalazine for active Crohn's disease.

Mesalazine (Pentasa) has also been compared with controlled ileal-release budesonide (Entocort CIR) in a randomised controlled trial in patients with active Crohn's disease of the terminal ileum with or without involvement of the right side of the colon [17]. In that trial, patients received either mesalazine (Pentasa) 2 g b.i.d or budesonide (Entocort CIR) 9 mg once daily for 16 weeks. Sixty-nine per cent of the budesonide-treated patients were in remission after 8 weeks as compared with only 45% of the mesalazine-treated group. The proportion of patients still in remission after 12 and 16 weeks showed a slight decrease in both arms, but budesonide continued to be statistically superior to mesalazine (62% vs 36% remission rates). In addition, 27 of the 61 patients randomised to receive mesalazine were withdrawn from the study because of worsening Crohn's disease as compared to only 10 of 63 budesonide-treated patients. Although the results appear to clearly demonstrate the superiority of budesonide over mesalazine, it should be noted that the remission rate in the budesonide-treated group was higher than that reported in any of the previous budesonide trials that have studied its use in very similar populations of patients with symptoms of active Crohn's disease [18–20]. Similarly, the remission rate observed in the Pentasa-treated group was somewhat lower at 16 weeks than that observed in the Singleton et al. [12] study. The absence of a placebo arm makes any conclusion regarding the absolute effectiveness of Pentasa problematic. There have also been several small studies that have compared mesalazine to conventional glucocorticoids, either prednisone or 6-methylprednisolone [21–24]. Scholmerich et al. found that 73% of the 30 patients randomised to mesalazine 2 g/day stopped therapy because of inadequate efficacy compared with 34% of the patients receiving 6-methylprednisolon [24]. However, the other three studies [21–23] showed no difference in response between mesalazine and conventional glucocorticoids. However, these studies were all small (between 17 and 35 patients per arm) and were not adequately powered to provide any conclusion regarding the equivalence of the two treatments.

The evidence presently available regarding the effectiveness of mesalazine for the treatment of active Crohn's disease is not consistent from one study to the next with respect to its effectiveness relative to placebo, budesonide or conventional glucocorticoids (Table 14.3). However, the studies appear to be consistent with respect to the absolute response rate that is observed when doses of 3.2 g/day or more are used. The proportion of patients responding to mesalazine is consistently between 36 and 47% in these trials [12, 16, 17, 21, 22]. Although there does seem to be some positive treatment effect the studies indicate only a modest effect with respect to remission rates, reductions in disease activity scores and improvements in quality of life scores after 8–16 weeks of therapy when all patients are considered. The unimpressive overall results may be due to the patient selection criteria used by the studies and the inherent heterogeneity of the

Table 14.3 Trials of mesalazine for active Crohn's disease.

Study	Study drug/daily dose	Control	Study duration (weeks)	Sample size Study drug	Sample size Control
Rasmussen, 1987	Pentasa/1.5 g	Placebo	16	30	37
Scholmerich, 1990	Not reported/2 g	Methyl-prednisolone	24	30	32
Martin, 1990	Salofalk/3 g	Prednisone	12	22	28
Mahida, 1990	Pentasa/1.5 g	Placebo	6	20	20
Singleton, 1993	Pentasa/1, 2 and 4 g	Placebo	8	80 (1 g) 75 (2 g) 75 (2 g)	80
Tremaine, 1994	Asacol/3.2 g	Placebo	16	20	18
Gross, 1995	Salofalk/4.5 g	Methyl-prednisolone	8	17	17
Thomsen, 1998	Pentasa/4 g	Budesonide 9 mg	16	61	63
Prantera, 1999	Asacol tablets/4 g Asacol microgranules/ 4 g	6-methyl-prednisolone	12	35 / 28	31

Study	Disease location	Proportion with improvement or remission Study drug	Control	Comments
Rasmussen, 1987	Small bowel +/− colon	0.40	0.30	Improvement determined by investigator's opinion
Scholmerich, 1990	Small bowel and /or colon	0.27	0.66	Improvement defined as not withdrawn for inadequate efficacy
Martin, 1990	Small bowel +/− colon	0.47	0.46	
Mahida, 1990	Small bowel and /or colon	0.40	0.35	
Singleton, 1993	TI +/− colon	0.43 (4 g/day) 0.24 (2 g/day) 0.23 (1 g/day)	0.18	
Tremaine, 1994	Colon +/− TI	0.45	0.22	Partial or complete response in 0.60 of study drug and 0.22 of control patients
Gross, 1995	Ileum and/or colon	0.40	0.56	Trend towards greater CDAI reduction on methyl-prednisolone
Thomsen, 1998	TI +/− right colon	0.36	0.62	
Prantera, 1999	TI +/− cecum	0.60 (tablets) 0.79 (micro-granules)	0.61	

Crohn's disease patient population. It may not be that mesalazine is ineffective but that physicians and investigators have not adequately defined subgroups of patients who are most likely to benefit from therapy. If mesalazine, which is primarily a topically active compound with little effect or penetration into the deeper layers of the gut wall, is to have any appreciable clinical benefit it is likely to be in patients with early or superficial disease. The inclusion in clinical trials of patients with extensive transmural inflammation and deep ulcers, fissures, fistulae and inflammatory masses may well have obscured a large potential benefit that might have been observed if only patients with more superficial disease or less advanced disease had been studied. Although the studies were all restricted to patients with mild to moderate disease, such patients can, and frequently do, have transmural involvement and complications that would make them less likely to respond to mesalazine.

The preparation of mesalazine that is used, the pharmacokinetic characteristics, the dose provided and the mode of administration (e.g. twice daily, three times daily or four times daily) may also be responsible for differences in study results and varying effectiveness across patient subgroups. There have been no head to head comparisons of the commonly available mesalazine preparations in the treatment of active CD. However, in a study by Prantera and colleagues [23] a new mesalazine micro-granule preparation was compared to mesalazine tablets and to 6-methylprednisolone. In that study 79% of patients receiving the mesalazine micro-granules achieved remission after 12 weeks compared with 60% of patients receiving the mesalazine tablets. The difference was not statistically significant but the results suggest that the type of mesalazine release preparation may influence clinical effectiveness. However, the very high remission rates seen in both mesalazine groups brings the validity of the results into question because these rates are considerably higher than those seen in almost all other mesalazine studies in active CD.

It appears that, where examined within a single trial, there is a dose-response effect, with doses of approximately 4 g/day required to achieve a measurable and statistically significant effect. The bulk of the evidence pertains to the use of the Pentasa preparation of mesalazine with few controlled data regarding the efficacy of other preparations. There are also no data regarding differences between different administration regimens and, as a result, it is difficult to advise patients as to whether the same total daily dose of medication when given as two or three divided doses is as effective as the usual four divided-dose regimens.

Given the complex pathogenesis of Crohn's disease and multiple pathways and mediators of inflammation, it would be extremely unlikely that a single drug with relatively limited mechanisms of actions would result in major improvements in active disease when given as monotherapy. Although a pure interpretation of the evidence would argue against it, for many clinicians mesalazine remains the first-line therapy in patients with mildly to moderately active CD where there is a desire to minimise potential for side effects, while recognising that the treatment effect is modest at best and that the therapy may not be the most effective choice available, and that a significant proportion of patients will not respond to therapy. If mesalazine is used, patients should be informed of the potential pros and cons of mesalazine therapy and must be monitored closely with the option to switch to alternative therapy, such as budesonide or systemic glucocorticoids, after a period of 2–4 weeks if improvement has not occurred or sooner if deterioration has occurred. For the 32–46% of patients who respond to such a strategy, they will avoid the use of glucocorticoids.

Maintenance of medically induced remission

Although the results of trials of mesalazine in the treatment of active disease have provided conflicting results and the trials that have suggested that mesalazine is effective have shown only a modest mean absolute clinical benefit, it was hoped that mesalazine, because of its excellent short- and long-term safety profile, would be an ideal candidate for long-term maintenance therapy for patients in medically induced remissions and for those who had recently undergone surgical resection. In fact, it could be predicted that mesalazine would have its greatest chance of therapeutic success in the post-operative setting where most, if not all, visibly involved bowel is resected and the remaining bowel is either minimally involved or free of macroscopic disease. Inflammation, if it were to recur, might begin in the superficial layers of mucosa and submucosa and, as a result, would be amenable to the effects of topically active agents such as mesalazine. The situation in patients with medically induced remissions is quite different and certainly less optimistic on theoretical grounds. This may explain some of the differences observed in the results achieved in the post-operative and medically induced remission patient populations. Following successful medical therapy of active Crohn's disease and induction of clinical remission, endoscopic remission is much less commonly achieved and the deep ulcers, fistulae, fissures and transmural inflammation seen prior to treatment commonly persist [25]. In this situation, as in the treatment of active disease, one would predict that the likelihood of achieving a demonstrable clinical effect with respect to the maintenance of remission through the use of a topically active agent such as mesalazine would be unlikely when much of the inflammatory activity is present in the deeper layers of the bowel wall.

The evidence from most of the trials that have been carried out in the setting of medically induced remission (Table 14.4) support the prediction that mesalazine would have, at most, a modest degree of efficacy [26–37]. Although the trials have produced important results, they have been quite heterogeneous in their design and, as a result, the question regarding the most accurate overall estimate of the efficacy of mesalazine remains to be answered. Several attempts have been made to calculate pooled estimates of efficacy or effectiveness by combining the results of all the published trials of mesalazine maintenance therapy using formal meta-analyses.

Similar to the varying results of the primary research papers, the results of the meta-analyses have varied somewhat as well. The meta-analysis of Camma et al. [38] demonstrated only a minimal overall significant risk difference between mesalazine and placebo, with no statistically significant risk difference found when only the studies including patients with medically induced remissions were examined. Two previous meta-analyses, which included a somewhat different sample of maintenance studies, demonstrated a more clinically and statistically significant benefit of mesalazine therapy. One meta-analysis [39] calculated a relative risk of relapse of 0.63 (95% CI 0.50–0.79) for patients receiving mesalazine, whereas the second by Messori et al. [40] calculated an odds ratio of 0.62 (95% CI 0.47–0.81) for relapse at 12 months. It is important to note that the Camma meta-analysis was performed more recently and, as a result, was based upon a larger body of data from published randomised trials. This, along with the details of the different analytical methods used and the different methods of presentation of the results, may account for the apparent differences among the meta-analyses. The meta-analyses have also shown some degree of heterogeneity among the individual study results, which may limit the validity of the pooled results

Table 14.4 Trials of mesalazine for relapse prevention.

Study (first author/year of publication)	Sample size Mesalazine	Sample size Control	Formulation and dose of mesalazine (g/day)	Maximum follow-up (months)	Risk of relapse (12 months) Mesalazine	Risk of relapse (12 months) Control
Wellmann, 1988	32	34	NR	18	0.32	0.40
International Mesalazine Study Group, 1990	101	105	Mesasal/Claversal 1.5	12	0.23	0.36
Bresci, 1991	20	18	NR 1.6	36	0.38	0.94
Brignola, 1992	21	22	Pentasa 2.0	4	0.52	0.59*
Prantera, 1992	64	61	Asacol 2.4	12	0.33	0.55
Gendre, 1993	80	81	Pentasa 2.0	24	0.28	0.40
Bresci, 1994	33	33	Eudragit-S Coated 2.4	48	0.16	0.29
Thomson, 1995	102	105	Mesasal/Claversal 3.0	12	0.30	0.30
Arber, 1995	28	31	Rafassal (Salofalk) 1.0	12	0.27	0.55
Modigliani, 1996	48	37	Pentasa 4.0	12	0.64	0.62
De Franchis, 1997	58	59	Claversal 3.0	12	0.58	0.52
Sutherland, 1997	87	93	Pentasa 3.0	11	0.31	0.42

*4-month follow-up.
NR = not reported.

reported in the meta-analyses. The heterogeneity of the trials with respect to their methodologies, mesalazine formulations, mesalazine doses and patient populations, has almost certainly resulted in the heterogeneous results observed. The heterogeneity of the patient populations, both between and within individual trials, is probably the most important factor in producing the variable outcomes that have been observed. Although this heterogeneity makes the determination of a single overall treatment effect problematic, it does provide opportunities to dissect out specific patient populations who may be most likely to benefit or who are expected to achieve the greatest therapeutic gain. The three meta-analyses that have been performed have included both studies of patients with medically and surgically induced remissions and some studies that have included a mixture of both patient populations [38–40]. Because the results of the original research and the meta-analyses are consistent in their conclusions that the relative risk reduction observed with the use of mesalazine is greater in the prevention of post-operative recurrence than it is in the prevention of relapses following medically induced remissions, the inclusion of both types of patients in a single trial or meta-analysis and the use of the resulting overall estimate of treatment effect would tend to underestimate the drug's effectiveness in the post-operative setting and overestimate it in the medical setting.

A subgroup of the patients with medically induced remissions for which the evidence that mesalazine is not effective in maintaining remission appears to be quite definite are those with remissions induced with the use of systemic corticosteroids. Modigliani *et al.* [33] demonstrated quite convincingly that mesalazine in the form of Pentasa given in a high dose (4 g/day) allowed a greater proportion of patients to successfully wean off prednisolone following recent acute treatment than did placebo. However, at the end of 1 year following initiation of treatment the proportions of patients who remained in remission over the entire period were no different in the two treatment arms. Similar results were found by De Franchis *et al.* [30] who randomised a total of 117 patients with remission induced by corticosteroid therapy to receive either placebo or mesalazine 3 g/day, but that study was terminated early because a slightly higher, but statistically insignificant, incidence of relapse was noted in the mesalazine arm. There are at least two possible explanations for these results. Firstly, it may be that the need for corticosteroids for the treatment of acute symptoms of Crohn's disease may be a marker for an aggressive form of the disease that would be less likely to respond to the modest and specific anti-inflammatory effects of mesalazine. Alternatively, it is possible that corticosteroid therapy in some way alters the disease and the inflammatory process thereby rendering it less responsive to other, less potent forms of anti-inflammatory drug therapy. In such instances immunosuppressive therapy such as azathioprine, 6-mercaptopurine or methotrexate may be necessary to achieve an adequate treatment effect [41, 42]. Differences among the trials with respect to the dose and form of mesalazine used, the proportion of patients with ileal disease and the duration of disease and duration of remission prior to initiation of maintenance therapy have also been suggested as being responsible for the varying results obtained from the reported trials. The trials have used doses of mesalazine varying between 1 [26] and 4 g/day [33] with most being in the range of 1.5–3 g/day [27–32, 34–37]. However, examination of the data reveals no evidence of a dose–response relationship.

In their meta-analysis, Camma *et al.* [38] performed a subgroup analysis of the results and found no differences in the estimates of efficacy between studies in which pH-dependent release formulations of mesalazine (Asacol, Mesasal, Salofalk and Rowasa) were used and those in which microsphere formulations (Pentasa) were used. They also performed a regression analysis to examine other potential confounding variables. They found that a higher proportion of patients with ileal disease and longer total disease duration both seemed to predict greater efficacy with maintenance mesalazine. Unfortunately, the analysis included studies with both medically and surgically induced remissions and did not examine the possibility of an interaction between the surgical/medical variable and other variables reported to have been significant in the overall group. An empirical review of the trials suggests that the increased benefit seen in patients with ileal disease is due primarily to inclusion of the post-operative trials, which, for the most part, demonstrated greater improvement in outcomes in the subgroup of patients with ileal disease.

The duration of remission has been suggested to be a potential prognostic factor and may provide a means for selecting patients who are most likely to obtain a clinically important reduction in relapse incidence. In their study of mesalazine (Pentasa) 2 g/day, Gendre et al. [31] divided patients into those who were at low risk of relapse and those who were at high risk of relapse as determined by the length of the remission prior to entry into the trial. They arbitrarily used a cut-off of 3 months with patients in remission less than that period of time considered being at high risk, and the remainder considered being at low risk of relapse. The 3-month cut-off successfully stratified the patient population with the placebo-treated patients in the low risk stratum having a relapse risk of 0.42 over 2 years and the high-risk stratum placebo-treated patients having a relapse risk of 0.71. Mesalazine was found to be effective in producing a statistically significant reduction in the risk of relapse only in the high-risk group with relapse risks of 0.71 in the placebo-treated patients and 0.55 in the mesalazine-treated patients. Although the 3-month cut-off for risk stratification appears to have been decided upon retrospectively, it should be noted that a similar reduction in relapse risk was noted in the smaller study of Bresci et al. [27]. In that study, only patients who had recently entered into remission on 4 weeks of cortico-steroid therapy were included. This would have effectively limited the study to those with duration of remission of less than 3 months, which is similar to the high relapse risk group of Gendre et al. (32).

Prevention of post-operative recurrence

Although the word 'prevention' is used to describe the outcome that is hoped for when maintenance or prophylactic therapies are used in Crohn's disease, there is no evidence that any therapy is capable of preventing relapse or recurrence. Crohn's disease will, almost by definition, recur following surgically or medically induced remissions if patients are followed long enough. If disease does not recur, one should question the diagnosis of Crohn's disease. Most studies have shown mesalazine to be effective in producing 'delay' of post-operative recurrence or 'reduction' in endoscopic severity but have not, in the truest sense, shown mesalazine to be effective for the 'prevention' of recurrence [35, 43–47]. The characteristics of the studies, which vary somewhat with respect to patient inclusion criteria, mesalazine formulation and dose, duration of follow-up and handling of dropouts, are summarised in Table 14.5. Another study by Caprilli et al. comparing two doses of mesalazine (Asacol), 2.4 and 4.0 g/day, in 101 patients after resection found a slight reduction in the frequency of endoscopic recurrence at 1 year, but this difference was accounted for by mild, clinically insignificant endoscopic recurrence [48]. Although there are some variations in trial design among the post-operative studies, they are more homogeneous than the studies that have been carried out in patients with medically induced remissions, and, as a result, the observed treatment effects tend to be more consistent among the studies. Camma et al. [38] estimated a pooled risk difference of 13.1% favouring mesalazine over placebo in the post-operative setting. However, the meta-analysis did not include the data from the Lochs [46] and Hanauer [45] studies, whose inclusion would likely have resulted in a lower estimated pooled risk difference. Although the Lochs' study of 318 patients showed no statistically significant reduction in post-operative recurrence over 18 months, there was a slight trend towards lower recurrence in the mesalazine-treated patients compared with placebo-treated patients (24.5% vs 31.4%) [46]. Consistent with the findings of the Camma meta-analysis, they also found that the benefit was greatest, and statistically significant, in the subgroup of patients with isolated small bowel disease. The Camma meta-analysis also found that mesalazine produced larger benefit in those with longer disease duration [38]. It should be noted, however, that this latter analysis was performed including studies of both surgically and medically induced remissions. Although the pooled risk difference of 13.1% is statistically significant, it would mean that, if the estimate were correct, approximately eight patients would need to be

Table 14.5 Trials of mesalazine for post-operative prophylaxis.

Study (first author/ year of publication)	Sample size Mesalazine	Sample size Placebo	Disease sites	Formulation and dose of mesalazine (g/day)	Time from surgery entry to study (weeks)
Caprilli, 1994	47	48[a]	SB, SB/C	Asacol 2.4	2
Brignola, 1995	44	43	SB, SB/C	Pentasa 3.0	4
McLeod, 1995	87	76	SB, SB/C, C	Rowasal/Salofalk 3.0	8
Sutherland, 1997	31	35	SB, SB/C	Pentasa 3.0	NR
Lochs, 2000	152	166	SB, SB/C, C	Pentasa 4.0	1.4
Hanauer, 2004	44	40	SB, SB/C	Pentasa 3.0	Before post-operative discharge

Study (first author/ year of publication)	Maximum length of follow-up (months)	Definition of recurrence	Proportion of patients with recurrence Mesalazine	Proportion of patients with recurrence Placebo
Caprilli, 1994	24	Typical endoscopic lesions (≥ 5 aphthous lesions)	0.30	0.60
Brignola, 1995	12	CDAI >150 and ≥ 100 higher than previous visit	0.16	0.23
McLeod, 1995	72	Symptomatic recurrence PLUS endoscopic/radiologic confirmation	0.26[b]	0.45[b]
Sutherland, 1997	11	CDAI >150 and ≥ 60 higher than baseline OR Investigator opinion/ corticosteroid therapy/ hospitalisation	0.10	0.23
Lochs, 2000	18	CDAI >250 OR CDAI >200 but more than 60 points greater than lowest post-operative value for two consecutive weeks OR Indication for surgery OR Development of a new fistula OR Occurrence of a septic complication	0.24	0.31
Hanauer, 2004	24	Score of two or more on clinical scoring system (mild symptoms or worse)	0.58	0.77

Legend:
SB = small bowel; SB/C = small bowel + cecum and/or ascending colon; C = colon.
a = open study (i.e. patients in control arm received no placebo).
b = 3year actuarial risk of recurrence.

treated in order to prevent one post-operative recurrence of Crohn's disease over a period of 12–36 months. It is not known if the calculated risk reduction is maintained over a more extended duration of therapy. The issue of whether a 13.1% reduction in the risk of recurrence is cost-effective is debatable and needs to be discussed in the context of the cost effectiveness of other commonly used medical interventions. Unfortunately, carefully conducted cost-effectiveness analyses, with results presented in terms of cost per quality-adjusted-life-year saved in order to allow such comparisons to be made, have not been performed. However, the effectiveness data do provide physicians with some helpful information to present to patients when discussing the issue of post-operative prophylaxis. There does appear to be a benefit associated with the use of mesalazine, but the overall benefit is modest when examined over a period of 1–3 years. There are some disease characteristics, such as small-intestinal disease site, which may predict a more favourable risk reduction associated with the use of mesalazine. The decision regarding the use of post-operative mesalazine prophylaxis should not be based on blanket recommendations, guidelines or policy statements. Without further information regarding its effect on subsequent requirement for corticosteroid, immunomodulatory or surgical therapy, the decision should be based upon individual patient and disease characteristics and patient preferences. Following surgery, patients often have their own goals and preferences regarding further use of medical therapy. Some patients are extremely risk-averse and are willing to 'do anything possible' to prevent a recurrence even if the risk reduction achieved with treatment is low. Other patients view surgery as a means of allowing them to discontinue medical therapy, even temporarily, and are willing to accept the increased risk of recurrence if it means that they will be 'drug free' for a period of time. Unfortunately, there are no data regarding the longer term outcomes, with respect to the need for corticosteroid, immunomodulatory or surgical therapy, for patients treated post-operatively with prophylactic mesalazine. It is quite possible that, given the modest treatment effect in reducing the risk of post-operative recurrence, mesalazine may have no effect on these other outcomes that are likely to be of even greater interest to patients, physicians and insurers than a delay in post-operative clinical recurrence.

References

1 Azad Khan AK, Piris J, Truelove SC. An experiment to determine the active therapeutic moiety of sulphasalazine. *Lancet* 1977;2:892–5.
2 Anthonisen P, Barany F, Folkenborg O, *et al.* The clinical effect of salazosulphapyridine (Salazopyrin r) in Crohn's disease. A controlled double-blind study. *Scand J Gastroenterol* 1974;9:549–54.
3 Malchow H, Ewe K, Brandes JW, *et al.* European cooperative Crohn's disease study (ECCDS): results of drug treatment. *Gastroenterology* 1984;86:249–66.
4 Rijk MC, van Hogezand RA, van Lier HJ, van Tongeren JH. Sulphasalazine and prednisone compared with sulphasalazine for treating active Crohn disease. A double-blind, randomized, multicenter trial. *Ann Intern Med* 1991;114(6):445–50.
5 Singleton JW, Summers RW, Kern F Jr, *et al.* A trial of sulfasalazine as adjunctive therapy in Crohn's disease. *Gastroenterology* 1979;77:887–97.
6 Summers RW, Switz DM, Sessions JT Jr, *et al.* National cooperative Crohn's disease study: results of drug treatment. *Gastroenterology* 1979;77:847–69.
7 Ursing B, Alm T, Barany F, *et al.* A comparative study of metronidazole and sulfasalazine for active Crohn's disease: the cooperative Crohn's disease study in Sweden: II. Result. *Gastroenterology* 1982;83:550–62.
8 Van Hees PA, van Lier HJ, Van Elteren PH, *et al.* Effect of sulphasalazine in patients with active Crohn's disease: a controlled double-blind study. *Gut* 1981;22:404–9.
9 Rasmussen SN, Binder V, Maier K, *et al.* Treatment of Crohn's disease with peroral 5-aminosalicylic acid. *Gastroenterology* 1983;85:1350–3.
10 Rasmussen SN, Lauritsen K, Tage-Jensen U, *et al.* 5-Aminosalicylic acid in the treatment of Crohn's disease. A 16-week double-blind, placebo-controlled, multicentre study with Pentasa. *Scand J Gastroenterol* 1987;22:877–83.
11 Mahida YR, Jewell DP. Slow-release 5-amino-salicylic acid (Pentasa) for the treatment of active Crohn's disease. *Digestion* 1990;45:88–92.
12 Singleton JW, Hanauer SB, Gitnick GL, *et al.* Mesalamine capsules for the treatment of active Crohn's disease: results of a 16-week trial. Pentasa Crohn's disease study group. *Gastroenterology* 1993;104:1293–1301.
13 Singleton JW, Hanauer S, Robinson M. Quality-of-life results of double-blind, placebo-controlled trial of mesalamine in patients with Crohn's disease. *Dig Dis Sci* 1995;40(5):931–5.
14 Singleton J. Second trial of mesalamine therapy in the treatment of active Crohn's disease. *Gastroenterology* 1994;107(2):632–3.
15 Hanauer SB, Stromberg U. Oral Pentasa in the treatment of active Crohn's disease: a meta-analysis of double-blind, placebo-controlled trials. *Clin Gastroenterol Hepatol* 2004;2(5):379–88.
16 Tremaine WJ, Schroeder KW, Harrison JM, Zinsmeister AR. A randomized, double-blind, placebo-controlled trial of the oral mesalamine (5-ASA) preparation, Asacol, in the treatment of symptomatic Crohn's colitis and ileocolitis. *J Clin Gastroenterol* 1994;19(4):278–82.
17 Thomsen OO, Cortot A, Jewell D, *et al.* A comparison of budesonide and mesalamine for active Crohn's disease. International budesonide–mesalamine study group. *N Engl J Med* 1998;339(6):370–4.

18. Campieri M, Ferguson A, Doe W, Persson T, Nilsson LG. Oral budesonide is as effective as oral prednisolone in active Crohn's disease. The global budesonide study group. *Gut* 1997;41(2):209–14.

19. Greenberg GR, Feagan BG, Martin F, et al. Oral budesonide for active Crohn's disease. Canadian inflammatory bowel disease study group. *N Engl J Med* 1994;331(13):836–41.

20. Rutgeerts P, Lofberg R, Malchow H, et al. A comparison of budesonide with prednisolone for active Crohn's disease. *N Engl J Med* 1994;331(13):842–5.

21. Gross V, Andus T, Fischbach W, et al. Comparison between high dose 5-aminosalicylic acid and 6-methylprednisolone in active Crohn's ileocolitis. A multicenter randomized double-blind study. German 5-ASA study group. *Z Gastroenterol* 1995;33(10):581–4.

22. Martin F, Sutherland L, Beck IT. Oral 5-ASA versus prednisone in short treatment of Crohn's disease: a multicentre controlled trial. *Can J Gastroenterol* 1990;4:452–7.

23. Prantera C, Cottone M, Pallone F, et al. Mesalamine in the treatment of mild to moderate active Crohn's ileitis: results of a randomized, multicenter trial. *Gastroenterology* 1999;116(3):521–6.

24. Scholmerich J, Jenss H, Hartmann F. Oral 5-aminosalicylic acid versus 6-methylprednisolone in active Crohn's disease. *Can J Gastroenterol* 1990;4:446–51.

25. Modigliani R, Mary JY, Simon JF, et al. Clinical, biological, and endoscopic picture of attacks of Crohn's disease. Evolution on prednisolone. Groupe d'Etude Therapeutique des Affections Inflammatoires Digestives. *Gastroenterology* 1990;98:811–8.

26. Arber N, Odes SH, Fireman Z, et al. A controlled double blind multicenter study of the effectiveness of 5-aminosalicylic acid in patients with Crohn's disease in remission. *J Clin Gastroenterol* 1995;20(3):203–6.

27. Bresci G, Petrucci A, Banti S. 5-aminosalicylic acid in the prevention of relapses of Crohn's disease in remission: a long-term study. *Int J Clin Pharmacol Res* 1991;11(4):200–2.

28. Bresci G, Parisi G, Banti S. Long-term therapy with 5-aminosalicylic acid in Crohn's disease: is it useful? Our four years experience. *Int J Clin Pharmacol Res* 1994;14(4):133–8.

29. Brignola C, Iannone P, Pasquali S, et al. Placebo-controlled trial of oral 5-ASA in relapse prevention of Crohn's disease. *Dig Dis Sci* 1992;37(1):29–32.

30. De Franchis R, Omodei P, Ranzi T, et al. Controlled trial of oral 5-aminosalicylic acid for the prevention of early relapse in Crohn's disease. *Aliment Pharmacol Ther* 1997;11(5):845–52.

31. Gendre JP, Mary JY, Florent C, et al. Oral mesalamine (Pentasa) as maintenance treatment in Crohn's disease: a multicenter placebo-controlled study. The Groupe d'Etudes Therapeutiques des Affections Inflammatoires Digestives (GETAID). *Gastroenterology* 1993;104(2):435–9.

32. International Mesalazine Study Group. Coated oral 5-aminosalicylic acid versus placebo in maintaining remission of inactive Crohn's disease. *Aliment Pharmacol Ther* 1990;4:55–64.

33. Modigliani R, Colombel JF, dupas JL, et al. Mesalamine in Crohn's disease with steroid-induced remission: effect on steroid withdrawal and remission maintenance, Groupe d'Etudes Therapeutiques des Affections Inflammatoires Digestives. *Gastroenterology* 1996;110(3):688–93.

34. Prantera C, Pallone F, Brunetti G, Cottone M, Miglioli M. Oral 5-aminosalicylic acid (Asacol) in the maintenance treatment of Crohn's disease. The Italian IBD study group. *Gastroenterology* 1992;103:363–8.

35. Sutherland LR, Martin F, Bailey RJ, et al. A randomized, placebo-controlled, double-blind trial of mesalamine in the maintenance of remission of Crohn's disease. The Canadian mesalamine for remission of Crohn's disease study group. *Gastroenterology* 1997;112(4):1069–77.

36. Thomson AB, Wright JP, Vatn M, et al. Mesalazine (mesasal/claversal) 1.5 g b.d. vs placebo in the maintenance of remission of patients with Crohn's disease. *Aliment Pharmacol Ther* 1995;9(6):673–83.

37. Wellmann W, Schroder U. New oral preparations for maintenance therapy in Crohn's disease. *Can J Gastroenterol* 1988;2A:71A–2A.

38. Camma C, Giunta M, Rosselli M, Cottone M. Mesalamine in the maintenance treatment of Crohn's disease: a meta-analysis adjusted for confounding variables. *Gastroenterology* 1997;113(5):1465–73.

39. Steinhart AH, Hemphill D, Greenberg GR. Sulfasalazine and mesalazine for the maintenance therapy of Crohn's disease: a meta-analysis. *Am J Gastroenterol* 1994;89(12):2116–24.

40. Messori A, Brignola C, Tralori G, et al. Effectiveness of 5-aminosalicylic acid for maintaining remission in patients with Crohn's disease: a meta-analysis. *Am J Gastroenterol* 1994;89(5):692–8.

41. Candy S, Wright J, Gerber M, Adams G, Gerig M, Goodman R. A controlled double blind study of azathioprine in the management of Crohn's disease. *Gut* 1995;37(5):674–8.

42 Feagan BG, Rochon J, Fedorak RN, et al. Methotrexate for the treatment of Crohn's disease. The North American Crohn's study group investigators. *N Engl J Med* 1995;332(5):292–7.

43 Brignola C, Cottone M, Pera A, et al. Mesalamine in the prevention of endoscopic recurrence after intestinal resection for Crohn's disease. Italian cooperative study group. *Gastroenterology* 1995;108(2):345–9.

44 Caprilli R, Andreoli A, Capurso L, et al. Oral mesalazine (5-aminosalicylic acid; Asacol) for the prevention of post-operative recurrence of Crohn's disease. Gruppo Italiano per lo Studio del Colon e del Retto (GISC). *Aliment Pharmacol Ther* 1994;8(1):35–43.

45 Hanauer SB, Korelitz BI, Rutgeerts P, et al. Postoperative maintenance of Crohn's disease remission with 6-mercaptopurine, mesalamine, or placebo: a 2-year trial. *Gastroenterology* 2004;127(3):723–9.

46 Lochs H, Mayer M, Fleig WE, et al. Prophylaxis of postoperative relapse in Crohn's disease with mesalamine: European cooperative Crohn's disease study VI. *Gastroenterology* 2000;118(2):264–73.

47 McLeod RS, Wolff BG, Steinhart AH, et al. Prophylactic mesalamine treatment decreases postoperative recurrence of Crohn's disease. *Gastroenterology* 1995;109(2):404–13.

48 Caprilli R, Cottone M, Tonelli F, et al. Two mesalazine regimens in the prevention of the post-operative recurrence of Crohn's disease: a pragmatic, double-blind, randomized controlled trial. *Aliment Pharmacol Ther* 2003;17(4):517–23.

15: Steroids or nutrition?

Miquel A. Gassull

Glucocorticoids in the treatment of IBD

Systemic administration of therapeutic doses of glucocorticoids (hydrocortisone, prednisone, prednisolone or methyl-prednisolone) to patients suffering from acute, moderate-severe, attacks of ulcerative colitis (UC) or Crohn's disease (CD) induce clinical response in 60–80% of cases [1–4]. Due to their marked anti-inflammatory activity and quick therapeutic action (within days) they are widely accepted as the treatment of choice in these situations. In addition it has the advantage of being an inexpensive therapy. Because of these 'virtues' it is considered one of the best examples of low cost and effective treatment. Steroids continue to be the most used and most useful drugs in the management of patients with acute attacks of IBD. They continue to be the standard against which new treatments are compared in IBD in clinical trials.

However, as in all drug-based therapy, steroids have also 'drawbacks'. These 'drawbacks' may have relevance in diseases such as CD and UC with a clinical course characterised by frequent relapses that may need repeated steroid treatments.

It is known that prolonged glucocorticoid administration leads to adrenal suppression. Moreover, unwanted aesthetic changes develop in patients on this treatment, including moon face, 'buffalo hump', striae, weight gain, acne, hirsutism and others [5, 6]. Although most of these side effects revert after discontinuing the treatment, steroids are not well accepted particularly by adolescents and youngsters with IBD, and especially when they have already experienced the effects of the glucocorticoid treatment once or twice.

In addition to these aesthetic side effects, there are severe metabolic consequences of steroid treatment. These include, hypocalcaemia, hyperglycaemia [7, 8] and protein hyper-catabolism [9, 10]. The latter may contribute to the development of malnutrition, which together with the inflammatory activity and enteral loss of proteins, are primary events leading also to growth arrest and sexual maturation delay in children and adolescents [11]. These are considered very severe complications of IBD in younger patients. Furthermore, growth failure in childhood will influence height in adult life. In Table 15.1 the side effects of steroids are shown.

Inflammatory bowel disease itself decreases bone mineral density [12] by the effect of increased cytokine expression [13]. In addition, several other factors related to the presence of active disease, such as malnutrition, dietary restrictions, lack of exercise or climatic factors (sun light exposure) are risk factors for metabolic bone disease [14, 15]. However, steroid treatment also contributes to the development of osteopenia in IBD, by decreasing bone formation and enhancing bone resorption by inhibiting intestinal calcium absorption, increasing renal calcium excretion and inducing parathormone secretion [16, 17]. As a consequence, steroids increase the risk of bone fractures and osteonecrosis [18], which although not frequent, when they do occur produce a serious handicap to the patient. All these facts are limiting factors for the repetitive use of corticosteroids, not only in elderly patients who may represent the highest risk group, but also in youngsters

Table 15.1 Corticosteroid side effects.

Weight gain
Moon face, buffalo hump
Striae, plethorae, acne
Adrenal atrophy
Impaired glucose tolerance, diabetes mellitus
Hypertension
Hypercholesterolemia
Osteoporosis
Aseptic necrosis of the bone
Electrolyte imbalance
Posterior sub-capsular cataract, glaucoma
Insomnia, psychosis
Neuropathy
Hyper-metabolism and negative nitrogen balance
Growth retardation
Proximal myopathy
Increased susceptibility to infections

and especially in children and adolescents in whom, as mentioned, it may further derange normal growth, especially in those suffering from CD [18]. In addition, the first treatment with glucocorticoids at a young age may negatively influence the bone mass in the future, because most of the bone loss occurs within the first 3 months of steroid use. Doses of 40 mg of prednisolone per day for 1 week produce a significant increase in urinary hydroxyproline and calcium excretion reflecting an increase in bone resorption [19]. At this time bone mass loss might be, at least in part, reversible after discontinuing the treatment, but repeated treatments for frequent relapses may lead to an irreversible osteopenia [20]. Even lower doses (10 mg/day) for longer periods (which is not an unusual practice) for 7 months resulted in a 34% reduction of trabecular bone volume [20]. Moreover, in a study of chronic low prednisone dose treatment (mean 5.6 mg/day) in patients with rheumatoid arthritis, a 2% per year loss of bone mineral density in the spine could be observed. Patients not receiving steroids did not show a significant change in bone mineral density [21, 22].

Adolescent IBD patients may reach a lower peak bone mass than a healthy population. In healthy people, peak bone mass is reached around the age of 30. Juvenile IBD patients, suffering the disease since an early age, will reach the fracture threshold (reflecting a lower peak bone mass) earlier in life than healthy controls. A group of paediatric CD patients has been described with vertebral compression fractures complicating osteoporosis [18, 23–26]. Because decreased bone mass is already an important problem in this young-age IBD population, the use of steroid treatment in such situations may have very serious consequences for their future.

Thus, steroid therapy-induced bone loss is dose and duration dependent, with a greater decrease in bone mass occurring during the first few months when administered at high doses. Even low steroid doses produce an accelerated loss of bone density. Bone mass should then be specifically protected in children, adolescents and elders, because they are recognised as high-risk populations. Adults should not be forgotten either, because they are in the most active and productive stage of their life. In Table 15.2 the mechanisms of corticosteroid-induced osteopenia are listed.

Steroids may also be dangerous when administered to patients with undiagnosed abdominal abscess, because it may result in an increased mortality due to septic complications [5, 27].

All of the above mentioned steroid 'drawbacks' preclude their use, at therapeutic doses or even at lower doses, either as long-term maintenance treatment or as established therapy in patients with frequent disease relapses (steroid dependent), which represent up to 50% of patients with CD [28]. This has stimulated the search for therapies other than steroids for treating these patients in steroid dependent cases.

Table 15.2 Mechanisms of steroid-induced osteopenia.

Decreased bone formation
1. Reduced synthesis of osteoblasts
2. Decreased osteoblasts proliferation
3. Impaired gonadal hormone production

Increased bone resorption
1. Decreased calcium absorption in the intestine
2. Increased urinary calcium excretion
3. Increased parathyroid hormone secretion
4. Decreased calcitonin synthesis
5. Enhanced osteoclastic activity
6. Excessive binding of macrophages to bone

The definition of steroid dependence is not well established. In general terms it was considered as such when patients tended to relapse two or three times within a given period of time (6 months or 1 year) after steroid discontinuation or when a low dose was reached when tapered. Although the concept has not been clearly and consistently defined, clinical experience has shown that when a patient suffers an early relapse when the drug has been discontinued after a correct tapering schedule, it is most likely that steroid dependence is present. This suggests that therapeutic measures leading to the use of alternative immunosuppressants to avoid the use of steroids should be taken at an earlier stage in such cases.

To spare steroids alternative drugs have been proposed, such as azathioprine, 6-MP [29], ciclosporine [30–33], methotrexate [34–36], mycophenolate mofetil [37], tacrolimus [38] and more recently the new biological therapies, especially anti-TNF-α antibodies [39]. Although these agents have proven to be useful, there are potential severe side effects [29–39]. Moreover, in a recent review, methotrexate has been shown to produce an osteopathy with loss of bone cortex, which is clinically characterised by the appearance of pain in the legs and a high probability of developing pathological fractures. Some of these fractures are often missed by conventional X-Ray and are only shown by bone scintigraphy [36].

Because of all these reasons, new less aggressive treatments influencing the immune response in chronic inflammatory conditions are being sought, especially to avoid or minimise corticosteroid therapy. One of these approaches is the use of nutrition as therapy in IBD.

Basis for the use of nutritional management as primary therapy in IBD

Nutrition was seen as a possible therapeutic tool in IBD due to various clinical observations:

1 Nutritional deficiencies (macro, micronutrients) are frequent in these patients; these include protein-energy malnutrition and various mineral, vitamin and trace element deficits [40–44]. The aetiology of such derangements is multi-factorial and includes anorexia, hyper-catabolism, extensive small intestinal involvement or resections, increased nutrient losses through the inflamed and ulcerated gut, the existence of fistulae, medical management (therapeutic fasting, steroids) and self (or doctor) imposed dietary restrictions. The consequences of protein-energy malnutrition in disease outcome are of the utmost importance in children and adolescents where, independently of those associated with steroid treatment, there may be growth failure and delay in sexual development [9, 11]. In adults they may lead to increased need for surgical treatment [40] and to complications related to surgery [45].

Sub-optimal levels of micronutrients are often found in children and adults with IBD. Symptoms related to such deficits are seldom evident (except for iron and folate). However, sub-optimal micronutrient status may favour disease self-perpetuation, because of impairment of tissue repair mechanisms, defective defence against free-radical damage and lipid peroxidation [46], as well as potential increase in mucosal dysplasia [47]. Although theoretically feasible, these possibilities have not been properly investigated. There are not, for instance, clinical trials showing the potential benefit of supplementing these patients with antioxidant micronutrients, either in inducing remission or preventing relapse of the disease [48].

2 Some foodstuffs may act as symptom-triggering antigens, especially in CD. This observation prompted the use of exclusion diets in which patients avoid eating the offending food(s). These have been shown to be of some use in a small percentage of patients [49]. On the other hand, it has not been demonstrated that the re-introduction of the foods that provoke symptoms actually cause a relapse of CD.

3 Insufficient amount of products of colonic metabolism of unabsorbed carbohydrates (mainly butyrate) or its defective oxidation by colonocytes, has been implicated in the pathogenesis of ulcerative colitis and pouchitis [50–56]. More recently a cross-over designed study in patients with refractory pouchitis has shown that the oral administration of inulin (an oligosaccharide fermentable in the colon) was able to induce clinical, endoscopic and histologic improvement [57]. Furthermore, the

administration of probiotic bacteria has been shown to be effective in such patients [58–62]. The nutritional approach to the maintenance treatment of UC has been studied. It has been shown that the relapse rate of quiescent disease treated with soluble dietary fibre (*Plantago ovata* seeds) was not different from that of patients given 5-ASA at the usual maintenance doses. Patients on fibre treatment increased butyrate production in the colon (as measured by stool analysis) as compared to those on 5-ASA [63]. The nutritional approach for the acute and maintenance therapy of UC, in addition to supporting the role of butyrate in the pathogenesis of the disease, opens a new therapeutic possibility for the long-term maintenance treatment of quiescent UC. The use of fermentable carbohydrates and probiotics has not shown any effectiveness in CD [64, 65].

4 Some common severe long-term complications, such as growth and sexual development failure (children and adolescents) and osteopenia (children and adults) are related, not only to the disease itself or its treatment (steroids), but are also strongly linked to the presence of malnutrition [9, 11, 16–19, 22]. As has been previously stressed, these are considered severe complications of the disease. Long-term nutritional support in this group of patients, especially in those suffering with CD, together with disease control, has been very helpful in recovering a more normal rate of growth [66, 67].

There is no evidence that either parenteral (TPN) or enteral (TEN) nutrition, when used as adjuvant therapy to steroid treatment, has any primary therapeutic effect on the outcome of patients with acute severe UC. The so called 'bowel rest' obtained by the use of TPN had no advantage in the treatment of these patients. However, those acutely ill patients given TEN (no bowel rest) coming to colectomy because of steroid unresponsiveness suffered significantly less complications related to surgery (sepsis, abdominal abscesses, etc.) as compared to those who received TPN [45]. These data confirm that enteral nutrition is the preferred modality of nutritional support in moderately severe ulcerative colitis.

5 Nutritional habits of some communities have been associated with a low incidence of UC and CD, suggesting that some components of their diets may favour a modulation of the inflammatory response [68]. This could be related to differences in the type of fat present in the diet [69] that would produce changes in the lipid composition in the membranes of the immune-competent cells, which, in turn, may influence, chemotaxis as well as eicosanoid, adhesion molecules and cytokine release [70–75]. *In vitro* and *in vivo* studies [70, 74–78] support this hypothesis. Trials have been carried out using different preparations of the n-3 long-chain polyunsaturated fatty acids (PUFA), eicosapentanoic and docosahexaenoic acids, in active or quiescent UC and CD, with negative results in most [79–86], with the exception of one study in CD [87]. However most clinical trials have problems of interpretation because of deficiencies in study design (cross-over), the use of a potentially active placebo, the use of a n-3 PUFA preparation that is possibly not well absorbed and heterogeneity in the groups studied. For all of these reasons, it has not been possible to obtain reliable information about the potential use of this nutritional approach in the treatment of either UC or CD. Clinical trials are necessary in order to ascertain the true effectiveness of this therapy and to identify the groups of patients that could benefit from it.

6 For the most part, the greatest interest in a nutritional approach to the management of IBD has been the possibility of using chemically defined enteral formula diets as primary treatment in CD. The first approach was made with the concept that introducing amino-acids (elemental diets), instead of intact proteins (polymeric diets) in the gut lumen would decrease the intestinal antigenic load, which in turn would diminish the chances of triggering or maintaining the abnormal or up regulated inflammatory bowel response [88]. In addition it has been reported that elemental diets decrease intestinal permeability in CD [89] and diminish the excretion of pro-inflammatory cytokines in the stools of these patients [90].

Randomised controlled trials, although with a small number of patients, showed very consistently that most, but not all, elemental diets achieved remission rates that were similar to corticosteroids, both in children and in adults [88, 89–106]. Also, studies have shown that some, but not all, polymeric diets, when used as a unique treatment, can also induce remission in active CD [94, 95, 98, 99, 107–111].

Because of some contradictory results observed in the published trials, together with the fact that most of them were carried out with a small sample of patients, a meta-analysis was performed to ascertain the effectiveness of enteral nutrition as compared to steroids [112]. It was shown that steroids induced remission in 80% of the cases whereas this occurred in about 60% of patients treated with enteral nutrition (including all type of diets). This percentage of remission is two to three times that obtained with placebo in early therapeutic trials in CD (20–30%). In addition, when most of the patients treated with elemental diets both in randomised and non-randomised clinical trials are pooled (549 patients), the mean remission rate obtained is 78.9%, similar to that with steroids (Fig 15.1). Moreover, when the same is done with polymeric diets (n = 124), the rate of remission is close to 70% (Fig 15.2). This strongly suggests that, at least in some groups of patients, enteral nutrition may be of primary therapeutic value.

The possibility that the amount and the type of the fat source could account for the therapeutic effect of enteral nutrition in CD was first pointed out by Fernandez-Bañares et al. in 1994 [113]. This hypothesis suggested that the fatty acids contained in the lipid source used and the quantity administered in the formula diet, may produce changes in the composition of the membrane phospholipids of the immune-competent cells. As previously mentioned, these changes in composition may influence cell membrane functions, such as cell-to-cell recognition, and modify the production of cytokine and eicosanoid as well as adhesion molecules [70–78].

Middleton et al. [103], in 1995, performed a meta-analysis relating the remission rate and the composition of the formula diets used as primary treatment in patients with CD. They pointed out that the response rate obtained with the formula diets was inversely correlated with the amount of long-chain triglycerides in the enteral formula. This finding was confirmed when we included more recent trials in the analysis.

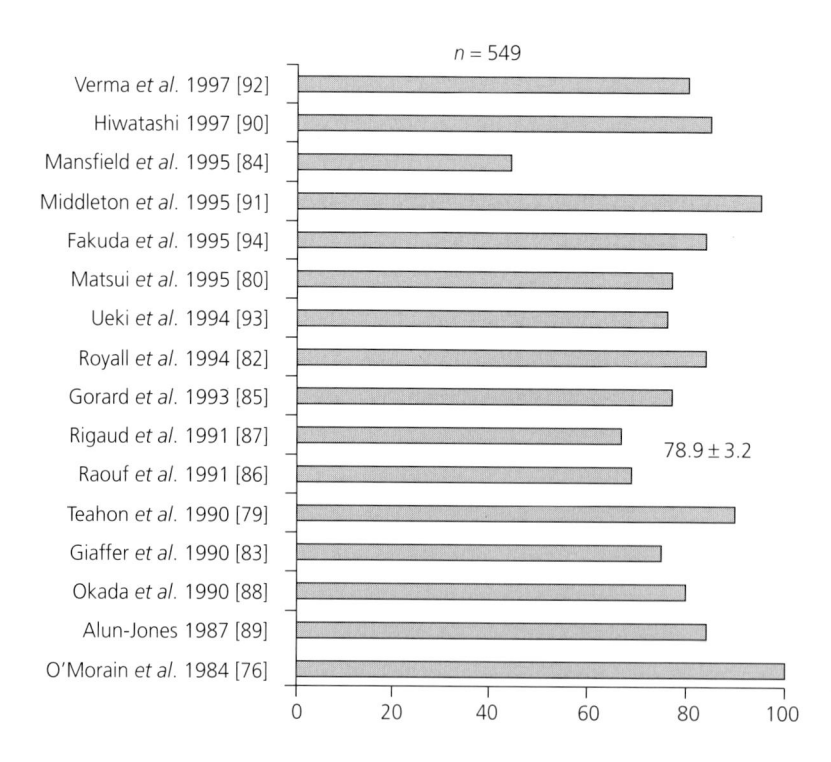

Fig 15.1 Mean (+/− sem) remisssion rate achieved in patients treated with elemental diets when randomised and non-randomised clinical trials are pooled (n = 549 patients) [76, 79–94].

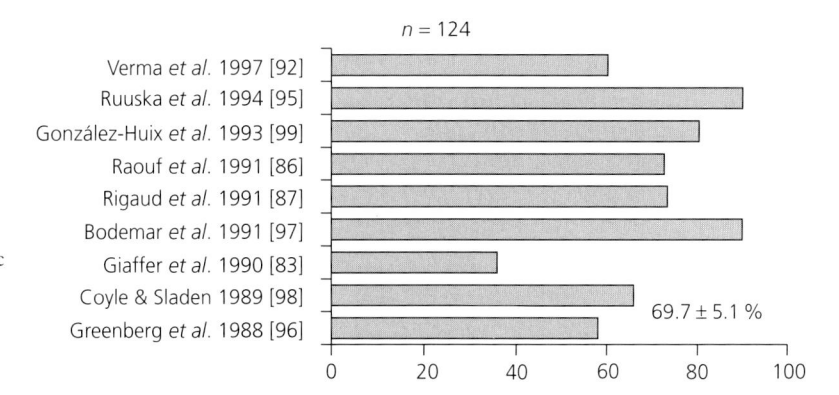

Fig 15.2 Mean (+/− sem) remisssion rate achieved in patients treated with polymeric diets when randomised and non-randomised clinical trials are pooled (*n* = 124 patients) [82, 83, 86, 87, 95–99].

Verma *et al.* 1997 [92]
Ruuska *et al.* 1994 [95]
González-Huix *et al.* 1993 [99]
Raouf *et al.* 1991 [86]
Rigaud *et al.* 1991 [87]
Bodemar *et al.* 1991 [97]
Giaffer *et al.* 1990 [83]
Coyle & Sladen 1989 [98]
Greenberg *et al.* 1988 [96]

n = 124

69.7 ± 5.1 %

More recently, in Japan, Hiwatashi *et al.* [102] also found that elemental diets with low-fat content are associated with the highest remission rate when administered as a primary treatment in active CD. They hypothesised that in addition to the low antigenic effect produced by the amino-acid mixture, the low-fat content would reduce intestinal motility, thus favouring an 'effective bowel rest'.

In a more recent study [114] the therapeutic role of fatty acid composition of the enteral diet in acute Crohn's disease was demonstrated by comparing two diets with identical caloric distribution but with different fat composition and source. Although the group treated with steroids achieved the usual 80% clinical remission rate, one of the diet treated groups (linoleic acid based) achieved a remission rate of 60%, whereas for the other diet-treated group (oleic acid-based) the remission rate was only 20%. Thus the fat source of the enteral diet appears to define its therapeutic effectiveness.

However, other factors related to the characteristics of the patients or the disease such as age, sex, race, disease location, severity of the attack, possible effect of previous treatments, genetic background, etc., may define specific subgroups of patients especially prone to respond to enteral nutrition. In this sense it is illustrative that as many as 72–85% of children with active CD respond to elemental diets, especially those with small bowel and ileocolonic disease [66]. This observation is of relevance, because it fits well with the observations in adults where it appears that enteral formula diets are also more effective in CD patients with small intestinal involvement as compared with those with colonic disease. Moreover, as already mentioned, conventional or fat-modified enteral formula diets in UC have not shown any primary therapeutic effectiveness. Large-scale trials are needed to help identify factors, such as small bowel involvement, that are predictive of response to enteral feeding in CD and to determine the optimal characteristics of the formulas used for feeding UC patients (and perhaps colonic CD).

Interesting data have been published about the role of enteral nutrition as maintenance treatment in CD. Hiwatashi reported retrospective data including long-term maintenance treatment of 410 CD patients [102]. Three hundred and twenty-two were treated with nocturnal elemental diets at home, administered through a self-intubated feeding tube, complementing a diet with low-fat foods. The control group were patients receiving drugs (mainly sulphasalazine) as maintenance treatment. Both the cumulative probability of remission and non-hospitalisation at 3000 days were significantly higher in the home enteral nutrition group than in the group of patients treated with drugs. Similar results were reported by Koga *et al.* [115] using polymeric instead of elemental diets. Both reports stress the fact that the higher the amount of calories administered daily (between 1200 and 1600) to these patients the greater the possibility of maintaining remission.

Wilschansky *et al.* [66] reported that children with CD who continued with nocturnal supplementary enteral nutrition with an elemental or semi-elemental liquid diet after resuming a normal diet, remained well longer than those who discontinued nocturnal supplements completely after achieving remission. In addition, height velocity for growth was significantly greater in those children receiving supplementary nocturnal enteral nutrition than in those of the control group. In addition, Walker-Smith has shown that mucosal histological improvement was observed in six out of seven children treated with enteral polymeric diets as primary therapy. In addition, in two of these children complete healing of the intestinal mucosa was demonstrated [116].

So far, objective data has shown:

1 Steroids are the most effective and the cheapest form of treatment in acute attacks of IBD. The high rate of severe side effects of this treatment precludes its use for long periods of time, even at low doses, in all cases. This is very important in some patient populations (children, adolescents and elders), where treatments should be especially short.

2 Alternative drugs to steroid treatment, although effective, should be incorporated in earlier stages of the treatment, and need to be closely monitored because they may be associated with serious side effects.

3 In randomised controlled trials (RCT), enteral nutrition is effective in greater than 60% in all type of patients with Crohn's disease (excluding fistulising and perianal disease). This percentage of effectiveness is very unlikely to be due to a placebo effect, since it is two to three times higher than that obtained by placebo in all classical studies. It is worth noting that when analysing the therapeutic effect of enteral nutrition in CD, only those patients achieving complete remission (as evaluated by different indices and biological parameters) have been taken into account. The term 'response' as representative of a certain decrease in the activity index has been very seldom used in these studies. In this sense the outcome criterion used in nutritional studies tends to be more stringent than that used in many drug RCTs.

4 Elemental diets decrease intestinal permeability in CD [89] and diminish the excretion of pro-inflammatory cytokines in the stools [90].

5 There may be, then, certain groups of patients with a more favourable response to the treatment with enteral diets (small intestinal involvement rather than colonic involvement only in CD). Conventional or fat modified enteral formula diets have not shown effectiveness in UC.

6 The analyses of the characteristics of the diets used in clinical trials suggest that the quantity and quality of the fat content, rather than the use of aminoacids as nitrogen source, may be a key factor in obtaining a more favourable response with this therapy. Low-fat-containing diets obtain the higher remission rates.

7 Soluble oligosaccharides have been shown to be effective in refractory pouchitis and soluble fibre has been shown to be effective in maintaining remission in UC.

Can nutrition be used in the year 2006 as primary treatment in inflammatory bowel disease?

It can be said, without fear of over-interpreting the data shown in this chapter that, rather than steroids, enteral nutrition is indicated, as first choice treatment in CD in children and adolescents. In addition to the observed clinical, biological and endoscopic anti-inflammatory effect, nutritional therapy will prevent or minimise growth failure, sexual development delay and osteopenia. This recommendation should apply not only to the first attack, but also in any relapse, especially when the activity could be classified as moderate.

For similar reasons, especially those related to maintaining bone mass, enteral nutrition can be seen as the first possible treatment in elderly patients with CD, mainly because there is a strong possibility that they may have previously received various long-term treatments with glucocorticoids.

Enteral diets should be tried in new onset attacks at all ages, because avoiding steroid side effects, in addition to being the aim of the doctor, is often a request of these patients, especially youngsters. In general, this should be the first therapeutic approach in all mild to moderate acute attacks, mainly when there is small intestine or ileocolonic involvement.

Also, this therapeutic approach may be a safer way of starting the treatment in patients with a possible undiagnosed abdominal abscess. It has been reported that steroid administration in such cases may increase mortality due to septic complications [5, 27].

Enteral nutrition can be used as maintenance treatment in children in whom, in addition to keeping the disease in remission, it maintains linear growth or results in catch-up linear growth. In fact, some reports also suggest that enteral nutrition, as a complement to a low-fat diet is a useful tool in maintaining remission in adults.

There is, at least one more situation in which enteral nutrition might be of great therapeutic value. In steroid-dependent disease the use of enteral nutrition provides the possibility of avoiding the use of immunosuppressive drugs and their potential side effects. Unfortunately, there are not enough data to support this indication.

One further point is the type of enteral diet to be used. From the data available, elemental (amino acid) or semi-elemental (small peptide) based diets, with very low-fat content, are the first choice to be used in acute CD as well as in maintenance treatment. However, polymeric diets (whole protein based), with low-fat content should be tried because most cases will respond to them. These diets have the advantage of being, for most patients, much more palatable and always much cheaper than elemental diets. Although data regarding the optimal type of lipids or fat source to be used in these diets are still not certain, it is obvious that the therapeutic effect does not rely only on one or two single fatty acids.

References

1. Truelove SC, Witts LJ. Cortisone and corticotrophin in ulcerative colitis. *Br Med J* 1959;1:387–94.
2. Truelove SC, Jewell DP. Intensive intravenous regimen for severe attacks of ulcerative colitis. *Lancet* 1974;1:1067–70.
3. Meyers S, Sachar DB, Goldberg JD, Janowitz HD. Corticotropin versus hydrocortisone in the intravenous treatment of ulcerative colitis: a prospective, randomized, double blind clinical trial. *Gastroenterology* 1983;85:351–7.
4. Margolin ML, Krumholz MP, Fochios SE, Korelitz BI. Clinical trials in ulcerative colitis II: historical view. *Am J Gastroenterol* 1988;83:227–43.
5. Malchow H, Eve K, Brandes JW, et al. European cooperative Crohn's disease study (ECCDS): result of drug treatment. *Gastroenterology* 1984;86:249–66.
6. Lennard-Jones JE. Corticosteroids and immunosuppressive drugs. In: Agnostides AA, Hodgson HJF, Kirsner JB, eds. *Inflammatory Bowel Disease*. London: Chapman & Hall; 1991:275–86.
7. Spencer JA, Kirsner JB, Mlynaryk P, Reed P, Palmer WL. Immediate and prolonged therapeutic effects of corticotrophin and adrenal steroids in ulcerative colitis: observations in 340 cases for periods up to 10 years. *Gastroenterology* 1962;42:113–28.
8. Sparsberg N, Kirsner JB. Long-term corticosteroid therapy for regional enteritis: an analysis of 58 courses in 54 patients. *Am J Dig Dis* 1966;1:865–80.
9. Winter HS. Special consideration in pediatric inflammatory bowel disease. In: Targan SR, Shanahan F, eds. *Inflammatory Bowel Disease: From Bench to Bedside*. Baltimore: Williams and Wilkins; 1994:701–10.
10. Williams GH, Dluhy G. Disease of the adrenal cortex. In: Fauci AS, Brawnwald E, Isselbacher KJ, et al., eds. *Harrison's Principles of Internal Medicine*. 14th ed. New York: McGraw-Hill; 1998:2035–60, chap 332.
11. Griffits AM, Nguyen P, Snmith C, MacMillan H, Sherman PM. Growth and clinical course of children with Crohn's Disease. *Gut* 1993;34:939–43.
12. Lamb EJ, Wong T, Smith DJ, et al. Metabolic bone disease is present at diagnosis in patients with inflammatory bowel disease. *Aliment Pharmacol Ther* 2002;16:1895–1902.
13. Vestergaard P. Prevalence and pathogenesis of osteoporosis in patients with inflammatory bowel disease. *Minerva Med* 2004;95:469–80.
14. Silvennoinen JA, Kartunnen TJ, Niemela SE, Manalius JJ, Lehtola JK. A controlled study of bone mineral density in patients with inflammatory bowel disease. *Gut* 1995;37:71–6.
15. Bjarnason I, Macpherson A, Mackintosh C, Buxton-Thomas M, Forgacs I, Moniz C. Reduced bone density in patients with inflammatory bowel disease. *Gut* 1997;40:228–33.
16. Canalis E. Mechanisms of glucocorticoid action in bone: implications to corticosteroid-induced osteoporosis. *J Clin Endocrin Metab* 1996;81:3441–7.
17. Adinoff AD, Hollister R. Steroid-induced fractures and bone loss in patients with asthma. *N Engl J Med* 1983309:265–8.

18 Schoon EJ, Wolffenbuttel BHR, Stockbrügger RW. Osteoporosis as a risk in inflammatory bowel disease. *Drugs of Today* 1999;35(Suppl A):17–28.

19 Hodsman AB, Toogood JH, Jennings B, et al. Differential effect of inhaled budesonide and oral prednisone in serum osteocalcin. *J Clin Endocrinol Metab* 1991;72:530–40.

20 Lo Cascio V, Bonicci E Imbimbo B, et al. Bone loss after glucocorticoid therapy. *Clacif Tiss Int* 1984;36:435–438.

21 Buckley LM, Leib ES, Caetularo KS, et al. Calcium and vitamin D3 supplementation prevents bone loss in the spine secondary to low-dose corticosteroids in patients with rheumatoid arthritis. *Ann Intern Med* 1996;125:961–8.

22 Valentine JF, Sninsky CA. Prevention and treatment of osteoporosis in patients with inflammatory bowel disease. *Am J Gastroenterol* 1999;94:878–83.

23 Gokhale R, Favus MJ, Karrison T, Sutton MM, Rich B, Kirschner B. Bone mineral density assessment in children with inflammatory bowel disease, *Gastroenterology* 1988;114:902–11.

24 Cowan FJ, Parker DR, Jenkins HR. Osteopenia in Crohn's disease. *Gut* 1995;73:225–56.

25 Semeao EJ, Stallings VA, Peck SN, Picolli DA. Vertebral compression fractures in pediatric patients with Crohn's disease. *Gastroenterology* 1997;112:1710–13.

26 Vakil N, Sparberg M. Steroid-related osteonecrosis in inflammatory bowel disease. *Gastroenterology* 1989;96:62–67.

27 Andus T, Targan SR. Glucocorticoids. In: Targan SR, Shanahan F, eds. *Inflammatory Bowel Disease: From Bench to Bedside*. Baltimore: Williams and Wilkins; 1994;487–502.

28 Munkholm P, Langholz E, Davidsen M, Binder V. Frequency of glucocorticoid resistance and dependency in Crohn's disease. *Gut* 1994;35:360–2.

29 Connell WR, Kamm MA, Ritchie JK, Lennard-Jones JE. Bone marrow toxicity caused by azathioprine in inflammatory bowel disease: 27-years of experience. *Gut* 1993;34:1081–5.

30 Carbonel F, Boruchowicz A, Duclos B, et al. Intravenous cyclosporine in attacks of ulcerative colitis: short and long-term responses. *Dig Dis Sci* 1996;41:2471–6.

31 Stack WA, Long RG, Hawkey CJ. Short- and long-term outcome of patients treated with cyclosporin for severe acute ulcerative colitis. *Aliment Prarmacol Ther* 1998;12:973–8.

32 Stange EF, Modigliani R, Pena AS, Wood AJ, Feutren G, Smith PR and the European Group of Crohn's Disease. European trial of cyclosporine in chronic active Crohn's disease. *Gastroenterology* 1995;109:774–82.

33 Fernandez-Bañares F, Bertran X, Esteve-Comas M, Cabre E, Menacho M, Gassull MA. Azathioprine is useful in the long-term maintaining remission induced by i.v. Cyclosporin in severe steroid-refractory ulcerative colitis. *Am J Gastroenterol* 1996;91:2498–9.

34 West SG. Methotrexate hepatotoxicity. *Rheumatic Disease Clinics of North America* 1997;23:883–915.

35 Cannon GW. Methotrexate pulmonary toxicity. *Rheumatic Disease Clinics of North America* 1997;23:917–37.

36 McKendry RJ. The remarkable spectrum of methotrexate toxicities. *Rheumatic Disease Clinics of North America* 1997;23:939–54.

37 Neurath MF, Wanitschke R, Peters M, Krummenauer F, Meyer zum Büschenfelde KH, Schlaak JF. Randomised trial of Mycophenolate Mofetil versus Azathioprine for treatment of chronic active Crohn's Disease. *Gut* 1999;44:625–8.

38 Fellermann K, Ludwig D, Stahl M, David-Walek T, Stange EF. Steroid unresponsive acute attacks of inflammatory bowel disease: immunomodulation by Tracolimus (FK 506). *Am J Gastroenterol* 1998;93:1860–6.

39 Anonimus. Infliximab (Remicade) for CD. *Med Lett Drugs Ther* 1999;41:19–20.

40 Gassull MA, Abad A, Cabre E, Gonzalez-Huix F, Giné JJ, Dolz C. Enteral tube feeding in inflammatory bowel disease. *Gut* 1987;27(Suppl):76–80.

41 Cabré E, Fernandez-Bañares F, Esteve M, Gassull MA. Micronutrients in inflammatory bowel disease. *J Clin Nutr Gastroenterol* 1989;4:100–102.

42 Fernandez-Bañares F, Abad-Lacruz A, Xiol X, et al. Vitamin status in patients with inflammatory bowel disease. *Am J Gastroenterol* 1989;84:744–8.

43 Fernandez-Bañares F, Mingorance MD, Esteve M, et al. Serum Zinc, Copper and Selenium levels in inflammatory bowel disease. *Am J Gastroenterol* 1990;85:1584–9.

44 Abad-Lacruz A, Fernandez-Bañares F, Cabre E, et al. The effect of total enteral tube feeding on the vitamin status of malnourished patients with inflammatory bowel disease. *Internat J Vit Nutr Res* 1988;58:428–35.

45 Gonzalez-Huix, Esteve M, Abad A, et al. Enteral vs parenteral nutrition as adjunct therapy in acute ulcerative colitis: a prospective randomized study. *Am J Gastroenterol* 1993;88:227–32.

46 Miralles-Barrachina O, Savoye G, Belmonte-Zalar L, et al. Low levels of Glutathione in endoscopic

47 Lashner BA, Provencher KS, Seidner DL, Knesebeck A, Brzezinski A. The effect of folic acid supplementation on the risk for cancer or dysplasia in ulcerative colitis. *Gastroenterology* 1997;112:29–32.

biopsies of patients with Crohn's colitis: the role of malnutrition. *Clin Nutr* 1999;18.

48 Fernandez-Bañares F. Papel de los metabolitos de oxigeno reactivos en la patogenia de la enfermedad inflamatoria intestinal. *Gastroenterol Hepatol* 1995;18:526–32.

49 Alun Jones V, Dickinson RJ, Workman E, Wilson AJ, Freeman AH, Hunter JU. Crohn's disease: maintenance of remission by diet. *Lancet* 1985;2:177–80.

50 Rombeau JL, Kripke SA. Metabolic effects of short-chain fatty acids. *JPEN* 1990;14(Suppl):18S–5S.

51 Royall D, Wolever TMS, Jeejeebhoy KN. Clinical significance of colonic fermentation. *Am J Gastroenterol* 1990;85:1307–12.

52 Scheppach W. Effects of short-chain fatty acids on gut morphology and function. *Gut* 1994;35:S35–38.

53 Vernia P, Cittadini M, Caprilli R, Torsoli A. Topical treatment of refractory distal ulcerative colitis sith 5-ASA and sodium butyrate. *Dig Dis Sci* 1995;40:305–7.

54 Chapman MAS, Grhan MF, Boyle MA, Hutton M, Rogers J, Williams NS. Butyrate oxidation is impaired in the colonic mucosa of sufferers of quiescent ulcerative colitis. *Gut* 1994;35:73–6.

55 Roediger WEW, Duncan A, Kapanidis O, Millard S. Reducing sulfur compounds of the colon impair colonocyte nutrition: implications for ulcerative colitis. *Gastroenterology* 1993;104:802–9.

56 Roediger WEW, Duncan A, Kapanidis O, Millard S. Sulphide impairement of butyrate oxidation in rat colonocytes: a biochemical basis for ulcerative colitis? *Clin Sci* 1993;85:623–7.

57 Welters CFM, Heineman E, Thunnissen FB, van den Bogaard AEJM, Soeters PB, Baeten CGMI. Effects of dietary inulin supplementation on inflammation of pouch mucosa in patients with ileal pouch-anal anastomosis. *Dis Colon Rectum* 2002;45:621–7.

58 Gionchetti P, Rizzello F, Venturi A, et al. Oral bacteriotherapy as maintenance treatment in patients with chronic pouchitis: a double-blind, placebo-controlled trial. *Gastroenterology* 2000;119:305–9.

59 Gionchetti P, Rizzello F, Helwig U, et al. Prophylaxis of pouchitis onset with probiotic therapy: a double-blind, placebo-controlled trial. *Gastroenterology* 2003;124:1202–9.

60 Mimura T, Rizzello F, Helwig U, et al. Once daily high dose probiotic therapy (VSL#3) for maintaining remission in recurrent or refractory pouchitis. *Gut* 2004;53:108–14.

61 Rembacken BJ, Snelling AM, Hawkey PM, Chalmers DM, Axon ATM. Non-pathogenic *Escherichia coli* versus mesalazine for the treatment of ulcerative colitis: a randomised trial. *Lancet* 1999;354:635–9.

62 Kruis W, Fric P, Pokrotnieks J, et al. Maintaining remission of ulcerative colitis with the probiotic *Escherichia coli* Nissle 1917 is as effective as with standard mesalazine. *Gut* 2004;53:1617–23.

63 Fernandez-Bañares F, Hinojosa J, Sanchez-Lombraña JL, et al. Randomized Clinical trial of *Plantago Ovata* seeds (Dietary Fiber) as compared with Mesalamine in maintaining remission in ulcerative colitis. *Am J Gastroenterol* 1999;94:427–33.

64 Prantera C, Scribano ML, Falasco G, Andreoli A, Luzi C. Ineffectiveness of probiotics in preventing recurrence after curative resection for Crohn's disease: a randomised controlled trial with *Lactobacillus GG*. *Gut* 2002;51:405–9.

65 Rutgeers P, D'Haens G, Baert F, et al. Randomized placebo controlled trial of a pro- and prebiotics (synbiotics cocktail) in maintenance of infliximab induced remission of luminal Crohn's disease. *Gastroenterology* 2004;126(Suppl 2):A467.

66 Wilchanski M, Sherman P, Pencharz P, Davis L, Corey M, Griffiths A. Supplementary enteral nutrition maintains remission in paediatric Crohn's disease. *Gut* 1996;38:543–8.

67 Kang A, Zamora SA, Scott RB, Parsons HG. Catch-up growth in children treated with home enteral nutrition. *Pediatrics* 1998;102:951–5.

68 Kromann N, Green A. Epidemiological studies in the Upernavik district, Greenland. *Acta Med Scand* 1980;208:401–6.

69 Bang H, Dyerberg J, Hjorne N. The composition of foon consumen by Greenland Eskimos. *Acta Med Scand* 1976;200:69–73.

70 De Caterina R, Cybulsky MI, Clinton SK, Gimbrone M, Libby P. The Omega-3 fatty acid docosahexanoate reduces cytokine-induced expression of proatherogenic and proinflammatory proteins in human endothelial cells. *Arterioscler Thromb* 1994;14:1829–36.

71 Lee T, Hoover R, Williams J, et al. Effect of dietary enrichment with eicosapentaenoic and docosahexaenoic acids on *in vivo* neutrophil and monocyte leucotriene generation and neutrophil function. *N Engl J Med* 1985;312:1217–24.

72 Cybulsky M, Grimbone MJ. Endothelial expression of a mononuclear leukocyte adhesion

73 De Caterina R, Libby P. Control of endothelial leucocyte adhesion molecules by fatty avids. *Lipids* 1996;31(Suppl):S57–S63.

74 Yeh SL, Chang KY, Huang C, Chen WJ. Effect of n-3 and n-6 fatty acids on plasma eicosanoid and liver antioxidant enzymes in rats receiving total parenteral nutrition. *Nutrition* 1997;13:32–6.

75 Kinsella LE. Lipids, membrane receptors and enzymes: effects of dietary fatty acids. *JPEN* 1990;14:200S–17S.

76 Enders S. Messengers and mediators: interactions among lipids, eicosanoids and cytokines. *Am J Clin Nutr* 1993;57(Suppl):798S–800S.

77 Calder PC. N-3 polyunsaturated fatty acids and immune cell function. *Advan Enzyme Regul* 1997;37:197–237.

78 Katz DP, Schwartz S, Askanazi J. Biochemical and cellular basis for potential therapeutic value of n-3 fatty acids derived from fish oil. *Nutrition* 1993;9:113–18.

79 Lorenz R, Weber PC, Szimnau P, Heldwein W, Strasser T, Oeschke K. Supplementation with n-3 fatty acids from fish oil in chronic inflammatory bowel disease: a randomized, placebo-controlled, double-blind cross-over trial. *J Intern Med Suppl* 1998;225:225–32.

80 Salomon P, Kornbluth AA, Janowitz HD. Treatment of ulcerative colitis with fish oil n-e omega fatty acid: an open trial.

81 Aslan A. Fish oil fatty acid supplementation in ulcerative colitis: a souble blind, placebo-controlled, crossover study. *Am J Gastroenterol* 1992;87:432–7.

82 Hawthorne AB. Treatment of ulcerative colitis with fish oil supplementation: a prospective 12-month randomised controlled trial. *Gut* 1992;33:922–8.

83 Stenson WF. Dietary supplements with fish oil in ulcerative colitis. *Ann Intern Med* 1992;116:609–14.

84 Greenfield SM. A randomozed controlled study of evening primrose oil and fish oil in ulcerative colitis. *Aliment Pharmacol Ther* 1993;7:159–66.

85 Loesche K, Uberschaer B, Pietsch A, *et al*. n-3 Fatty acids only delay early relapse of ulcerative colitis in remission. *Dig Dis Sci* 1996;41:2087–94.

86 Lorenz-Meyer H. Bauer P, Nicolay C, *et al*. Omega-3 fatty acids and low carbohydrate diet for maintenance in remission in Crohn's disease: a randomized controlled multicenter clinical trial. *Scan J Gastroenterol* 1996;31:778–85.

87 Belluzzi A, Brignola C, Campieri M, Pera A, Boschi S, Miglioli M. Effect of an enteric-coated fish-oil preparation on relapses in Crohn's disease. *N Engl J Med* 1996;334:1557–60.

88 O'Morain C, Segal AW, Levi AJ. Elemental diet as primary treatment of acute Crohn's disease: a controlled study. *Br Med J* 1984;228:1859–62.

89 Teahon K, Smethurst P, Pearson M, *et al*. The effect of elemental diet on intestinal permeability and inflammation in Crohn's disease. *Gastroenterology* 1991;101:84–9.

90 Ferguson A, Glen M, Ghoshi S. Crohn's disease: nutrition and nutritional therapy. *Ballieres Clin Gastroenterol* 1998;12:93–114.

91 Teahon K, Bjarnason I, Pearson M, Levi AJ. Ten years' experience with an elemental diet in the management of Crohn's disease. *Gut* 1990;31:1133–7.

92 Matsui U, Ueki M, Yamada M, et al. Indications and options of nutritional treatment for Crohn's disease: a comparison of elemental and polymeric diets. *J Gastroenterol* 1995;30(Suppl 8):95–7.

93 Seidman E. Nutritional therapy for Crohn's disease: lessons from the Ste.-Justine hospital experience. *Inflamm Bowel Dis* 1997;3:49–53.

94 Royall D, Jeejeebhoy KN, Baker JP, *et al*. Comparison of aminoacid vs peptide based enterl diets in active Crohn's disease: clinical and nutritional outcome. *Gut* 1994;35:783–7.

95 Giaffer MH, North G, Holdsworth CD. Controlled trial of polymeric versus elemental diet in the treatment of active Crohn's disease. *Lancet* 1990;335:816–19.

96 Mansfield JC, Giaffer MH, Holdsworth CD. Controlled trial of oligopeptide versus aminoacid diet in the treatment of active Crohn's disease. *Gut* 1995;36:60–6.

97 Gorard DA, Hunt JR, Payne-James JJ, *et al*. Initial response and subsequent course of Crohn's disease treated with elemental diet and prednisolone. *Gut* 1993;14:1198–1202.

98 Raouf AH, Hildrey V, Daniel J, *et al*. Enteral feeding as sole treatment for Crohn's disease: contriolled trial of whole protein v amino acid based feed and a case study of dietary challenge. *Gut* 1991;32:702–7.

99 Rigaud D, Cosnes J, Le Quintrec Y, René E, Gendre JP, Mignon M. Controlled trial comparing two types of enteral nutrition in treatment of active Crohn's disease: elemental vs polymeric diet. *Gut* 1991;32:1492–7.

100 Okada M, Yao T, Takenaka K, Imamura K, Maeda K, Fujita K. Controlled trial comparing elemental diet with prednisolone in the treatment of active Crohn's disease. *Hepato-gastroenterol* 1990;37:72–80.

101 Alun Jones V. Compariison of total parenteral nutrition and elemental diet in induction of remission of Crohn's disease: long-term maintenance of remission by personalized food exclusion diets. *Dig Dis Sci* 1987;32:100S–7S.

102 Hiwatashi N. Enteral nutrition for Crohn's disease in Japan. *Dis Colon Rectum* 1997;40(Suppl): S48–S53.

103 Middleton SJ, Rucker JT, Kirby GA, Riordan AM, Hunter JO. Long-chain triglycerides reduce the efficacy of enteral feeds in patients with active Crohn's disease. Clin Nurtr 1995;14:229–36.

104 Verma S, Brwn MH, Giaffer MH. Elemental versus polymeric diet in treatment of active Crohn's disease: a double blind randomised trial. *Gut* 1997;41 (Suppl 3):P832.

105 Ueki M, Matsui Y, Yamada M, *et al*. *Jpn J Gastroenterol* 1994;91:1415–25.

106 Fakuda Y, Kosaka T, Okui M, Hirakawa H, Shimoyama T. Efficacy of nutritional therapy for active Crohn's disease. *J Gastroenterol* 1995; 30(Suppl 8):83–7.

107 Ruuska T, Savilahti E, Maki M, Örmälä T, Visakorpi JK. Exclusive whole protein diet versus prednisolone in the treatment of acute Crohn's disease in children. *J Pediatr Gastroenterol Nutr* 1994;19:175–80.

108 Greenberg GR, Fleming CR, Jeejeebhoy KN, *et al*. Controlled trial of bowel rest and nutritional support in the management of Crohn's disease. *Gut* 1988;29: 1309–15.

109 Bodemar G, Nilsson L, Smedh K, Larson J. Nasogastric feeding with polymeric, whole protein low fat diet in Crohn's disease. *J Clin Nutr Gastroenterol* 1991;6:75–83.

110 Coyle BL, Sladen GE. Whole protein diet in the treatment of acute uncomplicated Crohn's disease. *J Hum Nutr Dietetics* 1989;2:25–30.

111 Gonzalez-Huix, F, de Leon R, Fernandez-Banares F, *et al*. Polymeric enteral diets as primary treatment of active Crohn's disease; a prospective steroid controlled trial. *Gut* 1993;34:778–82.

112 Fernandez-Bañares F, Cabré E, Esteve-Comas M, Gassull MA. How effective is enteral nutrition in inducing remission in active Crohn's disease? A meta-analysis of the randomized clinical trials. *JPEN* 1995;19:356–64.

113 Fernandez-Bañares F, Cabré E, Gonzalez-Huix F, Gassull MA. Enteral nutrition as primary therapy in Crohn's disease. *Gut* 1994;(Suppl 1):S55–9.

114 Gassull MA, Fernández-Bañares F, Cabré E, *et al*. Fat composition may be a clue to explain the primary therapeutic effect of enteral nutrition in Crohn's disease: results of a double blind randomised multicentre European trial. *Gut* 2002;51:164–8.

115 Koga H, Iida M, Aoyagi K, Matsui T, Fujishima M. Long-term efficacy of low residue diet for the maintenance of remission in patients with Crohn's disease. *Nippon Shokakibyo Gakkai Zasshi* 1993;90:2882–1888.

116 Walker-Smith JA. Mucosal healing in Crohn's disease. *Gastroenterology* 1998;114:419–20.

16: Do antibiotics have a role in Crohn's disease?

Séverine Vermeire and Paul Rutgeerts

Introduction

Patients with IBD require extensive treatment as a result of the chronic relapsing nature of their disease. Medical management includes oral and topical 5-aminosalicylates, systemic corticosteroids, budesonide, immunosuppressive agents, biological therapies like monoclonal anti-TNFα antibodies (infliximab) as well as antibiotic treatment. Antibiotics have been used empirically by many physicians for several years in the treatment of Crohn's disease (CD), although no causative micro-organism has been identified for CD and there is a lack of controlled trials to validate this approach. It is surprising that most of the studies concerning microbiological factors in Crohn's disease date from some 20 years ago. Studies of the flora using new techniques such as PCR are scarce. One of the reasons why these drugs were used initially is that the clinical picture of Crohn's disease, certainly when of acute onset, very much resembles that of an acute infectious episode. Moreover, Crohn's disease in its chronic phase is characterised by histologic lesions very similar to those detected in intestinal tuberculosis. Mycobacteria (especially *Mycobacterium paratuberculosis*) remain one of the putative causal agents of Crohn's disease and antimycobacterial strategies have been used.

Why antibiotics act beneficially on the clinical course of Crohn's disease is unclear, although several theories have been proposed [1]. It is possible that bacterial antigenic triggers initiate a heightened immune response and lead to inflammation. Besides their antibacterial action, some antibiotics such as metronidazole or quinolones also have potential immunosuppressive properties [2]. Enteric bacteria play a role in the pathogenesis of certain complications of Crohn's disease, including abscesses and fistulae, and antibiotics are used in the treatment of perianal fistulae, entero-enteric and entero-cutaneous fistulae. Bacterial overgrowth caused by strictures and blind loops responds well to antibiotic therapy. Furthermore, the fact that Crohn's lesions are mainly located in segments of the bowel harbouring extremely high bacterial counts and where the transit is slow, e.g. proximal to valves, suggests that bacteria play an important role [3]. There is more clinical evidence that bacteria may play a primary role in the aetiopathogenesis of Crohn's disease. Diversion of the faecal stream by split ileostomy settles the activity of severe Crohn's colitis although the effect may not last [4]. Endoscopic studies after surgery have suggested that bacteria are important in recurrence: patients with a terminal ileostomy proximal to the ileo-colonic anastomosis did not experience recurrent disease until the ileostomy was closed. Infusion of ileal contents in this protected segment of the bowel immediately caused inflammatory lesions [5]. The prominence and virulence of *E. coli* strains associated with the ileal mucosa in recurrent Crohn's disease after ileal resection was studied by a French group. They recovered *E. coli* from 65% of chronic lesions (resected ileum) and from 100% of the biopsy specimens of early lesions (post-operative endoscopic recurrence). *E. Coli* strains associated with ileal mucosa of patients with Crohn's disease adhered preferentially to differentiated Caco-2 cells, corresponding to mature intestinal cells. In addition

21.8% of the strains induced a cytolytic effect by synthesis of a α-hemolysin. Therefore, the combination of adhesive ability and synthesis of a cytotoxin would allow the bacteria to colonise intestinal epithelium, to damage intestinal cells and to participate in the inflammatory progress [6]. In a subsequent recent study from the same group, the prevalence of these adherent-invasive *E. coli* (AIEC) in the intestinal mucosa of patients with CD, UC and in controls was studied in detail [7]. The presence of *E. coli* virulence genes was assessed by polymerase chain reaction and DNA hybridisation. AIEC strains were found specifically in ileal mucosa of CD (21.7% of CD chronic lesions versus 6.2% of controls). In colonic specimens, AIEC strains were found in 3.7% of CD patients, 0% of UC patients and 1.9% of controls.

Metronidazole

Metronidazole is an imidazole component with activity against protozoa and most gram-negative and gram-positive anaerobic bacteria. It is the most widely used antibiotic in the treatment of Crohn's disease, especially in perianal disease. Metronidazole has an activity against protozoa such as *Giardia lamblia, Entamoeba histolytica* and *Trichomonas vaginalis*, for which the drug was first approved as an effective treatment. Anaerobic gram-negative bacteria that are sensitive to the drug include bacteroides and *Fusobacterium* spp. gram-positive anaerobic bacteria include *peptostreptococci* and *Clostridium* spp. However, higher percentages of resistance are found compared to gram-negative anaerobic spp. Metronidazole might also suppress cellular immunity [2]. Its effectiveness has first been reported in perianal disease [8] and the drug seems most effective in perianal complications of Crohn's disease, but no controlled trials are available to support this hypothesis. However, several uncontrolled trials and also clinical experience suggest efficacy for this indication [9–12]. Metronidazole is started at a dose of 20 mg/kg and usually the dose is reduced to 10 mg/kg when improvement or remission is achieved. A small study showed no advantage of adding metronidazole to sulphasalazine or steroids for the treatment of Crohn's disease [10].

Bernstein and colleagues reported complete healing in 10 of 18 patients with unremitting perianal Crohn's disease treated with metronidazole [11]. In a follow-up study, all patients had recurrence of their symptoms when the drug was discontinued, but promptly responded to reinstitution of full-dose therapy [12].

Two large trials have compared metronidazole to sulphasalazine and to placebo in small bowel and colonic CD. In a well-designed study in Sweden [13, 14], metronidazole 800 mg/day was compared with 3 g of sulphasalazine per day for active Crohn's disease. In this study lasting for 4 months, both drugs were equally effective. Only 25% of the metronidazole-treated patients entered remission, compared with 39% in the sulphasalazine group. Another 27.5% showed CDAI improvement after 4 months of therapy. A negative point of this study, however, is that no placebo group was included. A North American study randomised 105 patients to treatment with placebo or metronidazole, either 10 or 20 mg/kg/day for 4 months. Bearing in mind that only 56 patients (53%) completed the planned 16 weeks of follow-up, no difference was seen in achieving remission between the groups. However, a significantly higher decrease in inflammatory markers in serum and in CDAI score was observed in the metronidazole group (improvement of 97 points for metronidazole 20 mg/kg, 67 points for metronidazole 10 mg/kg, worsening of 1 point for placebo, $p = 0.002$). However, metronidazole was not effective in disease limited to the small bowel [15].

The efficacy of metronidazole in preventing recurrence after surgery was assessed in 60 patients receiving either metronidazole (20 mg/kg/day started within 7 days after ileocolonic resection) for 3 months or placebo. Endoscopic activity at the end of 3 months was investigated [16]. Although there was no difference in the overall endoscopic recurrence rate, severe lesions were found more frequently in the placebo group (43%) than in the metronidazole group (13%, $p = 0.02$). Symptomatic recurrence also seemed to be delayed by this therapy. In a recent study, the efficacy of ornidazole for the prevention of clinical recurrence of Crohn's disease after curative ileocolonic resection was assessed [17]. Ornidazole is thought to be associated with fewer side effects than metronidazole. Eighty patients were randomised to ornidazole 1 g/day or placebo started within 1 week of resection and continued for 1 year. The primary end-point was the proportion of patients with clinical recurrence at 1 year. Ornidazole significantly reduced the recurrence rate at 1 year from 15/40 (37.5%) in the placebo group to 3/38 patients (7.9%) in the ornidazole group ($p = 0.0046$; OR 0.14; 95% CI 0.037–0.546). Ornidazole also reduced endoscopic recurrence (secondary end-point) at 12 months from 26/33 (79.1%) in the placebo group to 15/28 (53.6%) in the ornidazole group ($p = 0.037$; OR 0.31; 95% CI 0.10–0.94). However, more patients discontinued therapy because of side effects in the ornidazole group ($n = 12$) than in the placebo group ($n = 5$) and also significantly more side effects occurred in the ornidazole group ($n = 26$) than in the placebo group ($n = 12$).

Side effects

Metronidazole is generally well tolerated but side effects occur in 1–20% of patients and include most often nausea, gastrointestinal intolerance, neurotoxicity and a metallic taste. Long-term treatment can give rise to peripheral neuropathy and is characterised by paresthesiae in the extremities [18]. The highest incidence of side effects is reported in patients treated for perianal disease, which normally requires very long treatment. In this sub-group up to 50–85% of patients reported intolerance. The adverse effects are reversible with discontinuation of the drug, although the neuropathy can occasionally last long after metronidazole is stopped.

Pregnancy

In humans, the antibiotic seems to be safe, although some mutations and teratogenicity are reported in animal studies. Available evidence suggests that the drug does not adversely affect foetal outcome. In a retrospective study comparing 1387 women who received metronidazole during pregnancy to the same number of controls, no differences in pregnancy outcome or birth defect occurrences were seen [19]. There is also no evidence that metronidazole is unsafe during breastfeeding. Although low levels of the drug are found in breast milk, these are less than the usual paediatric dosages and are very unlikely to have harmful effects. However, caution is required.

Ciprofloxacin

Ciprofloxacin is a quinolone derivative with a selective action against *E. coli* and aerobic *enterobacteriaceae*, and hence a selective suppressive agent for the intestinal microflora. Bacteroides and *Clostridium* spp. are not affected by this drug. Interestingly, ciprofloxacin has a very high concentration in faeces. Anecdotal reports on the benefit of this antibiotic in Crohn's disease were first reported in 1990 [20]. Ciprofloxacin has been used for both perianal disease and ileitis. In a number of open studies ciprofloxacin either alone or in combination with metronidazole was effective on symptoms [20], for controlling active disease [21] and for treating fistulae and abscesses [22].

A randomised controlled study from the French GETAID group investigated the efficacy of ciprofloxacin compared with mesalazine in treating active Crohn's disease [23]. Patients with a mild to moderate flare-up of Crohn's disease were randomised to receive ciprofloxacin 1 g/day or mesalazine 4 g/day for 6 weeks. Complete remission was observed in 10/18 patients (56%) treated with ciprofloxacin and 12/22 patients (55%) treated with mesalazine, the authors concluded that ciprofloxacin 1 g/day is as effective as mesalazine 4 g/day in treating mild to moderate relapses of Crohn's disease. The study was limited by the lack of a placebo control group since the efficacy of mesalazine in Crohn's disease is not well established.

A combination of metronidazole and ciprofloxacin has shown to be effective in the treatment of acute Crohn's disease as an alternative to steroids. Prantera *et al.* randomised 41 refractory or steroid-dependent Crohn's disease patients to either a combination of 1000 mg of ciprofloxacin and 1000 mg of metronidazole or methylprednisolone 0.70–1 mg/kg for 12 weeks [24]. Forty-five per cent (10/22) of patients achieved remission with antibiotic treatment versus 63% (12/19) with methylprednisolone. The best results occurred after

6 weeks of treatment. However, there were more side effects in the antibiotic arm and 6 patients withdrew because of side-effects in comparison with only 2 on steroids.

A double-blind multi-centre study of patients with active Crohn's disease randomised patients to ciprofloxacin and metronidazole, both 500 mg twice daily, or placebo for 8 weeks [25]. All patients received oral budesonide 9 mg once daily. Of the 130 patients who were randomised, 66 received placebo and 64 received antibiotics. At week 8, 33% of patients taking antibiotics were in remission as compared with 38% in the placebo group (not significant). The authors concluded that the addition of ciprofloxacin and metronidazole to budesonide is an ineffective intervention. Finally, a prospective study by Dejaco et al. [26] investigated the use of antibiotics as a bridging therapy. In this study, 52 patients were given an 8-week regimen of ciprofloxacin (500–1000 mg/day) and/or metronidazole (1000–1500 mg/day) and were started on azathioprine after 8 weeks of antibiotic treatment. Overall, 26 patients (50%) responded to antibiotic treatment, with complete healing in 25% of patients at week 8. The authors concluded that antibiotics are useful to induce a short-term response in perianal Crohn's disease, and may provide a bridging strategy to azathioprine, which seems to be essential for the maintenance of fistula improvement.

Side effects

Side effects are reported between 15 and 30% of patients. The severity of side effects depends on the dose and the duration of treatment. The most reported symptoms include gastrointestinal complaints. Skin eruptions, an increase in transaminase levels and even transient ischemic attacks have been described.

Broad spectrum antibiotics

In a study performed by Moss and co-workers, 44 patients were treated for at least 6 months with broad-spectrum antibiotics in combination with glucocorticosteroids or sulphasalazine. They reported improvement of X-ray abnormalities in 57% of patients [27]. Anecdotal reports also suggest benefit from treatment with trimethoprim-sulphamethoxazole in the treatment of Crohn's disease [28, 29].

Clarithromycin is a broad-spectrum macrolide antibiotic with a good tissue penetration. In an open-label study by Leiper et al., 25 patients with active CD were treated with oral clarithromycin 250 mg b.d. for 4 weeks, and continued to 12 weeks in patients who had shown a partial or complete response [30]. Twelve patients (48%) achieved remission (defined as a Harvey-Bradshaw index ≤ 4) at week 4, and 8 patients remained in remission on treatment at week 12. However, when the treatment with clarithromycin was stopped, 5 patients relapsed after a median of 5 months (range 4–9). Randomised controlled trials are needed before definitive conclusions can be made.

Antimycobacterial agents

Mycobacterium paratuberculosis has been identified in tissues from a higher proportion of Crohn's disease patients than controls, suggesting that it may be one of the causes of Crohn's disease. The possible involvement of *M. paratuberculosis* in Crohn's disease has led several investigators to use antimycobacterial therapy. However, several placebo-controlled trials have failed to show consistent benefit of combination approaches. Six placebo-controlled trials using antimycobacterial therapy have been carried out in Crohn's disease [31–36]. These are summarised in Table 16.1. Treatment ranged from 6 to 24 months, but significantly higher remission rates were not obtained at the end of the study in the treated patients compared to the placebo group, although trends were detected. In the trials where this was investigated, no healing of Crohn's lesions in the bowel was observed. A meta-analysis on the effect of antimycobacterial therapy in Crohn's disease concluded that this therapy was only effective in maintaining remission in patients who had had a course of corticosteroids combined with antimycobacterial therapy to induce remission. Treatment of Crohn's disease with antimycobacterial therapy does not seem to be effective without a course of corticosteroids to induce remission [37].

Table 16.1 Placebo-controlled trials of anti-mycobacterial therapy in Crohn's disease.

	Drug(s)	Number	Duration (months)	Remission
Elliot et al. Digestion 1982	Sulphadoxine + Pyrimethamin	51	12	33% vs 41.6%
Shaffer et al. Gut 1984	Rifampicin + Ethambutol	27	12	13 withdrawals
Basilisco et al. Curr Ther Res 1989	Rifabutin	24	6	42% vs 50%
Afdhal et al. Dig Dis Sci 1991	Clofazimine	49	12	48% vs 25%
Swift et al. Gut 1994	Rifampicin + Ethambutol + Isoniazide	126	24	NS
Prantera et al. Am J Ge 1994	E + C + D + R*	40	9	50% vs 22.2% no healing

*E = Ethambutol, C = Clofazimine, D = Dapsone, R = Rifampicine.

Two open trials also were negative. Quadruple antimycobacterial therapy for 9 months in 20 patients resulted in remission in 50% of patients [38]. Our centre studied 10 patients and specifically addressed tissue healing in Crohn's patients treated with rifabutin-ethambutol. None of the 10 patients treated for 6 months and none of five patients treated for 12 months showed clinical remission, and with repeated ileocolonoscopies no improvement or healing was observed in the neoterminal ileum [39]. A preliminary report on remission obtained with 3 months of either clarithromycin or placebo made the authors suggest that the beneficial effect might be due to the efficacy against *M. paratuberculosis* [40].

The combination of rifabutin with a macrolide antibiotic (clarithromycin or azithromycin) has been investigated in three open-label studies. The first by Gui et al. treated 52 patients with severe Crohn's disease with the combination of rifabutin and clarithromycin or azithromycin [41]. Six (11.5%) were intolerant of the medication and had to be excluded from the study. Patients were treated for a mean of 18.7 (range 6–35) months and followed up for 25.1 (range 7–41) months. Of the 19 patients who were steroid-dependent at the start of the study, only 2 continued to require steroids after the study. A reduction in the Harvey-Bradshaw Crohn's disease activity index occurred after 6 months of treatment ($p = 0.004$, paired Wilcoxon test) and was maintained at 24 months ($p < 0.001$). Inflammatory parameters, as measured by erythrocyte sedimentation rate and C-reactive protein, improved at 18 months ($p = 0.009$ and $p = 0.03$ respectively) compared with pre-treatment levels. There was also an increase in serum albumin levels at 12 months ($p = 0.04$). Patients with pan-intestinal disease responded better as a subgroup at 2 years compared with patients with less-extensive involvement ($p = 0.04$, Mann-Whitney). There was no difference in response to treatment with age, duration of disease, the presence of granulomas on histology or the occurrence of drug-induced side-effects. The results of this study suggest that combination therapy with rifabutin and macrolide antibiotics may improve the clinical course of Crohn's disease.

Shafran et al. treated 36 active CD patients, whose sera tested positive against p35 and p36 antigens (two recombinant proteins of *Mycobacterium avium* subsp. *paratuberculosis*), with rifabutin (150 mg b.i.d) and clarithromycin (250 mg b.i.d) and response was monitored over a period ranging from 4 to 17 months [42]. Seven patients (19.4%) withdrew from the study because of intolerance. Of the remaining 29 patients, 21 (58.3%) responded (defined as a 70 points decrease in the CDAI). Three patients (8.3%) noticed significant improvement, but required additional Crohn's medication to achieve and sustain improvement. Only 5 patients (13.8%) were non-responders. Finally, in the study by Borody and co-workers 12 patients with severe, obstructive or penetrating Crohn's disease failing maximal therapy were started on a combination of rifabutin (450 mg/day), clarithromycin (750 mg/day) and clofazimine (2 mg/kg/day) [43]. Six patients (50%) achieved complete clinical, colonoscopic and histologic remission of Crohn's disease. Four of these patients were able to cease treatment after 24–46 months, 3 of whom remained in total remission without treatment for up to 26 months and one patient relapsed after 6 months off treatment. A partial response was seen in 2 patients showing complete clinical remission with mild histologic inflammation.

Conclusion

The role of antibiotics in the treatment of Crohn's disease is not yet well defined. Clinicians sometimes have the impression that treatment with glucocorticosteroids makes patients more treatment-resistant and often treat their patients with first-line antibiotics. Antibiotics work in perianal disease although controlled trials are lacking. For active disease, a 40% remission rate is seen and is comparable with the efficacy of sulphasalazine or 5-ASA; however, more side effects are reported.

Only metronidazole for the treatment of Crohn's disease has been adequately studied in controlled trials but other antibiotic studies are pending. However, many more good clinical trials are needed, including the comparison of glucocorticosteroids and antibiotics for long-term. Also, placebo-controlled trials of metronidazole in perianal Crohn's disease are needed. The promising results with clarithromycin need confirmation. Whether antibiotics to prevent post-operative recurrence of Crohn's disease should be used requires further study. Long-term follow-up studies (1–2 years) are also needed.

References

1. Peppercorn MA. Is there a role for antibiotics as primary therapy in Crohn's ileitis? *J Clin Gastroenterol* 1993;17(3):235–7.
2. Miller JJ. The imidazoles as immunosuppressive agents. *Transplant Proc* 1980;12:300–3.
3. Rutgeerts P, Ghoos Y, Van Trappen G, et al. Ileal dysfunction and bacterial overgrowth in patients with Crohn's disease. *Eur J Clin Invest* 1981;11:199–206.
4. Harper PH, Truelove SC, Lee ECG, et al. Split ileostomy and ileocolostomy for Crohn's disease of the colon and ulcerative colitis: a 20-year survey. *Gut* 1983;24:106–13.
5. Rutgeerts P, Geboes K, Peeters M, et al. Effect of faecal stream diversion on recurrence of Crohn's disease in the neoterminal ileum. *Lancet* 1991;338:771–4.
6. Darfeuille-Michaud A, Neut C, Barnich N, et al. Presence of adherent *Escherichia coli* strains in ileal mucosa of patients with Crohn's disease. *Gastroenterol* 1998;115:1405–13.
7. Darfeuille-Michaud A, Boudeau J, Bulois P, et al. High prevalence of adherent-invasive *Escherichia coli* associated with ileal mucosa in Crohn's disease. *Gastroenterology* 2004;127:412–21.
8. Ursing B, Kamme C. Metronidazole for Crohn's disease. *Lancet* 1975;1:755–7.
9. Jakobovitis J, Shuster M. Metronidazole therapy for Crohn's disease and associated fistulae. *Am J Gastroenterol* 1984;79:533–40.
10. Blichfeldt P, Blomhoff JP, Myhre E, et al. Metronidazole in Crohn's disease: a double-blind cross-over clinical trial. *Scand J Gastroenterol* 1978;13:123–7.
11. Bernstein LH, Frank MS, Brandt LJ, et al. Healing of perineal Crohn's disease with metronidazole. *Gastroenterol* 1980;79:357–65.
12. Brandt LJ, Bernstein LH, Boley SJ, et al. Metronidazole therapy for perianal Crohn's disease: a follow-up study. *Gastroenterol* 1982;83:383–7.
13. Rosen A, Ursing B, Alm T, et al. A comparative study of metronidazole and sulfasalazine for active Crohn's disease: the cooperative Crohn's disease study in Sweden: I. Design and methodological considerations. *Gastroenterol* 1982;83:541–9.
14. Ursing B, Alm T, Barany F, et al. A comparative study of metronidazole and sulfasalazine for active Crohn's disease: the cooperative Crohn's disease study in Sweden: II. Result. *Gastroenterol* 1982;83:550–62.
15. Sutherland L, Singleton J, Sessions J, et al. Double blind, placebo controlled trial of metronidazole in Crohn's disease. *Gut* 1991;32:1071–5.
16. Rutgeerts P, Hiele M, Geboes K, et al. Controlled trial of metronidazole treatment for prevention of Crohn's recurrence after ileal resection. *Gastroenterol* 1995;108:1617–21.
17. Rutgeerts P, Van Assche G, D'Haens G, et al. Ornidazol for prophylaxis of postoperative Crohn's disease: final results of a double blind placebo-controlled trial. *Gastroenterology* 2005;128:256–61.
18. Duffy LF, Daum F, Fisher SE, et al. Peripheral neuropathy in Crohn's disease patients treated with metronidazole. *Gastroenterol* 1985;88:681–4.

19 Piper JM, Mitchel EF, Ray WA. Prenatal use of metronidazole and birth defects: no association. *Obstet Gynaecol* 1993;82:348–52.
20 Wolf JL. Ciprofloxacin may be useful in Crohn's disease. *Gastroenterol* 1990;98:A212.
21 Greenbloom SL, Steinhart AH, Greenberg GR. Combination ciprofloxacin and metronidazole for active Crohn's disease. *Can J Gastroenterol* 1998;12: 53–6.
22 Turunen U, Färkkilä V, Valtonen V, *et al*. Long-term outcome of ciprofloxacin treatment in severe perianal or fistulous Crohn's disease. *Gastroenterol* 1993;104:A793.
23 Colombel JF, Lemann M, Cassagnou M, *et al*. A controlled trial comparing ciprofloxacin with mesalazine for the treatment of active Crohn's disease. Groupe d'Etudes Therapeutiques des Affections Inflammatoires Digestives (GETAID). *Am J Gastroenterol* 1999;94:674–8.
24 Prantera C, Zannoni F, Scribano ML, *et al*. An antibiotic regimen for the treatment of active Crohn's disease: a randomized, controlled trial of metronidazole plus ciprofloxacin. *Am J Gastroenterol* 1996;91:328–32.
25 Steinhart AH, Feagan BG, Wong CJ, *et al*. Combined budesonide and antibiotic therapy for active Crohn's disease: a randomized controlled trial. *Gastroenterology* 2002;123:33–40.
26 Dejaco C, Harrer M, Waldhoer T, *et al*. Antibiotics and azathioprine for the treatment of perianal fistulas in Crohn's disease. *Aliment Pharmacol Ther* 2003;18: 1113–20.
27 Moss AA, Carbone JV, Kressel HY. Radiologic and clinical assessment of broad-spectrum antibiotic therapy in Crohn's disease. *Am J Roentgenol* 1978;131:787–90.
28 Danzi JT. Trimethoprim-sulphamethoxazole therapy of inflammatory bowel disease. *Gastroenterol* 1989; 96:A110.
29 Gradon JD, Zimbalist EH. Is trimethoprim-sulfamethoxazole helpful in Crohn's disease? *J Clin Gastroenterol* 1990;12:598–607.
30 Leiper K, Morris AI, Rhodes JM. Open label trial of oral clarithromycin in active Crohn's disease. *Aliment Pharmacol Ther* 2000;14:801–6.
31 Swift GL, Srivastava ED, Stone R, *et al*. Controlled trial of antituberculous chemotherapy for two years in Crohn's disease. *Gut* 1994;35: 363–8.
32 Prantera C, Kohn A, Mangiarotti R, *et al*. Antimycobacterial therapy in Crohn's disease: results of a controlled, double blind trial with a multiple antibiotic regimen. *Am J Gastroenterol* 1994;5: 513–8.
33 Elliot PR, Burnham WR, Berghouse LM, *et al*. Sulphadoxine-pyrimethamine therapy in Crohn's disease. *Digestion* 1982;23:132–4.
34 Shaffer JL, Hughes S, Linaker BD, *et al*. Controlled trial of rifampicin and ethambutol in Crohn's disease. *Gut* 1984;25:203–5.
35 Afdhal NH, Long A, Lennon J, *et al*. Controlled trial of antimycobacterial therapy in Crohn's disease. Clofazimine versus placebo. *Dig Dis Sci* 1991;36:449–53.
36 Basilisco G, Ranzi T, Campanini C, *et al*. Controlled trial of rifabutin in Crohn's disease. *Curr ther Res* 1989;46:242–50.
37 Borgaonkar MR, MacIntosh GD, Fardy JM. A meta-analysis of antimycobacterial therapy for Crohn's disease. *Am J Gastroenterol* 2000;95: 725–9.
38 Hampson SJ, Parker MC, Saverymuttu SH, *et al*. Quadruple antimycobacterial chemotherapy in Crohn's disease: results at 9 months of a pilot study in 20 patients. *Aliment Pharmacol Ther* 1989;3:343–52.
39 Rutgeerts P, Geboes K, Vantrappen G, *et al*. Rifabutin and ethambutol do not help recurrent Crohn's disease in the neoterminal ileum. *J Clin gastroenterol* 1992;15:24–8.
40 Graham DY, Al-Assi MT, Robinson M. Prolonged remission in Crohn's disease following therapy for *Mycobacterium paratuberculosis*. *Gastroenterol* 1995;108(A):826.
41 Gui GP, Thoms PR, Tizard ML, *et al*. Two-year outcomes analysis of Crohn's disease treated with rifabutin and macrolide antibiotics. *J Antimicrob Chemother* 1997;39:393–400.
42 Shafran I, Kugler L, El-Zaatari FA, *et al*. Open clinical trial of rifabutin and clarithromycin therapy in Crohn's disease. *Dig Liver Dis* 2002;34:22–8.
43 Borody TJ, Leis S, Warren EF, *et al*. Treatment of severe Crohn's disease using antimycobacterial triple therapy – approaching a cure? *Dig Liver Dis* 2002; 34:29–38.

17: The optimal use of infliximab in Crohn's disease
Geert D'Haens

Introduction

In recent years, a great deal of insight into the pathophysiology of Crohn's disease has been established. The pro-inflammatory cytokine TNF was shown to play a pivotal part in the orchestration and amplification of the inflammatory process and therefore received a lot of attention as a potential target for therapeutic intervention. Preliminary trials with the chimeric antibody infliximab, directed against TNF, immediately revealed the extreme potency of this novel agent. Further controlled and uncontrolled trials have confirmed the strong anti-inflammatory effects of infliximab and led to its rapid appearance on the international market. Whereas the mechanism of action of infliximab was originally believed to be the binding of biologically active TNF freely present in the lamina propria and expressed on inflammatory cells, it soon became clear that this binding phenomenon had to be followed by complement binding and activation, leading to apoptosis of the activated inflammatory TNF-bearing cells. This mechanism of action was elegantly demonstrated in a recent experiment by van den Brande *et al.* explaining the difference between infliximab and the recombinant p75 TNF receptor etanercept [1]. Whereas infliximab induced apoptosis of inflammatory cells, etanercept only bound to TNF without affecting the cells themselves. Besides infliximab, several other strategies that interfere with the biologic effects of TNF have been developed, such as recombinant soluble receptors targeting TNF and other (more humanised) antibodies inactivating TNF. These agents will not be discussed in this chapter.

Use of infliximab for active refractory Crohn's disease

Initially, infliximab was given as a single infusion at 5 mg/kg body weight for active luminal Crohn's disease. More than 80% of the patients who were enrolled in the initial trials had a response to this treatment (defined as a drop in the clinical score CDAI of more than 70 points) [2]. Endoscopic substudies revealed a remarkable degree of rapid mucosal healing and disappearance of inflammatory cells in biopsies collected from all segments of the colon and the terminal ileum [3, 4]. This initial response was observed in all patient subgroups to the same degree: whether patients were taking and failing immunosupressives, corticosteroids or aminosalicylates, whether they had undergone prior surgical resection and regardless of the location and type of Crohn's disease, all improved to the same degree [2]. *Post hoc* analysis of larger patient cohorts suggested a greater clinical improvement in patients with higher serum CRP levels, in patients with colonic disease and in patients using immunomodulatory drugs such as azathioprine, 6-mercaptopurine and methotrexate [5, 6]. It soon became clear, however, that the clinical benefit of infliximab treatment slowly disappeared 8–16 weeks following the first infusion, an observation that prompted further treatment with regular 'repeated' infliximab infusions as maintenance therapy [7]. The large ACCENT-1 trial randomised more than 500 patients who had an initial clinical response to a single 5 mg/infusion to: (1) further induction treatment with two additional 5 mg/kg infusions at week

2 and 6 followed by subsequent 8-weekly infusions of either 5 or 10 mg/kg or (2) subsequent placebo infusions at week 2 and 6 and further on every 8 weeks. Patients losing their initial response were given the option to 'step-up' to a higher dose level or to switch from placebo to active treatment. Clinical response improved from week 2 to week 10 in the 3-dose induction group (from 58 to 69%) compared to practically no improvement in the placebo group. Among patients who had an initial response but lost this response and crossed over to a higher dose, 90% regained a response when crossed over from 5 to 10 mg/kg and 80% when crossed over from 10 to 15 mg/kg. Fifty-three per cent of the patients receiving 10 mg/kg of infliximab as maintenance treatment still had a clinical response at the end of the year, versus 43% with 5 mg/kg and 17% with placebo, although many patients in the placebo group had received active medication on relapse during the trial. Virtually all corticosteroid-dependent patients could taper and discontinue their steroids completely after a mean period of 22 weeks. More than half of the patients treated with 10 mg/kg maintenance infusions every 8 weeks were found to have complete healing of the ulcerative lesions, significantly more than in the placebo group (only 1/17) [8]. Adverse events were relatively mild and uncommon: serious infections occurred in 3.8% (one case of tuberculosis), delayed hypersensitivity in 2.4%, acute infusion reactions in 1%. Although this trial could not really demonstrate the superiority of the three-dose induction regimen, it clearly showed the benefit of regular maintenance therapy in terms of clinical remission, improved quality of life, better endoscopic healing and fewer hospitalisations and need for surgical interventions [9].

While the ACCENT-1 trial was running, a rather large patient cohort was treated on an 'on-demand' base in a Belgian compassionate-use programme. Many of these patients developed infusion reactions during or after repeated administration and experienced a gradual loss of response to the treatment. The explanation of this phenomenon was found in the appearance of antibodies to infliximab (ATIs) in the majority of patients treated in this programme. The level of antibodies correlated with the risk of allergic reactions and loss of response.

Patients who were concomitantly using immunomodulatory medication generally had lower antibody titres [10].

Given the important consequences of loss of response to the patients' general well being and further therapeutic options, several strategies were examined in order to avoid this problem. Besides immunomodulation (which should be used in virtually all patients receiving infliximab) and 'automatic' retreatment (on an average every 8 weeks), pre-treatment with corticosteroids such as hydrocortisone has been shown to be effective. In an elegant trial by Farrell and colleagues, it was clearly demonstrated that antibody formation and allergic reactions were significantly reduced if patients received 200 mg of hydrocortisone IV prior to infliximab therapy [11]. Undoubtedly, further 'humanisation' of the anti-TNF antibody will further reduce the risk of antibodies and allergies.

Use of infliximab for fistulising Crohn's disease

For fistulising disease, a series of three infusions (week 0, 2 and 6) has been the recommended dose for induction of response, resulting in 'closure' of all fistulas (defined as discontinuation of purulent discharge) in 46% of patients, with a maximum effect at week 6 (52% of the patients). The onset of response was rapid, but the duration of this effect was in most cases limited to only 3 or 4 months [12]. Experience outside clinical trials confirmed this rather short-term effectiveness. For this reason, the initial trials were followed by a large maintenance trial for fistulising Crohn's disease, named 'ACCENT-2' [13]. Three hundred and six patients with actively draining enterocutaneous fistulas were treated with three induction infusions. Sixty-nine of them responded and were treated further with 5 mg/kg maintenance infusions or placebo every 8 weeks. Patients who lost response (defined as discontinuation of fistula drainage in more than 50% of fistulae) were switched from placebo to active treatment at 5 mg/kg or from 5 to 10 mg/kg. At the end of the trial (week 54), 46% of the patients on active retreatment had a fistula response versus 23% of those on placebo ($p = 0.001$). Complete response (all fistulae closed) was observed in 36% of patients on active treatment versus in 19% on placebo ($p = 0.009$). The most common adverse event was fistula-related abscess formation, observed in 13 patients on infliximab maintenance and in 19 patients on placebo.

In the absence of studies validating their use as surrogate markers for perianal fistulising disease, a number of studies looked at fistula healing using endosonography and magnetic resonance imaging. These studies revealed that the majority of fistulas had not completely disappeared after three infusions and that further treatments led to improved fistula outcome [14, 15].

Infliximab alone and infliximab as an adjunct to examination under anaesthesia and seton placement was compared in a group of 32 consecutive patients with fistulising Crohn's disease. The group with combined approach achieved a better initial response (100% vs 82.6%, $p = 0.014$), had lower recurrence rates (44% vs 79%, $p = 0.001$) and longer time to recurrence (13.5 months vs 3.6 months, $p = 0.0001$) compared with patients receiving infliximab alone [16]. It is clear that perianal and pelvic sepsis needs to be looked for and appropriately drained before infliximab therapy is initiated. Removal of seton drains can be considered when drainage has ceased completely, in the majority of cases after two to four infusions.

How safe is infliximab?

Several serious health problems with the use of infliximab have become apparent during the first years of its development, among which the reactivation of tuberculosis, the occurrence of immediate and late allergic reactions and the aggravation of congestive heart failure and demyelinating disorders have been the most significant ones. Reactivation of latent tuberculosis has even led to a few fatalities in the first years of anti-TNF therapies [17]. The human immune system indeed appears to need TNF to kill intra-cellular pathogens such as *mycobacterium tuberculosis*. Of all documented TB cases, 75% were diagnosed within the first three infusions and 97% within the first six infusions. It has since been recognised that this problem may occur with all types of anti-TNF treatment and that the problem can largely be prevented with strict measures: taking a history for prior tuberculosis exposure and using PPD skin tests and systematic chest X-rays have been standard recommendations that were added to the drug label and have reduced the incidence of TB reactivation to practically zero. Patients with signs of TB exposure can still be treated with infliximab, but need to receive prophylactic treatment with isoniazide (and pyridoxine) for 6–12 months.

Acute infusion reactions occur during or shortly after infusion and typically consist of fever, chills, nausea, dyspnoea and headaches. Delayed reactions, characterised by myalgias, arthralgias, fever, rash, pruritus, facial, hand or lip oedema, dysphagia, urticaria, sore throat and headache may occur 3–12 days after infusion. Although the mechanisms of these reactions are not yet clearly defined, emerging evidence indicates that these reactions may be associated with the immune response against infliximab and the development of antibodies to infliximab (ATIs). In a cohort study where patients were retreated on an 'on demand' basis, occurrence of these antibodies were measured in 61% of the patients after a mean of 3.9 infusions. The presence of ATI at concentrations more than or 8.0 μg/mL prior to an infusion was predictive of a shorter duration of response (35 days vs 71 days, $p < 0.001$) and carried a higher risk of infusion reactions (RR 2.40, $p < 0.001$). Concomitant immunosuppressive therapy suppressed the formation of ATI with 24/56 (43%) patients receiving immunosuppressives developing ATI as compared to 52/69 (75%) patients without immunosuppressives. This resulted in higher serum infliximab concentrations in the immunosuppressive group 4 weeks after the infusion ($p < 0.001$) [10].

Other factors that may be protective by helping to establish immune tolerance for the foreign infliximab protein include administration of corticosteroids, starting infliximab therapy with a 0, 2 and 6-week induction regimen, 'automatic' maintenance dose administration with infusions every 8 weeks or less, and avoiding long periods between infusions [18]. Treatment with 200 mg hydrocortisone prior to the infusion diminished the formation of ATI from 42 to 26% of patients, accompanied by a decrease in infusion reactions from 24 to 15%.

In this study, ATI positivity was associated with lower remission rates (0% vs 70%), lower clinical response rates (48% vs 86 %) higher rate of infusion reactions (40% vs 4.7%) and occurrence of severe infusion reactions (28% vs 0%) [11]. All together, it seems to be of paramount importance to prevent antibody formation with all possible means in order not to jeopardise future treatment in patients who are often refractory to other treatments.

Another safety problem is the deterioration of congestive heart failure. Initially, it was believed that infliximab could actually be used to treat heart failure, but the therapeutic trial investigating this problem had to be discontinued due to increased mortality in patients receiving infliximab. For this reason, infliximab should not be given to patients with congestive heart failure with NYHA classification 3 or 4.

Demyelinating neurological diseases such as multiple sclerosis have been reported to deteriorate with infliximab therapy. Only a few cases have been published, but extreme caution is warranted given the severity of this potential side effect.

Given the widespread use of infliximab worldwide, more attention is now being given to long-term toxicity. The TREAT registry included 5807 patients with Crohn's disease (2850 treated with infliximab and 2957 controls) at academic and community practices in the United States and was established to study long-term safety issues. For a mean follow up of 0.9 years no differences in mortality and cancer were observed. Tuberculosis and congestive heart failure after infliximab were not reported. Infusion reactions occurred in 5.4%, severe reactions in 0.16%. The incidence of serious infections was 1.27 per 100 patient-years within 3 months of an infliximab infusion compared to 0.85 per 100 patient years in controls. Multiple regression analysis showed that the severe infections were more associated with prednisone than with infliximab (RR = 2.32). In 66 reported pregnancies no differences in miscarriage rates and neonatal complications were reported. The study's preliminary conclusion stated that the safety of infliximab is similar to that of other Crohn's disease treatments [19].

Another cohort of 500 patients was studied at the Mayo clinic, with a median follow-up of 17 months [20]. Forty-three patients (8.6%) experienced at least one serious adverse event, 30 of which (6%) were considered at least possibly related to infliximab. Fifteen patients (3%) had serious infections (4 with fatal outcome), 2 (0.4%) had serious infusion reactions, 5 (1%) serum sickness-like disease, 3 (0.6%) drug-induced lupus, 2 (0.4%) cancers (1 fatal), 1 (0.2%) non-Hodgkin's lymphoma, 1 (0.2%) demyelination and 1 (0.2%) worsening of heart failure. The majority of infusion reactions occurred after the second infusion. Five deaths with potential association to infliximab were observed, corresponding to a mortality rate of 1%.

Further perspectives with infliximab

The following pertinent questions with regard to the use of infliximab in daily practice are emerging:
1 Should infliximab be used as a first-line agent in patients with newly diagnosed, extensive and severe disease or after failure of aminosalicylates?
2 Should infliximab always be given concomitantly with immunosupressives?
3 Should induction therapy with infliximab for active luminal disease always be followed by maintenance therapy?
4 Should induction therapy with infliximab for fistulising disease always be followed by maintenance therapy? How to follow and how long to treat patients with fistulising disease?
5 How long should maintenance therapy be continued?
6 What to do if patients lose their response to infliximab?
7 Is it safe to use infliximab shortly before surgery?
8 How can infusion reactions, delayed hypersensitivity and loss of activity be prevented?
9 What measures are to be taken before starting patients on infliximab?
10 What markers are available to determine if patients will respond to infliximab?

In the following section we will try to answer these questions based on the available literature and personal experience.

1 Should infliximab be used as a first-line agent in patients with newly diagnosed, extensive and severe disease or after failure of aminosalicylates?

Many clinicians nowadays would be inclined to start infliximab therapy up-front in patients who present with severe debilitating symptoms, including extra-intestinal manifestations such as pyoderma gangrenosum or ankylosing spondylitis and in patients with important endoscopic lesions or extensive involvement of the small bowel with or without malnutrition and growth retardation. Introduction of immunosuppressive therapy with 6-mercaptopurine was shown to be beneficial in a cohort of children with newly diagnosed Crohn's disease [21]. For this and other reasons, 'top-down' therapy with early introduction of biological therapy (in combination with immunosuppressives) with the potential benefit of healing the diseased mucosa, hence avoiding further complications, should be considered.

A recent trial in the Belgium and the Netherlands looked at this problem in 130 patients with newly diagnosed Crohn's disease who were randomised to receive 'classic' therapy with corticosteroids or 'top-down' therapy with three infusions of infliximab in combination with azathioprine. The latter strategy was found to be superior in terms of clinical response 6 and 12 months after diagnosis. Endoscopic healing was clearly more pronounced with infliximab and azathioprine. Further data from this pivotal trial will shed more light on the safety of this aggressive induction schedule and on its benefit with regard to quality of life and prevention of Crohn's-related complications. At this point in time, however, the use of infliximab as a first-line agent is not (yet) recommended and in the majority of countries not reimbursed for this indication.

In patients where aminosalicylates have failed as an induction therapy, especially in those with mild to moderate ileocaecal disease, a course of (topical) corticosteroids (budesonide) appears to be more appropriate than an immediate switch to infliximab. The high cost of infliximab and the limited availability of safety data beyond 10 years still justify the use of corticosteroids for a limited period of time, provided immunosupressives are added.

2 *Should infliximab always be given concomitantly with immunosupressives?*
Virtually all trials examining the issue of hypersensitivity reactions have demonstrated a significant reduction in the incidence of this problem if patients use concomitant immunosuppressive medication. A significant difference between the 'classic' immunomodulators azathioprine/6-mercaptopurine and methotrexate has not been demonstrated [22]. The question as to whether hydrocortisone prior to the infusions offers an additional benefit remains unanswered as yet, but patients who do not tolerate immunomodulators should definitely receive this treatment. Because antibody formation appears to be a problem of the first year of infliximab treatment predominantly, it was suggested that azathioprine could safely be discontinued after 1 year [23]. We carried out a comparative trial looking at a group of Crohn's disease patients who receive 6–8 weekly infliximab infusions as maintenance therapy, randomised to continued concomitant immunosuppression or to withdrawal of immunosuppression after at least 1 year of infliximab therapy. Preliminary analysis of the data could not show any benefit of continued concomitant immunosupression beyond 1 year [24]. As a consequence, current recommendations include immunosuppression during at least the first year of infliximab therapy.

3 *Should induction therapy with infliximab for active luminal disease always be followed by maintenance therapy?*
In patients who are not yet using immunomodulatory treatment, the initiation of infliximab should definitely be combined with the start of one of these drugs. Given the delay in time before antimetabolites begin to act, more than one 'induction' infusion may be needed as a 'bridge' to further maintenance therapy with azathioprine/6-MP or MTX. If patients are already using immunomodulation when infliximab is started, the question needs to be addressed whether this therapy is really 'optimal'. In many patients, the dose can be increased (dependent on body weight, 6-TGN blood levels or MCV of the red blood cells). Other patients may benefit from a switch from azathioprine/6-mercaptopurine to methotrexate. If all this has been done, remission can be induced with infliximab and the further course of the patient can be carefully observed. If early relapse occurs, the patient will probably need further maintenance infusions. In that case,

'automatic' re-infusion every 8 weeks (or even less if needed) is superior to treatment 'on demand'.

4 *Should induction therapy with infliximab for fistulising disease always be followed by maintenance therapy? How to follow and how long to treat patients with fistulising disease?*

MRI and endosonographic studies have demonstrated that cessation of drainage from fistulous openings does not mean that the internal track has healed. MRI scans seem to be a useful tool to guide infliximab therapy, because these scans beautifully show what is happening to the tracks: if inflammatory infiltration and fluid accumulation within the perianal tracks persist, further infliximab seems to be necessary until full healing has been attained [14]. Nonetheless, a number of patients will develop recurrent abscesses (often in the old fistula tracks) in spite of continued therapy. In these patients placement of seton drains for a prolonged period of time seems to be indicated. In patients with complete fistula healing but persistent fistulous openings, definitive closure with advancement flaps should be considered as a further therapeutic option. Data on the benefit of maintenance infusions beyond 1 year are still lacking.

5 *How long should maintenance therapy be continued?*

Nobody can give an evidence-based answer to this difficult question. A significant proportion of patients seem to gradually lose response with continued retreatments. Should every patient be treated up to that point? We do not have any markers indicating when therapy can safely be stopped, but endoscopic healing seems to be a reasonable goal to be achieved prior to discontinuation of therapy. Irrespective of endoscopic healing, a minimum of 1 year of maintenance therapy appears logical based on the available controlled data.

6 *What to do if patients lose their response to infliximab?*

A retrospective analysis in 56 patients revealed that the majority of patients continued to have a response, but that almost half of the patients needed an increase in dosage from 5 to 10 mg/kg and/or a shortened infusion internal (shorter than 8 weeks) [25]. It is probably not very beneficial to re-administer infliximab infusions at intervals shorter than 4–6 weeks. We were able to demonstrate that patients losing their response to 5 mg/kg infusions often have a response when the dose is increased to 10 mg/kg, and that further maintenance can be continued again with 5 mg/kg. In refractory patients alternative therapies should be considered such as surgery, corticosteroids, humanised anti-TNF antibodies or novel biologicals with different cytokine targets such as anti-IFN, anti-IL-6, anti IL-12 or anti-integrin antibodies.

7 *Is it safe to use infliximab before surgery?*

Two retrospective studies looked at perioperative complications in patients who underwent surgery and received infliximab treatment shortly before. The risk of complications was neither increased in the immediate post-operative period (within 30 days), nor after 90 days. It was concluded that infliximab can be used safely prior to surgery [26, 27]. The same groups of investigators failed to demonstrate, however, that the extent of the intestine to be resected was significantly reduced when infliximab was given prior to the resection.

8 *How can infusion reactions, delayed hypersensitivity and loss of activity be prevented?*

This issue has been discussed in the first part of this chapter. All patients should receive concomitant immuosuppressives if tolerated. If not, IV hydrocortione (200 mg) can be given shortly before the infusion. If infusion reactions occur nevertheless, the infusion needs to be discontinued for a while and antihistamines, acetaminophen and corticosteroids are given intravenously. Approximately 1 h later the infusion can be restarted at a much slower infusion rate. Patients who experienced infusion reaction in the past and patients with a long 'drug holiday' after the previous infusion should always receive antihistamines (even for several days) and corticosteroids prior to the infliximab infusions. The infusion should be started at a slower rate than usual. The vast majority of patients can be treated safely when all these measures are followed with care and caution.

9 *What measures are to be taken before starting patients on infliximab?*

It is important that patients realise that their Crohn's disease will not be 'cured' with infliximab therapy. Careful follow-up and continued concomitant therapies are necessary. A tuberculosis history and chest X-ray need to be obtained in all patients and

TB prophylaxis should be given to patients who have had prior exposure to this infection or have evidence of latent infection. In older patients, congestive heart failure needs to be ruled out. When patients receive treatment for fistulising Crohn's disease, we recommend either examination under general anaesthesia or MRI to exclude active per anal sepsis or abscess.

10 *What markers are available to determine if patients will respond to infliximab?*
Whereas initial controlled trials did not reveal any predictive factors, cohort studies suggested that higher CRP levels, colonic disease and use of immunomodulators were associated with a better response. The latter was not systematically confirmed by other publications. Also, smoking has not been consistently associated with better response [28]. Several genetic polymorphisms and serological markers that have been studied have not consistently been associated with a better response to anti-TNF therapy.

Conclusion

The anti-TNF approach in Crohn's disease has been a genuine success story. So far, infliximab is the only approved molecule for this indication, but undoubtedly newer antibodies will become available in the near future. Infliximab is also the only agent available for Crohn's disease with proven induction *and* maintenance benefits. It rapidly restores quality of life, induces mucosal healing and has a more than acceptable safety profile. In addition, maintenance therapy with infliximab has been shown to reduce the need for surgeries and hospitalisations. Potential opportunities for further optimalisation of anti-TNF drugs include replacement of intravenous administration by subcutaneous or enteral routes, reduction of infusion reactions with loss of response by further humanisation and development of an 'ideal' or 'individualised' maintenance schedule.

References

1. Van den Brande JM, Braat H, van den Brink GR, *et al*. Infliximab but not etanercept induces apoptosis in lamina propria T-lymphocytes from patients with Crohn's disease. *Gastroenterology* 2003;124:1774-85.
2. Targan SR, Hanauer SB, van Deventer SJ, *et al*. A short-term study of chimeric monoclonal antibody cA2 to tumor necrosis factor alpha for Crohn's disease. Crohn's disease cA2 study group. *N Engl J Med* 1997;337:1029-35.
3. D'Haens G, Van Deventer S, Van Hogezand R, *et al*. Endoscopic and histological healing with infliximab anti-tumor necrosis factor antibodies in Crohn's disease: a European multicenter trial. *Gastroenterology* 1999;116:1029-34.
4. Baert FJ, D'Haens GR, Peeters M, *et al*. Tumor necrosis factor alpha antibody (infliximab) therapy profoundly down-regulates the inflammation in Crohn's ileocolitis. *Gastroenterology* 1999;116(1):22-8.
5. Vermeire S, Louis E, Carbonez A, *et al*. Demographic and clinical parameters influencing the short-term outcome of anti-tumor necrosis factor (infliximab) treatment in Crohn's disease. *Am J Gastroenterol* 2002;97:2357-63.
6. Arnott ID, McNeill G, Satsangi J. An analysis of factors influencing short-term and sustained response to infliximab treatment for Crohn's disease. *Aliment Pharmacol Ther* 2003;17:1451-7.
7. Rutgeerts P, D'Haens G, Targan S, *et al*. Efficacy and safety of retreatment with anti-tumor necrosis factor antibody (infliximab) to maintain remission in Crohn's disease. *Gastroenterology* 1999;117:761-9.
8. Hanauer SB, Feagan BG, Lichtenstein GR, *et al*. ACCENT I study group. Maintenance infliximab for Crohn's disease: the ACCENT I randomised trial. *Lancet* 2002;359:1541-9.
9. Rutgeerts P, Feagan BG, Lichtenstein GR, *et al*. Comparison of scheduled and episodic treatment strategies of infliximab in Crohn's disease. *Gastroenterology* 2004;126:402-13.
10. Baert F, Noman M, Vermeire S, *et al*. Influence of immunogenicity on the long-term efficacy of infliximab in Crohn's disease. *N Engl J Med* 2003;348:601-8.
11. Farrell RJ, Alsahli M, Jeen YT, Falchuk KR, Peppercorn MA, Michetti P. Intravenous hydrocortisone premedication reduces antibodies to infliximab in Crohn's disease: a randomized controlled trial. *Gastroenterology* 2003;124:917-24.
12. Present DH, Rutgeerts P, Targan S, *et al*. Infliximab for the treatment of fistulas in patients with Crohn's disease. *N Engl J Med* 1999;340:1398-405.
13. Sands BE, Anderson FH, Bernstein CN, *et al*. Infliximab maintenance therapy for fistulizing Crohn's disease. *N Engl J Med* 2004;350:876-85.
14. Van Assche G, Vanbeckevoort D, Bielen D, *et al*. Magnetic resonance imaging of the effects of

14. infliximab on perianal fistulizing Crohn's disease. *Am J Gastroenterol* 2003;98:332–9.
15. van Bodegraven AA, Sloots CE, Felt-Bersma RJ, Meuwissen SG. Endosonographic evidence of persistence of Crohn's disease-associated fistulas after infliximab treatment, irrespective of clinical response. *Dis Colon Rectum* 2002;45:39–45.
16. Regueiro, M, Mardini H. Treatment of perianal fistulizing Crohn's disease with infliximab alone or as an adjunct to exam under anesthesia with seton placement. *Inflamm Bowel Dis* 2003;9:98–103.
17. Keane J, Gershon S, Wise RP, Mirabile-Levens E. Tuberculosis associated with infliximab, a tumour necrosis factor alpha-neutralizing agent. *N Engl J Med* 2001;345:1098–104.
18. Han PD, Cohen RD. Managing immunogenic responses to infliximab: treatment implications for patients with Crohn's disease. Managing immunogenic responses to infliximab: treatment implications for patients with Crohn's disease. *Drugs* 2004;64:1767–77.
19. Liechtenstein GR, Cohen RD, Feagan BG, *et al.* Safety of infliximab in Crohn's disease: data from the 5000 patients TREAT registry. *Gastroenterology* 2004;126:A-54.
20. Colombel JF, Loftus EV Jr, Tremaine WJ, *et al.* The safety profile of infliximab in patients with Crohn's disease: the Mayo clinic experience in 500 patients. *Gastroenterology* 2004;126:19–31.
21. Markowitz J, Grancher K, Kohn N, Lesser M, Daum F. A multicenter trial of 6-mercaptopurine and prednisone in children with newly diagnosed Crohn's disease. *Gastroenterology* 2000;119:895–902.
22. Noman M, Vermeire S, Van Assche G, *et al.* The effectiveness of immunosuppression to suppress the formation of antibodies to infliximab in Crohn's disease [Abstract]. *Gastroenterology* 2004;126:A54.
23. Tuvlin JA, Schaefer KG, Sane NP, Cohen RD, Hanauer SB. Infliximab is not a bridge to immunomodulators in Crohn's disease [Abstract]. *Gastroenterology* 2003;124:A518.
24. Van Assche G, D'Haens G, Baert F, *et al.* The clinical outcome of maintenance therapy with infliximab for luminal Crohn's disease is not affected by concomitant immunosupressives: results of a multicenter randomized infliximab maintenance/immunosuppressives discontinuation (IMID) trial [Abstract]. *Gastroenterology* 2005;128:A 26.
25. Shih CE, Bayless TM, Hariis ML. Maintenance of long term response to infliximab over 1 to 5 years in Crohn's disease including shortening dosing intervals or increasing dosage. *Gastroenterology* 2004;126:A-631.
26. Colombel JF, Loftus EV Jr, Tremaine WJ, *et al.* Early postoperative complications are not increased in patients with Crohn's disease treated perioperatively with infliximab or immunosuppressive therapy. *Am J Gastroenterol* 2004;99:878–83.
27. Marchal L, D'Haens G, Van Assche G, *et al.* The risk of post-operative complications associated with infliximab therapy for Crohn's disease: a controlled cohort study. *Aliment Pharmacol Ther* 2004;19:749–54.
28. Fefferman DS, Lodhavia PJ, Alsahli M, *et al.* Smoking and immunomodulators do not influence the response or duration of response to infliximab in Crohn's disease. *Inflamm Bowel Dis* 2004;10:346–51.

18: Designer drugs: from bench to bedside
Stephan R. Targan and Loren C. Karp

Introduction

For decades, virtually all of the agents used to treat inflammatory bowel disease were those approved for other inflammatory conditions such as rheumatoid arthritis and multiple sclerosis, or approved for situations requiring overall immune suppression, such as transplant rejection. Today, with a single exception, approved drugs that do have indications for Crohn's disease or ulcerative colitis are modifications of the steroids and aminosalicylic acid derivatives that have been used since the mid-twentieth century. The lack of specified treatments thus far reflects the available scholarship and the understanding of the aetiology of these diseases at the time. In recent years, however, following a tremendous increase in available model systems for investigation of inflammatory bowel disease, a number of pharmaceutical agents that have been designed to interfere with one or more specific pathogenic mechanism of intestinal inflammation have reached Phase III testing and one, infliximab, has been brought to the market with an indication for Crohn's disease.

The development of drugs with highly specific mechanisms of action can be approached in two ways. First, investigations, both animal-based and human-based, of the pathways of inflammation yield clues for development of biologic agents such as the various cytokine blockade therapies, and delivery systems such as the bacterial vehicles now being evaluated in all phases of clinical trials. The efficacy shown with some agents and vehicles in animal models does not always translate to human disease, and given the complexity of inflammatory bowel disease pathogenesis, there are many potential avenues to treatment.

Physiologic features, such as serum markers and genomic indicators, can be used to identify the patients most likely to respond to a particular intervention. Another benefit of evaluating new treatments by subgroup analysis is that much can be learned from drugs with lower efficacy and from the groups of patients who do not improve in an otherwise positive trial. The spectrum of biologic agents includes vaccines, recombinant molecules, antibodies, nucleic acid agents and gene therapies. In IBD, the emphasis has been on recombinant molecules, antibodies and nucleic acid agents, but in recent years, small molecules and vaccines have also shown potential.

Levine *et al.* demonstrated that the dominant molecules at the time of an acute flare-up of disease might be different from those during a chronic active state [1]. Therefore, response and non-response data from trials, and data from basic studies aimed at understanding the different pathways to inflammation in different diseases and at different stages of disease expression, should be combined with data from serum and genetic marker (immunophenotype) analysis. The combined information will target drugs or a designer 'cocktail' thereof on an individual patient basis, to the specific relevant pathways. Using all the available data generated from genomic, proteomic, phenomic, serotypic and clinical research will increase the likelihood that highly specific therapies that can interrupt the disease process, while preserving the essential functions of the immune system, can be developed.

In this chapter, we will discuss the biologic therapies now in use and in trials within the context of their mechanism of action, for their utility in treating IBD and as indicators of other mechanisms that can be exploited for drug development. We also present a review of physiological and genomic characteristics that define homogenous disease immunophenotypes, which can be used to predict treatment outcome, and to define treatments that will identify which patients are likely to develop severe, progressive disease and will, hopefully, point to new, preventative interventions.

IBD pathogenesis: targets of therapeutic intervention

Recent advances in basic research have provided new insights into the pathogenesis of IBD, and point to numerous potential avenues for therapeutic intervention (Fig 18.1). In general, IBD is a product of a dysregulated mucosal immune response to commensal bacterial products in a genetically susceptible host. We now know that among patients with IBD, serum responses to bacterial antigens are associated with the severity of the disease [2–4]. In patients who lack antibody responses to bacterial antigens and who have mild, non-progressive disease, it is likely that a single gene defect would generate a muted or mildly defective innate response and that the exposure to commensal bacteria would lead to a somewhat decreased protection from bacterial invasion. Decreased protection would then permit a slightly increased bacterial exposure, which would yield little to no increased adaptive immune response, resulting in a mild clinical phenotype and non-progressive disease. In contrast, patients who express high-level antibody response to multiple bacterial antigens may also have more (and/or more serious) genetic defects in the innate immune system, which would generate a severely modified innate immune response. Therefore, exposure to commensal bacteria and/or concomitant mucosal injury would lead to markedly decreased protection and a greatly increased bacterial exposure. Depending on the presence of any additional genetic defects, which either produce a defective T or B regulatory cell population or a potent effector T cell population

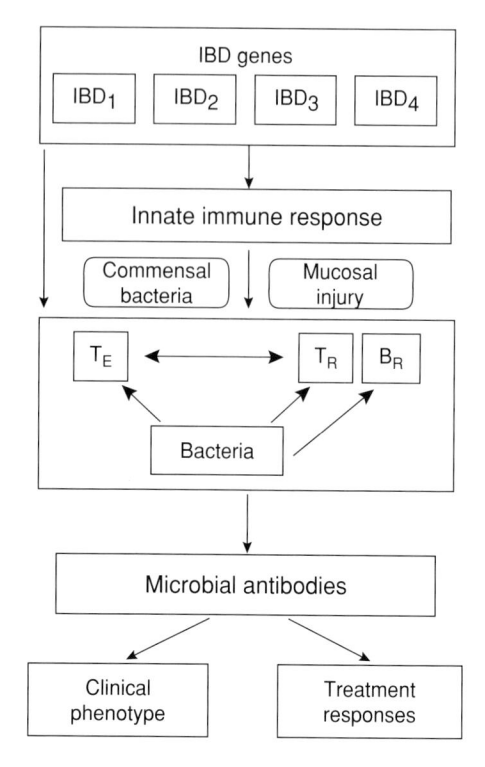

Fig 18.1 IBD pathogenesis.
Any one or a combination of genes regulate the host's immune response to any one or a combination of bacterial antigens, manifesting as serum antibodies, which can be used to define clinical phenotypes and then to choose the targeted therapies.

and/or abnormal cytokine regulation, these conditions would lead to a markedly increased Th1 adaptive immune response, which would be associated with very severe, rapidly progressive mucosal inflammation in humans and rodents. These concepts encompass multiple opportunities and targets for manipulation of the pathogenic process.

In recent years, geneticists have investigated several loci for associations with IBD. Most prominently, a susceptibility gene in chromosome 16 that codes for the NOD2/CARD15 protein has been associated with Crohn's disease [5, 6]. A complex interplay of genetic, microbial, and environmental factors results in a sustained mucosal immune response.

From an immunologic point of view, in healthy mucosal homeostasis, the intestinal mucosa is in a state of 'controlled' inflammation regulated by a delicate balance of pro-inflammatory and anti-inflammatory cytokines. Mucosal lymphocytes are activated to secrete interferon (IFN)-γ and interleukin (IL)-2 in response to antigens. IL-2 enhances T cell and B cell function. IFN-γ activates antigen presenting cells and macrophages to produce IL-12, resulting in a T helper (Th)-1 response, and increased production of IFN-γ, IL-2, and tumour necrosis factor (TNF). IFN-γ enhances macrophage production of TNF-α, IL-1, IL-6, IL-8, IL-12 and IL-18. In the healthy mucosa, down-regulatory cytokines, IL-10, and TGF-β control the magnitude of this response. In IBD, the control mechanisms fail, leading to tissue injury and clinical manifestation of the disease. TNF-α and IL-1, IL-6, IL-8 and IL-12 are categorised as pro-inflammatory cytokines and IL-4, IL-10, IL-11 and IL-13 are categorised as anti-inflammatory cytokines. Increased levels of IL-12 and IL-18 secreted by macrophages and dendritic cells result in a Th1-type inflammation in patients with Crohn's disease [7–9]. In contrast, ulcerative colitis patients are more likely to have a Th2-like phenotype, characterised by elevated production of IL-5 and the presence of auto-antibodies to perinuclear components of neutrophils [10]. Theoretically, therapies targeted at regulating pro-inflammatory cytokines, or amplifying anti-inflammatory factors would restore 'normal' mucosal homeostasis.

Biologic therapies for inflammatory bowel disease

Tumour necrosis factor inhibition

The therapeutic benefit of tumour necrosis factor inhibition is supported by several findings. Increased levels of TNF-α that correlate with disease activity are found in mucosal samples and in the stool of patients with CD [11]. Infliximab is a murine-human chimeric monoclonal antibody consisting of approximately 75% human protein and 25% murine protein. Clinically, approximately two-thirds of patients with Crohn's disease will experience improved symptoms after a single infusion of the anti-TNF-α antibody infliximab [12], which, at present, is the only biologic agent with Food and Drug Administration (FDA) approval in Crohn's disease. Use of infliximab is limited by the complications arising in association with the development of human antichimeric antibodies (HACAs) and delayed hypersensitivity reactions, which have led to the development of humanised antibodies to TNF. Such humanised anti-TNF biologic agents include CDP571, CDP870, etanercept, onercept and adalimumab.

CDP571 is a humanised anti-TNF-α monoclonal antibody, which despite an improvement in tolerability, has shown to have only moderate efficacy at 28 weeks [13–16]. However, sub-stratification of the study population did demonstrate that CDP571 was efficacious for the treatment of patients with elevated C-reactive protein (CRP) levels [15]. CDP571 does have potential for use in patients who have experienced a hypersensitivity response to infliximab. In an open trial of CDP571-treated patients who had developed HACAs to infliximab in previous treatment, no anti-CDP571 antibodies were detected and clinical response was observed in 41% of patients. Such observations highlight the potential benefit of further analysis of the subgroups within a trial population in a search for a particular 'niche' use for a drug and for clues to improve the biologic agent. Data suggest that another anti-TNF-α agent, CDP870 (pegylated anti-TNF-α monoclonal antibody fragment), like CDP571, may be useful in patients with elevated CRP levels who were found to be more likely to respond, although sustained response remains an issue [17].

Etanercept is a human protein, in which the Fc portion of an IgG1 human antibody is linked to human soluble p75 TNF receptors. Onercept is similar but uses a recombinant human soluble p55 TNF receptor. Both etanercept and onercept counteract the effect of TNF in the mucosa by binding to both soluble and membrane-bound TNF, which prevents it from binding to the host's TNF receptors. Etanercept, although an effective treatment for arthritis, is not a useful treatment in the majority of patients with Crohn's disease. The main difference in the effect of infliximab and etanercept is that etanercept does not upregulate T cell apoptosis, which may account for the difference in efficacy between the two [18]. Less is known about onercept, but preliminary findings are promising, as reduction in symptoms occurred quickly after treatment and two-thirds to three-quarters of the patients studied responded to treatment [19].

Adalimumab (Humira^{TM}). Adalimumab is an anti-TNF compound with similar properties to infliximab, but is different in that it is fully humanised. Preliminary data suggest that adalimumab may be a safe and effective substitute for infliximab-allergic patients. However, individuals who have been previously treated with other human antibodies may be sensitised to antibodies such as adalimumab [20].

In addition to monoclonal antibody modulators of TNF, small molecule compounds that interrupt mitogen-activated protein kinase (MAP-kinase) pathways are under investigation. One such small molecule in early phase trials is CNI-1493. CNI-1493 is a synthetic compound that blocks the production of several inflammatory cytokines, including TNF. Because it blocks production of multiple inflammatory mediators, it may be more active than products targeted to a specific cytokine. In addition, as it is a small molecule, it may be less likely to cause hypersensitivity reactions and likely will not induce formation of antibodies [15, 21].

Despite what some have described as the tremendous success of TNF blockade therapy, many patients do not respond. Furthermore the ACCENT trials showed that only 25% of patients who responded initially were still responding and steroid-free at 1 year after the initial treatment [22, 23]. Therefore, for the 75% of patients whose disease relapsed, there is a long way to go but detailed analysis of response rates in relation to genomic, immunologic and molecular data may help to show the way.

Regulatory cytokines

Cytokines known to down-regulate inflammation represent another category of agents that may have potential as therapeutics. IL-10 has been shown to decrease production of IFN-γ, IL-2 and IL-12 and is elevated in the mucosa of patients with IBD [24]. Despite evidence of the potential effectiveness of IL-10 in animal models, it was found to be ineffective for most patients in a large clinical trial [25, 26]. However, IL-10 has been used with some success, again in animal models, when delivered using bacteria-based and virus based vehicles. Studies have yet to be performed in humans.

IL-11, a cytokine with anti-inflammatory properties inhibits inflammation via suppression of NFκB, and subsequently IL-1 and TNF-α [27]. In a study of patients with Crohn's disease, recombinant IL-11 was shown to be effective, but, was associated with thrombocytosis at the effective doses. Topical IL-11 has shown more promise, without concomitant adverse effects in phase I studies.

Modulators of leukocyte adhesion molecules

This category of pathogenesis specific therapies includes antisense to ICAM-1 (ISIS 2302), anti-α4 integrin (natalizumab), and anti-α4β7 integrin (MLN-02). ISIS-2302 is designed to decrease levels of ICAM-1 protein expression. ISIS-2302 showed promise in animal models; however, the benefit did not translate to human studies [28, 29]. Natalizumab is the first anti-α4 compound within the class of selective adhesion molecules (SAM). The drug is designed to inhibit the migration of immune cells into chronically inflamed tissue where they may cause or maintain inflammation. Natalizumab was shown to be effective in the induction of clinical response and even remission. Patients in the trial experienced decreased CRP levels and improved quality of life measures [30]. MLN-02, is a monoclonal antibody to α4β7, which controls trafficking of lymphocytes to the intestine [31]. MLN-02 is an example of a treatment that may have been discarded based on general analysis, but its potential effect was found by subgroup analysis, which in this case showed that dosing was suboptimal. By the end of 1 year, 25% of subjects treated with these adhesion molecules were steroid free. It remains to be seen if this is the same 25% of patients who would have been steroid-free after 1 year of inflixmab. Whether the group is the same, and particularly interesting if it is not, these findings suggest such subgroup analysis might be quite fruitful.

Th1 inhibitors

As mentioned above, IFN-γ is a cytokine that augments Th1 responses, while decreasing Th 2 responses. Anti-IFN-γ has been tested in phase I and II trials [32]. In addition to decreased placebo effect in these studies, results showed that anti-IFN-γ was effective in Crohn's patients with high levels of C-reactive protein (CRP), which suggests that it may specifically act to decrease inflammation and may be a marker for a specific subset of patients with a distinct immunophenotype.

Anti-interleukin-12

Antibodies directed against interleukin-12 (IL-12) have been shown to be effective treatment for the intestinal inflammation in animal models of CD. In a small clinical trial, after 7 weeks of treatment, 75% of patients showed clinical improvement and 38% were in remission. Decreased secretion of IFN-γ, TNF-α and IL-12 was noted in the patients who clinically responded to anti-IL-12 therapy [33]. More work is needed to see how best to exploit the potential represented by this pathway.

Activators of immune function

Granulocyte-macrophage colony stimulating factor (GM-CSF) has received recent interest in the treatment of Crohn's disease. In a small trial, GM-CSF was found to be effective in achieving a clinical response and in some cases remission was achieved. The duration of effectiveness varied and discontinuation of treatment resulted in symptom flares [34].

Other anti-cytokine therapies

Daclizumab is a monoclonal antibody to IL2 receptor antagonists (IL-2rα). In early trials of patients with ulcerative colitis, blockade of IL2 binding with daclizumab was found to induce a clinical response, but mucosal healing assessed by endoscopy did not occur [35]. However, because it is thought that IL-2 may play a role in steroid-resistance, studies of basiliximab, another anti-IL-2 compound, were undertaken in steroid resistant patients in an open trial [36]. Nine of 10 patients achieved clinical remission along with improvement in histologic scores. Relapse occurred in most patients by 9 weeks, however, although remission could be once again induced with increased concomitant steroids or azathioprine. Basiliximab may find potential use as a bridge capable of inducing remission in steroid-resistant patients, who can then be maintained on azathioprine or other immune suppressant.

Visilizumab is an anti-CD3 compound, which has been shown to induce T cell apoptosis. Although early trials showed visilizumab to be effective in ulcerative colitis, adverse events, which may be dose-related, have led to studies to identify a lower effective dose [37].

Drug regimens designed by subgroup analysis based on response and non-response data

With the underlying motivation in pharmaceutical development being commercial, research is devoted primarily to agents likely to be applicable to a large audience. The consequences are two-fold. First, the population of patients with IBD, although increasing, is small compared to the population with gastrointestinal reflux disease, for example. Therefore, IBD drugs are a relatively lower priority. Secondly, when IBD drugs of potential do come to controlled trials, the tendency is to test a population of patients meeting quite general criteria for active Crohn's disease or ulcerative colitis. The data generated from these trials can be misleading. Although results from a trial may show non-responsiveness or poor efficacy in the study population as a whole, it is possible that the smaller group of patients for whom the treatment was effective represent those with a certain disease phenotype. It is now widely accepted that the terms 'Crohn's disease' and 'ulcerative colitis' actually represent numerous pathophysiologic distinct disorders, all of which manifest as intestinal mucosal inflammation. Because there are numerous pathways to mucosal inflammation, it follows that newly developed biologics, which target specific points in the inflammatory process, will work for some patients but not for others. Several examples have been presented in the preceding section of potential indications for a drug, which previously would have been discarded on the basis of efficacy data from trials using unselected populations of patients. Two such examples are CDP870 and CDP571, which may be useful in the population of patients with elevated CRP levels. In patients who experience delayed hypersensitivity reactions or develop HACAs to the chimeric antibody infliximab, some patients respond to therapy with humanised anti-TNF agents such as adalimumab without such reactions. As mentioned above, only 25% of patients who responded and were steroid-free after treatment with infliximab were still steroid free at 1 year [22]. Studying the 75% whose disease worsened has just as much merit as studying the 25% whose disease was ameliorated by treatment, in an attempt to evince clues to pathogenesis and for further refinement of the intervention. Much can be gained from merging the data from clinical trials with that from ongoing studies to sub-stratify patient populations based on genetic and immune markers.

Clinical subgroup analysis by immune and genetic markers – definition of immunophenotypes and implications for treatment

Genetic associations

Recent progress in the hunt for genes responsible for IBD has led to the identification of genetic associations with certain disease characteristics. First, disease characteristics have been reported to aggregate in families [38, 39] and associations between major histocompatibility genes and disease location and phenotypes have been shown in Crohn's disease [40]. Variants in the NOD2/CARD15 gene have been reported in 20–40% of European and American patients with Crohn's disease [5, 6]. NOD2 mediates the interaction between the innate immune response and the host as it recognises muramyl dipeptide, the smallest structure of peptidoglycan [41] and there have been several published reports of an association between mutations in NOD2 and a younger age of onset [42], small-bowel disease [40, 43] and fibrostenotic disease [44, 45]. NOD2/CARD15 variants as well as certain serological responses are both associated with small-bowel and fibrostenotic disease, but it has not yet been determined which has the stronger relationship to clinical phenotype. Mow *et al.* reported a stronger association between antibody expressions to bacterial antigens than that of NOD2, suggesting an environmental interaction [4]. Investigators have recently discovered allelic variants in the organic cationic transporter (OCTN) gene found in macrophages, T cells and colonic mucosal epithelial cells [46]. The variant located in the OCTN promoter renders it non-responsive to heat-shock proteins, which are induced in the host by bacterial structures. Among homozygotes of either of these genes (NOD2 and OCTN), there is an odds ratio of 2 for the development of CD, and in patients with both variants, the odds ratio of developing CD is in the range of 7–10. Through these and similar studies, we are beginning to develop associations between genomic information, clinical expression and disease behaviour.

Serologic associations

Numerous associations between serum markers and clinical expression of disease have already been made. For example, Crohn's disease patients with high serum levels of ASCA have more severe disease, as defined by fibrostenotic and internal perforating features, and are more likely to need small-bowel surgery [47]. In contrast, pANCA expression in Crohn's disease has been associated with a more benign disease course and ulcerative colitis (UC)-like features [44]. Crohn's disease patients can lose tolerance to *specific* bacterial antigens and patients can be clustered into four groups, depending on their antibody response patterns [2]. These clusters are (1) antibody responses against oligomannan (anti-*Saccharomyces cerevisiae*; ASCA), (2) antibody responses towards both *Escherichia coli* outer membrane protein C (anti-OmpC) and a CD-related protein from *Pseudomonas fluorescens* (anti-CD-related bacterial sequence {I2}), (3) antibody responses towards nuclear antigens (perinuclear antineutrophil cytoplasmic antibody; pANCA) or (4) low or no serological response to any of the tested antigens. These distinct antibody response patterns may indicate unique pathophysiological mechanisms in the progression of this complicated disease and may underlie the basis for the development of specific phenotypes.

A series of reports have helped to delineate further the relationship of these immunologic responses to disease phenotypes [4, 48]. It has recently been demonstrated that the greater the number of responses to different microbial antigens, and the magnitude thereof, the more severe the disease course. In contrast, patients who lack these immune responses have a more benign disease course. In a recent report, Arnott et al. [48] showed that progression of disease might be predicted by the number and magnitude of serologic responses to these microbial antigens in patients initially characterised as having 'inflammatory' disease. Indicators of disease progression, such as the need for surgery, fibrostenotic and internal perforating disease were associated with greater proportions and levels of immune responses. In contrast, a milder, uncomplicated disease course was associated with no or low serologic response.

In a recently published pilot study, patients with selected immune responses to I2 and OmpC responded better to antibiotics administered in addition to budesonide in a controlled trial of patients with CD [49]. These results suggest that the patients with the greatest immune responses to bacterial products are the best candidates for treatment with antibiotics. Furthermore, patients with medically resistant Crohn's disease patients who expressed serum antibodies to the bacterial antigen, I2, were shown to benefit from surgical diversion of the faecal stream, and those with no I2 reactivity did not benefit [50]. These results suggest that immune responses to bacterial components may serve as important markers of pathophysiologic abnormalities. The adaptive immune response to specific antigens implies that they are linked to specific pathophysiologic mechanisms and it follows that manipulation of these responses could be therapeutic. Furthermore, these immune responses might predict which patients would respond best to environmental manipulation including antibiotics, probiotics or diversion of the faecal stream.

An immunodominant flagellin, to which strong B cell and CD4$^+$ T cell responses occur in colitic mice, has recently been defined. In human studies, approximately 50% of patients with CD had serum reactivity to flagellin, whereas patients with ulcerative colitis, patients with other inflammatory GI diseases and control subjects had little or no reactivity to this flagellin [51]. Interesting results were derived from our studies among CD patients to determine the relationship of antibodies to flagellin to the previously-defined antibodies to microbial antigens. Among patients with increasing levels of reactivity to ASCA, OmpC and I2 (with a peak occurring in those who respond to all three), response to flagellin is greater, which is consistent with the concept that this subset of patients has a propensity to respond to multiple bacterial antigens. Nevertheless, high flagellin reactivity was seen across all antibody-defined subsets, demonstrating that anti-flagellin expression is independent of the other antibody responses.

As mentioned above, pANCA is predominantly associated with ulcerative colitis and may reflect cross reactivity to bacteria [52]. There is, however, a subset of patients with CD who also express pANCA [47, 53]. Crohn's disease patients with pANCA have both colitic and left-sided disease with features similar to ulcerative colitis. Nearly half of the population of CD patients who express pANCA but do not react to the other known antigens, react to flagellin, although the vast majority of pANCA$^+$ ulcerative colitis patients are not responsive to flagellin. Anti-flagellin expression appears to be associated with a specific CD subtype. Therefore, it may prove to be useful in categorising patients with indeterminate colitis; i.e. those that may be more Crohn's-like compared to those that may be more UC-like. Anti-flagellin expression may also be used in combination with pANCA to mark a subset of patients with colitic and/or colitic *and* small bowel disease, perhaps defining those patients likely to respond to manipulation of bacteria using either antibiotics or probiotics.

Expression of antibodies to flagellin presents a unique opportunity to investigate the underlying pathophysiologic mechanism related to this antigenic response, as it is the first antigen defined with dual effects on the immune system. Recent progress has been made in understanding the relationship between commensal microbe-associated molecular patterns and receptors that influence the innate immune compartment. Flagellins are important molecular components of complex structures on bacterial surfaces, important for both adhesion and motility [54] and they have been identified as the ligand for TLR5 [54, 55], which recognises flagellin from both gram-positive and gram-negative bacteria. Activation of nuclear factor κB (NFκB), required for induction of many Th1 cytokines, is the result of TLR5-flagellin interactions [54, 55]. In humans, CB flagellin induces different inflammatory mediators than does LPS in monocyte-derived dendritic cells [56].

Future investigations will need to determine whether anti-flagellin expression correlates with response to various therapeutic modalities and to identify any abnormalities of flagellin stimulation of the innate immune pathway and of Th1 responses.

Conclusion

At the interface between genetic, immunologic and clinical information, is advanced technology. Although serological associations with clinical manifestations represent phenomics, the findings must be correlated with genomic data. The combined phenomic and genomic results can then serve to stratify well characterised populations for proteomic analysis, which will help to discern which of the genomic and phenomic markers are reflective of the disease mechanism. Proteomics using high-resolution mass spectrometry will aid in the further refinement of targets for therapeutic design. Proteomic analysis will allow the correlation of differential protein expression among the different disease immunotypes and clinical phenotypes within IBD. We have demonstrated that there is a selective immune response and with this mass spectrometry technology, we will be able to determine which proteins are present in varying disease types as well as at different stages of disease and treatment. The amount of data generated by this method is massive. However, as patient subgroups become better defined by genetic, immunologic and clinical parameters, the information will not only be manageable but could also provide very clear pictures of pathogenetic elements and differences among the subgroups.

In the future, patient management should become far more efficient, with fewer discomforts for the patient, potentially altering the natural history of the disease. In a typical example (Fig 18.2), a patient would present with diarrhoea or pain of serveral week's duration. A battery of non-invasive tests would be administered to characterise the immuno-, geno-, proteo- phenotype of disease. An immunophenotypic diagnosis and prognosis would be made, and finally, a specific, targeted therapeutic plan would be designed and implemented that would ameliorate the patient's disease and prevent the progression to complications and surgery.

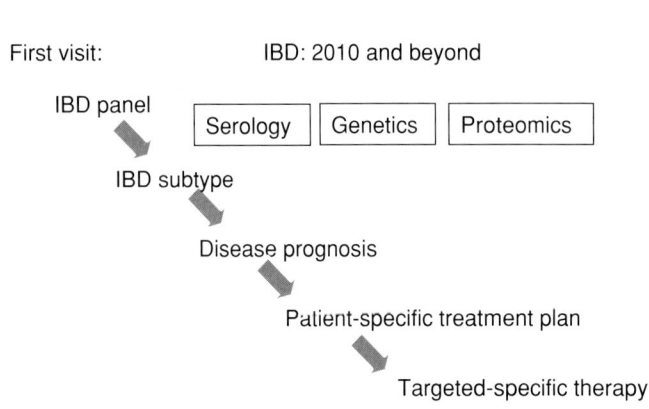

Fig 18.2 IBD 2010 and beyond. In the future, a patient will present with symptoms. A battery of non-invasive serum, genetic and proteomic analyses will yield the patient's specific IBD subtype and disease prognosis. The physician will then develop a patient-specific treatment plan, using targeted and designer drugs.

References

1. Jump RL, Levine AD. Mechanisms of natural tolerance in the intestine: implications for inflammatory bowel disease. *Inflamm Bowel Dis* 2004;10(4):462–78.
2. Landers CJ, Cohavy O, Misra R, *et al.* Selected loss of tolerance evidenced by Crohn's disease-associated immune responses to auto- and microbial antigens. *Gastroenterology* 2002;123(3):689–99.
3. Mow WS, Landers CJ, Steinhart AH, *et al.* High-level serum antibodies to bacterial antigens are associated with antibiotic-induced clinical remission in Crohn's disease: a pilot study. *Dig Dis Sci* 2004;49(7–8): 1280–6.
4. Mow WS, Vasiliauskas EA, Lin YC, *et al.* Association of antibody responses to microbial antigens and complications of small bowel Crohn's disease. *Gastroenterology* 2004;126(2):414–24.
5. Hugot JP, Chamaillard M, Zouali H, *et al.* Association of NOD2 leucine-rich repeat variants with susceptibility to Crohn's disease. *Nature* 2001; 411(6837):599–603.
6. Ogura Y, Bonen DK, Inohara N, *et al.* A frameshift mutation in NOD2 associated with susceptibility to Crohn's disease. *Nature* 2001;411(6837): 603–6.
7. Monteleone G, Trapasso F, Parrello T, *et al.* Bioactive IL-18 expression is up-regulated in Crohn's disease. *J Immunol* 1999;163(1):143–7.
8. Pizarro TT, Michie MH, Bentz M, *et al.* IL-18, a novel immunoregulatory cytokine, is up-regulated in Crohn's disease: expression and localization in intestinal mucosal cells. *J Immunol* 1999;162(11): 6829–35.
9. Strober W, Ludviksson BR, Fuss IJ. The pathogenesis of mucosal inflammation in murine models of inflammatory bowel disease and Crohn disease. *Ann Intern Med* 1998;128(10):848–56.
10. Pallone F, Monteleone G. Regulatory cytokines in inflammatory bowel disease. *Aliment Pharmacol Ther* 1996;10(Suppl 2):75–9; discussion 80.
11. Braegger CP, Nicholls S, Murch SH, Stephens S, MacDonald TT. Tumour necrosis factor alpha in stool as a marker of intestinal inflammation. *Lancet* 1992;339(8785):89–91.
12. Targan SR, Hanauer SB, van Deventer SJ, *et al.* A short-term study of chimeric monoclonal antibody cA2 to tumor necrosis factor alpha for Crohn's disease. Crohn's disease cA2 study group. *N Engl J Med* 1997;337(15):1029–35.
13. Mamula P, Cohen SA, Ferry GD, *et al.* CDP571, a humanized anti-tumor necrosis factor-alpha monoclonal antibody in pediatric Crohn's disease. *Inflamm Bowel Dis* 2004;10(6):723–30.
14. Sandborn WJ, Feagan BG, Hanauer SB, *et al.* An engineered human antibody to TNF (CDP571) for active Crohn's disease: a randomized double-blind placebo-controlled trial. *Gastroenterology* 2001; 120(6):1330–8.
15. Sandborn WJ, Feagan BG, Radford-Smith G, *et al.* CDP571, a humanised monoclonal antibody to tumour necrosis factor alpha, for moderate to severe Crohn's disease: a randomised, double blind, placebo controlled trial. *Gut* 2004;53(10):1485–93.
16. Stack WA, Mann SD, Roy AJ, *et al.* Randomised controlled trial of CDP571 antibody to tumour necrosis factor-alpha in Crohn's disease. *Lancet* 1997;349(9051):521–4.
17. Winter TA, Wright J, Ghosh S, Jahnsen J, Innes A, Round P. Intravenous CDP870, a PEGylated Fab' fragment of a humanized antitumour necrosis factor antibody, in patients with moderate-to-severe Crohn's disease: an exploratory study. *Aliment Pharmacol Ther* 2004;20(11–12):1337–46.
18. Van den Brande JM, Braat H, van den Brink GR, *et al.* Infliximab but not etanercept induces apoptosis in lamina propria T-lymphocytes from patients with Crohn's disease. *Gastroenterology* 2003;124(7): 1774–85.
19. Rutgeerts P, Lemmens L, Van Assche G, Noman M, Borghini-Fuhrer I, Goedkoop R. Treatment of active Crohn's disease with onercept (recombinant human soluble p55 tumour necrosis factor receptor): results of a randomized, open-label, pilot study. *Aliment Pharmacol Ther* 2003;17(2):185–92.
20. Youdim A, Vasiliauskas EA, Targan SR, *et al.* A pilot study of adalimumab in infliximab-allergic patients. *Inflamm Bowel Dis* 2004;10(4):333–8.
21. Hanauer SB, Sandborn W. Management of Crohn's disease in adults. *Am J Gastroenterol* 2001;96(3): 635–43.
22. Hanauer SB, Feagan BG, Lichtenstein GR, *et al.* Maintenance infliximab for Crohn's disease: the ACCENT I randomised trial. *Lancet* 2002;359(9317): 1541–9.
23. Hanauer SB, Wagner CL, Bala M, *et al.* Incidence and importance of antibody responses to infliximab after maintenance or episodic treatment in Crohn's disease. *Clin Gastroenterol Hepatol* 2004;2(7):542–53.
24. Podolsky DK. Inflammatory bowel disease. *N Engl J Med* 2002;347(6):417–29.
25. Fedorak RN, Gangl A, Elson CO, *et al.* Recombinant human interleukin 10 in the treatment of patients with mild to moderately active Crohn's disease. The interleukin 10 inflammatory bowel disease cooperative

25. study group. *Gastroenterology* 2000;119(6): 1473–82.
26. Schreiber S, Fedorak RN, Nielsen OH, et al. Safety and efficacy of recombinant human interleukin 10 in chronic active Crohn's disease. Crohn's disease IL-10 cooperative study group. *Gastroenterology* 2000; 119(6):1461–72.
27. Trepicchio WL, Bozza M, Bouchard P, Dorner AJ. Protective effect of rhIL-11 in a murine model of acetaminophen-induced hepatotoxicity. *Toxicol Pathol* 2001;29(2):242–9.
28. Bennett CF, Kornbrust D, Henry S, et al. An ICAM-1 antisense oligonucleotide prevents and reverses dextran sulfate sodium-induced colitis in mice. *J Pharmacol Exp Ther* 1997;280(2):988–1000.
29. Yacyshyn BR, Bowen-Yacyshyn MB, Jewell L, et al. A placebo-controlled trial of ICAM-1 antisense oligonucleotide in the treatment of Crohn's disease. *Gastroenterology* 1998;114(6):1133–42.
30. Ghosh S, Goldin E, Gordon FH, et al. Natalizumab for active Crohn's disease. *N Engl J Med* 2003;348(1): 24–32.
31. Farstad IN, Halstensen TS, Kvale D, Fausa O, Brandtzaeg P. Topographic distribution of homing receptors on B and T cells in human gut-associated lymphoid tissue: relation of L-selectin and integrin alpha 4 beta 7 to naive and memory phenotypes. *Am J Pathol* 1997;150(1):187–99.
32. Rutgeerts P, Reinisch W, Colombel JF, et al. Preliminary results of a phase I/II study of Huzaf, an anti-IFN monoclonal antibody, in patients with moderate to severe active Crohn's disease. *Gastroenterology* 2002;122:A61.
33. Mannon PJ, Fuss IJ, Mayer L, et al. Anti-interleukin-12 antibody for active Crohn's disease. *N Engl J Med* 2004;351(20):2069–79.
34. Dieckgraefe BK, Korzenik JR. Treatment of active Crohn's disease with recombinant human granulocyte-macrophage colony-stimulating factor. *Lancet* 2002;360(9344):1478–80.
35. Van Assche G, Dalle I, Noman M, et al. A pilot study on the use of the humanized anti-interleukin-2 receptor antibody daclizumab in active ulcerative colitis. *Am J Gastroenterol* 2003;98(2):369–76.
36. Creed TJ, Norman MR, Probert CS, et al. Basiliximab (anti-CD25) in combination with steroids may be an effective new treatment for steroid-resistant ulcerative colitis. *Aliment Pharmacol Ther* 2003;18(1):65–75.
37. Plevy SE, Salzberg BA, Regueiro M, et al. A humanized anti-CD3 monoclonal antibody, visilizumab, for the treatment of steroid refractory ulcerative colitis: preliminary results of a phase I study. *Gastroenterology* 2003;123:A7.
38. Bayless TM, Tokayer AZ, Polito JM, 2nd, Quaskey SA, Mellits ED, Harris ML. Crohn's disease: concordance for site and clinical type in affected family members –potential hereditary influences. *Gastroenterology* 1996;111(3):573–9.
39. Taylor KD, Rotter JI, Yang H. Genetics of inflammatory bowel disease. In: Targan SR, Karp LC, Shanahan F, eds. *Inflammatory Bowel Disease: From Bench to Bedside*. 2nd ed. Dordrecht: Kluwer Academic Publishers; 2003:21–65.
40. Ahmad T, Armuzzi A, Bunce M, et al. The molecular classification of the clinical manifestations of Crohn's disease. *Gastroenterology* 2002;122(4): 854–66.
41. Inohara N, Ogura Y, Fontalba A, et al. Host recognition of bacterial muramyl dipeptide mediated through NOD2. Implications for Crohn's disease. *J Biol Chem* 2003;278(8):5509–12.
42. Lesage S, Zouali H, Cezard JP, et al. CARD15/NOD2 mutational analysis and genotype-phenotype correlation in 612 patients with inflammatory bowel disease. *Am J Hum Genet* 2002;70(4):845–57.
43. Cuthbert AP, Fisher SA, Mirza MM, et al. The contribution of NOD2 gene mutations to the risk and site of disease in inflammatory bowel disease. *Gastroenterology* 2002;122(4):867–74.
44. Abreu MT, Taylor KD, Lin YC, et al. Mutations in NOD2 are associated with fibrostenosing disease in patients with Crohn's disease. *Gastroenterology* 2002; 123(3):679–88.
45. Helio T, Halme L, Lappalainen M, et al. CARD15/NOD2 gene variants are associated with familially occurring and complicated forms of Crohn's disease. *Gut* 2003;52(4):558–62.
46. Peltekova VD, Wintle RF, Rubin LA, et al. Functional variants of OCTN cation transporter genes are associated with Crohn disease. *Nat Genet* 2004;36(5): 471–5.
47. Vasiliauskas EA, Kam LY, Karp LC, Gaiennie J, Yang H, Targan SR. Marker antibody expression stratifies Crohn's disease into immunologically homogeneous subgroups with distinct clinical characteristics. *Gut* 2000;47(4):487–96.
48. Arnott IDR, Landers CJ, Nimmo EJ, Drummond HE, Targan SR, Satsangi J. Reactivity to microbial components in Crohn's disease is associated with severity and progression. *Am J Gastroenterol* 2004; 99(12):2376–84.
49. Mow WS, Landers CJ, Steinhart AH, et al. High level serum antibodies to bacterial antigens is associated with antibiotic induced clinical remission in Crohn's disease: a pilot study. *Dig Dis Sci* 2004;49(7–8): 1280–6.

50. Spivak J, Targan SR, Vasiliauskas EA, et al. Antibodies to I2 predict clinical response to fecal diversion in CD. *Gastroenterology* 2004;124: 528A.
51. Lodes MJ, Cong Y, Elson CO, et al. Bacterial flagellin is a dominant antigen in Crohn disease. *J Clin Invest* 2004;113(9):1296–306.
52. Seibold F, Brandwein S, Simpson S, Terhorst C, Elson CO. pANCA represents a cross-reactivity to enteric bacterial antigens. *J Clin Immunol* 1998;18(2): 153–60.
53. Vasiliauskas EA, Plevy SE, Landers CJ, et al. Perinuclear antineutrophil cytoplasmic antibodies in patients with Crohn's disease define a clinical subgroup. *Gastroenterology* 1996;110(6): 1810–9.
54. Liaudet L, Deb A, Pacher P, et al. The Flagellin-TLR5 axis: therapeutic opportunities. *Drug News Perspect* 2002;15(7):397–409.
55. Hayashi F, Smith KD, Ozinsky A, et al. The innate immune response to bacterial flagellin is mediated by toll-like receptor 5. *Nature* 2001;410(6832): 1099–103.
56. Means TK, Hayashi F, Smith KD, Aderem A, Luster AD. The toll-like receptor 5 stimulus bacterial flagellin induces maturation and chemokine production in human dendritic cells. *J Immunol* 2003;170(10): 5165–75.

19: Current controversies in the surgical management of Crohn's disease

W.M. Chambers, I. Lindsey and N.J. Mortensen

Introduction

Areas of controversy related to the surgical treatment of Crohn's disease include the suitability of patients with Crohn's and indeterminate colitis for pouch surgery, the treatment of perianal Crohn's disease, the application of laparoscopic surgery to Crohn's patients and the limiting of post-surgical recurrence.

Pouch surgery in Crohn's disease

When compared with pouch surgery for ulcerative colitis the results seen for Crohn's disease are worse. Although many clinicians see Crohn's disease as a contraindication to pouch surgery some feel that in selected patients results can be acceptable. Certainly, the course of these patients is variable and pouch failure is not inevitable.

Panis *et al*. [1] in 1996 published literature on pouch surgery for selected Crohn's patients (those with colonic Crohn's with no evidence of perianal or small bowel involvement) and found no difference in complications when these were compared with ulcerative colitis patients undergoing pouch surgery at a mean follow up of 59 months. At 5-year follow-up there was also no difference in stool frequency, continence, leak or need for pads between the two groups. It was argued by others that some of the patients involved in this study had indeterminate colitis rather than Crohn's [2].

Regimbeau *et al*. [3] reported 10-year follow up results from the same centre. Forty-one patients were studied 26 of whom had a pre-operative diagnosis of Crohn's disease. Mean follow up was 113 months. Twenty-seven per cent of patients experienced Crohn's disease-related complications and 7 out of 41 (17%) experienced pouch perineal fistulas. Of 20 patients followed for more than 10 years, 2 patients had their pouch excised. The authors felt the long-term results justified offering pouch surgery to selected Crohn's patients.

This was a view supported by Hartley *et al*. [4] analysing outcome in patients from the Cleveland Clinic who had pouch surgery for apparent ulcerative colitis and who were subsequently found to have Crohn's disease. Of these patients 12% lost their pouch with a median follow-up of 46 months. The authors concluded that the secondary diagnosis of Crohn's disease after pouch formation was associated with protracted freedom from clinically evident Crohn's disease, low pouch loss rate and good functional outcome.

However, Braveman *et al*. [5], reporting results from the Lahey Clinic, found that patients undergoing pouch surgery who were subsequently found to have Crohn's disease experienced significant morbidity and they decided on the basis of their results not to recommend the routine application of ileal pouch anal anastomoses in any subset of patients with known Crohn's disease. Median follow-up was 153 months and complications occurred in 93% of 32 patients. This included perianal abscess or fistula in 63%, pouchitis in 50% and stricture in 38%. Pouch failure occurred in 29%. Pre-operative perianal disease did not predict pouch failure.

Thus major centres differ in their opinions on this issue. Majority opinion is still against pouch surgery for known Crohn's disease. The risk of recurrent Crohn's disease in the pouch, with loss of distensibility and function, of abscess formation and fistulation, and of subsequent pouch excision and short-bowel syndrome have been documented from experience with both the Kock pouch [6] and ileal-anal pouch [7–11].

Despite these risks and, given the existing evidence, patients with colonic Crohn's might feel that they are prepared to take the risk of undergoing pouch surgery for their condition if it offers the possibility of avoiding a permanent stoma.

Pouch surgery in indeterminate colitis

Although a diagnosis of indeterminate colitis is not a contraindication to construction of a pouch, adequate steps must be taken to exclude Crohn's disease, because at the present time such surgery is generally regarded as contraindicated. Sometimes, after reviewing all available information the diagnosis is still not clear-cut, leaving a small proportion of patients overall (reported as 2–8% in series from major centres) with the label 'indeterminate colitis' [12–14]. The majority of such cases behave like ulcerative colitis, and the risk of manifesting as Crohn's disease is small (0–15%) [7, 12, 13, 15–17].

When pouches are made for indeterminate colitis rates of operative morbidity and pouchitis are similar to those in ulcerative colitis. Failure of the pouch (diversion or excision) is greater than in ulcerative colitis. This relates to the manifestation of Crohn's disease in the anus or small bowel in a minority of patients [13]. Those who retain their pouches have similar function to those in ulcerative colitis. This is generally supported in the literature, although one series from the Lahey Clinic has suggested an increased risk of perineal complications in indeterminate colitis pouches [15].

Yu et al. [17] reporting long-term results from the Mayo Clinic stated that indeterminate colitis patients had significantly more pouch failure (27% vs 11%) than ulcerative colitis patients. During the 10-year follow up period 15% of indeterminate colitis patients had their diagnosis changed to Crohn's disease against 2% of UC patients. When the outcomes of these newly diagnosed patients were considered separately the rate of complications for the remaining patients with indeterminate colitis was identical to that from ulcerative colitis patients. Crohn's disease, whether it developed after surgery for ulcerative colitis or indeterminate colitis, was associated with a poor outcome.

It is argued that patients with indeterminate colitis can be offered pouches fairly confidently; the likelihood being their outcome will be similar to ulcerative colitis patients. Even if the patient ends up having Crohn's disease they usually have a good outcome if the surgeon avoids pouch surgery for indeterminate colitis in patients with a clinical suspicion of Crohn's disease [7].

However, pre-operative clinical features do not always correlate with outcome. The indeterminate colitis patient being offered pouch surgery must be adequately counselled as to their risk.

Improving pre-operative decision making

The non-committal pathology report

A pathology report of 'indeterminate colitis' from colonoscopy biopsies means that features of both ulcerative colitis and Crohn's disease are present histologically, and the pathologist cannot commit to either diagnosis. Faced with such a report one must take into account clinical and radiological evidence [18] in order to correctly label the patient's condition. Careful review of further discriminating features after initial pathological uncertainty will allow many cases of indeterminate colitis to be reclassified as either ulcerative colitis or Crohn's disease with reasonable confidence [12]. When clinical features of Crohn's disease are present, such features, along with a histological diagnosis of indeterminate colitis, can predict a poor outcome for restorative proctocolectomy compared to those without them [7, 13]. The patient with a short history provides a particular difficulty.

The most important clinical features of Crohn's disease include the absence of rectal disease and presence of small-bowel or anal disease. A past history of perianal fistula or fissure was found in a substantial proportion of patients who eventually turned out to have Crohn's disease [7]. However, anal disease does not necessarily mean Crohn's disease: around 10% of patients with ulcerative colitis coming to restorative proctocolectomy have an anal lesion, often a low fistula or a fissure [18]. A high fistula, rectovaginal fistula or anal ulcer is more suspicious for Crohn's disease. There must be a thorough examination of the patient, including a search for any extra-intestinal manifestations. The small and large bowel needs to be examined carefully to exclude any features of Crohn's disease. Information from all other possible sources should be pursued, including biopsy and surgical specimens for pathological review as well as clinical, endoscopic and radiological information from other doctors or hospitals. Often colonoscopies have been performed elsewhere or by someone other than the surgeon undertaking the restorative proctocolectomy. If the surgeon is uncertain, he or she should repeat the colonoscopy. Intubation of the terminal ileum at colonoscopy and biopsy is mandatory. Usually the small bowel will have been imaged at some stage, but if not, or if not for some time, then an up-to-date small-bowel enema provides important information.

Staging surgery and deferring definitive pouch construction

Where there is no doubt about the diagnosis, the surgeon and the pathologist should conduct a combined intra-operative macroscopic 'confirmation' of the pre-operative diagnosis of ulcerative colitis in the opened colectomy specimen prior to proctectomy. However, if there is any pre-operative suspicion of Crohn's disease it is unwise to proceed directly to restorative proctocolectomy and the patient should undergo three-stage surgery. A colectomy with ileostomy is performed, giving the pathologist a better specimen on which to make an accurate diagnosis. Restorative proctocolectomy may still be performed at a later date. If Crohn's disease seems likely or is confirmed, then completion proctectomy with ileostomy or ileorectal anastomosis, if the rectum is spared, may be contemplated. There is little evidence as to whether three-stage surgery reduces the incidence of a false-positive diagnosis of ulcerative colitis, or whether surgical morbidity or pouch function is adversely affected. Some surgeons recommend routine staging of surgery in order to be as sure as possible of the diagnosis [8].

However, the situation may not become any clearer after colectomy. This is particularly the case when emergency colectomy has been performed for severe uncontrolled colitis. The severity of the pathological changes frequently obscures any discriminating histological features [19]. A sizeable proportion of Crohn's disease patients undergoing inadvertent restorative proctocolectomy had previously undergone emergency colectomy for severe colitis [12, 18].

Once the colectomy has been performed the rectal stump may yield further useful information. In general terms, the defunctioning of the rectum in UC causes worsening of proctitis, whereas in Crohn's disease proctitis may improve [20]. Multiple biopsies of the rectum should be undertaken. It is important to be aware that the diverted ulcerative colitis rectum can develop histological features of Crohn's disease [21], and that a previously spared rectum in Crohn's disease may become inflamed, underlining the importance of the pre-existing mucosal state [20].

Occasionally surgery cannot be staged preferentially, for example, the patient may wish to avoid a stoma. If there is diagnostic doubt, careful intra-operative macroscopic inspection of the opened colon prior to proctectomy with or without frozen section may be valuable. Pathologists are usually against the use of frozen section in the assessment of inflammatory bowel disease. However, we suggest there is an important role for frozen section in selected circumstances [21].

When the macroscopic appearances of the opened colon lead to diagnostic doubt, we would recommend frozen section from the following sites:
1 *The largest lymph node*: The presence of well-formed granulomas would support a diagnosis of Crohn's disease. Poorly formed granulomas are not enough.
2 *A transmural section of the most severely affected area*: This will assess the presence and pattern of transmural inflammation. Characteristically, in Crohn's disease there are multiple discrete

lymphoid aggregates throughout the full thickness of the bowel wall, particularly on the external border of the muscularis propria. In fulminant ulcerative colitis inflammation may be seen deep into the mucosa, but this is a diffuse inflammatory cell infiltrate at the sites of severe ulceration, and discrete lymphoid aggregates are not seen here.

3 *Macroscopically normal bowel between focal lesions*: This is to look for continuity of mucosal disease. This is often the most useful sample. The only recognised and acceptable 'skip' lesions in ulcerative colitis are in the appendix [22] and the caecal patch lesion [23]. Minor changes should be ignored and the pathologist should be prepared to give one of three firm answers: 'definite ulcerative colitis', 'definite Crohn's disease' or 'I do not know'.

Given that the appearances of the defunctioned rectum in ulcerative colitis may be confused with Crohn's disease [14], there is no role for frozen section of a diverted proctectomy specimen to determine whether a pouch should or should not be constructed.

In tertiary colorectal referral centres there are a high proportion of one- and two-stage pouch procedures. In this setting, careful intra-operative macroscopic evaluation with or without frozen section becomes more important.

Anal fistula in Crohn's disease

These occur in 6–34% of patients with Crohn's disease particularly in those with colonic or rectal disease. Fistulas may be directly secondary to fistulating disease of the anorectum or may be incidental to the Crohn's disease and be of cryptogenic origin.

Treatment may be surgical or non-surgical. The aim of treatment is to cure the fistula and, where possible, minimise recurrence while preserving continence. In Crohn's disease the last goal is important given the prevalence of diarrhoea and short gut in the patients, the reduced rectal compliance secondary to proctitis and the perhaps already impaired continence due to previous anal surgery, anal stenosis and the direct local effects of anal Crohn's disease.

Low fistulae

With low fistulae (sub-cutaneous, inter-sphincteric and low trans-sphincteric fistulae) the controversy revolves around whether these can be simply laid open or not. Most surgeons would lay open a non-Crohn's fistula at these levels, but some consider that special consideration ought to be given to the Crohn's patient and that no sphincter muscle, external or internal, be divided at all. There are two schools of thought. The conservative school is based on the apparent natural history of Crohn's fistulae. In many cases fistulae pursue a relatively benign course; in natural history studies, 15–50% of fistulae seem to heal spontaneously at 2 years [24, 25]. However, reopening or development of new fistulae occurred in up to 44% within 18 months of healing [25], although it may be difficult to distinguish between a healed fistula and a fistula in remission. In one study, fewer than 5% of patients came to proctectomy at 10 years because of fistulous disease [24]. Another concern is the apparent high rate of non-healing of perineal wounds, up to 40% in some studies [26–29]. Furthermore, of course, continence may be impaired, resulting in an incidence of 'iatrogenic' requirement for proctectomy.

However, others have reported successful results with aggressive therapy, questioning the wisdom that local surgery should be avoided in these patients. Sangwan *et al.* reported laying open 35 low fistulae without functional deterioration [30]. This was supported by data from Williams *et al.* [31] and Sohn *et al.* [32]. Wound healing eventually occurred in the majority of cases, although often this was delayed to between 3 and 6 months. The risk of proctectomy for incontinence was very low.

For a disease such as Crohn's that is incurable, where surgery remains palliative, when several other factors contributing to incontinence may be present, and when other therapeutic options are becoming available, it is wise to be conservative.

High fistulae

Laying open these fistulas leaves the patient incontinent because the tract will involve a large amount of external sphincter. After acute suppuration has been dealt with many treatment options exist to choose from, none of which is particularly successful.

Observation

Even if no action is taken, some fistulae will close spontaneously [24, 25]. However, there is a large reactivation rate.

Medical therapy

Medical therapy is appealing in principle, because continence is not jeopardised.

Steroids and aminosalicylates

Closure of a fistula is rare among patients receiving standard therapy only, such as 5-aminosalicylic acid (5-ASA) or corticosteroids. Steroids may prevent the healing of fistulas [33, 34]. Patients with perianal Crohn's disease seem resistant to steroids [35]. It is unclear whether oral aminosalicylates are effective but topical aminosalicylates may be helpful in reducing associated rectal inflammation [34, 36].

Antibiotics

Some antibiotics, including metronidazole and ciprofloxacin, have been anecdotally successful in treating fistulae but have not been properly studied in controlled clinical trials [37, 38].

Immunomodulatory drugs

Some success has been achieved with immunomodulatory agents. There are no controlled trials with fistula closure as the primary end point showing the efficacy of azathioprine or 6-mercaptopurine. Their use in this setting is based on a meta-analysis of 5 controlled studies in which fistula closure was a secondary end point [39].

Intravenous ciclosporin was shown in two small uncontrolled studies to close fistulae, but they recurred on switching to oral ciclosporin [40, 41]. In another small, uncontrolled study, methotrexate closed one-third of fistulae [42].

Newer drugs such as mycophenylate mofetil and tacrolimus have also been used in this context. Fickert et al. [43] used mycophenolate mofetil to treat a small number of patients who had failed treatment with azathioprine, with some success in all cases. However, another study showed less optimistic results. Of 11 patients who had failed treatment with 6-mercaptopurine or azathioprine, mycophenelate was of benefit in only 3 patients [44]. In a study of tacrolimus with either 6-mercaptopurine or azathioprine 7 out of 11 patients treated had a complete response and 4 a partial response [45]. A more recent randomised placebo-controlled trial of tacrolimus found that the drug was not significantly more effective than placebo in causing fistula remission, although it was significantly more likely to result in some improvement [46].

Infliximab

A randomised, placebo-controlled, double-blind trial of infliximab, a chimeric monoclonal antibody to tumour necrosis factor (TNF) for the treatment of Crohn's enterocutaneous or perianal fistulae in 94 patients [47] showed a 50% reduction in the number of draining fistulae in 68% of infliximab-treated patients as compared with 26% for placebo-treated patients ($P = 0.002$). Fistula closure was achieved in 55% as compared with 13% for placebo ($P = 0.001$). Many of these responses were rapid and dramatic. Although infliximab was seen to close fistulas, the median duration of response following the 3-dose induction regimen was only 12 weeks.

To evaluate the efficacy of infliximab maintenance therapy for patients with Crohn's fistulas a multi-centre, double blind, randomised, placebo-controlled trial, ACCENT II, [48] was conducted. This showed that of 282 patients who received infliximab at 0, 2 and 6 weeks, 195 had a response at 10 and 14 weeks. A complete response was seen in 48% of patients at week 14. All patients regardless of response were then randomly assigned to receive placebo or infliximab every 8 weeks and were followed for 54 weeks. The primary analysis was the time to loss of response among patients who had a response at week 14. The time to loss of response was significantly longer in those who received infliximab maintenance therapy. At week 54, 36% in the infliximab maintenance group had a complete absence of a draining fistula compared to 19% of patients in the placebo maintenance group.

Rutgeerts et al. [49] recently published guidelines for optimising anti-TNF treatment and recommended that, as the majority of patients relapse if not re-treated, maintenance doses of infliximab at 8-week intervals are indicated. They stated further that if episodic therapy on relapse is undertaken, as opposed to a regular 8-week regime, maintenance therapy with azathioprine/6-mercaptopurine or methotrexate is mandatory.

Safety problems with antibody treatment have been a concern. The Mayo Clinic reported its experience of 500 patients [50] who received a median three doses of infliximab and were followed up for a median of 17 months. Serious adverse events related to infliximab were observed in 6% of patients. Acute infusion reactions occurred in 3.8%, serum sickness in 2.8%. Three patients developed drug-induced lupus. One patient developed a new demyelinating disorder, and 8.2% had an infectious event attributed to infliximab. Three malignancies were detected, possibly related to infliximab, as were 5 deaths (1%).

In the ACCENT II trial adverse events occurred at the same rate in the placebo maintenance and the infliximab groups. The most common serious adverse event was worsening Crohn's disease. Infections requiring antibiotics occurred in a third of patients. Infusion reactions occurred more often in the infliximab group (4% vs 1%, $p < 0.001$).

Fibrin glue

This has been used to treat other fistulae such as enterocutaneous, non-Crohn's fistulae with some success. Although encouraging short-term results have been achieved in non-Crohn's fistula, with published cure rates of 33–85%, the smaller experience in Crohn's disease is not as good. In five small series [51–55] only 3 out of 26 patients treated were cured (12%), although there was a symptomatic improvement in a proportion of the remaining patients. The role of fibrin glue in the setting of Crohn's disease is not yet defined. No controlled trials are reported as yet.

Surgical therapy

Long-term draining seton

The long-term draining seton has gained popularity in recent years. The aim here is to control the fistula and prevent recurrent sepsis. Faucheron et al. reported on 41 patients with setons and noted a recurrent sepsis rate of 30% requiring an additional seton, as well as a 39% recurrence rate with simple removal [56]. The incontinence rate was 12% and ultimately 12% came to proctectomy, mainly for severe disease. White et al. reported on 16 patients with long-term setons, and noted a recurrent sepsis rate of 11% [57]. No recurrent sepsis developed in two patients, who's setons fell out. Williams et al. published his experience in treating 23 Crohn's fistulae [58]. Recurrent sepsis developed in 75% of 12 patients in whom the seton was removed or fell out, but in 48% of patients sepsis was controlled, allowing the seton to be removed in a minority. Minor incontinence was seen in 26%, and 13% of patients came to proctectomy for severe progressive disease. More recently, Buchanan et al. [59] published long-term follow-up data on six Crohn's disease patients whose complex fistulae were treated with a loose seton. All had at least 10-years follow-up and at this stage five of six patients had relapsed. They stated that the success rate of loose setons falls over time.

It appears that draining setons have a very useful role to play, allowing control of recurrent sepsis with preservation of continence rather than fistula cure. However, recurrent sepsis may occur despite drainage, and the setons may fall out, making recurrence more likely. Significant rates of minor incontinence occur, perhaps related to the diarrhoeal disease, or possibly an unintended cutting seton effect in some. Their precise role as definitive therapy is less clear.

Cutaneous advancement flap

Cutaneous flap advancement has been used recently in small numbers to treat Crohn's disease and non-Crohn's trans-sphincteric fistulae [60, 61]. The rationale is the same as that for endoanal advancement flap, while avoiding the problem of mucosal ectropion. With modest follow-up, four out of nine Crohn's fistulae (44%) were healed. One theoretical concern might be the risk of poor skin healing with flap failure and it would be contraindicated in the presence of otherwise active disease. Its place in the treatment of Crohn's fistula in not defined.

Mucosal advancement flap

A mucosal advancement flap has several attractions. A trans-sphincteric fistula can be closed with minimal risk to continence and a perineal wound, with its associated pain and poor healing, is avoided. The increasing use of flaps has developed because of the concern that aggressive laying open of high fistulae results in a high risk of incontinence, with subsequent need for proctectomy. Rectal advancement flaps have been used in patients with non-Crohn's trans-sphincteric and rectovaginal fistula with good success. The results in Crohn's fistulae are less encouraging. Table 19.1 documents the reported series of rectal advancement flaps for anorectal fistulae in Crohn's disease. Successful closure rates vary from 43 to 92% [62–71]. Makowiec et al. reported a series of 20 flaps where primary closure of the fistula was achieved in 95% [62]. These patients were then closely followed for recurrence over 2 years. Twenty-five per cent of patients experienced recurrence, and if the appearance of new fistulae is included it was even higher. Incontinence was minimal. In this study, recurrence was strongly associated with the presence of colonic rather than small-bowel Crohn's disease. Rectal disease activity is thought to influence surgical success, and there is general agreement that a flap ought not to be attempted in the presence of macroscopic proctitis, which should be controlled medically.

Summary

In the face of numerous treatment options and with little quality evidence to choose between strategies, the following treatment algorithm was published by the American Gastroenterological Association [72]. Fistula treatment should begin with drainage of abscesses and dilatation of ano-rectal strictures. Simple fistulas (low, single external opening and no associated rectovaginal fistula) with no evidence of rectal inflammation can be treated medically with antibiotics and azathioprine or infliximab, or by fistulotomy after formal assessment using an examination under anaesthetic (EUA), and endoanal ultrasound (EUS) or magnetic resonance imaging (MRI). If there is evidence of rectal inflammation treatment should be medical with antibiotics, azathioprine

Table 19.1 Reported series of rectal advancement flaps for anorectal Crohn's fistula.

Study (First author, reference)	Number	Primary failure	Recurrence	Follow-up (months)
Makowiec [62]	20	1/20	4/20	12 (median)
Jones [63]	6	2/6	2/4	3–67
Lewis [64]	6	1/6	–	2–24
Fry [65]	3	0/3	–	–
Joo [66]*	8	–	–	–
Ozuner [67]*	47	–	15/47	31 (median)
Kodner [68]*	24	–	7/24	–
Sonoda [69]*	44	–	22/44	17 (median)
Mizrahi [70]*	28	–	16/28	40 (median)
Hyman [71]	14	4/14	3/14	
Total	200	8/49 (16%)	69/181 (38%)	–

* Report mixed rectovaginal and anorectal fistulae: 50% anorectal fistulae [67]; 33% anorectal fistulae [68]; 25% anorectal fistulae [66]; anorectal fistulae 63% [69]; anorectal fistulae 56% [70].

and infliximab or tacrolimus considered in selected patients. A loose seton may also be employed.

Complex fistulas (high, and/or with multiple external openings, rectovaginal fistula and anorectal stricture) should be assessed as above and treated initially with antibiotics, infliximab, azathioprine or 6-mercaptopurine, followed by maintenance therapy with azathioprine or 6-mercaptopurine, in some cases combined with infliximab. Placement of loose setons or the use of advancement flaps is reserved for those patients who fail medical therapy. Advancement flaps should not be attempted in the presence of macroscopic rectal inflammation. Tacrolimus or ciclosporin can be considered in selected patients who fail multi-modal treatment, including infliximab, before proceeding to faecal diversion or proctectomy.

It should always be borne in mind that Crohn's disease is incurable, and as such all therapies are palliative and must be conservative. The aim should be to control the patient's symptoms with the least risk to continence, aiming for maximal rectal conservation. However, in cases where function is poor because of severe Crohn's disease, about 10% of patients will ultimately be better served by proctectomy and permanent ileostomy.

Laparoscopic surgery for Crohn's disease

Patients with Crohn's disease are likely to require surgery at some stage and may often require more than one operation. Laparoscopic surgery has several potential benefits in a Crohn's setting. Limiting the extent of such surgery has always been a goal because Crohn's patients tend to heal badly. Reducing the surgical insult (with a reduced size of incision) may result in less impairment of the patient's immunological system, which is already compromised in Crohn's patients, especially if being treated with immunosuppressive drugs. Smaller incisions may also result in fewer adhesions. Cosmesis is an important concern to many patients and is better with laparoscopic surgery. Additionally, there may be the benefits of quicker recovery time and shorter hospital stay.

However, it is controversial as to whether the potential benefits of the laparoscopic approach are so great as to compensate for the extra technical difficulty involved and with this the potential for increased complications. Morbidity and mortality outcomes remain the most important end points in judging between open and laparoscopic surgery. It is clearly also important to show that long-term outcomes in terms of disease recurrence are also similar.

Considering papers produced over the last 5 years describing different authors' experience of laparoscopic surgery for bowel resection in Crohn's disease, most actually describe laparoscopically assisted surgery rather than pure laparoscopic surgery. The most common operation described is ileocaecal resection. The majority of the publications detail retrospective series or case control studies with only one prospective randomised trial existing.

Milsom *et al.* [73] reported a prospective randomised trial from the Cleveland Clinic of 60 patients undergoing surgical resection for Crohn's disease. Thirty-one patients were assigned to the laparoscopic group and 29 to the open group; all had isolated Crohn's disease of the terminal ileum with or without caecal involvement. Length of incision was 5cm in the laparoscopic group and 12 cm in the open group. Lung function recovered faster in the laparoscopic group. There was no significant difference in the time to return of bowel movement, the amount of morphine equivalents, or major complications. Minor complications were lower in the laparoscopic group. The length of stay was shorter by a day in the laparoscopic group (5 vs 6). All patients followed an identical and highly controlled peri-operative protocol.

Eighteen papers were identified from the literature [74–91] describing series of laparoscopic bowel resections for Crohn's disease in the last 5 years. Reviewing these, the following general comments can be made. Surgical time for laparoscopic operations tends to be longer than for open operations. Conversion rates from laparoscopic to open range from 4–29%, the median percentage quoted being 14.6%. Complications were not significantly different between the laparoscopic and open groups where such a comparison could be made (10 papers). Post-operative analgesic requirements, time to return of bowel function and hospital stay all tended to be lower for the laparoscopic patients. Return to bowel function was typically 2–3 days earlier in the laparoscopic patients and hospital discharge tended to be 3 days earlier in this group.

There is a lack of consensus as to whether patients with large fixed masses, complex fistulas or recurrent Crohn's disease are suitable for the laparoscopic approach, but most of the authors would attempt such cases and accept that the conversion rate to open would be higher than in more straightforward patients. Laparoscopic surgery has been successfully used to treat children and adolescents [74, 88, 91]. No paper showed differences in disease recurrence rates between the groups. Less symptomatic bowel obstruction was seen in the laparoscopic group in 30 months of follow up in one paper [87], perhaps suggesting fewer adhesions in this group. Two papers suggest lower costs in the laparoscopic group [84, 89].

In a recent review, Milsom [92] suggested it was possible that many of the short-term benefits of laparoscopic surgery over open surgery will be removed or at least considerably reduced when progressive multi-modal peri-operative management is used. If this is the case the principal arguments for laparoscopic surgery will be cosmesis and the possible reduction in long-term complications relating to a larger abdominal wound in open surgery. Multi-centre randomised trials with lengthy follow-up would of course answer such questions definitively. However, recruitment to such trials may be difficult if patients feel cosmesis to be a high priority and cannot be shown current evidence of a clear downside to the laparoscopic approach.

Sylla *et al.* [93], in comprehensive review article, have recently looked at the possible immunological benefits of laparoscopic surgery. Surgical trauma results in deleterious alterations in immune function. Laparoscopic surgery is associated with less pronounced perturbations in immune function than open surgery. This was seen for a number of pro-inflammatory and acute phase proteins. However, documented post-operative alterations have not been definitely associated with specific differences in clinical outcome. They conclude that the evaluation of peri-operative immune function warrants further investigation.

Minimising post-surgical recurrence

5-ASA agents and other therapies

Surgery has little effect on the rate of recurrence after resection for Crohn's disease. Recurrence remains a major problem with about 50% of patients relapsing by 10 years and a significant proportion demonstrating endoscopic preanastomotic recurrence within months of the primary operation. It was once believed that wide surgical resection might influence recurrence, but this has not been shown to be the case. Recurrence is lowest where there is no anastomosis and an end ileostomy and highest after ileorectal anastomosis.

To improve recurrence rates interest has been shown in adjuvant medical therapy after surgical resection. Most interest is in the 5-ASA agents. The results of trials using various 5-ASA formulations have been inconclusive and such prophylactic therapy remains controversial.

Five of seven placebo-controlled trials of the prophylactic effects of mesalamine compounds failed to show any benefit [94–98]. In one study there was less severe recurrence in the mesalamine group. The largest placebo-controlled study showed a reduction in the risk of relapse of 19% (45–26%) after 3 years prophylaxis with 4 g of a coated, pH-dependent release formulation [99]. The results of this trial eclipsed previous studies and it was recommended that adjuvant therapy be adopted.

However, recent data have emerged casting doubt on the efficacy of prophylaxis. A meta-analysis of published studies concluded that the risk reduction was 0.13 with mesalamine (95% CI 0.05–0.21) [100]. Additionally, the results of what was hoped would be the definitive trial of prophylaxis have been published [101]. The trial addressed some of the perceived shortcomings of previous studies: all patients were entered within 10 days of resection, the maximum recommended dose for the micro-sphere formulation of mesalamine (Pentasa) was used, and in a preparation that released the drug along the whole length of the small bowel. Three hundred and eighteen patients were randomised to receive 4 g of Pentasa or placebo. On an intention-to-treat analysis, the recurrence rate in the active arm was 24.5% and 31.4% in the placebo arm ($P = 0.1$).

What should be made of these results? If we conclude that routine use of 5-ASA prophylaxis is not indicated, are there selected subsets of patients who may benefit and can we target them? What are the other alternatives? Although theoretically attractive, it is difficult to identify early relapsers or high-risk patients. Those with more extensive disease, and inflammatory rather than fibrostenosing disease, should *a priori* be given the possible benefit of adjuvant therapy until further evidence becomes available.

What other prophylactic options are available? Metronidazole (20 mg/kg or 400 mg bd for 3 months) and metronidazole-like drugs have been studied, with a significant reduction in clinical relapse at 12 months but not sustained over time [102]. Budesonide 6 mg has been compared to placebo in a double-blind randomised trial of 129 patients after ileal or ileocaecal resection for Crohn's disease [103]. There was no significant difference in endoscopic recurrence between the two groups at 12 months. This parallels pooled budesonide data in maintenance of medical remission [104]. Although recurrence was reduced with budesonide for those in whom the indication for surgery was disease activity rather than fibrostenotic disease (32% vs 65%, $P = 0.047$), it may be statistically unjustified to draw any subset conclusions from a negative study. Although methotrexate and azathioprine have been shown to be effective in preventing relapse after medically induced remission, the post-surgical data that are available are in most cases disappointing [105, 106]. Alves *et al.* [107] found that patients following a second resection for Crohn's who were treated with azathioprine, 6-mercaptopurine or methotrexate had a significantly lower level of clinical recurrence at 3 years (25% vs 60%, $P < 0.05$) than those given either salicylates or no treatment. This difference lost significance at a mean follow up time of 80 months. 6-mercaptopurine has been shown in a double blind randomised multicentre trial to be more effective than placebo in preventing clinical recurrence over 2 years (50% vs 77%, $P < 0.05$) [98]. Because recurrence rates are highest in smokers, especially young females,

probably the best thing we can do for patients is to encourage smokers to give up [108]. Ex-smokers quickly adopt the recurrence risk profile of non-smokers [109].

Stapled ileocolic anastomoses

It has been suggested that the anastomotic configuration after ileal or ileocaecal resection for Crohn's disease may influence the rate of symptomatic or surgical recurrence. The rationale for this lies in the known high early preanastomotic recurrence as documented by endoscopy [110, 111] and the notion that a standard end-to-end anastomosis produces the narrowest lumen and so may make anastomotic recurrence more likely to be symptomatic. This is, however, controversial. Scott reported on a series of 102 anastomoses constructed over 20 years [112]. In the first 12 years, an end-to-side ileocolic anastomosis was used. Thereafter, a side-to-side configuration was preferred. It was thought that by producing a larger lumen, symptomatic recurrence might be reduced or delayed. Although the median follow-up was dissimilar, on an actuarial assessment there was no difference in recurrence. Similarly Cameron *et al.*, in a prospective randomised study, found no difference between end-to-end and side-to-end anastomosis [113].

Conversely, in a multi-centre randomised trial on the effectiveness of post-resection 5-ASA agents in reducing recurrence, a trend to less recurrence was seen in those who had anastomoses other than end-to-end, and this reached significance in those on a 5-ASA agent using multivariate analysis [114]. A report from Mayo and Birmingham retrospectively comparing so-called wide-lumen stapled anastomosis to a matched group who had undergone sutured end-to-end anastomosis showed fewer symptomatic recurrences (24% vs 57%) and a significantly ($P = 0.017$) lower cumulative re-operation rate for the wide stapled anastomosis [115]. Further trials will be reporting shortly.

It is difficult to be clear about the claimed advantage of leaving a wider anastomotic lumen. Some surgeons express concern at stapling in Crohn's disease due to the often thickened bowel wall, but there is no evidence for an increase in anastomotic leaks.

References

1. Panis Y, Poupard B, Nemeth J, Lavergne A, Hautefeuille P, Valleur P. Ileal pouch/anal anastomosis for Crohn's disease. *Lancet* 1996;347: 854–7.
2. Phillips RKS. Ileal pouch-anal anastomosis for Crohn's disease. *Gut* 1998;43:303–4.
3. Regimbeau JM, Panis Y, Pocard M, et al. Long-term results of ileal pouch-anal anastomoses for colorectal Crohn's disease. *Dis Colon Rectum* 2001;44:769–78.
4. Hartley JE, Fazio VW, Remzi FH, et al. Analysis of the outcome of ileal pouch-anal anastomoses in patients with Crohn's disease. *Dis Colon Rectum* 2004;47: 1808–15.
5. Braveman JM, Schoetz DJ, Marcello PW, et al. The fate of the ileal pouch in patients developing Crohn's disease. *Dis Colon Rectum* 2004;47:1613–19.
6. Kock NG, Myrvold HE. Progress report on the continent ileostomy. *World J Surg* 1980;4:143–8.
7. Hyman NH, Fazio VW, Tuckson WB, Lavery IC. Consequences of ileal pouch-anal anastomosis for Crohn's colitis. *Dis Colon Rectum* 1991;34:653–7.
8. Lucarotti ME, Freeman BJC, Warren BF, Durdey P. Synchronous proctocolectomy and ileoanal pouch formation and the risk of Crohn's disease. *Br J Surg* 1995;82:755–6.
9. Grobler SP, Hosie KB, Thompson H, Keighley MRB. Outcome of restorative proctocolectomy when the diagnosis is suggestive of Crohn's disease. *Gut* 1993; 34:1384–8.
10. Sagar PM, Dozois RR, Wolff BG. Long-term results of ileal pouch-anal anastomosis in patients with Crohn's disease. *Dis Colon Rectum* 1996;39:893–8.
11. Deutsch AA, McLeod RS, Cullen J, Cohen Z. Results of the pelvic-pouch procedure in patients with Crohn's disease. *Dis Colon Rectum* 1991;34:475–7.
12. Wells AD, McMillan I, Price AB, Ritchie JK, Nicholls RJ. Natural history of indeterminate colitis. *Br J Surg* 1991;78:179–81.
13. McIntyre PB, Pemberton JH, Wolff BG, Dozois RR, Beart RW. Indeterminate colitis: long-term outcome in patients after ileal pouch-anal anastomosis. *Dis Colon Rectum* 1995;38:51–5.
14. Warren BF, Shepherd NA, Bartolo DCC, Bradfield JWB. Pathology of the defunctioned rectum in ulcerative colitis. *Gut* 1993;34:514–16.
15. Koltun WA, Schoetz DJ, Roberts PL, Murray JJ, Coller JA, Veidenheimer MC. Indeterminate colitis predisposes to perineal complications after ileal pouch-anal surgery. *Dis Colon Rectum* 1991;34: 857–60.
16. Pishori T, Dinnewitzer A, Zmora O, et al. Outcome of patients with indeterminate colitis undergoing a double-stapled ileal pouch-anal anastomoses. *Dis Colon Rectum* 2004;47:717–21.
17. Yu CS, Pemberton JH, Larson D. Ileal pouch-anal anastomoses in patients with indeterminate colitis: long term results. *Dis Colon Rectum* 2000;43: 1487–96.
18. Nicholls RJ, Bartolo DCC, Mortensen NJ McC. *Restorative Proctocolectomy.* 1st ed. Oxford: Blackwell Scientific Publications, 1993.
19. Tytgat GNJ, Bartelsman JFW, van Deventer SJH. What is indeterminate colitis? In: *Inflammatory Bowel Diseases.* Falk Symposium 85.
20. Edwards CM, George BD, Warren BF. Diversion colitis a new light through old windows. *Histopathology* 1999;34:1–5.
21. Warren BF, Shepherd NA. The role of pathology in pelvic ileal reservoir surgery. *Int J Colorectal Dis* 1992;7:68–75.
22. Davison AM, Dixon MF. The appendix as a 'skip lesion' in ulcerative colitis. *Histopathology* 1990;16: 93–5.
23. D'Haens G, Geboes K, Peeters M, Baert F, Ectors N, Rutgeerts P. Patchy caecal inflammation associated with distal ulcerative colitis: a prospective endoscopic study. *Am J Gastroenterol* 1997;92: 1275–9.
24. Buchmann P, Keighley MRB, Allan RN, Thompson H, Alexander-Williams J. Natural history of perianal Crohn's disease. Ten year follow-up: a plea for conservatism. *Am J Surg* 1980;140:642–4.
25. Makowiec F, Jehle EC, Starlinger M. Clinical course of perianal fistulas in Crohn's disease. *Gut* 1995;37: 696–701.
26. Hellers G, Bergstrand O, Ewerth S, Holmström B. Occurrence and outcome after primary treatment of anal fistulae in Crohn's disease. *Gut* 1980;21: 525–7.
27. Bernard D, Morgan S, Tassé D. Selective surgical management of Crohn's disease of the anus. *Can J Surg* 1986;29:318–321.
28. Levien DH, Surrell J, Mazier WP. Surgical treatment of anorectal fistula in patients with Crohn's disease. *Surg Gynaecol Obstet* 1989;169:133–6.
29. Baker WN, Milton-Thompson GJ. Management of anal fistulas in Crohn's disease. *Proc R Soc Med* 1974;67:58.
30. Sangwan YP, Schoetz DJ Jr, Murray JJ, Roberts PL, Coller JA. Perianal Crohn's disease: results of local surgical treatment. *Dis Colon Rectum* 1996;39: 529–35.
31. Williams JG, Rothenberger DA, Nemer FD, Goldberg SM. Fistula-in-ano in Crohn's disease: results of aggressive surgical treatment. *Dis Colon Rectum* 1991;34:378–84.

32. Sohn N, Korelitz BI, Weinstein MA. Anorectal Crohn's disease: definitive surgery for fistulas and recurrent abscesses. *Am J Surg* 1980;139:394-7.
33. Singh B, Mortensen NJ, Jewell DP, George B. Perianal Crohn's disease. *Br J Surg* 2004;91:801-14.
34. Lichtenstein GR. Treatment of fistulizing Crohn's disease. *Gastroenterology* 2000;119:1132-47.
35. Gelbmann CM, Rogler G, Gross V, et al. Prior bowel resections, perianal disease, and a high initial Crohn's disease activity index are associated with corticosteroid resistancein active Crohn's disease. *Am J Gastroenterol* 2002;97:1438-45.
36. Basu A, Wexner SD. Perianal Crohn's disease. *Curr Treat Options Gastroenterol* 2002;5:197-206.
37. Brandt LJ, Bernstein LH, Boley SJ, Frank MS. Metronidazole therapy for perineal Crohn's disease: a follow-up study. *Gastroenterology* 1982;83:383-7.
38. Solomon MJ, McLeod RS, O'Connor BI, Steinhart AH, Greenberg GR, Cohen Z. Combination ciprofloxacin and metronidazole in severe perianal Crohn's disease. *Can J Gastroenterology* 1993;7:571-3.
39. Pearson DC, May GR, Fick GH, Sutherland LR. Azathioprine and 6-mercaptopurine in Crohn disease: a meta-analysis. *Ann Intern Med* 1995;123:132-42.
40. Hanauer SB, Smith MB. Rapid closure of Crohn's disease fistulas with continuous intravenous cyclosporin A. *Am J Gastroenterol* 1993;88:646-9.
41. Present DH, Lichtiger S. Efficacy of cyclosporin in treatment of fistula of Crohn's disease. *Dig Dis Sci* 1994;39:374-80.
42. Mahadevan U, Marion JF, Present DH. The place for methotrexate in the treatment of refractory Crohn's disease [Abstract]. *Gastroenterology* 1997;112(Suppl):A1031.
43. Fickert P, Hinterleitner TA, Wenzl HH, Aichbichler BW, Petritsch W. Mycophenolate mofetil in patients with Crohn's disease. *Am J Gastroenterol* 1998;93:2529-32.
44. Hassard PV, Vasiliaus kas EA, Kam LY, Targan SR, Abreu MT. Efficacy of mycophenolate mofetil in patients failing 6-mercaptopurine or azathioprine therapy for Crohn's disease. *Inflamm Bowel Dis* 2000;6:16-20.
45. Lowry PW, Weaver AL, Tremaine WJ, sandborn WJ. Combination therapy with oral tacrolimus (FK506) and azathioprine or 6-mercaptopurine for treatment-refractory Crohn's disease perianal fistulae. *Inflamm Bowel Dis* 1999;5:239-45.
46. Sandborn WJ, Present DH, Isaacs KL, et al. Tacrolimus for the treatment of fistulas in patients with Crohn's disease: a randomized, placebo controlled trial. *Gastroenterology* 2003;125:380-8.
47. Present DH, Rutgeerts P, Targan S, et al. Infliximab for the treatment of fistulas in patients with Crohn's disease. *New Engl J Med* 1999;340:1398-1405.
48. Sands BE, Anderson FH, Bernstein CN, et al. Infliximab maintenance therapy for fistulizing Crohn's disease. *N Engl J Med* 2004;350:876-85.
49. Rutgeerts P, Van Assche G, Vermeire S. Optimizing anti-TNF treatment in inflammatory bowel disease. *Gastroenterology* 2004;126:1593-1610.
50. Colombel JF, Loftus EV, Tremaine WJ, et al. The safety profile of infliximab in patients with Crohn's disease: the Mayo clinic experience in 500 patients. *Gastroenterology* 2004;126:19-31.
51. Cintron JR, Park JJ, Orsay CP, Pearl RK, Nelson RL, Abcarian H. Repair of fistulas-in-ano using autologous fibrin tissue adhesive. *Dis Colon Rectum* 1999;42:607-13.
52. Abel ME, Chiu YS, Russell TR, Volpe PA. Autologous fibrin glue in the treatment of rectovaginal and complex fistulas. *Dis Colon Rectum* 1993;36:447-9.
53. Venkatesh KS, Ramanujam P. Fibrin glue in the treatment of recurrent anorectal fistulas. *Dis Colon Rectum* 1999;42:1136-9.
54. Lindsey I, Smilgin-Humphreys MM, Cunningham C, Mortensen NJ, George BD. A randomized, controlled trial of fibrin glue vs. conventional treatment for anal fistula. *Dis Colon Rectum* 2002;45:1608-15.
55. Zmora O, Mizrahi N, Rotholtz N, et al. Fibrin glue sealing in the treatment of perineal fistulas. *Dis Colon Rectum* 2003;46:584-9.
56. Faucheron J-L, Olivier S-M, Guibert L, Parc R. Long-term seton drainage for high anal fistulas in Crohn's disease sphincter-saving operation? *Dis Colon Rectum* 1996;39:208-11.
57. White RA, Eisenstat TE, Rubin RJ, Salvati EP. Seton management of complex anorectal fistulas in patients with Crohn's disease. *Dis Colon Rectum* 1990;33:587-9.
58. Williams JG, MacLeod CA, Rothenberger DA, Goldberg SM. Seton treatment of high anal fistulae. *Br J Surg* 1991;78:1159-61.
59. Buchanan GN, Owen HA, Torkington J, Lunniss PJ, Nicholls RJ, Cohen CR. Long term outcome following loose-seton technique for external sphincter preservation in complex anal fistula. *Br J Surg* 2004; 91:476-80.
60. Robertson WG, Mangione JS. Cutaneous advancement flap closure: alternative method for treatment of complicated anal fistulas. *Dis Colon Rectum* 1998;41:884-7.
61. Del Pino A, Nelson RL, Pearl RK, Abcarian H. Island flap anoplasty for treatment of transsphincteric fistula-in-ano. *Dis Colon Rectum* 1996;39:224-46.

62 Makowiec F, Jehle EC, Becker HD, Starlinger M. Clinical course after transanal advancement flap repair of perianal fistula in patients with Crohn's disease. *Br J Surg* 1995;82:603–6.

63 Jones IT, Fazio VW, Jagelman DG. The use of transanal rectal advancement flaps in the management of fistulas involving the anorectum. *Dis Colon Rectum* 1987;30:919–23.

64 Lewis P, Bartolo DCC. Treatment of trans-sphincteric fistulae by full thickness anorectal advancement flaps. *Br J Surg* 1990;77:1187–89, 97.

65 Fry RD, Shemesh EI, Kodner IJ, Timmcke A. Techniques and results in the management of anal and perianal Crohn's disease. *Surg Gynaecol Obstet* 1989;68:42–8.

66 Joo JS, Weiss EG, Nogueras JJ, Wexner SD. Endorectal advancement flap in perianal Crohn's disease. *Am Surg* 1998;64:147–50.

67 Ozuner G, Hull TL, Cartmill J, Fazio VW. Long-term analysis of the use of transanal rectal advancement flaps for complicated anorectal/vaginal fistulas. *Dis Colon Rectum* 1996;39:10–14.

68 Kodner IJ, Mazor A, Shemesh EI, Fry RD, Fleshman JW, Birnbaum EH. Endo rectal advancement flap repair of rectovaginal and other complicated anorectal fistulas. *Surgery* 1993;114:682–90.

69 Sonoda T, Hull T, Piedmonte MR, Fazio VW. Outcomes of primary repair of anorectal and rectovaginal fistulas using the endorectal advancement flap. *Dis Colon Rectum* 2002;45:1622–88.

70 Mizrahi N, Wexner SD, Zmora O, et al. Endorectal advancement flap: are there predictors of failure? *Dis Colon Rectum* 2002;45:1616–21.

71 Hyman N. Endoanal advancement flap repair for complex anorectal fistulas. *Am J Surg* 1999;178:337–40.

72 Sandborn WJ, Fazio VW, Feagan BG, Hanauer SB. AGA technical review on perianal crohn's disease. *Gastroenterology* 2003;125:1508–30.

73 Milsom JW, Hammerhofer KA, Bohm B, Marcello P, Elson P, Fazio VW. Prospective randomized trial comparing laparoscopic vs. conventional surgery for refractory ileocolic Crohn's disease. *Dis Colon Rectum* 2001;44:1–8.

74 von Allmen D, Markowitz JE, York A, Mamula P, Shepanski M, Baldassano R. Laparoscopic-assisted bowel resection offers advantages over open surgery for treatment of segmental Crohn's disease in children. *J Paediatr Surg* 2003;38:963–5.

75 Evans J, Poritz L, MacRae H. Influence of experience on laparoscopic ileocolic resection for Crohn's disease. *Dis Colon Rectum* 2002;45:1595–1600.

76 Hamel CT, Pikarsky AJ, Wexner SD. Laparoscopically assisted hemicolectomy for Crohn's disease: are we still getting better? *Am Surg* 2002;68:83–6.

77 Luan X, Gross E. Laparoscopic assisted surgery for Crohn's disease an initial experience and results. *J Tongji Med Univ* 2000;20:332–5.

78 Tabet J, Hong D, Kim CW, Wong J, Goodacre R, Anvari M. Laparoscopic versus open bowel resection for Crohn's disease. *Can J Gastroenterol* 2001;15:237–42.

79 Huilgol RL, Wright CM, Solomon MJ. Laparoscopic versus open ileocolic resection for Crohn's disease. *J Laparoendosc Adv Surg Tech A* 2004;14:61–5.

80 Bergamaschi R, Pessaux P, Arnaud JP. Comparison of conventional and laparoscopic ileocolic resection for Crohn's disease. *Dis Colon Rectum* 2003;46:1129–33.

81 Hasegawa H, Watanabe M, Nishibori H, Okabayashi K, Hibi T, Kitajima M. Laparoscopic surgery for recurrent Crohn's disease. *Br J Surg* 2003;90:970–3.

82 Benoist S, Panis Y, Beaufour A, Bouhnik Y, Matuchansky C, Valleur P. Laparoscopic ileocecal resection in Crohn's disease: a case-matched comparison with open resection. *Surg Endosc* 2003;17:814–18.

83 Shore G, Gonzalez QH, Bondora A, Vickers SM. Laparoscopic vs conventional ileocolectomy for primary Crohn disease. *Arch Surg* 2003;138:76–9.

84 Duepree HJ, Senagore AJ, Delaney CP, Brady KM, Fazio VW. Advantages of laparoscopic resection for ileocecal Crohn's disease. *Dis Colon Rectum* 2002;45:605–10.

85 Bemelman WA, Slors JF, Dunker MS, et al. Laparoscopic-assisted vs. open ileocolic resection for Crohn's disease: a comparative study. *Surg Endosc* 2000;14:721–5.

86 Msika S, Iannelli A, Deroide G, et al. Can laparoscopy reduce hospital stay in the treatment of Crohn's disease? *Dis Colon Rectum* 2001;44:1661–6.

87 Alabaz O, Iroatulam AJ, Nessim A, Weiss EG, Nogueras JJ, Wexner SD. Comparison of laparoscopically assisted and conventional ileocolic resection for Crohn's disease. *Eur J Surg* 2000;166:213–17.

88 Diamond IR, Langer JC. Laparoscopic-assisted versus open ileocolic resection for adolescent Crohn disease. *J Pediatr Gastroenterol Nutr* 2001;33:543–7.

89 Young-Fadok TM, HallLong K, McConnell EJ, Gomez Rey G, Cabanel RL. Advantages of laparoscopic resection for ileocolic Crohn's disease: improved outcomes and reduced costs. *Surg Endosc* 2001;15:450–4.

90 Motson RW, Kadirkamanathan SS, Gallegos N. Minimally invasive surgery for ileo-colic Crohn's disease. *Colorectal Dis* 2002;4:127–31.

91 Dutta S, Rothenberg SS, Chang J, Bealer J. Total intracorporeal laparoscopic resection of Crohn's disease. *J Pediatr Surg* 200;38:717–19.

92 Milsom JW. Laparoscopic surgery in the treatment of Crohn's disease. *Surg Clin N Am* 2005;85:25–34.

93 Sylla P, Kirman I, Whelan RL. Immunological advantages of advanced laparoscopy. *Surg Clin N Am* 2005;85:1–18.

94 Florent CH, Cortot A, Quandale P, *et al*. Placebo-controlled clinical trial of mesalazine in the prevention of early endoscopic recurrences after resection for Crohn's disease. *Eur J Gastroenterol Hepatol* 1996;8:229–33.

95 Fiasse R, Fontaine F, Vanheurverzwyn R. Prevention of Crohn's disease recurrence after intestinal resection with Eudragid-L-coated 5-aminosalicylic acid. Preliminary results of a one-year double-blind placebo-controlled study [Abstract]. *Gastroenterology* 1991;100:A208.

96 Sutherland LR, Martin F, Bailey RJ, Fedorak RN, Poleski M, Dallaire C. A randomised, placebo-controlled, double-blind trial of mesalamine in the maintenance of remission of Crohn's disease. *Gastroenterology* 1997;112:1069–77.

97 Lochs H, Mayer M, Fleig WE, Mortensen PB, Bauer P. Prophylaxis of postoperative relapse in Crohn's disease with mesalazine (Pentasa) in comparison to placebo. *Gastroenterology* 1997;112(Suppl 4):A1027.

98 Hanauer SB, Korelitz BI, Rutgeerts P, *et al*. Postoperative maintenance of Crohn's disease remission with 6-mercaptopurine, mesalamine, or placebo: a 2-year trial. *Gastroenterology* 2004;127:723–9.

99 McLeod RS, Wolff BG, Steinhart AH, *et al*. Prophylactic mesalamine treatment decreases postoperative recurrence of Crohn's disease. *Gastroenterology* 1995;109:404–13.

100 Camma C, Giunta M, Roselli M, Cottone M. Mesalamine in the maintenance treatment of Crohn's disease: a meta-analysis adjusted for confounding. *Gastroenterology* 1997;113:1465–73.

101 Lochs H, Mayer M, Fleig WE, *et al*. Prophylaxis of postoperative relapse in Crohn's disease with mesalamine: European cooperative Crohn's disease study VI. *Gastroenterology* 2000;118:264–73.

102 Rutgeerts P, Peeters M, Hiele M, *et al*. A placebo-controlled trial of metronidazole for recurrence prevention of Crohn's disease after resection of the terminal ileum [Abstract]. *Gastroenterology* 1992;102:A688.

103 Hellers G, Cortot A, Jewell D, *et al*. Oral budesonide for prevention of postsurgical recurrence in Crohn's disease. *Gastroenterology* 1999;116:294–300.

104 Feagan B, Greenberg GR, Löfberg R, Ferguson A, Persson T. Budesonide controlled ileal release prolongs remission in Crohn's disease (CD): a pooled analysis [Abstract]. *Gastroenterology* 1997;112:A970.

105 Feagan B, McDonald JW, Hopkins M, Wong C, Koval J. A randomised controlled trial of methotrexate (MTX) as a maintenance therapy for chronically active Crohn's disease (CD) [Abstract]. *Gut* 1999;45(Suppl):A131.

106 Pearson DC, May GR, Fick G, Sutherland LR. Azothiaprine and 6-mercaptopurine in Crohn's disease: a meta-analysis. *Ann Intern Med* 1995;123:132–42.

107 Alves A, Panis Y, Joly F, Pocard M, Lavergne-Slove A, Bouhnik Y, Valleur P. Could immunosuppressive drugs reduce recurrence rate after second resection for Crohn disease? *Inflamm Bowel Dis* 2004;10:491–5.

108 Sutherland LR, Ramcharan S, Bryant H, Fick G. Effect of cigarette smoking on recurrence of Crohn's disease. *Gastroenterology* 1990;98:1123–8.

109 Cottone M, Rosselli M, Orlando A, *et al*. Smoking habits and recurrence in Crohn's disease. *Gastroenterology* 1994;106:643–8.

110 Rutgeerts P, Geboes K, Vantrappen G, Kerremans R, Cenegrachts JL, Coremans G. Natural history of recurrent Crohn's disease at the ileocolonic anastomosis after curative surgery. *Gut* 1984;25:665–72.

111 Olaison G, Smed LK, Sjodahl R. Natural course of Crohn's disease after ileocolic resection: endoscopically visualised ileal ulcers preceding symptoms. *Gut* 1991;33:331–5.

112 Scott NA, Sue-Ling HM, Hughes LE. Anastomotic configuration does not affect recurrence of Crohn's disease after ileocolonic resection. *Int J Colorect Dis* 1995;10:67–9.

113 Cameron JL, Hamilton SR, Coleman J, Sitzman JV, Bayless TM. Patterns of ileal recurrence in Crohn's disease: a prospective randomised study. *Ann Surg* 1992;215:546–52.

114 Caprilli R, Corrao G, Taddei G, *et al*. Prognostic factors for postoperative recurrence of Crohn's disease. *Dis Colon Rectum* 1996;39:335–41.

115 Munoz-Juarez M, Yamamoto T, Wolff BG, Keighley MR. Wide-lumen stapled anastomoses vs. conventional end-to-end anastomoses in the treatment of Crohn's disease. *Dis Colon Rectum* 2001;44:20–5.

20: Perianal Crohn's disease

Carl J. Brown and Robin S. McLeod

Introduction

Gabriel described the presence of multi-nucleated giant cells in the tissues of patients with rectal fistulae nearly 10 years prior to the sentinel description of Crohn's disease by Crohn, Ginzberg and Oppenheimer [1, 2]. Although the significance of this discovery was not appreciated at the time, subsequently Bissell was able to show an association between 'regional enteritis' and perianal disease [3]. It is now accepted that perianal disease occurs frequently and is a cause of morbidity in patients with Crohn's disease.

There is great variation in the reported frequency of perianal lesions. These discrepancies are likely due to differences in the intensity of the search made for anal lesions and in the definition of what constitutes perianal Crohn's disease. In addition, most reviews have been performed retrospectively. Rates ranging from 32 to 80% have been reported [4–7]. Although the rates vary from series to series, there is consistency in reporting a higher frequency of perianal lesions in patients with colonic or rectal disease. In a retrospective study, Fielding reviewed 167 patients and found that 80% had perianal complications [4]. The National Crohn's Cooperative Disease Study (NCCDS) was a prospective study that reported on the prevalence of perianal disease [6]. Only fissures, fistulae and abscesses were considered. Overall, of the 569 patients entered into the study, 36% gave a history of perianal disease before randomisation, including 14% who had perianal complications at the time of randomisation. During the study, an additional 70 (12%) developed perianal complications. Palder et al. reported that 200 of 325 (62%) paediatric patients with Crohn's disease developed perianal manifestations [8]. This included skin tags in 35%, fissures in 51%, fistulae in 15% and abscesses in 13%. Approximately three-quarters of these patients with perianal disease had a perianal symptom as part of their initial presentation.

There is a wide range of perianal manifestations of Crohn's disease. Buchmann and Alexander-Williams classified perianal disease into the following categories: (1) skin lesions, including maceration, erosion, ulceration, superficial abscess formation and skin tags; (2) anal canal lesions, including fissure, ulcer and stenosis; and (3) fistulae, encompassing low, high and recto-vaginal fistulae [9]. In this classification, skin lesions are usually considered to be due to diarrhoea and local irritation resulting in maceration and subsequent ulceration and subcutaneous abscess formation. Non-operative management only is required. Anal canal lesions and fistulae will be reviewed in this chapter.

Measurement of perianal Crohn's disease severity

In 1995, Irvine proposed the Perianal Disease Activity Index (PDAI) as a tool to assess perianal disease severity [10]. This instrument includes five elements of perianal disease and each item is evaluated using a five-point Likert scale (Table 20.1). This tool has been validated against physician (MDGA) and patient (PGA) global assessments. In a recent review,

Table 20.1 Perianal disease activity index (PDAI) [10].

Categories affected by fistulae		Score
Discharge	No discharge	0
	Minimal mucous discharge	1
	Moderate mucous or purulent discharge	2
	Gross faecal soiling	3
Pain/restriction of activities	No activity restriction	0
	Mild discomfort, no restriction	1
	Moderate discomfort, some limitations of activity	2
	Marked discomfort, marked limitations	3
	Severe pain, severe limitations	4
Restriction of sexual activity	No restriction of sexual activity	0
	Slight restriction of sexual activity	1
	Moderate limitations of sexual activities	2
	Marked limitations of sexual activities	3
	Unable to engage in sexual activities	4
Type of perianal disease	No perianal disease/skin tags	0
	Anal fissure/mucosal tear	1
	<3 perianal fistulae	2
	≥3 perianal fistulae	3
	Anal sphincter ulcerations or fistulae with significant undermining of skin	4
Degree of induration	No induration	0
	Minimal induration	1
	Moderate induration	2
	Substantial induration	3
	Gross fluctuance/abscess	4

this instrument was said to be the gold standard for evaluating severity of perianal disease [11], and it has been utilised in recent prospective trials [12, 13].

Pikarsky et al. [14] have suggested an alternative to the PDAI, citing its weakness in determining prognosis when considering surgical interventions for perianal Crohn's disease. They describe the Perianal Crohn's Disease Activity Index (PCDAI), an assessment designed to assess severity and predict postoperative outcome in patients undergoing surgery for perianal Crohn's disease (Table 20.2). A retrospective analysis of 28 patients undergoing a variety of surgical procedures was used to validate the scoring system against a subjective assessment of patient outcome assessed by the attending surgeon. They found that pre-operative scores greater than 20 (of a possible 55) were associated with poor outcomes after surgical intervention. Further prospective evaluation of this instrument is necessary to determine its utility in clinical and research applications.

An assessment tool designed specifically to measure fistula healing was developed by Present et al. (Table 20.3) [15]. There are two endpoints: improvement, which is defined as a decrease from baseline in the number of open-draining fistulae of 50% for at least two consecutive visits (at least 4 weeks); and remission, defined by closure of all fistulae that were draining at baseline for at least two consecutive visits. Although the choice of 50% or more fistula closure at two consecutive visits may provide an objective measure of 'improvement' in drug trials, it is uncertain whether it indicates eradication of the fistula given the natural history of fistula-in-ano. The long-term utility of this measure has never been assessed. However, this tool has been

Table 20.2 Perianal Crohn's disease activity index (PCDAI) [14].

Feature	Score
Abscess	
None or	1
First occurrence, single abscess or	3
First occurrence, multiple abscess or	4
First recurrence, single or multiple abscess	5
Maximum score	**8**
Fistula	
None	0
Short-term (<30 day) fistula or	1
Long-term (>30 day) fistula or	2
Persistent post-surgery fistula or	3
Recurrent fistula	3
Multiple fistula	3
Recto-vaginal/recto-urethral fistula	4
Recurrent recto-vaginal/recto-urethral fistula	6
Maximum fistula score	**14**
Ulcer and Fissure	
None	0
Short-term (<30 day) ulcer/fissure or	1
Long-term (>30 day) ulcer/fissure or	2
Single ulcer/fissure or	1
Multiple ulcers/fissures	2
Maximum ulcer/fissure score	**4**
Stenosis	
None	0
Short-term (<30 day) stenosis or	1
Long-term (>30 day) stenosis	2
Recurrent stenosis	4
Maximum stenosis score	**6**
Incontinence Score*	
No incontinence or	0
Incontinence score of 1–6 or	1
Incontinence score of 7–14 or	3
Incontinence score >14	5
Maximum incontinence score	**5**
Concomitant Disease†	
None or	0, 0, 0
Moderate or	3, 2, 1
Severe	4, 3, 2
Active fistula	4, 3, 2
Maximum concomitant disease score	**18**

*From Jorge and Wexner, 1993 [103].
†For rectal, colonic and small bowel disease, respectively.

Table 20.3 Fistulae drainage assessment [15].

Endpoints	Definition
Improvement	Improvement defined as a decrease from baseline in the number of open draining fistulae of 50% for at least two consecutive visits (at least 4 weeks)
Remission	Remission defined as closure of all fistulae that were draining at baseline for at least two consecutive visits (at least 4 weeks)

Closure of individual fistulae defined as no fistula drainage despite gentle finger compression.

used in studies of antibiotics, azathioprine and infliximab in perianal Crohn's disease and appears to be gaining wide acceptance [12, 15].

Anal fissures, ulcers and haemorrhoids

Anal fissure

Anal canal lesions include fissures and ulcers. Fissures tend to be broad-based and deep with undermining of the edges. There may be associated large skin tags and a cyanotic hue to the surrounding skin. They may be multiple and placed eccentrically around the anal canal. Fissures or ulcers such as these are often associated with rectal disease. Often these ulcers are asymptomatic. If there is pain, one must be suspicious of associated sepsis. If sepsis is suspected, examination under anaesthesia and possible drainage is recommended.

Most patients with fissures associated with Crohn's disease are managed medically. Patients having frequent bowel movements may benefit from the management of active proximal disease or, in the absence of disease, anti-diarrhoeal agents. Local therapies, including nitro-glycerine and diltiazem ointment, may be prescribed. There is evidence that these agents are effective in treating anal fissure in patients without Crohn's disease [16]. However, it is unclear if patients with fissures associated with Crohn's disease will derive similar benefits. Occasionally, fissures in these patients may be idiopathic in nature. Typically, these fissures occur in the posterior midline and are not associated with rectal disease. Local therapies may be helpful in these patients. In patients with multiple ulcers, particularly those associated with rectal disease, medical therapies such as infliximab and ciclosporin (q.v.) may be helpful.

Sphincterotomy should be reserved for patients with unremitting symptoms despite optimal medical management. Small case series have demonstrated successful fissure healing in 67–88% after surgical intervention [17, 18]. However, these are results observed in a small group of highly selected patients accrued over 25 years and should not be generalised to patients with ulcers due to their Crohn's disease. Careful patient selection is key, reserving surgical treatment for patients with idiopathic fissures (i.e. posterior midline) with no signs of sepsis and no active Crohn's disease of the rectum.

Anal stenosis

Patients with Crohn's disease may develop anal stenosis as a result of recurrent sepsis and fissures. Buchmann and Alexander-Williams demonstrated that 27 of 54 patients with anal fissure would develop significant 'induration' or frank anal stenosis at a 10-year follow-up [19]. However, despite the occasionally severe narrowing of the anal outlet, many patients have minimal or no symptoms because their stool is only semi-formed and can still pass. In patients who require treatment, digital anal dilation or dilation with Hagar dilators is the preferred treatment [20]. Advancement flaps may not heal, tend to cause further stenosis and therefore should be avoided. Patients with severe symptomatic recurrent stenosis despite multiple dilations are best treated with proctectomy [21].

Haemorrhoids

Patients with Crohn's disease will occasionally develop symptomatic haemorrhoids. In 1977, Jeffery et al. reported a 41% complication rate after 26 procedures for haemorrhoids in patients with Crohn's disease [22]. These complications included non-healing and anal stenosis. Furthermore, 30% of these patients required a proctectomy as a direct result of these haemorrhoidectomy complications. Based on this report, conservative treatment has been the rule in these patients. A more recent study by Wolkomir et al. demonstrated a 76% successful healing rate after haemorrhoidectomy in patients with Crohn's disease [18]. However, this was a small series and none of these patients had active disease at the time of surgery. To date, there have been no reports on haemorrhoid banding or stapled haemorrhoidectomy in patients with Crohn's disease.

It is a very rare circumstance that a patient with Crohn's disease has perianal symptoms that are truly related to haemorrhoids. More commonly, these symptoms are actually a result of perianal manifestations of the Crohn's disease (undiagnosed fistula, skin tags, etc.) or irritation resulting from frequent loose bowel movements. The primary goal of therapy in these patients should be to focus on controlling these symptoms, and it is the opinion of the authors that haemorrhoidectomy is never indicated.

Abscess and fistula

Abscesses and fistulae in Crohn's disease are vexing problems that often require a combined medical and surgical approach. Considerable research in this area over the past decade has advanced the diagnostic and treatment options to treat these difficult manifestations.

Diagnosis and classification

Perianal abscesses and fistulae in patients with Crohn's disease are classified using the same anatomical relationships as those seen in otherwise healthy patients. Abscesses are described as perianal, inter-sphincteric, ischiorectal or supralevator (Fig 20.1). Similarly, fistula-in-ano are described using the Parks classification (Fig 20.2) as superficial, inter-sphincteric, trans-phincteric, supra-sphincteric or extra-sphincteric [23]. Fistulae may also be categorised as simple or complex. Simple fistulae are generally those that are low lying with only one external opening. However, complex fistulae exhibit at least one of the following qualities that make them more complicated to treat: 'high' tract incorporating a significant amount of anal sphincter, recto-vaginal fistulae, multiple fistulae and concurrent abscess.

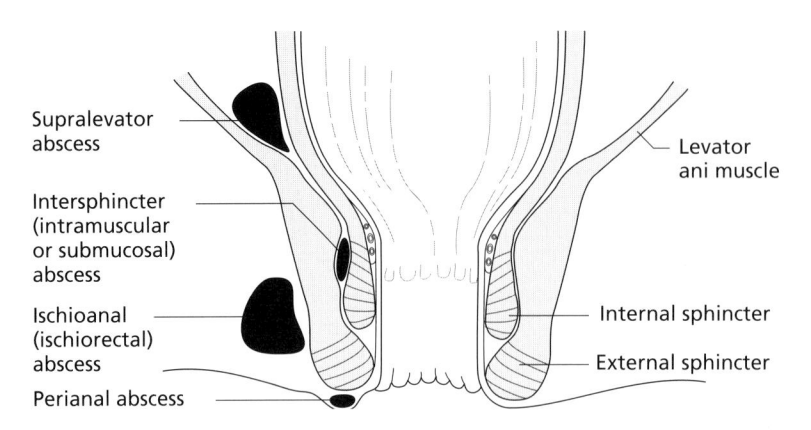

Fig 20.1 Anatomical classification of abscesses of the ano-rectum.

Clinical evaluation

Perianal abscess is a common problem and is seen in many patients without Crohn's disease. However, because perianal disease may precede intestinal manifestations [24], a high degree of suspicion is required in patients who present for treatment of their perianal lesions and have atypical lesions or symptoms related to their gastrointestinal tract. Patients with suspicious bowel habit or abdominal complaints should be assessed with small bowel follow-through, CT scan and/or colonoscopy. Other diseases that must be considered in the differential diagnosis are sexually transmitted diseases, perianal leukaemia, perianal tuberculosis and anal cancer and appropriate investigations must be undertaken to rule out these diseases. In patients with perianal lesions who have known endoscopic and histologic evidence of ulcerative colitis, one should be suspicious of the diagnosis of Crohn's disease.

Although examination of the perianal area is often the key component of the evaluation, patients may experience significant discomfort, making examination difficult. In those instances examination under anaesthesia (EUA) is indicated.

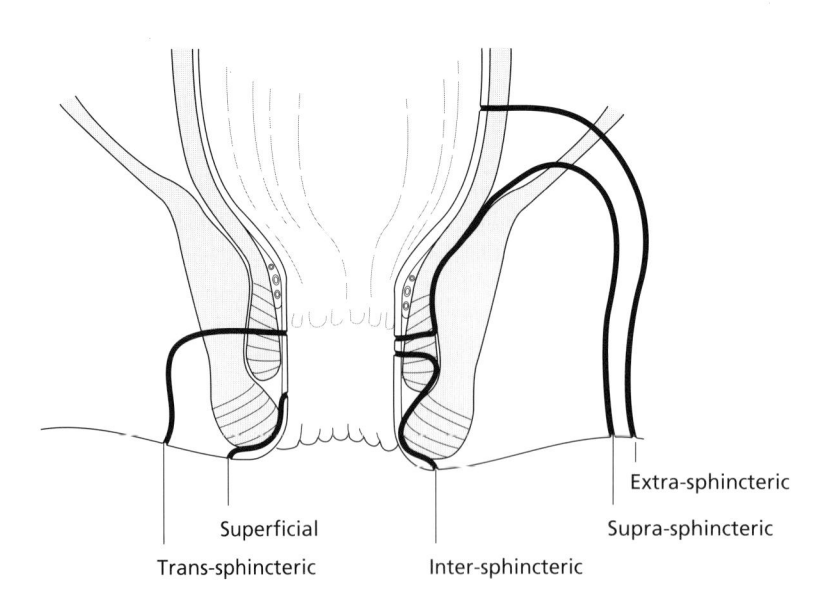

Fig 20.2 Parks' classification of fistula-in-ano.

Examination under anaesthetic

Examination under anaesthetic can be both diagnostic and therapeutic in patients with perianal abscesses and fistulae. It is indicated in patients who (1) are unable to be assessed clinically due to discomfort or pain (2) have complex perineal disease that cannot be assessed fully in the clinic or (3) have a suspected abscess that requires drainage. Abscesses should be suspected in all patients who have perianal disease and who complain of pain in previously asymptomatic fissures and fistulae.

EUA should be performed under general anaesthesia with the patient positioned in either lithotomy or prone jacknife position. Frequently, the perineum of a patient with severe perianal disease is diffusely indurated making identification of small abscesses challenging (Fig 20.3). Probing with an 18-gauge needle can help identify the abscess cavity. Examination under anaesthetic is 80–100% sensitive in identifying superficial abscesses [25–27]. However, Schaefer et al. and Beets-Tan et al. demonstrated that 14–35% of supralevator abscesses identified by magnetic resonance imaging (MRI) could be missed by an initial EUA, even when performed by an experienced colorectal surgeon [26, 27].

Fistulae should be suspected in all patients with Crohn's disease who have had a perineal infection. External openings are usually identifiable by a slight puckering of the skin. The fistula may be identified by cannulation with a malleable probe. If the internal opening is not easily identified with probing, the external opening can be injected with methylene blue, milk or hydrogen peroxide. These substances will fill the tract and can be observed bubbling out through the internal opening. These techniques have been shown to be more than 90% sensitive in identifying the fistula tract [25, 26].

Fistulography and computed tomography

The use of fistulography in the evaluation of perianal Crohn's disease has been found to be inferior to EUA and occasionally misleading [28]. Early assessment of fistula in Crohn's disease with computed tomography showed similarly poor results [29]. The introduction of endorectal ultrasound and magnetic resonance imaging has replaced fistulography and CT scan in the evaluation of perianal disease.

Endorectal ultrasound

Since the early 1990s, endorectal ultrasound (EUS) has been utilised to assess perianal abscess and fistula [30]. Recent studies using surgical evaluation as a comparison have demonstrated accuracy of over 90% [25, 31]. Technical improvements such as the adjunctive use of a transvaginal probe and the utilisation of hydrogen peroxide injected into the external opening of the fistula have led to improved diagnostic capabilities of EUS (Fig 20.4) [31–35].

EUS has been criticised for its inter-operator variability and questionable ability to augment surgical assessment. Furthermore, it may not be possible to use it outside of the operating room if painful abscesses are present. However, Solomon used EUS

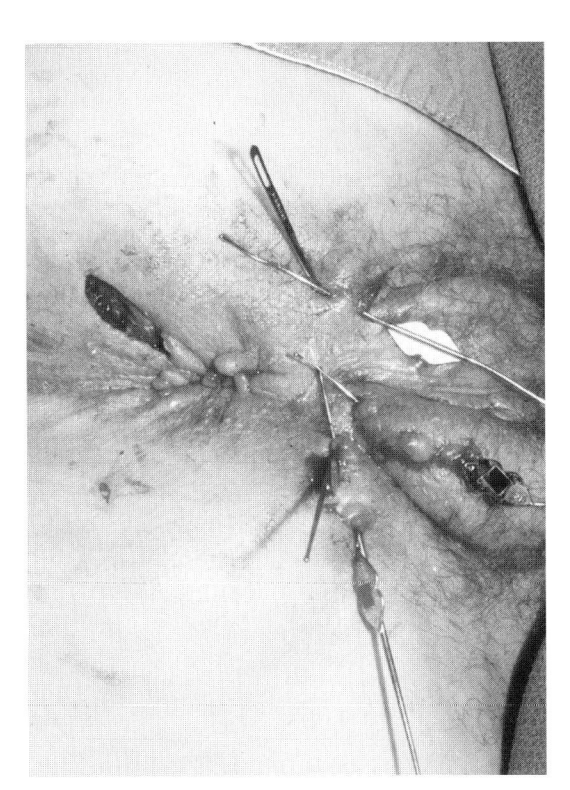

Fig 20.3 Patient with Crohn's disease with complex perineal fistula.

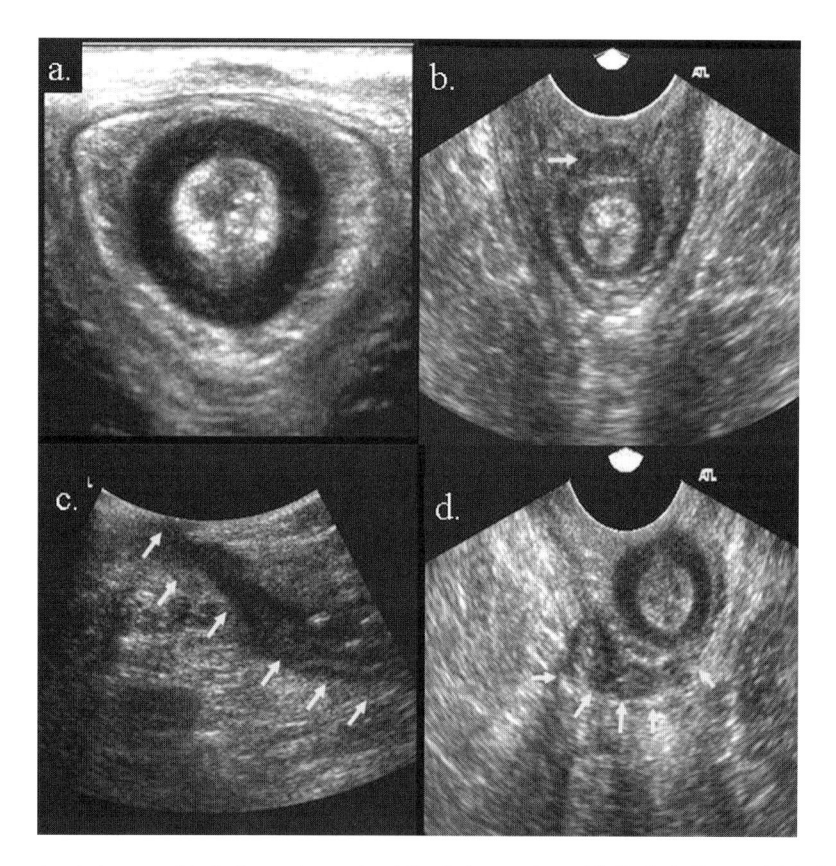

Fig 20.4 Transperineal ultrasound (us) of complex perianal fistula in a patient with Crohn's disease. (a) Axial US image of normal anal canal, demonstrating both internal (hypodense dark ring) and external (hyperdense white ring) sphincter. (b) Axial image of the mid anal canal taken with a transvaginal probe on the perineum shows an intersphincteric fluid collection (arrows) anteriorly. (c) Fistula tract elucidated by placing probe over external opening (EO) at skin. The tract runs deep away from the EO towards its connection with the anal canal, shown on a different image. (d) Axial image shows a transphincteric tract which originated slightly higher in the anal canal at an opening in the posterior midline. After passing through the external anal sphincter, the tract (arrows) runs obliquely to the right side and to the EO, shown on a different image. (Images courtesy of Dr. Stephanie Wilson, University of Toronto.)

to assess patients with Crohn's disease and suspected perianal disease and found that endorectal ultrasound changed patient management in 61% of patients [36]. The key advantages of endorectal ultrasound are that it is inexpensive, portable and has potential for intra-operative use in conjunction with EUA [37]. The disadvantage is that it is operator-dependent. Optimally, EUS should be performed in the operating room by the operating surgeon. It has the potential to become more prevalent as surgeons gain experience with this modality, although there is a distinct possibility that EUS will be supplanted by MRI.

Magnetic resonance imaging

In 1992, Luniss reported a cohort of 16 patients with suspected anal fistula, 13 of whom had had a previously negative EUA. He showed that magnetic resonance imaging (MRI) accurately assessed the fistula status in 14 of 16 patients when compared to subsequent surgical evaluation [38].

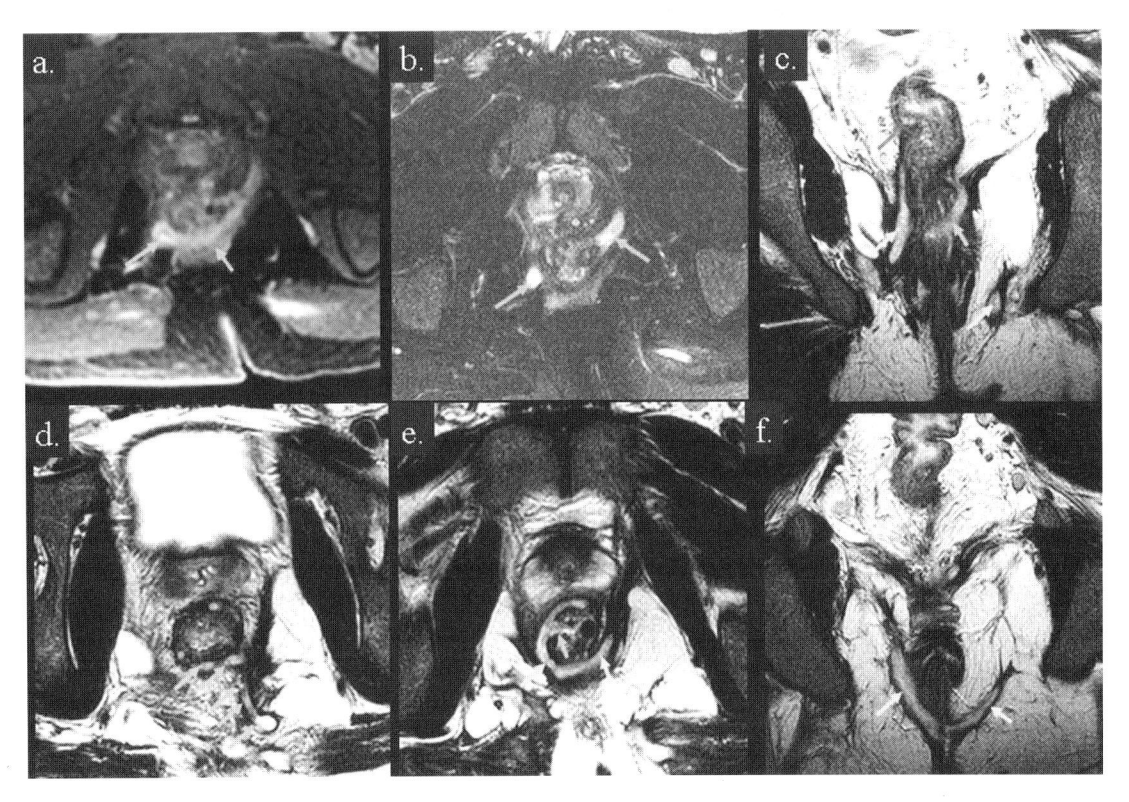

Fig 20.5 MRI of complex Crohn's perianal fistula. MRI of pelvis in 29-year old male with complex perianal fistula. (a) Axial T1 fast saturated image, intersphincteric and transsphincteric component of fistula with gadolinium enhancement of tract wall. (b) Axial T2 fat saturated image, two fistula tracts extending inferiorly just lateral to external sphincter. (c) Coronal image, fistula traversing sphincter (internal opening on left side of image), then extending inferiorly in two bilateral tracts in the ischioanal fat (two arrows). Mucosal thickening of the rectum is noted (right arrow). (d) Axial image, cephalad to internal opening, arrows demonstrate fistula extension across levator muscles into supralevator space. (e) Axial image, internal opening extending into intersphincteric space and continuing in horseshoe fashion around anus (two arrows). (f) Coronal image, abnormally thick rectum (top arrow) suggesting active Crohn's disease and two fistula tracts extending caudad to skin (two arrows). (Images courtesy of Dr. Masoom Haider, University of Toronto.)

Since this initial report, MRI results have been shown to change surgical management in up to 21% of patients [25, 26, 39]. Buchanan *et al.* showed that in patients with recurrent fistula-in-ano, surgeons who acted on auxiliary MRI information had lower fistula recurrence rates than those who ignored the MRI findings (16% vs 57%, $p = 0.008$) [39]. This study did not specifically recruit patients with Crohn's disease, but the results provide reasonable evidence that MRI can help delineate the anatomy of complicated fistulae. Moreover, Beets-Tan *et al.* demonstrated that MRI was more likely to provide clinically important information in patients with perianal Crohn's disease than patients without Crohn's disease undergoing EUA for fistula-in-ano (40% vs 15%, $p < 0.05$) [26].

MRI images display the course of fistula with characteristic hyper-intensity on T2-weighted images (Fig 20.5). MRI assessment of perianal fistulae is usually reported using a classification similar to that described by Parks *et al.* [40, 41]. However, a recent report has proposed an MRI classification

Table 20.4 MRI-based score for severity of perianal Crohn's disease [42].

Number of fistula tracks	
None	0
Single, unbranched	1
Single, branched	2
Multiple	3
Location	
Extra- or inter-sphincteric	1
Trans-sphincteric	2
Supra-sphincteric	3
Extension	
Infralevatoric	1
Supralevatoric	2
Hyper-intensity on T2-weighted images	
Absent	0
Mild	4
Pronounced	9
Collections (cavities >3 mm in diameter)	
Absent	0
Present	4
Rectal wall involvement	
Normal	0
Thickened	2

of perianal disease severity specific to Crohn's disease (Table 20.4) [42]. These authors report good inter-observer concordance, but in a small number of patients were unable to clearly link clinical improvement with significantly improved MRI scores. Further assessment of this classification scheme is necessary before drawing any conclusions about its utility.

In summary, the current diagnostic approach to perianal disease should start with thorough clinical assessment with early EUA in patients with suspected perineal sepsis or fistula. In patients with unremitting or recurrent sepsis and/or fistula, suspected abscess with no obvious drainable site and complex fistulous disease, evaluation with endorectal ultrasound or MRI is indicated prior to the surgical assessment of the perineum. The addition of either EUS or MRI to surgical evaluation of the perineum has been shown to have near-uniform success in mapping perianal fistulae and abscesses in these patients [25]. As expertise with these modalities varies from centre to centre, it is important to work closely with a local radiologist or ultrasonographer to determine which will yield the best results.

Treatment options for perianal abscess and fistula in Crohn's disease

Abscess

Generally, abscesses are treated the same whether the patient does or does not have Crohn's disease. Simple abscesses may be drained under local or general anaesthetic and should consist of incision, unroofing and drainage. Incision and drainage results in healing in 68–79%, but recurrence of perineal sepsis occurs in up to 70% of patients at 3 years follow-up [43, 44]. Primary fistulotomy should be avoided except in very superficial fistulae, but concurrent seton placement may prevent recurrent abscess formation. There is no role for treating abscesses with antibiotics alone, although combination metronidazole and ciprofloxacin therapy may be a useful adjunct to surgical drainage, especially if there is cellulitis [45].

Fistulae

Fistulae in patients with Crohn's disease tend to be the most difficult perianal lesions to treat. Often, both medical and surgical modalities must be employed. Initial treatment will depend on the symptoms, the complexity of the fistula and whether there is associated rectal disease.

Simple fistulae

Simple fistulae are generally those that are low-lying with only one external opening. They are usually seen in patients without rectal involvement. Even in Crohn's disease, they make up the majority of fistulae. Although many gastroenterologists treat simple fistulae with repeated courses of antibiotics when the patient becomes symptomatic, these fistulae are usually amenable to fistulotomy, and the fistula can be eradicated without risk of incontinence or delayed wound healing. A recent review summarised the results of 21 studies of conventional fistulotomy for low perianal fistulae [46]. Although the healing rates ranged from 8 to 100%, 18 of the 21 trials demonstrated healing rates better than 59%. It is important that the extent of fistulous disease and the presence of associated sepsis be properly evaluated by means of an examination with the patient under anaesthesia and the rectum be evaluated by means of an endoscopic examination before undertaking fistulotomy.

Complex fistulae

Although simple fistulae can usually be treated definitively by means of surgical intervention, complex fistulae or fistulae occurring in the presence of active rectal disease must be approached cautiously. These include fistulae with multiple external openings or tracts as well as those that are high. Although it is unusual that these complex fistulae can be eradicated surgically, EUA should be performed in most patients. Occasionally, fistulae are not as complex as they appear. For example, multiple external openings can be seen where there is a single fistula tract that is amenable to fistulotomy. This is especially true in 'neglected' perianal disease where abscesses have drained spontaneously. Although surgery continues to play an important role in the treatment of complex fistulae, the recent addition of tumour necrosis factor antibodies (anti-TNF) as an effective medical treatment has shifted the emphasis of therapy from primarily surgical to a combined medical and surgical approach [15].

Medical treatment

Despite a lack of controlled clinical trials, metronidazole and ciprofloxacin are mainstays of treatment in perianal fistulous disease. Although early small case series showed either improvement or complete healing of fistulae in 50–100% of patients [47–49], this is not the outcome for most patients. The improvement with antibiotics is usually related to control of sepsis, and thus is contingent on continued antibiotic use in most patients. Use of metronidazole often leads to glossitis and metallic taste and prolonged use can lead to peripheral neuropathy [50].

There is some evidence that azathioprine, a purine analogue that inhibits DNA synthesis and acts as an immunosuppressant, is effective in healing fistula in Crohn's disease. The concomitant use of azathioprine and antibiotics appears to facilitate ongoing remission of perianal fistulising disease, even when the antibiotics are discontinued [12]. There are seven randomised controlled trials of azathioprine or mercaptopurine versus placebo in patients with Crohn's disease in which perianal fistulising disease outcomes are described [51–57]. Improvement in perianal fistulae was not a primary outcome in any of these trials. However, Pearson et al. conducted a subgroup analysis on these trials as part of a larger meta-analysis of all randomised controlled trials of azathioprine or 6-mercaptopurine versus placebo for Crohn's disease [58]. In this analysis, the authors combined data available from five of these trials and found a pooled odds ratio of 4.44 (95% confidence interval 1.50–13.20) favouring fistula healing, with a cumulative response rate of 54%. Although this was a secondary outcome of the included studies, these results are cited as important evidence that immunomodulators are effective in the treatment of perianal Crohn's disease. However, there may be a publication bias where only trials that showed a positive result reported this outcome, and trials with negative results were not reported.

A recent large retrospective case series of 94 patients with perianal Crohn's disease demonstrated a discouraging response rate of 29% in patients treated with either azathioprine or 6-mercaptopurine [59]. Furthermore, the presence of fistula was a predictor of poor response in this series (cumulative 24-month probability of response 0.14 vs 0.54, $p = 0.0001$), and the authors concluded that immunomodulators should not be used if the primary objective is healing of perianal disease. Furthermore, up to 15% of patients treated with azathioprine or mercaptopurine will experience potentially serious adverse events (e.g. leucopenia, allergic reactions, infections and pancreatitis) [60].

Ciclosporin is another immunosuppressant that is used primarily in transplant populations, but has been used to treat patients with Crohn's disease. It inhibits T cell activation and suppresses interleukin

2 production. In 1993, Hanauer and Smith reported on the use of continuous intravenous ciclosporin (4 mg/kg/day) in 5 patients with a total of 12 perianal fistulae, who were unresponsive to previous therapy including surgery, antibiotics and azathioprine or 6-MP [61]. Although the initial response was prompt and uniform (10/12 fistulae had resolution of drainage at a mean of 7.9 days) relapses were common once patients were switched over to oral ciclosporin. Relapses were seen in 5 of 10 fistulae. Present and Lichtiger reported on 16 patients, 10 of who had perirectal fistulae and 2 who had recto-vaginal fistulae [62]. All patients were given a 2-week course of intravenous ciclosporin followed by orally administered medication. Four of the patients with perirectal disease and one with a recto-vaginal fistula were said to have closed their fistulae after 2 weeks. After a mean follow-up of 12 months, 7 of the 10 patients with perirectal fistula remained on ciclosporin with half improved and half having closure of the fistulae. Both of the patients with recto-vaginal fistulae relapsed with one requiring surgery. Recently, Çat et al. reported their results in 20 patients with perianal disease refractory to multiple medical treatments (antibiotics, steroids and/or azathioprine) [63]. One week of intravenous ciclosporin followed by conversion to oral therapy resulted in 80% of patients having complete or partial response within 30 days. However, after mean follow-up of 5 months the failure rate increased to 50%.

Tacrolimus (FK-506), a drug with a similar mechanism of action, has been tested in a placebo-controlled trial. Sandborn et al. randomised 48 patients with fistulising Crohn's disease to a 10-week course of either 0.2 mg/kg/day of tacrolimus or placebo [64]. Most of the patients had perianal disease ($n = 42$). In this subgroup, patients treated with tacrolimus were more likely to experience closure of more than 50% of the fistulae for at least 4 weeks compared to patients treated with placebo (45% vs 9%, $p = 0.01$). Overall, complete fistula remission was similar between the groups (10% vs 8%, $p = 0.86$). Moreover, side effects including headache, insomnia, paresthesiae and transient elevated creatinine were observed more frequently in the tacrolimus group (mean 5.2 vs 2.3, $p = 0.009$).

This study followed patients for only 10 weeks, so long-term outcome is still uncertain. Lama et al. reported on 10 patients with fistulising Crohn's disease (seven with perianal fistulae) refractory to infliximab therapy [65]. At 6–18 months follow-up, nine of 10 patients achieved partial or complete response with a lower initial dose of tacrolimus (0.05 mg/kg/day), which was then adjusted to achieve whole blood levels of 5–15 ng/ml. These results suggest tacrolimus may be an option for patients with perianal fistulae, particularly if they have failed more conventional medical therapies.

Recently, there has been great interest in infliximab, a chimeric murine/human monoclonal antibody against tumour necrosis factor α, in treating perianal fistula. In 1999, Present et al. published results of a randomised controlled trial comparing placebo to infliximab infusions in 94 patients with Crohn's fistulae [15]. After infusions of placebo or infliximab (either 5 or 10 mg/kg at 0, 2 and 6 weeks), closure of at least 50% of the fistulae was observed in 68% of the patients in the low dose and 56% of patients in the high dose infusion groups compared to 26% in the placebo group. Although results for patients with perianal disease were not reported separately, the majority of the trial participants (94% of the placebo group and 89% of the treatment group) had perianal fistulae.

Sands et al. subsequently identified 195 patients (175 with perianal fistulae) who achieved closure of at least 50% of fistulae at week 10 and 14 after the aforementioned 5 mg/kg infliximab infusion protocol [66]. They randomised these patients to either maintenance doses of 5 mg/kg of infliximab every 8 weeks (starting at week 14) or placebo. At 54 weeks of follow up, the median time to loss of response was significantly longer in the infliximab group (median 40 weeks vs 14 weeks, $p < 0.001$). At 54 weeks, the infliximab maintenance therapy group had more patients with a continued response to treatment (46% vs 23%, $p = 0.001$) and complete remission of fistulae (36% vs 19%, $p = 0.009$) compared to placebo. No significant differences in adverse events were noted. A recent subgroup analysis of women with recto-vaginal fistulae showed an encouraging 44.8% (13/29) fistula closure rate at 14 weeks [67].

There is emerging evidence that multi-drug regimens of infliximab with either azathioprine/mercaptopurine or methotrexate, a folate analogue and inhibitor of dihydrofolate reductase, may be more effective [68, 69]. However, these small case series should be interpreted with caution, particularly when the auxiliary drug has not been proven to be independently effective in controlled trials and follow up is often short.

Despite these early encouraging results with infliximab, there are reasons for reservation regarding the long-term potential of infliximab. Only one randomised trial has reported the outcome in patients after 1 year of treatment [66]. There is no evidence that measuring fistula improvement using the fistula drainage assessment (Table 10.2) really predicts long term eradication of the fistulae. Although the natural history of fistulae is that they drain and then close, the improvement in drainage reported by Present *et al.* does not mean that the fistula is going to heal. In fact, there have been several recent reports demonstrating persistent fistula tracts on both EUS and MRI after apparent clinical response [40, 42, 70, 71]. Van Assche *et al.* assessed eight patients in clinical remission after 6–10 weeks of infliximab treatment. They demonstrated that all of these patients had persistent inflammation along fistula tracts on MRI [42]. Similarly, Rasul *et al.* followed 35 patients treated with infliximab for perianal fistula. The authors conducted transperineal ultrasound 56 weeks after initiation of treatment in patients on maintenance doses of infliximab or within 8 weeks of discontinuation of infliximab therapy. Despite clinical remission in 43% of patients, transperineal ultrasound demonstrated complete radiologic healing in only 11% of patients [72]. These radiological findings suggest that clinical remission with infliximab does not equate to fistula healing in most patients.

However, just because infliximab does not heal fistulae does not mean that it is not useful. The main goal of treatment in complex fistulae is to prevent abscess formation. Therefore, if infliximab eliminates drainage, it may be worthwhile. To maintain this effect, repeated doses of infliximab are necessary. This strategy is associated with risks. There are reports of increased rates of potential life-threatening infections, including pneumonia, tuberculosis, listerosis, aspergillosis and histoplasmosis [73–76]. Chronic immunosuppression with anti-TNF α may increase the risk of malignancies, particularly non-Hodgkins lymphomas [77–80]. Moreover, the development of antibodies to infliximab has been linked to increased infusion reactions and diminishing efficacy [81]. Until large population-based studies with prolonged follow-up are reported, the long-term benefits and consequences of repeated dose infliximab treatment in perianal fistulising Crohn's disease can only be speculated upon [82]. In the meantime, clinicians and patients must carefully weigh the risks and benefits of this expensive therapy.

Surgical treatment

Even with the emergence of multiple promising medical treatment options, early surgical evaluation and treatment in these patients continues to be an important component of the multi-disciplinary approach to complex perianal fistulae in Crohn's disease. In fact, a recent study on the natural history of fistulising Crohn's disease reports that 72% of patients with perianal fistula will require surgical treatment [83]. Before initiating any form of therapy, an examination with the patient under anaesthesia should be undertaken to evaluate carefully the extent of disease and the presence of associated sepsis. Undetected abscesses should be drained. Some patients with multiple fistulae may have less complex disease with all the tracts emanating from one internal opening. In these cases, the fistula may be treated definitively with excellent results (Fig 20.6). If the fistula is complex, the tracts should be identified and unroofed and curetted of all infected granulation tissue. This tissue should be sent for histological assessment to rule out the rare association of cancer with Crohn's disease fistulae [84]. Although these measures may not necessarily allow for complete healing of the fistula, they may lead to partial healing of the tracts and significantly decreased drainage. Drains and setons can be inserted on a long-term basis to prevent re-accumulation of pus. As with medical treatment, the goal is usually the prevention of sepsis.

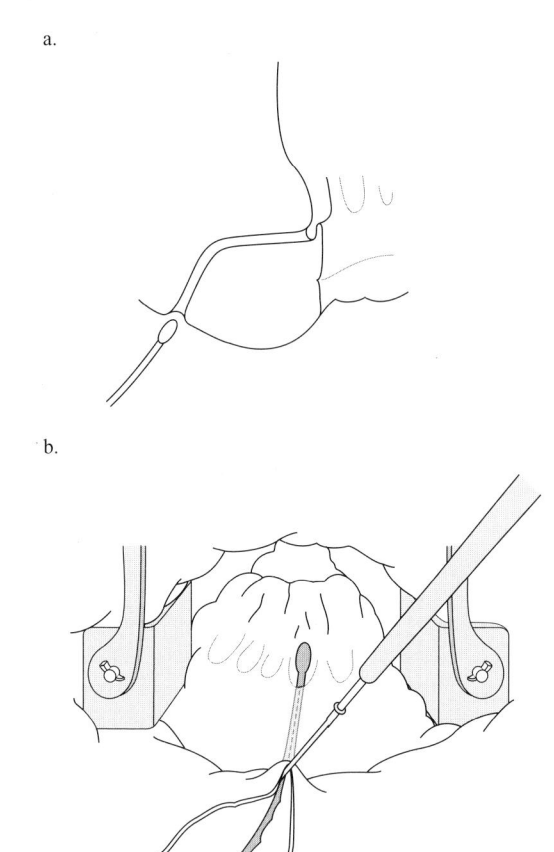

Fig 20.6 A transphincteric fistula arising from a crypt at the dentate line, passing through both the internal and external sphincters with an external opening in the perianal skin covered. (b) A fistulotomy can be performed by passing a probe through the external opening to the internal opening. Then the tract can be laid open by dividing the overlying tissue. It is unnecessary and usually unwise to remove the tract. The wound is packed and allowed to heal secondarily.

Topstad *et al.* [84] reported a combined surgical and medical approach in patients with perianal disease receiving infliximab treatment. They demonstrated an 86% response rate and a 67% complete response after a mean follow-up of 10 months in patients who had EUA combined with abscess drainage, seton placement or faecal diversion prior to the initiation of infliximab treatment. Similarly, Regueiro and Mardini [85] showed better response, lower fistula recurrence rates and increased time to recurrence in patients who underwent EUA prior to initiation of infliximab therapy.

Should medical measures fail, be refused by a patient or be contraindicated, other measures may be required. Construction of a loop or split ileostomy to divert the faecal stream may be of benefit in some patients [86–88]. Although initial improvement in the local perianal disease usually occurs, the ileostomy does not lead to healing of the fistula. In our series of 12 patients treated with a diverting ileostomy for proctitis or anorectal sepsis, all had temporary remission of their disease [88]. Five required proctocolectomy because of exacerbation of their disease and none has had successful closure of the ileostomy. Harper and colleagues reported that 21 (72%) of 29 patients with anorectal Crohn's disease treated with split ileostomy had early improvement [86]. In another series reported by Zelas and Jagelman, 22 patients underwent ileostomy for anorectal disease and only 6 remained well for 3–5 years [87]. Although a recent report claims successful restoration of bowel continuity in 8 of 17 (47%) patients [89], the preponderance of evidence indicates that less than 20% of patients will ever achieve this goal [86, 90, 91]. Despite this, there may be some merit in constructing a diverting ileostomy. First, the general status, including the nutritional status, of the patient often improves and the perianal sepsis resolves to some extent. Therefore, at least in theory, a subsequent proctectomy or other definitive procedure can be performed with less morbidity. Second, some patients may be loath to have definitive surgery as an initial procedure and a loop or split ileostomy allows them to adjust psychologically to a stoma without committing themselves to a permanent stoma.

Proctectomy may be necessary in patients who are refractory to other medical and surgical measures. It is unusual for proctectomy to be required to treat perianal disease alone. Patients almost always have associated severe rectal involvement. Farmer *et al.* reported that perianal disease was a significant indication for surgery in only 12–19% of patients with ileocolonic or colonic Crohn's disease [92].

Before performing a proctectomy, it is important that the patient be in optimal condition because this operation is associated with a relatively high morbidity, particularly perianal wound problems. Thus, pre-operative measures to decrease local sepsis and improve healing should be undertaken. To decrease local sepsis, a staged procedure may be planned. This may mean a subtotal colectomy or defunctioning ileostomy initially. A recent case series of 12 patients suggests that perineal sinus can be avoided when primary closure of complicated perineal wounds is undertaken using myocutaneous flaps [93]. Although pre-operatively many patients are loath to have an ileostomy, the quality of life for these patients is usually excellent. Thus, this should not be considered a failure of treatment, but rather a part of the combined medical and surgical approach to this disease.

Primary surgical intervention may be warranted in patients who have a high fistula not amenable to fistulotomy. The use of anal flap advancement has been reported recently with some success. This involves undermining the anal mucosa at the site of the fistula, curetting or excising the tract at the internal opening, suturing the muscularis layer closed at the internal opening, excising a rim of mucosa at the site of the fistula and then closing the defect with the mucosal flap (Fig 20.7). Clearly, this should not be attempted if the rectum has active Crohn's disease. The results of this technique are variable, with success rates of 25–100% reported [43, 94–100]. The number of patients in each series is small, and further evaluation is needed. Similarly, Marchesa *et al.* have reported a sleeve advancement procedure, which is essentially a perineal approach to a short segment full thickness rectal resection [101]. In this small series, eight of 13 (65%) patients had healed their fistula at 1-year follow-up. Further evaluation of these novel techniques is necessary before wide adoption.

Recto-vaginal fistulae

The presence of a recto-vaginal fistula is often an ominous sign indicating severe rectal disease Despite encouraging reports with infliximab and other immunosuppressants, patients with recto-vaginal fistula have a poor response to any intervention. This is because the recto-vaginal septum is thin and once the tract epithelialises, it will not heal. However, in selected patients, local repair of the fistula may be undertaken (Fig 20.7). Medical treatment may have a role in inducing a remission of the rectal disease so that a local repair can be undertaken, or improving the consistency of stool so there is less discharge through the fistula opening.

Whether a local repair is advocated depends on two factors: patient symptoms and the disease status of the rectum. If the fistula is small and low-lying, the patient may experience relatively minor symptoms and no treatment other than medical management of any rectal disease is indicated, although spontaneous closure of the fistula for long periods would be unusual. However, if the patient has persistent faecal or purulent discharge from the vagina or has gross incontinence, treatment is indicated. However, in these patients the presence of rectal Crohn's disease is a contraindication to attempting a local repair. If the fistula is very symptomatic and the rectal disease is severe, proctectomy is indicated. These patients usually have very complex perianal disease, and proctectomy is rare in patients with an isolated recto-vaginal fistula.

In the Cleveland Clinic experience, 40% of patients were amenable to local repair of the recto-vaginal fistula [102]. In these patients, repair was successful after one attempt in 54% and 68% overall. The type of repair performed largely depends on the preference of the individual surgeon. Our preference, where possible, is to perform a mucosal flap advancement via the rectum. Meticulous surgical technique is mandatory. We also recommend temporary fecal diversion with a loop ileostomy in most patients, although in the Cleveland Clinic series, protection with a stoma did not affect outcome. If patients are carefully selected, excellent results may be achieved.

Management of perianal abscess and fistula in Crohn's disease

In all patients with suspected abscess or fistula, a detailed clinical history and physical examination must be performed. In particular, a flexible or rigid

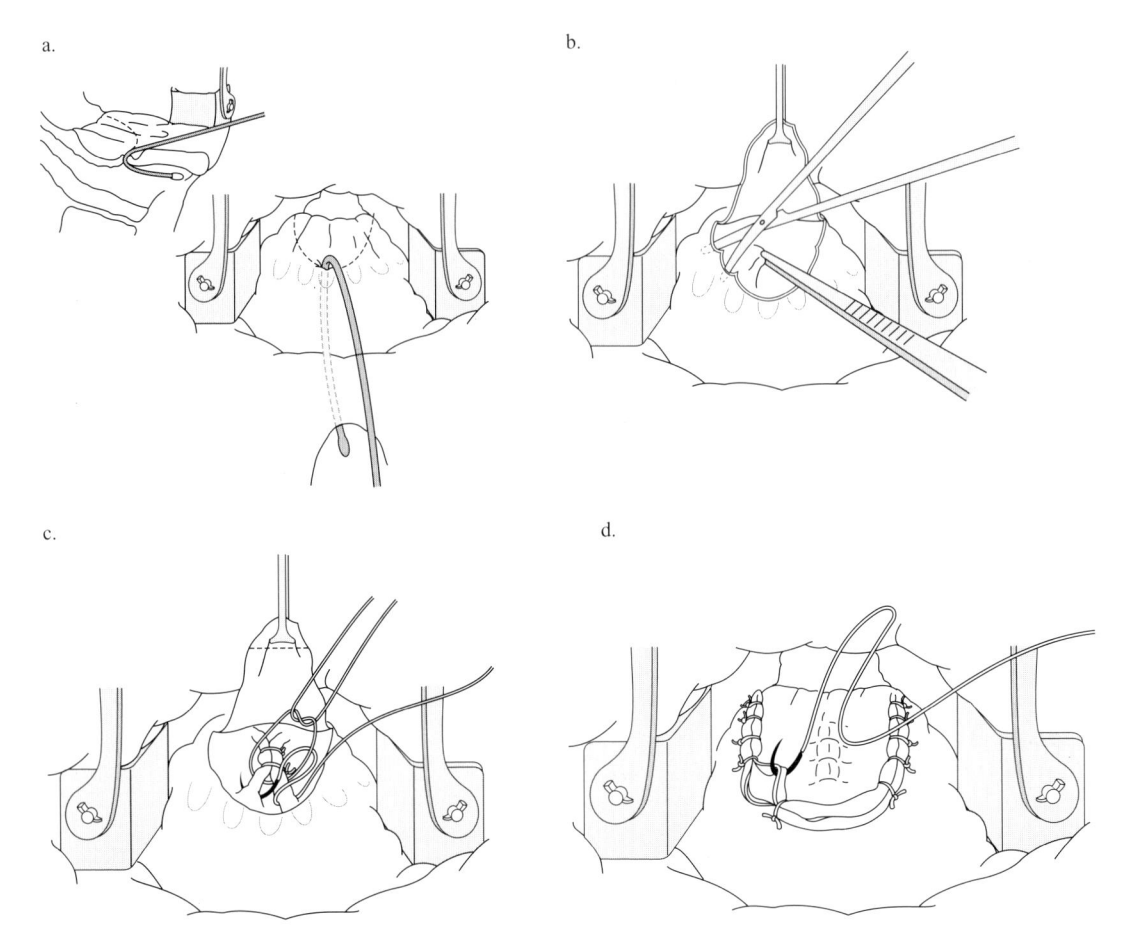

Fig 20.7 (a) The opening to the recto-vaginal fistula is identified just above the dentate line. (b) A flap of mucosa and internal sphincter is raised beginning just below the opening of the fistula and extending until the flap can be brought down beyond the fistulous opening without tension. The flap should be rhomboid in shape to blood supply is adequate. (c) The fistula tract is curetted, then closed with several interrupted sutures. Closure of the fistula on the vaginal side is unnecessary. (d) The mucosal flap is brought down and sutured so the fistula is completely covered.

sigmoidoscopy must be performed to determine if there is any rectal disease. If there are any gastrointestinal symptoms, the entire gastrointestinal tract should be evaluated. Finally, the perianal region should be examined to determine if there is ongoing sepsis. If severe, further examination may not be possible. However, in patients with a simple perianal abscess, drainage is all that is necessary. This may be performed under local or general anaesthetic. In patients with apparent simple low fistula, fistulotomy is recommended to most patients as the likelihood of eliminating the fistula is high and the risk of incontinence is low. In other words, patients with straightforward perianal disease may be treated the same as patients who do not have Crohn's disease. The routine use of antibiotics or the institution of any other medical therapy is unnecessary in these patients.

For patients with a single fistula but one that is high and not amenable to a fistulotomy, anal flap advancement can be considered. However, this procedure should only be considered in select patients with single internal openings, no or quiescent rectal disease, normal sphincter function and good nutritional status. Similar criteria should be used when considering local procedures for treatment of recto-vaginal fistula. Other options include closure with fibrin glue or long-term insertion of a seton.

In patients with more complex disease (i.e. multiple fistula with or without rectal disease), the goal of therapy should be controlling and preventing recurrence of perianal sepsis and sphincter preservation. Thus, a key to the initial evaluation is to determine the severity of the patient's symptoms. If the patient has minimal symptoms, it may be better to counsel the patient against having further treatment because it is unlikely that the fistulae can be eradicated.

An examination under anaesthesia is indicated in most patients with complex disease. This will allow drainage of the abscesses and delineation of the anatomy of fistula tracts. If possible, fistulotomies can be performed or unroofing of abscess cavities and insertion of setons. In this group of patients an MRI performed pre-operatively may be of value. Combination ciprofloxacin and metronidazole may help to control perineal sepsis in these patients, once the abscesses are drained.

Once perineal sepsis is controlled, then additional therapeutic measures can be considered. In most patients, infliximab is the treatment of choice. Other treatment modalities include ciclosporin and tacrolimus. However, the evidence supporting the effectiveness of the latter therapies is limited. Although azathioprine is often used in combination with infliximab for maintenance therapy, again there are limited data supporting its effectiveness. Although initial reports of infliximab closing fistula were impressive, it seems now that most fistulae do not heal and continuous repeated infusions are necessary. Patients who have long-standing perianal disease with significant scarring are much less likely to respond to infliximab and other treatment (defunctioning or proctectomy) should be considered if there is no response after a few infusions of infliximab. If setons are inserted prior to initiation of infliximab therapy, it is usually recommended that they be removed after two or three infusions (6–8 weeks). However, it is often difficult to know when to remove them because the data suggest that infliximab may eliminate drainage and close the fistula openings but does not heal the fistula tract completely. Thus, there is a risk of recurrence of an abscess when they are removed. If patients do not respond to infliximab therapy, ciclosporin or tacrolimus may be tried but alternatively, the setons may be left in long-term to prevent abscess recurrence.

If patients continue to have problems with persistent sepsis or recurrent abscess formation, then proctectomy may be required. A defunctioning stoma often results in temporary eradication of the sepsis but rarely results in healing of the fistulas and re-establishment of gastrointestinal continuity is not possible. However, a defunctioning procedure often is of value as it allows patients to come to terms with a stoma and may decrease the likelihood of a perineal wound infection if proctectomy is performed subsequently. Either a loop ileostomy or colostomy can be performed, the choice depending on whether there is significant colonic disease. Both procedures can be performed laparoscopically, which decreases the morbidity and pain of the procedure. Most patients will have a good quality of life if sepsis is controlled. If this cannot be accomplished, proctectomy should be considered because most patients will have an excellent quality of life with a stoma. Surgery should not be considered a failure of treatment.

Patients with Crohn's disease who develop a recto-vaginal fistula, particularly in the presence of other perianal fistulae or proctitis usually require proctectomy. Local repair is only offered to patients who have minimal associated perianal disease, no rectal disease and good health otherwise. Fistulotomy should never be performed because it will almost always lead to significant problems with incontinence even in seemingly low fistula.

Summary

A significant number of patients with Crohn's disease will experience at least one perianal manifestation. Although these problems can be very morbid, there are a number of emerging medical and surgical therapies that are improving the lives of many of these patients. In the rush to embrace these new treatments, gastroenterologists and surgeons must be vigilant in identifying both beneficial and adverse outcomes, carefully balancing them when recommending treatments for these people. Because of the variable patterns of disease seen in Crohn's disease as well as the individual concerns of patients, treatment must be individualised. Optimally, care should be given with a team approach including gastroenterologists, surgeons and allied health professionals such as wound-care nurses and enterostomal therapists.

References

1. Crohn BB, Ginzberg L, Oppenheimer GD. Regional ileitis, a pathological and clinical entity. *J Am Med Assoc* 1932;99:1323–9.
2. Gabriel WB. Results of an experimental and histological investigation into seventy-five cases of rectal fistulae. *Proc R Soc Med* 1921;14:156–61.
3. Bissell AD. Localized chronic ulcerative colitis. *Ann Surg* 1934;99:957–66.
4. Fielding JF. Perianal lesions in Crohn's disease. *J R Coll Surg Edinb* 1972;17:32–7.
5. Marks CG, Ritchie JK, Lockhart-Mummery HE. Anal fistulas in Crohn's disease. *Br J Surg* 1981;68:525–7.
6. Rankin GB, Watts HD, Melnyk CS, Kelley ML Jr. National cooperative Crohn's disease study: extraintestinal manifestations and perianal complications. *Gastroenterology* 1979;77:914–20.
7. Hobbiss JH, Schofield PF. Management of perianal Crohn's disease. *J R Soc Med* 1982;75:414–7.
8. Palder SB, Shandling B, Bilik R, Griffiths AM, Sherman P. Perianal complications of pediatric Crohn's disease. *J Pediatr Surg* 1991;26:513–5.
9. Buchmann P, Alexander-Williams J. Classification of perianal Crohn's disease. *Clin Gastroenterol* 1980;9:323–30.
10. Irvine EJ. Usual therapy improves perianal Crohn's disease as measured by a new disease activity index. McMaster IBD study group. *J Clin Gastroenterol* 1995;20:27–32.
11. Sostegni R, Daperno M, Scaglione N, Lavagna A, Rocca R, Pera A. Review article: Crohn's disease: monitoring disease activity [Review] [35 refs]. *Aliment Pharmacol Ther* 2003;17(Suppl 2):11–7.
12. Dejaco C, Harrer M, Waldhoer T, Miehsler W, Vogelsang H, Reinisch W. Antibiotics and azathioprine for the treatment of perianal fistulas in Crohn's disease. *Aliment Pharmacol Ther* 2003;18(11–12):1113–20.
13. Jeshion WC, Larsen KL, Jawad AF, et al. Azathioprine and 6-mercaptopurine for the treatment of perianal Crohn's disease in children. *J Clin Gastroenterol* 2000;30(3):294–8.
14. Pikarsky AJ, Gervaz P, Wexner SD. Perianal Crohn disease: a new scoring system to evaluate and predict outcome of surgical intervention. *Arch Surg* 2002;137(7):774–7.
15. Present DH, Rutgeerts P, Targan S, et al. Infliximab for the treatment of fistulas in patients with Crohn's disease. *N Engl J Med* 1999;340(18):1398–405.
16. Nelson R. A systematic review of medical therapy for anal fissure. *Dis Colon Rectum* 2004;47:422–31.
17. Fleshner PR, Schoetz DJ Jr, Roberts PL, Murray JJ, Coller JA, Veidenheimer MC. Anal fissure in Crohn's disease: a plea for aggressive management. *Dis Colon Rectum* 1995;38:1137–43.
18. Wolkomir AF, Luchtefeld MA. Surgery for symptomatic hemorrhoids and anal fissures in Crohn's disease. *Dis Colon Rectum* 1993;36:545–7.
19. Buchmann P, Keighley MR, Allan RN, Thompson H, Alexander-Williams J. Natural history of perianal Crohn's disease. Ten year follow-up: a plea for conservatism. *Am J Surg* 1980;140:642–4.
20. Bernard D, Morgan S, Tasse D. Selective surgical management of Crohn's disease of the anus. *Can J Surg* 1986;29(5):318–21.
21. Linares L, Moreira LF, Andrews H, Allan RN, Alexander-Williams J, Keighley MR. Natural history and treatment of anorectal strictures complicating Crohn's disease. *Br J Surg* 1988;75(7):653–5.
22. Jeffery PJ, Parks AG, Ritchie JK. Treatment of haemorrhoids in patients with inflammatory bowel disease. *Lancet* 1977;1:1084–5.
23. Parks AG, Gordon PH, Hardcastle JD. A classification of fistula-in-ano. *Br J Surg* 1976;63:1–12.
24. Gray BK, Lockhart-Mummery HE, Morson BC. Crohn's disease of the anal region. *Gut* 1965;6:515–24.
25. Schwartz DA, Wiersema MJ, Dudiak KM, et al. A comparison of endoscopic ultrasound, magnetic resonance imaging, and exam under anesthesia for evaluation of Crohn's perianal fistulas. *Gastroenterology* 2001;121(5):1064–72.
26. Beets-Tan RG, Beets GL, van der Hoop AG, et al. Preoperative MR imaging of anal fistulas: does it really help the surgeon? *Radiology* 2001;218:75–84.
27. Schaefer O, Lohrmann C, Langer M. Assessment of anal fistulas with high-resolution subtraction MR-fistulography: comparison with surgical findings. *J Magn Reson Imaging* 2004;19:91–8.

28. Kuijpers HC, Schulpen T. Fistulography for fistula-in-ano. Is it useful? *Dis Colon Rectum* 1985;28:103–4.
29. Schratter-Sehn AU, Lochs H, Vogelsang H, Schurawitzki H, Herold C, Schratter M. Endoscopic ultrasonography versus computed tomography in the differential diagnosis of perianorectal complications in Crohn's disease. *Endoscopy* 1993;25: 582–6.
30. Choen S, Burnett S, Bartram CI, Nicholls RJ. Comparison between anal endosonography and digital examination in the evaluation of anal fistulae. *Br J Surg* 1991;78:445–7.
31. Stewart LK, McGee J, Wilson SR. Transperineal and transvaginal sonography of perianal inflammatory disease. *AJR Am J Roentgenol* 2001;177: 627–32.
32. Sloots CE, Felt-Bersma RJ, Poen AC, Cuesta MA, Meuwissen SG. Assessment and classification of fistula-in-ano in patients with Crohn's disease by hydrogen peroxide enhanced transanal ultrasound. *Int J Colorect Dis* 2001;16(5):292–7.
33. Navarro-Luna A, Garcia-Domingo MI, Rius-Macias J, Marco-Molina C. Ultrasound study of anal fistulas with hydrogen peroxide enhancement. *Dis Colon Rectum* 2004;47:108–14.
34. Poen AC, Felt-Bersma RJ, Eijsbouts QA, Cuesta MA, Meuwissen SG. Hydrogen peroxide-enhanced transanal ultrasound in the assessment of fistula-in-ano. *Dis Colon Rectum* 1998;41:1147–52.
35. Moscowitz I, Baig MK, Nogueras JJ, et al. Accuracy of hydrogen peroxide enhanced endoanal ultrasonography in assessment of the internal opening of an anal fistula complex. *Tech Coloproctol* 2003;7: 133–7.
36. Solomon MJ. Fistulae and abscesses in symptomatic perianal Crohn's disease. *Int J Colorect Dis* 1996; 11(5):222–6.
37. Rieger N, Tjandra J, Solomon M. Endoanal and endorectal ultrasound: applications in colorectal surgery. *ANZ J Surg* 2004;74:671–5.
38. Lunniss PJ, Armstrong P, Barker PG, Reznek RH, Phillips RK. Magnetic resonance imaging of anal fistulae. *Lancet* 1992;340:394–6.
39. Buchanan G, Halligan S, Williams A, et al. Effect of MRI on clinical outcome of recurrent fistula-in-ano. *Lancet* 2002;360:1661–2.
40. Bell SJ, Williams AB, Wiesel P, Wilkinson K, Cohen RC, Kamm MA. The clinical course of fistulating Crohn's disease. *Aliment Pharmacol Ther* 2003;17(9): 1145–51.
41. Morris J, Spencer JA, Ambrose NS. MR imaging classification of perianal fistulas and its implications for patient management. *Radiographics* 2000;20: 623–35.
42. Van Assche G, Vanbeckevoort D, Bielen D, et al. Magnetic resonance imaging of the effects of infliximab on perianal fistulizing Crohn's disease. *Am J Gastroenterol* 2003;98(2):332–9.
43. Makowiec F, Jehle EC, Becker HD, Starlinger M. Perianal abscess in Crohn's disease. *Dis Colon Rectum* 1997;40(4):443–50.
44. Michelassi F, Melis M, Rubin M, Hurst RD. Surgical treatment of anorectal complications in Crohn's disease. *Surgery* 2000;128(4):597–603.
45. Solomon MJ, McLeod RS, O'Connor BI, Steinhart H, Greenberg GR, Cohen Z. Combination ciprofloxacin and metronidazole in severe perianal Crohn's disease. *Can J Gastroenterol* 1993;7: 571–3.
46. Sandborn WJ, Fazio VW, Feagan BG, Hanauer SB, American Gastroenterological Association Clinical Practice Committee. AGA technical review on perianal Crohn's disease [Review] [223 refs]. *Gastroenterology* 2003;125(5):1508–30.
47. Turunen U, Farkkila M, Valtonen V. Long-term outcome of ciprofloxacin treatment in severe perianal or fistulous Crohn's disease [Abstract]. *Gastroenterology* 1993;104:793.
48. Bernstein LH, Frank MS, Brandt LJ, Boley SJ. Healing of perineal Crohn's disease with metronidazole. *Gastroenterology* 1980;79:357–65.
49. Jakobovits J, Schuster MM. Metronidazole therapy for Crohn's disease and associated fistulae. *Am J Gastroenterol* 1984;79:533–40.
50. Brandt LJ, Bernstein LH, Boley SJ, Frank MS. Metronidazole therapy for perineal Crohn's disease: a follow-up study. *Gastroenterology* 1982;83: 383–7.
51. Rhodes J, Bainton D, Beck P, Campbell H. Controlled trial of azathioprine in Crohn's disease. *Lancet* 1971; 2:1273–6.
52. Klein M, Binder HJ, Mitchell M, Aaronson R, Spiro H. Treatment of Crohn's disease with azathioprine: a controlled evaluation. *Gastroenterology* 1974;66: 916–22.
53. Summers RW, Switz DM, Sessions JT Jr, et al. National cooperative Crohn's disease study: results of drug treatment. *Gastroenterology* 1979;77:847–69.
54. Willoughby JM, Beckett J, Kumar PJ, Dawson AM. Controlled trial of azathioprine in Crohn's disease. *Lancet* 1971;2:944–7.
55. Ewe K, Press AG, Singe CC, et al. Azathioprine combined with prednisolone or monotherapy with prednisolone in active Crohn's disease. *Gastroenterology* 1993;105:367–72.

56 Rosenberg JL, Levin B, Wall AJ, Kirsner JB. A controlled trial of azathioprine in Crohn's disease. *Am J Dig Dis* 1975;20:721–6.

57 Present DH, Korelitz BI, Wisch N, Glass JL, Sachar DB, Pasternack BS. Treatment of Crohn's disease with 6-mercaptopurine. A long-term, randomized, double-blind study. *N Engl J Med* 1980;302:981–7.

58 Pearson DC, May GR, Fick GH, Sutherland LR. Azathioprine and 6-mercaptopurine in Crohn disease: a meta-analysis. *Ann Intern Med* 1995;123:132–42.

59 Lecomte T, Contou JF, Beaugerie L, *et al.* Predictive factors of response of perianal Crohn's disease to azathioprine or 6-mercaptopurine. *Dis Colon Rectum* 2003;46(11):1469–75.

60 Schwartz DA, Herdman CR. Review article: The medical treatment of Crohn's perianal fistulas. *Aliment Pharmacol Ther* 2004;19:953–67.

61 Hanauer SB, Smith MB. Rapid closure of Crohn's disease fistulas with continuous intravenous cyclosporin A. *Am J Gastroenterol* 1993; 88:646–9.

62 Present DH, Lichtiger S. Efficacy of cyclosporine in treatment of fistula of Crohn's disease. *Dig Dis Sci* 1994;39:374–80.

63 Cat H, Sophani I, Lemann M, Modigliani R, Solue JC. Cyclosporin treatment of anal and perianal lesions associated with Crohn's disease. *Turk J Gastroenterol* 2003;14(2):121–7.

64 Sandborn WJ, Present DH, Isaacs KL, *et al.* Tacrolimus for the treatment of fistulas in patients with Crohn's disease: a randomized, placebo-controlled trial. *Gastroenterology* 2003;125(2):380–8.

65 Gonzalez LY, Abreu LE, Vera MI, de la RJ, Fernandez-Puga N, Escartin P. Long-term oral tacrolimus in refractory to infliximab fistulizing Crohn's disease: comments from Spanish experience. *Gastroenterology* 2004;126:942–3.

66 Sands BE, Anderson FH, Bernstein CN, *et al.* Infliximab maintenance therapy for fistulizing Crohn's disease. *N Engl J Med* 2004;350:876–85.

67 Sands BE, Blank MA, Patel K, van Deventer SJ. Long-term treatment of rectovaginal fistulas in Crohn's disease: response to infliximab in the ACCENT II Study. *Clin Gastroenterol Hepatol* 2004;2:912–20.

68 Ochsenkuhn T, Goke B, Sackmann M. Combining infliximab with 6-mercaptopurine/azathioprine for fistula therapy in Crohn's disease. *Am J Gastroenterol* 2002;97:2022–5.

69 Schroder O, Blumenstein I, Schulte-Bockholt A, Stein J. Combining infliximab and methotrexate in fistulizing Crohn's disease resistant or intolerant to azathioprine. *Aliment Pharmacol Ther* 2004;19:295–301.

70 van Bodegraven AA, Sloots CE, Felt-Bersma RJ, Meuwissen SG. Endosonographic evidence of persistence of Crohn's disease-associated fistulas after infliximab treatment, irrespective of clinical response. *Dis Colon Rectum* 2002;45(1):39–45; discussion 45–6.

71 Rasul I, Wilson SR, MacRae H, Irwin S, Greenberg GR. Clinical and radiological responses after infliximab treatment for perianal fistulizing Crohn's disease [see comment]. *Am J Gastroenterol* 2004;99(1):82–8.

72 Rasul I, Wilson SR, MacRae H, Irwin S, Greenberg GR. Clinical and radiological responses after infliximab treatment for perianal fistulizing Crohn's disease [see comment]. *Am J Gastroenterol* 2004;99(1):82–8.

73 Keane J, Gershon S, Wise RP, *et al.* Tuberculosis associated with infliximab, a tumor necrosis factor alpha-neutralizing agent. *N Engl J Med* 2001;345:1098–104.

74 Warris A, Bjorneklett A, Gaustad P. Invasive pulmonary aspergillosis associated with infliximab therapy. *N Engl J Med* 2001;344:1099–100.

75 Nakelchik M, Mangino JE. Reactivation of histoplasmosis after treatment with infliximab. *Am J Med* 2002;112:78.

76 Morelli J, Wilson FA. Does administration of infliximab increase susceptibility to listeriosis? *Am J Gastroenterol* 2000;95:841–2.

77 Fiocchi C. Closing fistulas in Crohn's disease – should the accent be on maintenance or safety? *N Engl J Med* 2004;350:934–6.

78 Adams AE, Zwicker J, Curiel C, *et al.* Aggressive cutaneous T-cell lymphomas after TNFalpha blockade. *J Am Acad Dermatol* 2004;51:660–2.

79 Ljung T, Karlen P, Schmidt D, *et al.* Infliximab in inflammatory bowel disease: clinical outcome in a population based cohort from Stockholm county. *Gut* 2004;53:849–53.

80 Bickston SJ, Lichtenstein GR, Arseneau KO, Cohen RB, Cominelli F. The relationship between infliximab treatment and lymphoma in Crohn's disease. *Gastroenterology* 1999;117:1433–7.

81 Baert F, Noman M, Vermeire S, *et al.* Influence of immunogenicity on the long-term efficacy of infliximab in Crohn's disease. *N Engl J Med* 2003;348:601–8.

82 Sandborn WJ, Faubion WA. Biologics in inflammatory bowel disease: how much progress have we made? *Gut* 2004;53:1366–73.

83. Schwartz DA, Loftus EV Jr, Tremaine WJ, et al. The natural history of fistulizing Crohn's disease in Olmsted county, Minnesota. *Gastroenterology* 2002; 122(4):875–80.
84. Ky A, Sohn N, Weinstein MA, Korelitz BI. Carcinoma arising in anorectal fistulas of Crohn's disease. *Dis Colon Rectum* 1998;41:992–6.
85. Regueiro M, Mardini H. Treatment of perianal fistulizing Crohn's disease with infliximab alone or as an adjunct to exam under anesthesia with seton placement. *Inflamm Bowel Dis* 2003;9(2):98–103.
86. Harper PH, Truelove SC, Lee EC, Kettlewell MG, Jewell DP. Split ileostomy and ileocolostomy for Crohn's disease of the colon and ulcerative colitis: a 20 year survey. *Gut* 1983;24:106–13.
87. Zelas P, Jagelman DG. Loop illeostomy in the management of Crohn's colitis in the debilitated patient. *Ann Surg* 1980;191:164–8.
88. Grant DR, Cohen Z, McLeod RS. Loop ileostomy for anorectal Crohn's disease. *Can J Surg* 1986;29: 32–5.
89. Regimbeau JM, Panis Y, Cazaban L, et al. Long-term results of faecal diversion for refractory perianal Crohn's disease. *Colorectal Dis* 2001;3:232–7.
90. Winslet MC, Andrews H, Allan RN, Keighley MR. Fecal diversion in the management of Crohn's disease of the colon. *Dis Colon Rectum* 1993;36:757–62.
91. Yamamoto T, Allan RN, Keighley MR. Effect of fecal diversion alone on perianal Crohn's disease. *World J Surg* 2000;24(10):1258–62; discussion 1262–3.
92. Farmer RG, Hawk WA, Turnbull RB Jr. Indications for surgery in Crohn's disease: analysis of 500 cases. *Gastroenterology* 1976;71:245–50.
93. Hurst RD, Gottlieb LJ, Crucitti P, Melis M, Rubin M, Michelassi F. Primary closure of complicated perineal wounds with myocutaneous and fasciocutaneous flaps after proctectomy for Crohn's disease. *Surgery* 2001; 130:767–72.
94. Fry RD, Shemesh EI, Kodner IJ, Timmcke A. Techniques and results in the management of anal and perianal Crohn's disease. *Surg Gynecol Obstet* 1989; 168(1):42–8.
95. Williamson PR, Hellinger MD, Larach SW, Ferrara A. Twenty-year review of the surgical management of perianal Crohn's disease. [Review] [15 refs]. *Dis Colon Rectum* 1995;38(4):389–92.
96. Kangas E. Anal lesions complicating Crohn's disease. *Ann Chir Gynaecol* 1991;80:336–9.
97. McKee RF, Keenan RA. Perianal Crohn's disease – is it all bad news? *Dis Colon Rectum* 1996;39: 136–42.
98. Williams JG, Rothenberger DA, Nemer FD, Goldberg SM. Fistula-in-ano in Crohn's disease. Results of aggressive surgical treatment. *Dis Colon Rectum* 1991;34:378–84.
99. Scott HJ, Northover JM. Evaluation of surgery for perianal Crohn's fistulas. *Dis Colon Rectum* 1996;39: 1039–43.
100. Fuhrman GM, Larach SW. Experience with perirectal fistulas in patients with Crohn's disease. *Dis Colon Rectum* 1989;32:847–8.
101. Marchesa P, Hull TL, Fazio VW. Advancement sleeve flaps for treatment of severe perianal Crohn's disease. *Br J Surg* 1998;85(12):1695–8.
102. Hull TL, Fazio VW. Surgical approaches to low anovaginal fistula in Crohn's disease. *Am J Surg* 1997; 173:95–8.
103. Jorge JM, Wexner SD. Etiology and management of fecal incontinence. *Dis Colon Rectum* 1993;36: 77–97.

21: What is dysplasia?

Karel Geboes

Introduction

Since the first descriptions of colorectal cancer (CRC) in ulcerative colitis (UC) [1, 2] one of the major considerations regarding UC is its propensity for developing into cancer because this accounts for 1/6 of all deaths in UC patients. Approximately 1% of all colorectal cancer cases occur in the background of chronic idiopathic inflammatory bowel diseases (IBD). In hereditary and sporadic cancer, polypoid and flat adenomas identify individuals at risk. As early as 1949, Warren and Sommers postulated that a structural precursor to carcinoma existed also in longstanding ulcerative colitis. It was suggested that CRC could develop either from pre-existing adenomatous polyps or from regenerative epithelial hyperplasia [3]. In 1967 'pre-cancerous' changes were described in the mucosa of colectomy specimens of patients operated for carcinoma in UC [4]. The occurrence of 'pre-cancer' was confirmed in retrospective studies and was later referred to as 'dysplasia' [5]. Similar changes were reported in Crohn's disease [6, 7]. Overall, dysplasia is detected in surgical specimens from 87% of patients with Crohn's disease and CRC and in 70% of UC patients with CRC [8]. Dysplasia is therefore used as a marker for early detection of neoplasia in patients with IBD. However, the practical application and the cost-effectiveness of surveillance programmes are not entirely satisfactory. The lesions are often not identifiable at endoscopy. Furthermore, there are problems with inter- and intra-observer variability among pathologists, and uncertainties in the clinical interpretation of dysplasia. Therefore, a precise definition of 'dysplasia' and reliable criteria for its detection are needed.

Definition of dysplasia

Dysplasia is a morphological term that etymologically means 'malformation'. It is derived from classic Greek and is composed of two elements, 'dys' which is 'bad' or 'wrong' and 'plasis' which means 'form'. The origin and nature of a malformation can be variable. It can be a macroscopic or microscopic lesion and congenital (hereditary or not) or acquired. If acquired, the nature of the dysplastic transformation can be regenerative (due to healing and repair following damage), or neoplastic (degenerative) [9]. When used for microscopic epithelial changes, dysplasia is often defined as a lesion 'in which part of the epithelium is replaced by cells showing varying degrees of 'atypia'. The latter term is usually restricted to cytological abnormalities, while 'dysplasia' encompasses also changes in architecture and aberrant differentiation [10]. Changes in architecture and cytology such as the appearance of immature cells (altered differentiation) are phenomena that occur during healing and repair and might also be considered as dysplasia according to this definition. Yet, these alterations have no clinical consequences. A purely morphological definition of dysplasia is therefore not appropriate. A more precise definition of 'dysplasia' has been proposed by an international 'inflammatory bowel disease – dysplasia morphology study group'. According to this definition, IBD-associated dysplasia is used for lesions showing 'unequivocal, non-invasive (confined within the basement membrane), neoplastic transformation of the epithelium excluding all reactive changes' [11]. This definition stresses the nature and origin of the lesion, but its identification still relies upon the recognition of morphological features resulting from cytological and architectural changes in routinely processed and haematoxylin and eosin stained sections. More recently, it has been proposed to replace the term 'dysplasia' by 'intra-epithelial neoplasia'. This is implemented in the World Health Organization classification of neoplasia of the gastrointestinal tract [12]. The background for this proposal is that this term defines more clearly the nature and the extent of the lesion and allows recommendations for diagnostic and therapeutic measures.

Precursor lesions and carcinogenesis

Morphology

The normal intestine contains proliferating epithelial cells in the distal compartment of the crypts, while the surface is covered by mature, differentiated cells. The latter cells cease dividing and withdraw permanently from the cell cycle. Normally there is a balance between cell proliferation, growth arrest and differentiation and loss of mature cells by programmed cell death. The development and progression of cancer involves processes that allow cellular immortalisation. In a first step, colorectal epithelium shows expansion of the proliferative compartment from the lower crypt to the upper part where undifferentiated cells accumulate. This phenomenon is observed in 'aberrant crypt foci' and 'adenomas', the precursor lesions of sporadic and hereditary CRC. In these classical examples of 'dysplasia', the morphology of the neoplastic epithelium reflects abnormal proliferation and affects nuclei and cytoplasm of cells and the architecture of crypts. The various histopathologic entities can be arrayed in stages of increasing abnormality. This arrangement is compatible with a multi-step process, the adenoma (polyp)-cancer sequence in which initially normal cells pass through a succession of increasingly abnormal stages on their way to becoming fully neoplastic. In IBD, dysplasia is the earliest phase in the development of CRC, which can be recognised by routine morphology.

The molecular era

The 'adenoma-carcinoma' sequence has gained a molecular basis. Changes in nuclear DNA-content and gross chromosomal alterations are identified with flow cytometry, image cytometry and fluorescent *in situ* hybridisation (FISH). Mutations and/or loss of heterozygosity (LOH) of genes can be detected with polymerase chain reaction (PCR). The expression of abnormal proteins or the aberrant expression of proteins resulting from mutations can be demonstrated with immunohistochemistry. These techniques have been applied to colorectal cancer, including ulcerative colitis-associated CRC. The development of CRC is marked by an accumulation of genetic defects and the morphological spectrum of the precursor lesions is a continuum reflecting the stepwise accumulation of these defects [13]. Three major pathways can be identified: chromosomal instability, micro-satellite instability and the methylator pathway [14]. Chromosomal instability (CIN) is the result of a defect in pathways that direct the segregation of genetic material during cell division. It is characterised by losses and/or gains of genetic material. Abnormal amounts of DNA (aneuploidy) are the result. Micro-satellite instability (MSI) is the result of defects in pathways that maintain the integrity of genomic sequences such as mutations of enzymes that direct the DNA-based mismatch repair process (hypermutability). These cases are diploid. The methylator pathway overlaps CIN and MSI and is characterised by hypermethylation of key regulatory genes resulting in their inactivation. CIN accounts for nearly 85% of sporadic CRC. Approximately 10–15% of sporadic CRC are characterised by MSI. Genetic alterations occur in two major classes of genes: proto-oncogenes and tumour suppressor genes. Loss or inactivation of the APC (adenomatous polyposis coli), a tumour suppressor gene involved in the migration of enterocytes, is an early step in the formation of aberrant dysplastic crypts and sporadic adenomas. APC abnormalities may also lead to disruption of normal cell–cell adhesion by altered binding to E-cadherin. Activating mutations of the K-ras proto-oncogene (involved in cell proliferation) occur at an early stage. They confer polypoid growth to developing adenomas. The DCC (deleted in colon cancer) suppressor gene is involved in cell differentiation. Abnormalities occur in the transition from early to late adenoma. P53 mutations are a late event. Inactivation of p53 mediates the progression to carcinoma. It is in this way that stepwise molecular alterations result in the progression of aberrant crypt foci to small polypoid adenoma and to advanced adenoma and cancer.

Molecular mechanism underlying IBD-related carcinogenesis

Genetic instability and IBD-related dysplasia

The molecular pathway leading to the formation of IBD-associated dysplasia and CRC has particularly been studied for ulcerative colitis (Table 21.1). The origin of the genomic instability in IBD-associated CRC can be linked to the inflammation. The risk of CRC increases with duration and extension of the disease and may be reduced with anti-inflammatory therapies. Inflammation in IBD generates abundant reactive oxygen species that can damage DNA, increase p53 mutation and promote telomere shortening, which in turn causes the accumulation of chromosomal aberrations through a mechanism of chromatin bridge breakage and fusion. Carcinogenesis in IBD appears to follow a 'colitis–dysplasia–carcinoma' pathway. In IBD-associated CRC, aneuploidy and CIN are detected in approximately 85% of UC-related cases and in nearly 76% of Crohn's disease-related cases. Aneuploidy is closely related with the development of dysplasia [15–17]. Its presence is not necessarily associated with inflammation. Its detection may, therefore, be more objective than the assessment of dysplasia. It has been detected in samples from non-neoplastic and neoplastic colitic mucosa. Absence of aneuploidy may have a strong negative predictive value (high degree of protection) [18]. Some carcinomas are, however, unassociated with aneuploidy and in other cases there is a transition from aneuploidy to carcinoma without dysplasia [19]. Aneuploidy alone is neither necessary nor sufficient to cause transition towards malignancy and it may also occur later in the process of colonic

Table 21.1 Molecular abnormalities in ulcerative colitis cancer and sporadic cancer.

	Ulcerative colitis				Sporadic colorectal cancer		
	Non-neoplastic mucosa	Hyperplastic polyp	Dysplasia	Cancer	Hyperplastic polyp	Adenoma	Cancer
Aneuploidy	3–5%	—	20–25%	76–85%	—	85%	85%
MSI	+		+	2–9%	20%[4]	8–25%	10–15%
APC mut[1]/LOH[2]	—	11%	10–30%	10–80%	0%	60–90%	60–90%
K-ras mut	0	19%	40%	30%	13%	40–60%[3]	50–60%
DCC mut/LOH			35%	12%		±70%	65%
p53 mut/LOH	5%	27%	33–63%	70–80%	20%	15–20%	70–80%
BCL$_2$ up-regulation		3–5%	±35%	23%	2%	±80%	50–60%
Cyclin D$_1$ up-regulation	7%		40%	30%		±30%	20–64%
p21 down-regulation			23%	50%		10%	25–40%
p27 down-regulation				100%			30%
p16 hyper-methylation	15%	13%	35–50%	100%	20%	5%	10%
Beta-catenin dysregulation			8%	45–50%		46%	70–90%

Results are based on a selection of studies.
[1] mut = mutation.
[2] LOH = Loss or heterozygosity.
[3] In large adenomas.
[4] Depending on histology.

carcinogenesis in UC [20, 21]. Comparable results are obtained with FISH [22]. Changes in DNA content can thus occur before or after the emergence of the morphological features of dysplasia. Overall MSI is observed in 2.4–14% of UC-related CRC cases. The data show no major differences compared with those obtained for sporadic CRC [23, 24]. Abnormalities occur in colitic non-neoplastic mucosa and in dysplastic lesions.

Dysplasia and defects in genes in control of cell proliferation and cell death

The frequency of APC tumour suppressor gene and ras oncogene mutations in UC-associated cancers is lower and mutations are a late event compared to familial polyposis (FAP) and sporadic CRC [25–28]. K-ras mutations have been particularly found in so-called villous, hypermucinous mucosa in UC [29]. Inactivation of p53 by mutation and loss of heterozygosity (LOH) seems an early event in UC-associated CRC [30, 31]. Both p53 mutations and k-ras mutations can be detected in non-neoplastic mucosa and neoplastic mucosa in UC. Overexpression of the B-cell leukaemia/lymphoma (bcl2) proto-oncogene product, associated with inhibition of apoptosis is less common in UC-associated cancer [32]. In UC-related dysplasia and CRC overexpression of cyclin D1 (involved in the passage through the G1/S phase of the cell cycle) occurs in association with β-catenin nuclear expression whereas $p21^{waf1}$, $p27^{kip1}$ and $p16^{ink4a}$ (inhibitors of cyclin D1) are down regulated [33, 34].

Dysplasia and defects in genes in control of cell and tissue structure

Cancer development is also associated with abnormalities in genes coding for proteins involved in the preservation of cell shape, cell cohesion and tissue structure and integrity. Aberrant expression of cytokeratins (involved in cell shape) was reported in Crohn's disease-associated carcinoma and dysplasia [35]. Expression of CD44v6, a cell adhesion receptor, has been described in IBD in association with proliferation. The data are comparable with those observed in colorectal adenomas [36–38]. Adhesion molecules like e-cadherins and β-catenin are involved in cell signalling, cell–cell adhesion, cell differentiation and migration and related to polarity. Loss of polarity is one of the features used to diagnose dysplasia. Reduced expression of e-cadherin and β-catenin has been reported in ulcerative colitis and Crohn's disease [39, 40]. Loss of e-cadherin expression is also found in ulcerative colitis-associated cancers [32]. P-cadherins, on the contrary, are up-regulated in Crohn's disease and ulcerative colitis, especially in dysplastic tissue [41]. Up-regulation of cyclooxygenase 2 (COX-2), involved in the expression of regulators of apoptosis such as bcl2 protein, in cellular adhesion to extra-cellular matrix proteins and in angiogenesis, is observed in active UC (approx 11%) and in UC-associated neoplasia [38–53%]. In sporadic CRC, COX-2 expression is increased in almost 85% of cases [42, 43].

Diagnosis of dysplasia in IBD

Macroscopic diagnosis

Macroscopically, IBD-associated dysplasia occurs in colitic mucosa. It should be distinguished from sporadic adenomas occurring in a bowel segment that is entirely free from disease. Over 95% of dysplastic foci occur in flat mucosa. It is difficult to identify these lesions macroscopically [44]. Chromoendoscopy and magnifying chromoendoscopy can increase the diagnostic yield [45]. The elevated lesions, approximately 5% of the IBD-associated dysplastic lesions are conventionally referred to by the acronym DALM (dysplasia-associated lesion or mass) [46]. They are a heterogeneous group. Dysplastic polyps with a well-defined stalk, encountered in a diseased region can be regarded as a sporadic adenoma if the mucosa of the stalk and surrounding mucosa is not dysplastic. This has lead to the introduction of the term ALM (adenoma-like mass) or adenoma-like DALM for these lesions (Fig 21.1). They must be distinguished from genuine DALMs, which are poorly circumscribed elevated lesions surrounded by flat dysplastic mucosa. It is, however, not yet clear whether all adenoma-like DALMs are similar. Molecular studies show indeed that some ALM lesions are closer to genuine

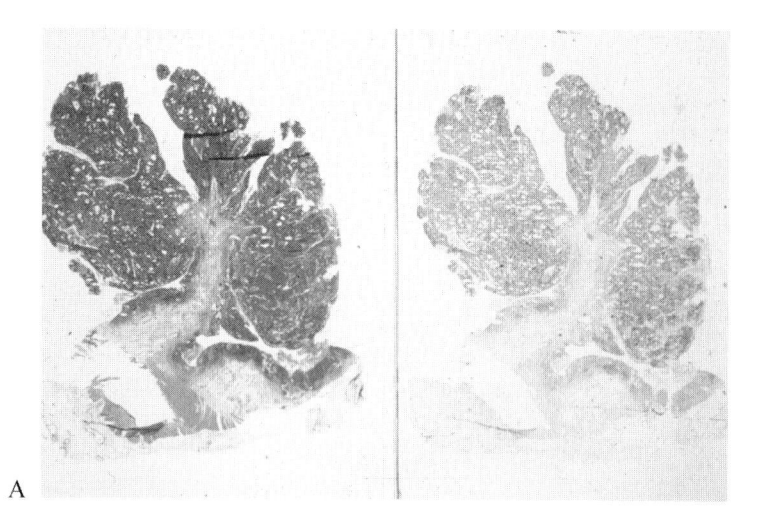

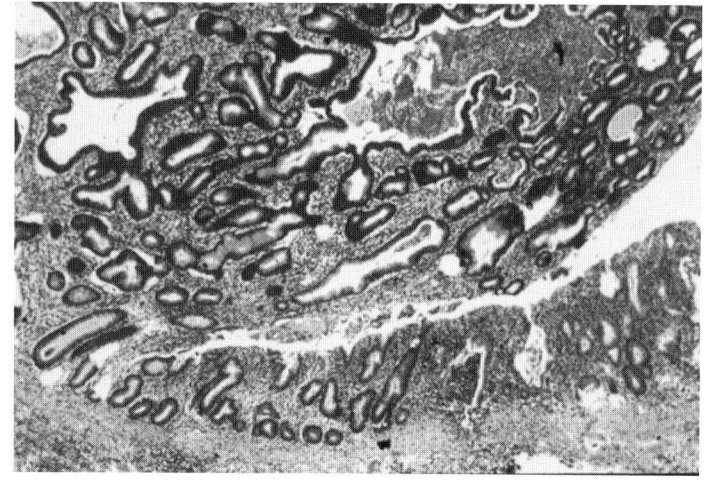

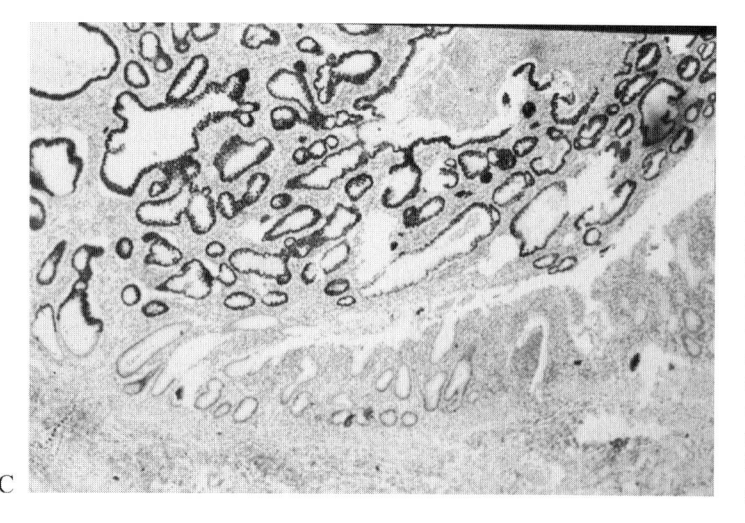

Fig 21.1 Polypoid dysplasia in ulcerative colitis. (a) This is a low-power micro-photograph of a section of the lesion stained with haematoxylin and eosin (right panel). The left panel shows a serial section stained with antibodies directed against p53. The polypoid lesion shows diffuse nuclear positivity. (b) This is a high-power micro-photograph of the same lesion stained with haematoxylin and eosin showing the transition between the colitic-non-dysplastic mucosa surrounding the elevated lesion and dysplasia. (c) This is a serial section stained with antibodies against p53. The lesion can be considered to be an adenoma-like mass based on histology, although it shows aberrant expression of p53.

DALMs. Molecular markers may ultimately afford a more objective means of making the distinction between DALMs and ALMs.

Microscopy

The diagnosis of IBD-associated dysplasia relies mainly on microscopy. The mucosa can be negative for dysplasia, indefinite or positive. When a biopsy is diagnosed as negative for dysplasia, it must be realised that dysplasia in IBD shows a patchy distribution and sampling error is a significant problem with random biopsies from unremarkable mucosa. Thirty-three to 64 biopsies are required to detect dysplasia with 90 and 95% probabilities, respectively, and with 20–40 biopsies less than 0.1% of the colorectal mucosa is covered [20, 47]. Current practice guidelines recommend that 2–4 biopsy specimens be taken from every 10 cm of diseased bowel in addition to macroscopically atypical lesions [48]. The sampling problems might be solved by chromoendoscopy and targeted biopsies. A variety of other factors affect the interpretation of biopsy specimens. It may be impossible to classify some epithelial changes either unequivocally negative or positive for dysplasia. The most important of these patterns is a failure of the crypt epithelium to differentiate into normal mature cells. Such cases are classified as indefinite. The importance of this category is that, although it may occasionally be a hedge for ignorance, it signals the equivocal nature of a lesion and implies that further biopsies should be obtained [49]. A biopsy can only be diagnosed as positive for dysplasia when the lesion is unequivocally present. Generally, the histological features of dysplasia in IBD are comparable with those seen in colonic adenomas in non-colitic patients [11]. A villous, hypermucinous mucosa and hyperplastic polyps may represent a second type of lesion with increased risk for developing CRC.

In the classical adenomatous type, the morphological spectrum of lesions forms a continuum. However, in practice, dysplasia is divided into different categories according to the severity of the alterations, because of different implications for patient management. A distinction can be made between three grades (mild, moderate or severe) or two grades (Table 21.2). In the most commonly used classification, two grades are distinguished [11]. The category 'low-grade dysplasia' includes cases of mild and moderate dysplasia. The category 'high-grade dysplasia' includes some cases of moderate dysplasia (those with prominent architectural alteration) and all cases of severe dysplasia and carcinoma *in situ*. The grade of dysplasia is determined by the features of the most dysplastic portion. The two grade classification appears to be reproducible, although in general the agreement is better for high-grade dysplasia [50].

Architectural features include thickening of the mucosa, lengthening and distortion of the crypts with excessive budding and increased size [11, 49, 51]. In contrast with the budding that occurs in regenerated mucosa, which is usually associated with a reduced number of crypts, in dysplasia the crypts may be increased in number and much more closely approximated. Dysplastic crypts are further often enlarged and lined by tall columnar cells in which there is frequently some mucus differentiation. The dysplastic process will usually involve the surface epithelium, although cells at the surface may show minimal lesions. They may appear normal except for their large size and their tall, high columnar (non-goblet) shape. Mucin tends to be in columnar cells rather than in the usual goblet cells. It appears sometimes as small mucin droplets. Stains for acid mucopolysaccharides show that the mucin is of the intestinal type. This can be regarded as a failure of crypt epithelium to differentiate into mature cell types. There may be marked reduction in the number of goblet mucus cells and sometimes 'dystrophic' or 'upside-down' goblet cells appear. These are goblet cells in which the mucin droplet is located in the basal rather than apical portion of the cell (abnormal polarity of goblet cells – mucin below,

Table 21.2 Biopsy classification of dysplasia in inflammatory bowel disease [11].

Negative
Indefinite
Positive
Low-grade dysplasia
High-grade dysplasia

rather than above the nucleus). In some cases abnormal double layers of goblet cells are seen. Occasionally, excessive numbers of Paneth or endocrine cells are present. In both of these cases the cytoplasmic granules may be perinuclear, in contrast to their usual supra- and sub-nuclear locations, respectively [11]. Nuclear changes are morphologically similar to those seen in tubular adenomas: hyperchromatic and enlarged with nuclear crowding and frequent overlapping. The nuclei are also typically stratified, particularly near the base of the crypts, although still largely confined to the basal half of the cell. Mitotic figures may be present in the upper part of the crypt, and even in the surface (which is abnormal). In low-grade dysplasia the nuclei remain confined to the basal half of the cells [52] (Fig 21.2). High-grade dysplasia is associated with true stratification of neoplastic cells and marked distortion of crypt architecture. Crypts may be tightly packed with branching and lateral budding, often yielding a complex architecture (Fig 21.3). There is intraglandular bridging of epithelium to form a cribriform pattern of back-to-back glands, and frequently a villiform surface configuration. The latter can also be seen in non-dysplastic long-standing ulcerative colitis, and should not be over-interpreted. Cytological changes usually involve the surface and crypt epithelium. Goblet cell mucin is diminished or depleted and 'dystrophic' goblet cells may again be seen. Nuclear stratification extends into the superficial (luminal) parts of the cells. Other criteria include a greater degree of cytological variance, prominent hyperchromatism, pleomorphism, overlapping vesicular nuclei and loss of nuclear polarity. The nuclei often

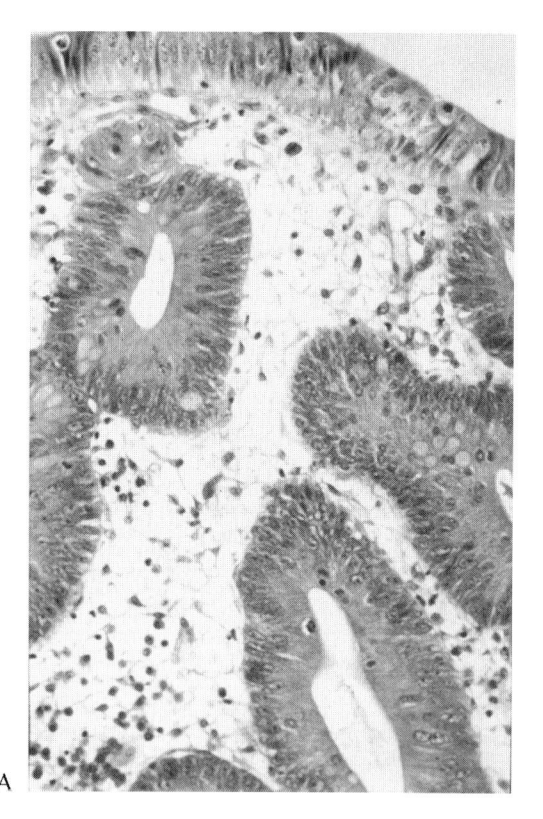

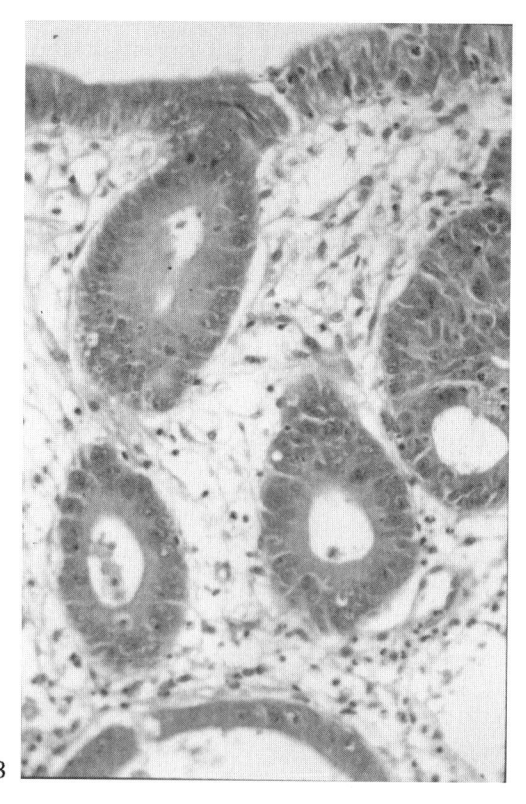

Fig 21.2 (a) This shows low-grade dysplasia: the pattern is characterised by the presence of tall columnar cells on the surface and in the crypts and by mitotic figures on the surface. (b) This represents low-grade dysplasia in the left half and high-grade dysplasia with loss of polarity of the epithelial cells in the right half of the picture.

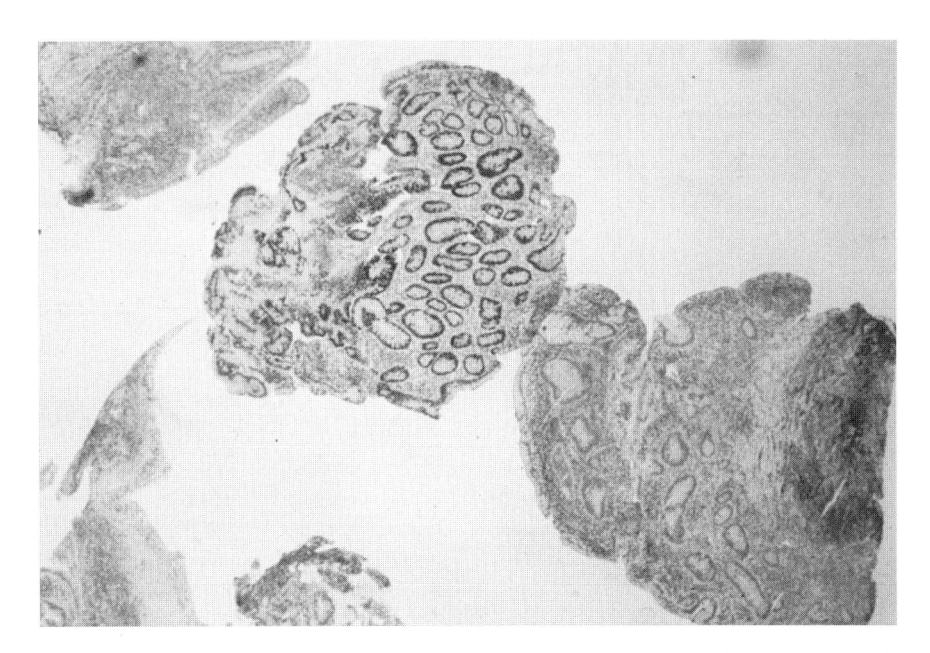

Fig 21.3 Immunohistochemical staining with an antibody directed against p53 shows one biopsy sample with positively staining nuclei. Compared with the negatively staining, non-dysplastic colitic samples, the positive sample shows also crowding of crypts.

vary markedly in size, shape and staining characteristics [11, 49, 51]. Mitotic figures can appear on the surface and peri-crypt fibroblasts become dispersed. In general, inflammation is not a prominent feature in dysplasia, but the absence of active inflammation in an area of equivocal atypia is not proof of its neoplastic nature [53].

Ancillary techniques and the diagnosis of dysplasia in IBD

Because of the diagnostic problems related to dysplasia, the use of markers has been proposed to improve the reliability of the diagnosis. The value of staining for carcinoembryonic antigen (CEA) and CA19-9 seems limited [54, 55]. Staining for Sialosyl-Tn antigen shows a shift in mucinous production preceding the occurrence of dysplasia in ulcerative colitis by several years. Sialyl-Tn antigen (STn) expression is independent of and may precede aneuploidy. Like aneuploidy, it is expressed more widely throughout the colon than dysplasia [56]. Further prospective studies are needed to confirm the findings [57]. Staining for proliferating nuclear antigen (PCNA), AgNOR (argyrophylic proteins associated to nucleolar organiser regions) and Ki-67 allows one to delineate dysplastic from non-dysplastic lesions, but the results are influenced by inflammation making the utility of the test in practice uncertain [58].

Additional techniques can be useful for the solution of differential diagnostic problems between 'genuine' dysplasia and reparative phenomena. At present molecular techniques do not yet offer an alternative for the microscopic diagnosis of dysplasia. A search for genetic alterations in order to define dysplasia more precisely can offer support for the diagnosis if positive, but a negative finding does not exclude the possibility of dysplasia. Furthermore, the results obtained with additional techniques must be interpreted with caution. Absence or decrease of e-cadherin protein expression occurs in ulcerative colitis-associated CRC and in sporadic CRC. However, it is not constantly present in all ulcerative colitis-associated cancers and has been observed also in benign ulcerative lesions in UC [39].

Aneuploidy, MSI, LOH of p53 and k-ras mutations can be present before the appearance of dysplasia, but the natural history and cancer risk of these alterations is not known. Dysplasia and the genetic defects associated with cancer development are different phenomena identified with entirely different techniques. Although a combination of routine morphology and new techniques for markers can help to identify dysplasia, the search for additional markers by itself can only support a diagnosis of dysplasia if positive, or help identify the cancer risk in patients in whom routine morphology fails to detect dysplasia. For example, p53 over-expression in non-dysplastic mucosa has been shown to carry a five times increased risk for the subsequent development of dysplasia [59].

Differential diagnosis

Polypoid IBD-associated dysplasia and sporadic adenomas occurring in IBD patients and polypoid dysplasia and inflammatory polyps

The differential diagnosis between sporadic adenomas and polypoid IBD-associated neoplasia is based upon clinical and pathologic features. Sporadic adenomas are more common in older patients, having no disease activity and a relatively short disease history. Histologically there is often a mixture of normal and dysplastic crypts at the surface of the polyps in IBD-associated polypoid dysplasia. The presence of stalk dysplasia, if the lesion is pedunculated and the presence of dysplasia in flat mucosa adjacent to a dysplastic polyp favour a diagnosis of IBD-associated polypoid dysplasia [60–62]. Inflammation of the lamina propria is uncommon in sporadic adenomas. Presence of immunostaining for p53 and lack of bcl2 and nuclear β-catenin immunostaining favour a diagnosis of DALM over sporadic adenoma, but confirmation is needed [63]. Qualitative differences in the expression of survivin have been reported in DALM and LOH at 3p (the von Hippel-Landau gene) is less common in ALM than in DALM.

The differential diagnosis between polypoid IBD-associated dysplasia and inflammatory pseudopolyps or dysplasia in inflammatory pseudopolyps is another problem. In general, dysplasia in inflammatory polyps is rare [11]. The major problem is that these polyps frequently contain areas of residual regeneration and it may be difficult to make a clear distinction between unequivocally neoplastic changes and regeneration. The presence of a mucosal defect (erosion or ulceration) close by can suggest regeneration. In cases of doubt, multiple biopsies from the lesion and the surrounding mucosa can help to solve the problem.

Polypoid dysplasia and hyperplastic polyps

Hyperplastic polyps in the colon have long been regarded as benign. However, there is growing evidence implicating at least a subset of hyperplastic polyps in the development of CRC in the non-IBD population. Hyperplastic polyps may also develop in UC and in Crohn's disease. It is unclear if these are biologically similar to the sporadic type or represent a separate type of hypermucinous dysplasia. Hyperplastic polyps from UC patients have been shown to be genotypically similar to sporadic hyperplastic polyps from age- and sex-matched patients without UC. This study, however, supported the theory that hyperplastic polyps may have neoplastic potential [64].

'Genuine' dysplasia and reparative lesions

IBD is characterised by episodes of remission with a decrease of inflammation and restoration of the goblet cell population, and active disease associated with mucin depletion. Abnormal mucin secretion is also a feature of dysplasia. Whereas high-grade dysplasia can usually be reliably distinguished, the distinction between repair and low-grade dysplasia may present a serious problem. It is important to solve this properly, given the clinical consequences. A better knowledge of the repair phenomena occurring in the intestine can be of great help. In the gastrointestinal tract, the repair of injured surfaces can occur rapidly and does not necessarily require increased proliferation. This process, known as 'restitution', involves migration of cells from the crypts onto the surface. Migrating cells appear at first flattened, and subsequently increase in height to cuboidal and columnar. Absence of mucus and a low number of goblet cells are common, as the cells are not yet fully differentiated [65]. Promotion of cell migration occurs also in IBD, as illustrated by the reduced expression of e-cadherins [39]. The process can be regarded as an exaggeration of the normal migration. Even in the normal situation the surface epithelial cells are constantly replaced by new cells, formed in the proliferative compartment in the distal part of the crypts and these cells will undergo terminal differentiation during their migration towards the intercryptal surface [66]. The initial restitutive phase of regeneration can be readily distinguished from dysplasia. Surface and crypt epithelial cells are attenuated, cuboidal or low columnar. The nuclei are elongated but orientated in the same plane as the cell. As the cells become more cuboidal, the nuclei appear rounded and vesicular with prominent nucleoli (Fig 21.4). Sometimes a transition from more cuboidal cells in the upper part of the crypts towards attenuated cells on the surface can be observed. In the basal part of the crypts the number of cells can be increased (compensatory hyperproliferation). In addition, the presence of inflammation orients also to reactive changes. The major findings are summarised in Table 21.3.

In IBD, epithelial cell damage is not limited to the intercryptal surface. Crypt epithelial cells are usually extensively involved as illustrated by the presence of cryptitis, numerous crypt abscesses and crypt destruction in the active phase of the diseases. Repair of the extensive epithelial damage, therefore, also requires 'increased proliferation' [67]. Normal cell proliferation and increased proliferation following damage occur in the distal part of the crypts. Increased proliferation is characterised by an increased number of mitoses and expansion of the proliferative compartment. Newly formed cells show dark cytoplasmic staining. Nuclear chromatin increases so that the nuclei are normo- or hyperchromatic. This can be accompanied by elongation and mild stratification. However, mitoses are still confined to the crypts. The presence of atypical mitoses is of limited value, although they are more common in neoplasia. They were shown to occur in chronic inflammation (19%) as well as in dysplasia (34%) and cancer (49%) [68]. Alterations of surface epithelial cells are limited as there is still a normal maturation towards the surface. This implies preservation of the basal position of the nuclei and of nuclear polarity and absence of cellular pleomorphism. Immunohistochemistry using antibodies directed against Ki67, a nuclear protein expressed in all active phases of the cell cycle (G1, S, G2 and M) can be used for the distinction between reparative and neoplastic processes. Restriction of Ki67 staining to the lower third of the crypts is never seen in dysplasia. However, extension of Ki67 staining beyond the lower third is characteristic for repair and common in active UC. Therefore, this staining has only a low negative predictive value.

In general, the cytologic alterations due to reparative phenomena can usually be readily correlated with a marked increase in inflammatory cells such as neutrophils, lymphocytes and plasma cells. However, there may be a problem when the patient receives active treatment. Some of the recently developed treatment modalities may indeed decrease the inflammatory reaction before completion of reparative phenomena. This discrepancy can result in a pattern showing little or no inflammatory activity and marked regeneration. The latter represents pseudodysplasia and should not be mistaken for dysplasia [69].

Natural history

The natural history of dysplasia is not known. One paradigm proposes that carcinogenesis follows a progression from no dysplasia to low-grade dysplasia, high-grade dysplasia and carcinoma. This is however, a theoretical model. In some patients CRC develops without any prior dysplasia. In other patients no progression from low- to high-grade dysplasia is seen before the development of cancer. Furthermore, it is important to realise that patients may already have CRC at the time dysplasia is discovered. However, the results of several studies show that approximately 32% of the patients with high-grade dysplasia develop CRC after some follow-up period. Furthermore, data from different centres in the United Kingdom and the United States show a 5–10 years progression rate from low-grade to high-grade dysplasia and cancer that varies between

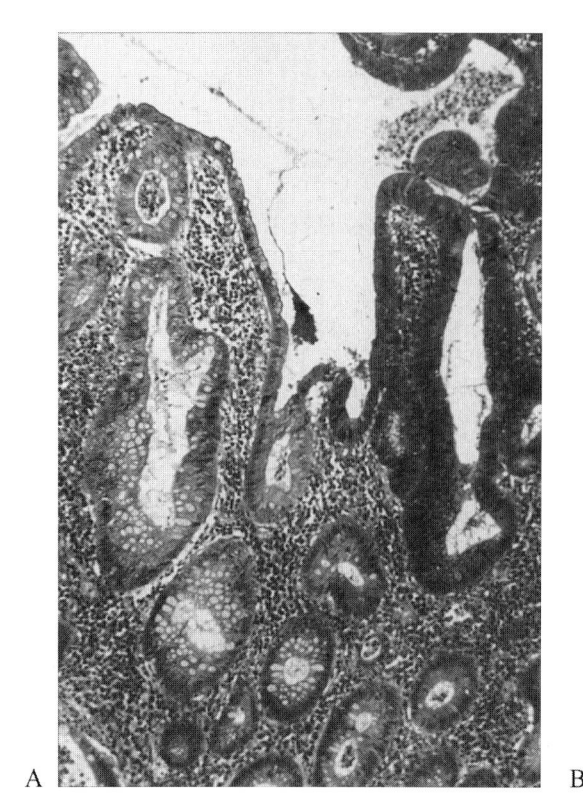

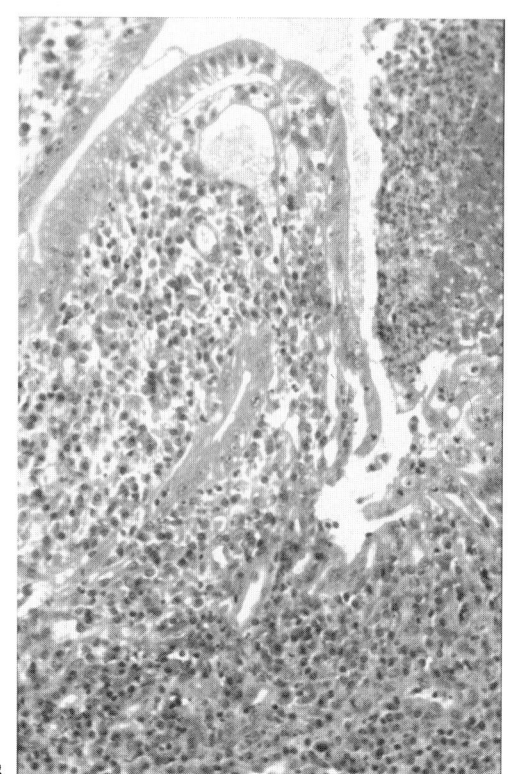

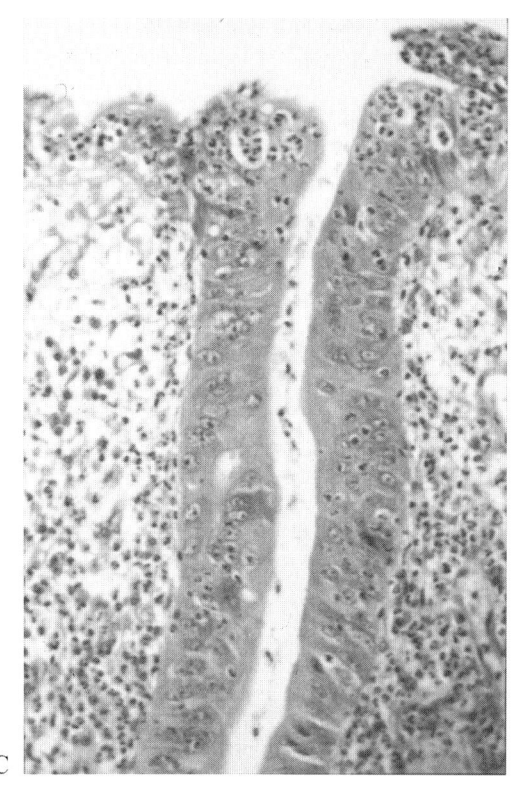

Fig 21.4 (a) This is a low-power micro-photograph showing active ulcerative colitis with restitution of the epithelium in the left half and epithelial dysplasia (cells with darkly staining cytoplasm) in the right half. (b) This shows active ulcerative colitis with restitution of the surface and crypt epithelium-flattened cells. (c) This shows low-grade dysplasia with active inflammation. Dysplastic cells are still high columnar cells.

Table 21.3 Microscopic features of adenoma, IBD-associated dysplasia and reparative phenomena in IBD.

	Features of adenoma	Dysplasia in IBD Low	Dysplasia in IBD High	Repair in IBD Low	Repair in IBD High
Inflammation	−	−	++		
Cytological features					
Cells flattened–low cuboidal cells	−	−	−/+	++	
High columnar cells	+	+	+	+	−
Dystrophic goblet cells	?	?	+	+	−
Abnormal mucin secretion	+	+	+	+	−/+
Mucin depletion	±	+	+	+	+
Nuclei enlargement (elongation) of nuclei	+	++	+	++	−/+
Crowding of nuclei	+	++	+	++	−/+
Stratification of nuclei	−/+	++	−/+	++	−/+
Hyperchromatism	−/+	+	−/+	+	−/+
Coarse chromatin	−	++	−	++	−/+
Polymorphism	−	++	−	++	−
Loss of polarity	−	+	−	++	−
Rounded–vesicular nuclei	−	+	−	+	±
Prominent nucleoli	−	+	−	+	−/+
Frequent mitoses	±	+	+/−	+	±
Abnormal location of mitoses	+	++	+	+	−
Glandular architecture lengthening of crypts	+	+	+	+	−
Enlargement of crypts	+	+	+	+	−/+
Branching of crypts	+	++	+	++	−/+
Bridging and budding of crypts	−	++	+	++	+
Back-to back-orientation of crypts	−	++	+	++	−
Increased number of crypts	+	++	+	++	−
Villiform surface	−	+	+	+	−/+

10 and 50%. Flat low-grade dysplasia would carry a greater risk [52]. The cancer risk and natural history of single marker abnormalities remain to be assessed.

Conclusion

IBD-associated dysplasia or intra-epithelial neoplasia is the earliest phase in the development of colorectal cancer in IBD, which can be recognised with routine morphology. It is an unequivocal neoplastic lesion characterised by cytological and architectural abnormalities of the epithelial cells. These abnormalities are the result of a stepwise accumulation of multiple defects in genes in control of cell proliferation, cell death and cell and tissue structure [70]. Genetic defects that can be identified with molecular techniques can occur in non-neoplastic colitic mucosa before the appearance of the alterations of cell shape and size and tissue structure, which are characteristic for dysplasia. Dysplasia appears often as a flat lesion, probably because k-ras mutations are less common than in sporadic adenomas. The precise natural history of dysplasia is not known, but the likelihood of progression to malignancy is high [71]. Different pathways are involved in the development of CRC in IBD. Therefore, a diagnosis of dysplasia should rely upon morphology, but may eventually be performed in combination with a panel of markers.

References

1 Crohn B, Rosenberg H. The sigmoidoscopic picture of chronic ulcerative colitis (non-specific). *Am J Med Sci* 1925;170:220–8.

2 Bargen JA. Chronic ulcerative colitis associated with malignant disease. *Arch Surg* 1928;17:561–76.

3 Dawson IMP, Pryse-Davies J. The development of carcinoma of the large intestine in ulcerative colitis. *Br J Surg* 1959;47:113–28.

4 Morson BC, Pang LS. Rectal biopsy as an aid to cancer control in ulcerative colitis. *Gut* 1967;8:423–34.

5 Myrvold HE, Kock NG, Ahren C. Rectal biopsy and precancer in ulcerative colitis. *Gut* 1974;15:301–4.

6 Cantwell JD, Kettering RF, Carney JA, Ludwig J. Adenocarcinoma complicating regional enteritis: report of a case and review of the literature. *Gastroenterology* 1968;54:599–604.

7 Simpson S, Traube J, Riddell RH. The histologic appearance of dysplasia (precarcinomatous change) in Crohn's disease of the small and large intestine. *Gastroenterology* 1981;81:492–501.

8 Sigel JE, Petras RE, Lashner BA, Fazio VW, Goldblum JR. Intestinal adenocarcinoma in Crohn's disease: a report of 30 cases with a focus on coexisting dysplasia. *Am J Surg Pathol* 1999;23:651.

9 Geboes K, Rutgeerts P. Dysplasia in inflammatory bowel diseases: definition and clinical impact. *Can J Gastroenterol* 1999;13:671–8.

10 Tannock IF, Hill RP. Glossary. In: Tannock IF, Hill RP, eds. *The Basic Science of Oncology*. 3rd ed. New York: McGraw-Hill; 1998: 497.

11 Riddell RH, Goldman H, Ransohoff DF, *et al*. Dysplasia in inflammatory bowel disease: standardized classification with provisional clinical applications. *Human Pathol* 1983;14:931–68.

12 Hamilton SR, Vogelstein B, Kudo S, *et al*. Carcinoma of the colon and rectum. In: Hamilton SR, Aaltonen IA, eds.*Tumours of the Digestive System. WHO Classification of Tumors*. Lyon: IARC Press; 2000: 113–4.

13 Fearon ER, Vogelstein B. A genetic model for colorectal tumourigenesis. *Cell* 1990;61:759–67.

14 Jass JR, Whitehall VL, Young L, Leggett BA. Emerging concepts in colorectal neoplasia. *Gastroenterology* 2002;86:1467–95.

15 Melville DM, Jass JR, Shepherd NA, *et al*. Dysplasia and deoxyribonucleic acid aneuploidy in the assessment of precancerous changes in chronic ulcerative colitis. Observer variation and correlations. *Gastroenterology* 1988;95:668–75.

16 Löfberg R, Broström O, Karlen P, Tribukait B, Öst A. Colonoscopic surveillance in long-standing total ulcerative colitis – a fifteen year follow-up study. *Gastroenterology* 1990;99:1021–31.

17 Löfberg R, Befrits R, Sjökvist U, *et al*. Colorectal cancer in colonic Crohn's disease – high frequency of DNA-aneuploidy [Abstract]. *Gut* 1996;39:A165.

18 Chen R, Rabinovitch PS, Crispin DA, *et al*. DNA fingerprinting abnormalities can distinguish ulcerative colitis patients with dysplasia and cancer from those who are dysplasia/cancer free. *Am J Pathol* 2003;162:665–72.

19 Befrits R, Hammarberg C, Rubio C, Jaramillo E, Tribukait B. DNA aneuploidy and histologic dysplasia in long-standing ulcerative colitis: a 10-year follow-up study. *Dis Colon Rectum* 1994;37:313–9.

20 Rubin CE, Haggitt RC, Burmer GC, *et al*. DNA-aneuploidy in colonic biopsies predicts future development of dysplasia in ulcerative colitis. *Gastroenterology* 1992;103:1611–20.

21 Karlen P, Löfberg R, Broström O, Tribukait B. Absolute cumulative risk of developing DNA-aneuploidy in longstanding extensive ulcerative colitis [Abstract]. *Gastroenterology* 1993;104:A720.

22 Willenbucher RF, Zelman SJ, Ferrell LD, Moore DH, II, Waldman, FM. Chromosomal alterations in ulcerative colitis-related neoplastic progression. *Gastroenterology* 1997;113:791–801.

23 Suzuki H, Harpaz N, Tarmin L, *et al*. Microsatellite instability in ulcerative colitis-associated colorectal dysplasias and cancers. *Cancer Res* 1994;54:4841–4.

24 Cawkwell L, Sutherland F, Murgatroyd H, *et al*. Defective hMSH2/hMLH1 protein expression is seen infrequently in ulcerative colitis associated colorectal cancer. *Gut* 2000;46:367–9.

25 Burmer GC, Levine DS, Kulander BG, Haggitt RC, Rubin CE, Rabinovitch PS. c-ki-ras mutations in ulcerative colitis and sporadic colon carcinoma. *Gastroenterology* 1990;99:416–20.

26 Chen J, Compton C, Cheng E, Fromowitz F, Viola MV. c-Ki-ras mutations in dysplastic fields and cancers in ulcerative colitis. *Gastroenterology* 1992;102:1983–7.

27 Redston M, Papadopoulos N, Caldas C, Kinzler KW, Kern SE. Common occurrence of APC and K-ras gene mutations in the spectrum of colitis-associated neoplasias. *Gastroenterology* 1995;108:383–92.

28 Tarmin L, Yin J, Harpaz N, *et al*. APC gene mutations in ulcerative colitis associated dysplasias and cancers versus sporadic colon neoplasms. *Cancer Res* 1995;55:2035–8.

29 Andersen SN, Lovig T, Clausen OP, Bakka A, Fausa O, Rognum TO. Villous, hypermucinous mucosa in longstanding ulcerative colitis shows high frequency of K-ras mutations. *Gut* 1999;45:686–92.

30 Burmer GC, Rabinovitch PS, Haggitt RC, *et al*. Neoplastic progression in ulcerative colitis: histology, DNA content and loss of p53 allele. *Gastroenterology* 1992;103:1602–10.

31 Brentnall TA, Crispin DA, Rabinovitch PS, *et al*. Mutations in the p53 gene: an early marker of

neoplastic progression in ulcerative colitis. *Gastroenterology* 1994;107:369–78.
32. Ilyas M, Tomlinson IP. Genetic pathways in colorectal cancer. *Histopathology* 1996;28:389–99.
33. Loeb KR, Loeb LA. Genetic instability and the mutator phenotype: studies in ulcerative colitis. *Am J Pathol* 1999;154:1621–6.
34. Wong NACS, Harrison DJ. Colorectal neoplasia in ulcerative colitis – recent advances. *Histopathology* 2001;39:221–34.
35. Cuvelier C, Bekaert E, De Potter C, Pauwels C, De Vos M, Roels H. Crohn's disease with adenocarcinoma and dysplasia. Macroscopical, histological, and immunohistochemical aspects of two cases. *Am J Surg Pathol* 1989;13:187–96.
36. Mulder JW, Wielenga VJ, Polak MM, *et al.* Expression of mutant p53 protein and CD44 variant proteins in colorectal tumourigenesis. *Gut* 1995;36:76–80.
37. Rosenberg WM, Prince C, Kaklamanis L, *et al.* Increased expression of CD44v6 and CD44v3 in ulcerative colitis but not colonic Crohn's disease. *Lancet* 1995;345:1205–9.
38. Fromont-Hankard G, Cezard JP, Aigrain Y, Navarro J, Peuchmaur M. CD44 variant expression in inflammatory colonic mucosa is not disease specific but associated with increased crypt cell proliferation. *Histopathology* 1998;32:317–21.
39. Karayiannakis AJ, Syrigos KN, Efstathiou J, *et al.* Expression of catenins and E-cadherin during epithelial restitution in inflammatory bowel disease. *J Pathol* 1998;185:413–8.
40. Walsh SV, Loda M, Torres CM, *et al.* p53 and β catenin expression in chronic ulcerative colitis-associated polypoid dysplasia and sporadic adenomas: an immunohistochemical study. *Am J Surg Pathol* 1999;23:963–9.
41. Jankowski JA, Bedford FK, Boulton RA, *et al.* Alterations in classical cadherins associated with progression in ulcerative and Crohn's colitis. *Laboratory Invest* 1998;78:1155–67.
42. Sakuma K, Fujimor T, Hirabayashi K, Terano A. Cyclooxygenase (COX) -2 immunoreactivity and relationship to p53 and Ki-67 expression in colorectal cancer. *J Gastroenterol* 1999;34:189–94.
43. Agnoff SN, Brentnall TA, Crispin DA, *et al.* The role of cyclooxygenase 2 in ulcerative colitis associated neoplasia. *Am J Pathol* 2000;157:737–45.
44. Tytgat GN, Dhir V, Gopinath N. Endoscopic appearance of dysplasia and cancer in inflammatory bowel disease. *Eur J Cancer* 1995;31:1174–7.
45. Kiesslich R, Neurath MF. Surveillance colonoscopy in ulcerative colitis: magnifying chromoendoscopy in the spotlight. *Gut* 2004;53:165–7.
46. Blackstone MO, Riddell RH, Rogers BH, Levin B. Dysplasia-associated lesion or mass (DALM) detected by colonoscopy in long-standing ulcerative colitis: an indication for colectomy. *Gastroenterology* 1981;80:366–74.
47. Rosenstock E, Farmer RG, Petras R, Sivak MV Jr, Rankin GB, Sullivan BH. Surveillance for colonic carcinoma in ulcerative colitis. *Gastroenterology* 1985;89:1342–6.
48. Kornbluth A, Sachar DB. Ulcerative colitis practice guidelines in adults. American College of Gastroenterology, Practice Parameters Committee. *Am J Gastroenterol* 1997;92:204–11.
49. Morson BC. Precancer and cancer in inflammatory bowel disease. *Pathology* 1985;17:173–80.
50. Batts KP, Haggitt RC. Dysplasia in ulcerative colitis and Crohn's disease: clinical pathology and current surveillance methods. In: Targan SR, Shanahan F, eds. *Inflammatory Bowel Disease, From Bench to Bedside.* Baltimore: Williams & Wilkins; 1994:631–42.
51. Faintuch J, Levin B, Kirsner JB. Inflammatory bowel diseases and their relationship to malignancy. *Crit Rev Oncol /Hematology* 1985;2:323–53.
52. Itzkowitz SH, Harpaz N. Diagnosis and management of dysplasia in patients with inflammatory bowel diseases. *Gastroenterology* 2004;126:1634–48.
53. Pascal RR. Dysplasia and early carcinoma in inflammatory bowel disease and colorectal adenomas. *Human Pathol* 1994;25:1160–71.
54. Isaacson P. Tissue demonstration of carcinoembryonic antigen (CEA) in ulcerative colitis. *Gut* 1976;17:561–7.
55. Allen DC, Foster H, Orchin JC, Biggart JD. Immunohistochemical staining of colorectal tissues with monoclonal antibodies to ras oncogene p21 product and carbohydrate determinant antigen 19-9. *J Clin Pathol* 1987;40:157–62.
56. Karlen P, Young E, Broström O, *et al.* Sialyl-Tn antigen as a marker of colon cancer risk in ulcerative colitis: relation do dysplasia and aneuploidy. *Gastroenterology* 1998;115:1395–404.
57. Itzkowitz SH, Young E, Dubois D, *et al.* Sialosyl-Tn antigen is prevalent and precedes dysplasia in ulcerative colitis: a retrospective case-control study. *Gastroenterology* 1996;110:694–704.
58. Noffsinger AE, Miller MA, Cusi MV, Fenoglio-Preiser CM. The pattern of cell proliferation in neoplastic and nonneoplastic lesions of ulcerative colitis. *Cancer* 1996;78:2307–12.
59. Lashner BA, Shapiro BD, Hussain A, Goldblum JR. Evaluation of the usefulness of testing for p53 mutations in colorectal cancer surveillance for ulcerative colitis. *Am J Gastroenterol* 1999;94:456–62.

60 Stolte M, Schneider A. Differential diagnosis of adenomas and dysplasias in patients with ulcerative colitis. In: Tytgat GNJ, Bartelsman JFWM, van Deventer SJH, eds. *Inflammatory Bowel Diseases*. Dordrecht: Kluwer Academic Publishers;1995: 133–44.

61 Torres C, Antonioli D, Odze RD. Polypoid dysplasia and adenomas in inflammatory bowel disease: a clinical, pathologic, and follow-up study of 89 polyps from 59 patients. *Am J Surg Pathol* 1998;22:275–84.

62 Suzuki K, Muto Y, Shinozaki M, *et al*. Differential diagnosis of dysplasia-associated lesion or mass and coincidental adenoma in ulcerative colitis. *Dis Colon Rectum* 1998;41:322–7.

63 Selaru FM, Xu Y, Yin J, *et al*. Artificial neural networks distinguish among subtypes of neoplastic colorectal lesions. *Gastroenterology* 2002;122:606–13.

64 Odze RD, Brien T, Brown CA, Hartman CJ, Wellman A, Fogt F. Molecular alterations in chronic ulcerative colitis-associated and sporadic hyperplastic polyps: a comparative analysis. *Am J Gastroenterol* 2002;97:1235–42.

65 Dignass AU, Tsunekawa S, Podolsky DK. Fibroblast growth factors modulate intestinal epithelial cell growth and migration. *Gastroenterology* 1994;106:1254–62.

66 Hall C, Youngs D, Keighley MR. Crypt cell production rates at various sites around the colon in Wistar rats and humans. *Gut* 1992;33:1528–31.

67 Biasco G, Paganelli GM, Miglioli M, Barbara L. Cell proliferation biomarkers in the gastrointestinal tract. *J Cellular Biochem* 1992;16G(Suppl):73–8.

68 Rubio CA, Befrits R. Atypical mitoses in colectomy specimens from patients with long standing ulcerative colitis. *Anticancer Res Earch* 1997;17:2721–6.

69 Hyde GM, Warren BF, Jewell DP. Histological changes following intravenous cyclosporin in the treatment of refractory severe ulcerative colitis may mimic dysplasia [Abstract]. *Gut* 1998;42:A43.

70 O'Sullivan J, Bronner MP, Brentnall TA, *et al*. Chromosomal instability in ulcerative colitis is related to telomere shortening. *Nat Genet* 2002;32:280–4.

71 Warren S, Sommers SC. Pathogenesis of ulcerative colitis. *Am J Pathol* 1949;25:657–79.

22: Colonoscopic surveillance – if and when?

Urban Sjöqvist and Robert Löfberg

Introduction

The increased risk of intestinal cancer is one of the major problems in the long-term management of patients with inflammatory bowel disease (IBD). The risk of colorectal cancer (CRC) in longstanding ulcerative colitis (UC) has been particularly in focus since the recognition of this complication in a series of cases reported by Bargen in 1928 [1], and management strategies have been controversial ever since. There are difficulties in correctly assessing the individual cancer risk and hence, there are also problems in taking appropriate actions to prevent the development of CRC. A large retrospective population-based study of 2509 UC-patients [2] showed that death due to CRC was the main cause of the excess long-term mortality, thus emphasising the clinical importance of the problem. During the last decade, some large, well-defined population-based studies have provided accurate estimates of the cancer risk in IBD, making it easier to predict individual prognosis. Our knowledge has improved regarding the identification of certain factors indicating a particularly high cancer risk, and some protective factors have also been elucidated. Furthermore, long-term experience of colonoscopic surveillance programmes is now available and the pros and cons of this approach to reduce the cancer risk have been scrutinised.

Overall cancer risk

From large population-based studies performed in Sweden and the United Kingdom it appears that the elevated, overall cancer-risk among patients with UC [2–4] and Crohn's disease (CD) [2, 3] is due predominantly to an increase of intestinal cancer. However, in an epidemiological study of malignancies in CD [5], a slight excess risk was found for small bowel carcinoma and urinary bladder carcinoma, but not for CRC. Although the absolute number is small, a subgroup of patients having UC and the hepatobiliary complication primary sclerosing cholangitis (PSC), runs a significantly increased risk of developing carcinoma of the bile ducts [6, 7] and pancreatic malignancies [8].

Small bowel carcinoma in Crohn's disease

The incidence of small bowel carcinoma among patients with CD is low, but as it is extremely uncommon in an age-matched population, the relative risk becomes significantly increased, as shown in some population-based studies [5, 9–11]. Long duration of CD seems to be the most important determinant for this malignant complication [12, 13].

Colorectal cancer risk in ulcerative colitis

The risk of CRC is most appropriately assessed by the use of actuarial, life-table methods, when duration of disease is taken into account and the absolute cumulative risk is calculated [4, 14]. Such calculations should also compensate for proctocolectomy and death from causes other than CRC. Relative risk comparisons, given the rarity of CRC in the younger age groups of the general population, are of limited value. Several larger population-based studies from different geographical regions have taken those considerations into account and provided consistent, independent results regarding the cumulative CRC-risk in UC. A study of 486 patients with extensive UC (i.e. involvement proximal to the splenic flexure) from three different geographical areas in England and Sweden [4] followed for a minimum of 17 years, estimated the CRC-risk to be 11.6% (CI 6.4–16.8) after 25 years from the onset of disease. This increase is approximately six to ten times higher than expected in the general population. In non-extensive UC the risk was only marginally raised (left-sided and distal UC) and not increased at all in patients with proctitis. Remarkably similar results were obtained from a large epidemiological study from Uppsala, Sweden [14] of 679 patients having extensive disease. After 25 years, the cumulative risk was 12% among patients aged 15–39 years at onset. The cumulative cancer risk in patients with left-sided UC at the time of diagnosis was less than 5% after 30 years, except for those patients who got the diagnosis between 15 and 29 years of age who had a 12 % risk. As it is well known that patients with distal and left-sided UC at time of initial diagnosis may often progress to more extensive involvement, it could be anticipated that a large proportion of patients in this latter group had extensive disease at the time of cancer development. In a population study from Israel [15], the cumulative risk was 13.8% in extensive UC after 20 years of duration. A prospective study from Copenhagen [16] could not demonstrate any CRC-risk increase at all for a defined UC-cohort, while another recent Danish study [17], covering the entire country, has provided CRC-risk estimates for UC more in line with those previously reported. In a recent meta-analysis [18] the estimated CRC-risk in all patients with UC was found to be 2% at 10 years, 8% at 20 years and 18% at 30 years, irrespective of disease extent.

Colorectal cancer risk in Crohn's disease

There are conflicting results of the magnitude of the risk of CRC in CD. Several reports have failed to demonstrate a risk [5, 9, 19–21] while others have demonstrated [22–26] an increased CRC-risk in these patients. There have been two population-based studies, both from Sweden, addressing the CRC-risk in CD. In 1251 patients with CD, diagnosed between 1955 and 1984 in Stockholm County, the occurrence of CRC was not increased with a standardised morbidity ratio of 0.89 (CI 0.29–2.07) [5]. The other one from Uppsala, ($n =$ 1655), demonstrated that CD patients having substantial/extensive colonic involvement and long duration of the disease had more than five times increase of the relative risk of CRC [25]. This report as well as one reported from Birmingham, England [26, 27], showed that patients with extensive CD of the colon had an absolute cumulative risk of 8% after 22 years of disease duration, quite similar to the risk level previously found in extensive UC [4]. In a recent population-based study from Canada [11], the risk of developing CRC was 2.64 (95% CI 1.69–4.12) for CD-patients, quite similar to that found for patients with UC (2.75; 95% CI 1.91–3.97) in that study. This study was, however, performed using administrative data and hence charts were not reviewed. No other population-based studies have assessed the CRC-risk in CD-patients with colonic involvement, but there are reasons to believe that the problem with CRC in Crohn's colitis may become more of a clinical reality as an increasing proportion of this patient group receives long-term immunosuppressive treatment and thereby avoiding or considerably delaying major surgical intervention (i.e. proctocolectomy) [28]. An association between longstanding anorectal CD and distal rectal and anal cancers has been reported from St Mark's Hospital [29].

Clinical risk factors for colorectal cancer in IBD

Several clinical factors indicating an increased CRC-risk have been identified. From most of the larger population-based studies it is apparent that the two major risk factors for malignant transformation of the colorectal mucosa in UC are extensive disease (maximal involvement at any time during the disease history being proximal to the splenic flexure) and long duration (>8 years) [4, 14, 15]. Although young age at onset of UC is associated with a high cumulative CRC-risk [14, 30], this risk may not be an independent risk factor as such, but rather inter-related to an observed long duration of UC [14, 30]. In patients with extensive UC the presence of concomitant PSC has also been demonstrated to be an independent risk factor for colorectal neoplasia [6, 31]. This association has subsequently been confirmed in several other reports [32–34], but was not reported in studies from the Mayo Clinic [35, 36]. In a recent study, familial CRC was associated with a more than two-fold risk of CRC (RR = 2.5, 95% CI 1.4-4.4) in patients with IBD [37], in line with a previous reported study [38]. Notably, patients with a first-degree relative with CRC diagnosed before 50 years of age had an even higher relative risk of 9.2 (95% CI 3.7–23).

Protective factors for colorectal cancer in IBD

5-amino salicylic acid

Patients in a state of chronic continuous disease activity were found to run a higher risk for CRC in a study from Oxford [39], to some extent being contradicted by a later Swedish case-control study indicating that patients with a high inflammatory activity had a decreased risk [40], as had those patients taking sulphasalazine for maintenance treatment for more than 3 months (RR = 0.38; 95% CI 0.2–0.7). Results in line with the latter observations were also found in a population-based study from Leicestershire [41] where UC-patients non-compliant with long-term sulphasalazine therapy had a significantly increased absolute cumulative risk of CRC (40% vs 10% after 20 years of duration). In fact, regular therapy with 5-ASA (>2 g/day) was found to reduce the CRC-risk by 75% (OR 0.25, 95% CI 0.13–0.48) in a recent case-control study of 102 cases of UC patients with CRC [42]. The risk reduction for those patients taking mesalazine was even greater (81% (OR 0.19, 95% CI 0.06–0.61).

The data from Copenhagen [16], indicating that an aggressive medical and surgical approach reduces CRC-risk, may be in line with those observations.

The protective virtues of sulphasalazine and mesalazine in this respect are unclear. Aspirin and other NSAIDs reduce the risk of sporadic CRC and adenomas [43], as well as polyp formation in FAP (familial adenomatosis polyposis) [44–47]

and it might therefore be tempting to assume that the 5-ASA compound in sulphasalazine and mesalazine might have the same properties (e.g. ASA-like actions by cyclooxygenase inhibition). A non-pharmacological explanation might be that patients compliant with 5-ASA medication visit the gastroenterologist when experiencing changes in symptoms, thus lowering the risk of CRC [42].

Ursodeoxycholic acid

Ursodeoxycholic acid (UDCA), a natural bile acid, used primarily in the treatment of primary billiary cirrhosis, but also in PSC, has been in focus ever since Earnest et al. reported that dietary UDCA decreased the incidence of experimental colonic carcinogenesis in a rat azoxymethane model [48]. In a retrospective study, comprising 59 patients with UC and PSC, Tung et al. showed that the use of UDCA was associated with a lower risk of colonic dysplasia compared to patients not taking the compound (OR 0.18, $P = 0.005$) [49]. This protective effect remained after adjusting for duration of colitis, and age at onset. Surprisingly, no protective effect of sulphasalazine was seen in this study. Recently, Pardi et al. [50], in a prospective study, analysed the outcome of colonic neoplasia in 52 UC/PSC patients who were initially enrolled in an ursodiol, placebo controlled trial, investigating UDCA:s role in improving liver function in these patients [51]. Those originally assigned to receive UDCA had a relative risk of 0.26 for developing colorectal dysplasia or cancer (95% CI 0.06–0.92; $P = 0.034$).

UDCA has been demonstrated to have several anticarcinogenic properties, one of which is the reduction of the colonic concentration of deoxycholic acid, recognised as a strong cancer promoter [52, 53].

Folic acid

Low folate intake has been associated with an increased risk of developing adenomas and CRC in the general population [54, 55]. A case-control study examining the effects of folic acid use, in patients with pancolitis followed in a surveillance programme, suggested that folate supplementation was associated with a 62% (OR 0.38, 95% CI 0.12–1.2, NS) lower incidence of neoplasia as compared to individuals not receiving supplementation [56]. Another case-control study showed that the risk of dysplasia or cancer was significantly decreased by 18% for each 10 ng/mL increase in blood cell folate [57] and another study gives further supporting evidence for the routine use of daily folate supplementation [58].

Immunomodulating drugs

Very few reports have discussed possible chemoprotective properties of immunomodulating drugs (azathioprine, 6-mercaptopurine and glucocorticosteroids). Patients treated with azathioprine or 6-mercaptopurine do not appear to have an increased risk of CRC compared to controls [59]. On the other hand, no CRC protective properties of these two drugs have been shown in UC [49, 58]. For glucocorticosteroids, one study [42] has shown a beneficial effect of systemically administered steroids (OR 0.26, 95% CI 0.01–0.7), while other studies [49, 58] have not shown such an effect.

Management strategies for colorectal cancer in IBD

It might be argued that the increased risk of CRC in colonic IBD is not high enough compared to the general population (less than 1% of cases of CRC in the general population [60], in Sweden about 5000 new cases/year), to warrant any specific action from physicians handling the patient. On the other hand, it might be regarded as sufficiently high to necessitate expedient prophylactic proctocolectomy within a certain time frame of 3–10 years of onset. The latter option was frequently advocated and performed for extensive UC during the 1960s and 1970s [61]. Indeed, the only large study failing to show an increased risk of CRC in UC used an aggressive surgical approach (e.g. colectomy) where 35% of the patients were treated surgically during the first 5 years of disease [16]. This handling of the patients now receives limited support. High-risk patients with IBD are usually in remission with a satisfactory quality of life and are reluctant to accept surgery as a means of CRC prevention. It should also be remembered that well over 80% of the patients do not develop CRC and, furthermore, the morbidity of colectomy and ileostomy of the ileal-pouch anal anastomosis (IPAA) type operation must be considered when treatment options are evaluated.

Managing the patients within the frame of 'routine clinical care', including vigilance if clinical symptoms of CRC occur, has also been suggested [62]. Such an approach is deemed to achieve, at best, a 50% 5-year survival as seen in sporadic CRC, and is thus not very attractive. The standard approach at most IBD centres in order to manage the increased CRC-risk, at least in UC, has become colonoscopic surveillance.

Colonoscopic surveillance in ulcerative colitis

Based on the concept of a dysplasia-to-carcinoma sequence in UC [63, 64] and on the development of the flexible fibre-endoscope, programmes for surveillance of high-risk patients were introduced in the early 1970s [65–67]. By performing colonoscopies with multiple biopsies from different parts of the colon and rectum at regular intervals, those programmes were aimed at detecting mucosal dysplasia, or carcinoma in early stages. The ultimate goal has been to decrease CRC morbidity and mortality in UC. Some of the larger studies have confirmed the association between colorectal dysplasia and carcinoma in UC [65], as well as the sequential development of lower grades of dysplasia into high-grade dysplasia (HGD) and, ultimately, to invasive carcinoma [63, 65, 68]. The need for total colonoscopies has been underlined by the frequent initial finding of dysplasia or dysplasia associated lesion or mass (DALM) only in the proximal colon. It must also be remembered that dysplasia is not always found in association with a carcinoma. Studies of resected colonic specimens and studies in large surveillance programmes [68–70] show that no dysplasia (either adjacent to or distant from the tumour) is detected in up to 25% of the patients. The sensitivity of dysplasia as a marker for CRC-development is thus only 75%, but if the endoscopic examinations are performed at regular intervals the risk of missing a carcinoma before it becomes incurable by surgical resection is small [59, 66, 71].

The St Mark's group in London has been the pioneer centre in the field of colonoscopic surveillance, and their most recent report [68] has provided us with the largest clinical experience so far. In 322 patients with extensive UC entered between 1971 and 1992, colonoscopic examinations contributed to the detection of 11 asymptomatic CRC and 12 further patients underwent colectomy due to findings of dysplasia. However, six symptomatic interval tumours also occurred, partly because of compliance problems. One of the most important findings in this study was the 5-year predictive value of low-grade dysplasia (LGD) as a marker for cancer or high-grade dysplasia of 54% using the classification by Riddell et al. [64]. In contrast, only one early CRC plus abundant cases with LGD were the somewhat disappointing results in an ambitious study from Leeds [71]. However, there were several patients with advanced CRC among defaulters and among patients not followed within the frame of the surveillance programme, emphasising the importance of compliance as one of the mainstays for a successful follow-up. Based on the experience from a dedicated prospective surveillance programme in Stockholm initiated in 1973 [66], the yield of findings leading to surgical intervention seems to be between 0.5 and 1% of colonoscopies carried out per year. This figure is in accordance with that expected based on recent epidemiological CRC risk assessments. Compliance in this programme has been high and, so far, with more than 140 patients with extensive UC followed for up to 29 years, there are still no deaths due to CRC (P. Karlén, personal communication).

The fundamental issue of surveillance of UC-patients is the impact on cancer morbidity, and mortality. In many of the hitherto reported surveillance programmes, the technical feasibility of the concept has indeed been proven [66, 68, 71–73], and moreover, non-randomised studies have indicated that surveyed UC-patients have much less risk of dying from CRC compared to non-surveyed patients [72, 74]. Some authors [75–77] have criticised surveillance programmes for being an ineffective and costly way of managing the increased CRC-risk in UC. Instead, the poorly defined management 'routine clinical control', including colonoscopy only when symptoms suggestive of cancer occur, has been advocated. As controlled studies comparing colonoscopic surveillance with the passive handling policy of 'routine clinical control' will never be performed due to practical and ethical reasons, another way to address the potential value of surveillance is to perform case-control studies. The result from a joint study from the Stockholm-Uppsala area indicates a frequency-response related, protective effect of colonoscopic surveillance on CRC-mortality in UC [78]. Furthermore, theoretical decision-type analysis supports the concept since patients selected for colectomy based on findings of LGD at colonoscopy will have almost the same life expectancy as patients undergoing prophylactic colectomy 10 years after onset [79].

Aims and prerequisites for successful colonoscopic surveillance

By performing complete colonoscopies with multiple biopsies from the entire colon and rectum at regular intervals, a surveillance programme for UC aims at detecting mucosal dysplasia, in order to select the high-risk CRC-prone individuals for prophylactic colectomy. The ultimate goal with colonoscopic surveillance is to decrease CRC morbidity and to eliminate the excess CRC mortality. Surveillance is only effective if all patients running the highest risk of CRC are included (e.g. those with extensive, longstanding UC and colonic CD, and in particular, those with early onset and concomitant PSC).

The patients enrolled must be fully informed about the possible consequences of findings of dysplasia. Furthermore, patient compliance is of utmost importance in a successful surveillance. It is important to adhere to a strict protocol with predefined criteria for surgery (high-grade dysplasia, certain DALM-lesions, or repeated low-grade dysplasia in multiple locations and/or at repeated examinations).

The optimal timing for initiating surveillance is around 10 years after first onset of symptoms [65,

67, 68, 71, 72], as this is the point when the CRC risk starts to increase [4, 14, 15, 30, 80]. However, in patients with PSC, in whom the IBD onset may be hard to estimate, as the disease is often quiescent, it may be wise to start surveillance as soon as extensive UC has been diagnosed [81].

The intervals between colonoscopies should not exceed 2 years, and annual examinations are recommended by some experts [82]. Biannual investigations between 8 and 20 years of duration have been adopted in the Swedish studies [66, 83], with annual colonoscopies from that point.

Dysplasia may be patchy and unevenly distributed throughout the colon leading to problems with sampling errors. Even if 20–40 biopsies are taken less than 0.1% of the colorectal mucosa is covered [65]. Still, the experience from several prospective colonoscopic programmes shows that biopsies taken from 6 to 10 different sites throughout the colon and rectum is sufficient to detect dysplasia, and thereby the risk of missing an incurable CRC is low [65, 66, 68, 71–74].

Colonoscopic surveillance in colonic Crohn's disease

Only limited experience exists from prospective colonoscopic surveillance of patients with longstanding, extensive colonic CD. In fact, the only study published so far [84] reported on 259 patients with chronic Crohn's colitis of duration of 8 years or more who were followed for 18 years by colonoscopic surveillance (mean 2.6 examinations per patient). This screening and surveillance programme detected dysplasia or CRC in 16% of the patients (10 with indefinite, 23 with low-grade and four high-grade dysplasias and five CRC). Furthermore, age more than 45 years at the time of colonoscopy was associated with increased risk of neoplasia. After a negative colonoscopy, the probability of finding neoplasia by the fourth surveillance examination was 22% and comparable to those reported from UC-patients undergoing surveillance [85, 86]. The authors recommended that all patients with extensive Crohn's colitis of long duration (>8 years) should undergo colonoscopic surveillance.

The reports on cancer frequency in UC based on histopathological records should be subjected to critical histological re-evaluation as suggested in a retrospective study [87]. That study, in fact, showed that CRC in Crohn's colitis had increased and that colonoscopic surveillance was warranted.

The number of patients having CD involving the large bowel with no major resection or colectomy are likely to increase in the future as an effect of improved and more aggressive medical therapy (azathioprine, 6-mercaptopurine and infliximab). Furthermore, the incidence of CD is steadily increasing, especially the colonic form, with a reported overall incidence of 4.6 per 100,000 inhabitants, and with an age-specific peak incidence between 20 and 30 years [88].

It may thus be appropriate to consider surveillance with multiple biopsies for detection of histopathological dysplasia in this subgroup of patients with CD.

Colonoscopy in CD-patients, with colorectal involvement, may be difficult because of colonic strictures. Thinner calibre paediatric colonoscope may help to improve the percentage of complete examinations. Besides technical difficulties with stricturing, there is up to 12% chance that the stricture is of malignant nature [89]. Ongoing prospective programmes are needed to determine guidelines regarding surveillance examinations in CD. Based on the discussion above, it would be wise to apply a UC-based colonoscopic strategy at least in patients with Crohn's colitis of long duration.

Surveillance schedule

Screening colonoscopy

The optimal timing for initiating surveillance is around 8–10 years after first onset of symptoms [65, 67, 68, 71, 72], as this is the point when the CRC risk starts to increase [4, 14, 15, 30, 80]. However, in patients with PSC, in whom the IBD onset may be hard to estimate as the disease is often quiescent, it may be wise to start surveillance as soon as extensive UC has been diagnosed [81]. Patients having disease beyond the splenic flexure, but not necessarily a total colitis should also be offered a colonoscopy at this point (e.g. 10 years).

Surveillance colonoscopy

When to perform the surveillance colonoscopy obviously depends on the histopathological report from the initial screening colonoscopy. The following guidelines based on the findings from the pathologist are used at our centre:

No dysplasia, indefinite, probably negative (probably reactive) changes and indefinite, unknown changes

After a negative screening or surveillance colonoscopy, the intervals between colonoscopies should not exceed 2 years, and annual examinations are recommended by some experts [82]. Biannual investigations between 8 and 20 years of duration have been adopted in the Swedish studies [66, 83], with annual colonoscopies from that point.

Indefinite, probably positive (probably dysplastic) changes

The significance of indefinite changes, probably positive for dysplasia is not clear. In some studies the predictive value of such findings are rather limited for future development of dysplasia of higher grades [66, 73]. In a recent study [90] the authors found that dysplasia of any grade, including indefinite, probably dysplastic changes, was an indication for colectomy due to a high probability of co-existent carcinoma. Yearly examinations for these patients are recommended.

Low-grade dysplasia

Managing LGD in flat mucosa is the most controversial part of colonoscopic surveillance in patients with UC. Once, confirmed by an experienced pathologist, some authors recommend proctocolectomy [68, 91–93] due to the fact that many patients may already harbour a CRC and are at risk of progressing to more severe forms of neoplasia.

However, two recent studies [94, 95] challenge the predictive value of LGD as a marker for CRC or progression to more severe forms of neoplasia, and instead of colectomy the authors recommend increased surveillance. The following approach is a compromise:

If LGD is detected at a single location, and confirmed by an experienced pathologist, increased surveying vigilance is advocated with re-examinations annually. In the case of confirmed multi-focal LGD, a further colonoscope should be performed within 3–6 months. If repeated findings of multi-focal LGD are then confirmed, the patient should be advised to have a proctocolectomy.

High-grade dysplasia, DALM and colorectal cancer

Findings of a carcinoma, a DALM with HGD or LGD, or HGD in flat mucosa, are indications for proctocolectomy [66, 71]. When adjusted to Dukes stage there is no apparent difference in 5-year survival between sporadic CRC and UC-associated cancer. The carcinomas in UC are often flat, multiple and poorly differentiated [96] and they may often be advanced if found in a symptomatic stage. Colonoscopic surveillance has the potential of detecting UC-associated CRC without preceding dysplasia at an early stage, provided that the surveillance intervals are strictly adhered to [66, 68, 73]. A DALM with only indefinite changes needs to be handled with care as more severe dysplasia, or even carcinoma may be hidden underneath the epithelium. Closer surveillance or recommendation for colectomy is advised.

Polyps in UC

If macroscopic lesions are detected, special attention is warranted and additional biopsies should be sampled in order to exclude a DALM [65, 66, 71, 97]. Pedunculated adenomas found in a dysplasia-free, surrounding mucosa may be managed as in non-colitis patients (e.g. snare-polypectomy) [98], whereas sessile polyps should be regarded as a potential DALM, at least in patients over 40–45 years

[83]. However, in a recent study [99] of 24 UC-patients with DALMs, the authors proposed the same management as for sporadic polyps (e.g. snare polypectomy) because no patient developed CRC or dysplasia elsewhere in the colon and rectum. Long-term follow-up data from this study were recently reported [100] with a median follow-up time of 71.8 months. The 24 patients with adenoma-like DALMs were compared with 49 non-UC patients with sporadic polyps (both groups had been treated with snare polypectomy). There was no significant difference between the two groups regarding polyp formation in this long-term follow-up study and the authors concluded that adenoma-like DALMs may be treated with polypectomy (instead of colectomy) and continued endoscopic surveillance. An algorithm for the management of neoplastic polyps in patients with IBD has been suggested [101] and is further discussed in Chapter 26. In patients with substantial numbers of post-inflammatory pseudopolyps, a safe surveillance may never be offered and instead, prophylactic colectomy should be discussed.

Conclusions

The increased risk of CRC in longstanding UC is one of the major problems in the long-term management of these patients. The realisation that widespread dysplastic lesions in the colorectal mucosa preceded the development of invasive carcinoma, forms the mainstay for colonoscopic surveillance. Examinations with multiple biopsies, at regular intervals, can be used as an instrument to select high-risk patients for prophylactic colectomy before cancer occurs or, if cancer is detected, at a potentially curable stage. Although controlled studies comparing the impact on CRC mortality among surveyed versus non-surveyed UC-patients are lacking, several prospective follow-up programmes demonstrate both the technical feasibility of such an approach and a low frequency of lethal cancers. Despite obvious shortcomings in the interpretation of histopathological dysplasia, it is still the only acceptable way of CRC-prevention in these patients. As well as an experienced, specialised gastrointestinal pathologist, other prerequisites for a successful surveillance include a fully informed and compliant patient and strict criteria for surgery (e.g. CRC, HGD, DALM and repeated, confirmed LGD). A combination of enhanced colonoscopic surveillance, using markers that are more sensitive (than dysplasia) may in the future be the optimal way, to manage the increased CRC risk in patients with longstanding UC.

References

1 Bargen JA. Chronic ulcerative colitis associated with malignant disease. *Arch Surg* 1928;17:561–76.
2 Ekbom A, Helmick CG, Zack M, Holmberg L, Adami HO. Survival and causes of death in patients with inflammatory bowel disease: a population-based study. *Gastroenterology* 1992;103(3):954–60.
3 Ekbom A, Helmick C, Zack M, Adami HO. Extracolonic malignancies in inflammatory bowel disease. *Cancer* 1991;67(7):2015–9.
4 Gyde SN, Prior P, Allan RN, *et al*. Colorectal cancer in ulcerative colitis: a cohort study of primary referrals from three centres. *Gut* 1988;29(2):206–17.
5 Persson PG, Karlen P, Bernell O, *et al*. Crohn's disease and cancer: a population-based cohort study. *Gastroenterology* 1994;107(6):1675–9.
6 Broome U, Lofberg R, Veress B, Eriksson LS. Primary sclerosing cholangitis and ulcerative colitis: evidence for increased neoplastic potential. *Hepatology* 1995; 22(5):1404–8.
7 Mir-Madjlessi SH, Farmer RG, Sivak MV Jr. Bile duct carcinoma in patients with ulcerative colitis. Relationship to sclerosing cholangitis: report of six cases and review of the literature. *Dig Dis Sci* 1987; 32(2):145–54.
8 Bergquist A, Ekbom A, Olsson R, *et al*. Hepatic and extrahepatic malignancies in primary sclerosing cholangitis. *J Hepatol* 2002;36(3):321–7.
9 Munkholm P, Langholz E, Davidsen M, Binder V. Intestinal cancer risk and mortality in patients with Crohn's disease. *Gastroenterology* 1993;105(6): 1716–23.
10 Mellemkjaer L, Johansen C, Gridley G, Linet MS, Kjaer SK, Olsen JH. Crohn's disease and cancer risk (Denmark). *Cancer Causes Control* 2000;11(2):145–50.
11 Bernstein CN, Blanchard JF, Kliewer E, Wajda A. Cancer risk in patients with inflammatory bowel disease: a population-based study. *Cancer* 2001;91(4): 854–62.
12 Lashner BA. Risk factors for small bowel cancer in Crohn's disease. *Dig Dis Sci* 1992;37(8):1179–84.

13 Senay E, Sachar DB, Keohane M, Greenstein AJ. Small bowel carcinoma in Crohn's disease. Distinguishing features and risk factors. *Cancer* 1989;63(2):360–3.

14 Ekbom A, Helmick C, Zack M, Adami HO. Ulcerative colitis and colorectal cancer: a population-based study. *N Engl J Med* 1990;323(18):1228–33.

15 Gilat T, Fireman Z, Grossman A, et al. Colorectal cancer in patients with ulcerative colitis. A population study in central Israel. *Gastroenterology* 1988;94(4):2870–7.

16 Langholz E, Munkholm P, Davidsen M, Binder V. Colorectal cancer risk and mortality in patients with ulcerative colitis. *Gastroenterology* 1992;103(5):1444–51.

17 Mellemkjaer L, Olsen JH, Frisch M, Johansen C, Gridley G, McLaughlin JK. Cancer in patients with ulcerative colitis. *Int J Cancer* 1995;60(3):330–3.

18 Eaden JA, Abrams KR, Mayberry JF. The risk of colorectal cancer in ulcerative colitis: a meta-analysis. *Gut* 2001;48(4):526–35.

19 Binder V, Hendriksen C, Kreiner S. Prognosis in Crohn's disease – based on results from a regional patient group from the county of Copenhagen. *Gut* 1985;26(2):146–50.

20 Gollop JH, Phillips SF, Melton LJ, 3rd, Zinsmeister AR. Epidemiologic aspects of Crohn's disease: a population based study in Olmsted County, Minnesota, 1943–1982. *Gut* 1988;29(1):49–56.

21 Kvist N, Jacobsen O, Norgaard P, et al. Malignancy in Crohn's disease. *Scand J Gastroenterol* 1986;21(1):82–6.

22 Greenstein AJ, Sachar DB, Smith H, Janowitz HD, Aufses AH Jr. A comparison of cancer risk in Crohn's disease and ulcerative colitis. *Cancer* 1981;48(12):2742–5.

23 Weedon DD, Shorter RG, Ilstrup DM, Huizenga KA, Taylor WF. Crohn's disease and cancer. *N Engl J Med* 1973;289(21):1099–103.

24 Gyde SN, Prior P, Macartney JC, Thompson H, Waterhouse JA, Allan RN. Malignancy in Crohn's disease. *Gut* 1980;21(12):1024–9.

25 Ekbom A, Helmick C, Zack M, Adami HO. Increased risk of large-bowel cancer in Crohn's disease with colonic involvement. *Lancet* 1990;336(8711):357–9.

26 Gillen CD, Andrews HA, Prior P, Allan RN. Crohn's disease and colorectal cancer. *Gut* 1994;35(5):651–5.

27 Gillen CD, Walmsley RS, Prior P, Andrews HA, Allan RN. Ulcerative colitis and Crohn's disease: a comparison of the colorectal cancer risk in extensive colitis. *Gut* 1994;35(11):1590–2.

28 Sachar DB. Cancer in Crohn's disease: dispelling the myths. *Gut* 1994;35(11):1507–8.

29 Connell WR, Sheffield JP, Kamm MA, Ritchie JK, Hawley PR, Lennard-Jones JE. Lower gastrointestinal malignancy in Crohn's disease. *Gut* 1994;35(3):347–52.

30 Devroede GJ, Taylor WF, Sauer WG, Jackman RJ, Stickler GB. Cancer risk and life expectancy of children with ulcerative colitis. *N Engl J Med* 1971;285(1):17–21.

31 Broome U, Lindberg G, Lofberg R. Primary sclerosing cholangitis in ulcerative colitis – a risk factor for the development of dysplasia and DNA aneuploidy? *Gastroenterology* 1992;102(6):1877–80.

32 Brentnall TA, Haggitt RC, Rabinovitch PS, et al. Risk and natural history of colonic neoplasia in patients with primary sclerosing cholangitis and ulcerative colitis. *Gastroenterology* 1996;110(2):331–8.

33 D'Haens GR, Lashner BA, Hanauer SB. Pericholangitis and sclerosing cholangitis are risk factors for dysplasia and cancer in ulcerative colitis. *Am J Gastroenterol* 1993;88(8):1174–8.

34 Kornfeld D, Ekbom A, Ihre T. Is there an excess risk for colorectal cancer in patients with ulcerative colitis and concomitant primary sclerosing cholangitis? A population based study. *Gut* 1997;41(4):522–5.

35 Loftus EV Jr, Sandborn WJ, Tremaine WJ, et al. Risk of colorectal neoplasia in patients with primary sclerosing cholangitis. *Gastroenterology* 1996;110(2):432–40.

36 Nuako KW, Ahlquist DA, Sandborn WJ, Mahoney DW, Siems DM, Zinsmeister AR. Primary sclerosing cholangitis and colorectal carcinoma in patients with chronic ulcerative colitis: a case-control study. *Cancer* 1998;82(5):822–6.

37 Askling J, Dickman PW, Karlen P, et al. Family history as a risk factor for colorectal cancer in inflammatory bowel disease. *Gastroenterology* 2001;120(6):1356–62.

38 Nuako KW, Ahlquist DA, Mahoney DW, Schaid DJ, Siems DM, Lindor NM. Familial predisposition for colorectal cancer in chronic ulcerative colitis: a case-control study. *Gastroenterology* 1998;115(5):1079–83.

39 Edwards FC, Truelove SC. The course and prognosis of ulcerative colitis: IV. Carcinoma of the colon. *Gut* 1964;5:15–22.

40 Pinczowski D, Ekbom A, Baron J, Yuen J, Adami HO. Risk factors for colorectal cancer in patients with ulcerative colitis: a case-control study. *Gastroenterology* 1994;107(1):117–20.

41 Moody GA, Jayanthi V, Probert CS, Mac Kay H, Mayberry JF. Long-term therapy with sulphasalazine protects against colorectal cancer in ulcerative colitis: a retrospective study of colorectal cancer risk and compliance with treatment in Leicestershire. *Eur J Gastroenterol Hepatol* 1996;8(12):1179–83.

42 Eaden J, Abrams K, Ekbom A, Jackson E, Mayberry J. Colorectal cancer prevention in ulcerative colitis: a case-control study. *Aliment Pharmacol Ther* 2000;14(2):145–53.

43 Gwyn K, Sinicrope FA. Chemoprevention of colorectal cancer. *Am J Gastroenterol* 2002;97(1): 13–21.

44 Labayle D, Fischer D, Vielh P, *et al.* Sulindac causes regression of rectal polyps in familial adenomatous polyposis. *Gastroenterology* 1991;101(3):635–9.

45 Winde G, Gumbinger HG, Osswald H, Kemper F, Bunte H. The NSAID sulindac reverses rectal adenomas in colectomized patients with familial adenomatous polyposis: clinical results of a dose-finding study on rectal sulindac administration. *Int J Colorectal Dis* 1993;8(1):13–7.

46 Nugent KP, Farmer KC, Spigelman AD, Williams CB, Phillips RK. Randomized controlled trial of the effect of sulindac on duodenal and rectal polyposis and cell proliferation in patients with familial adenomatous polyposis. *Br J Surg* 1993;80(12):1618–9.

47 Tonelli F, Valanzano R, Dolara P. Sulindac therapy of colorectal polyps in familial adenomatous polyposis. *Dig Dis* 1994;12(5):259–64.

48 Earnest DL, Holubec H, Wali RK, *et al.* Chemoprevention of azoxymethane-induced colonic carcinogenesis by supplemental dietary ursodeoxycholic acid. *Cancer Res* 1994;54(19): 5071–4.

49 Tung BY, Emond MJ, Haggitt RC, *et al.* Ursodiol use is associated with lower prevalence of colonic neoplasia in patients with ulcerative colitis and primary sclerosing cholangitis. *Ann Intern Med* 2001;134(2):89–95.

50 Pardi DS, Loftus EV Jr, Kremers WK, Keach J, Lindor KD. Ursodeoxycholic acid as a chemopreventive agent in patients with ulcerative colitis and primary sclerosing cholangitis. *Gastroenterology* 2003;124 (4):889–93.

51 Lindor KD. Ursodiol for primary sclerosing cholangitis. Mayo primary sclerosing cholangitis-ursodeoxycholic acid study group. *N Engl J Med* 1997;336(10):691–5.

52 Batta AK, Salen G, Holubec H, Brasitus TA, Alberts D, Earnest DL. Enrichment of the more hydrophilic bile acid ursodeoxycholic acid in the fecal water-soluble fraction after feeding to rats with colon polyps. *Cancer Res* 1998;58(8):1684–7.

53 Rodrigues CM, Kren BT, Steer CJ, Setchell KD. The site-specific delivery of ursodeoxycholic acid to the rat colon by sulfate conjugation. *Gastroenterology* 1995; 109(6):1835–44.

54 Freudenheim JL, Graham S, Marshall JR, Haughey BP, Cholewinski S, Wilkinson G. Folate intake and carcinogenesis of the colon and rectum. *Int J Epidemiol* 1991;20(2):368–74.

55 Giovannucci E, Stampfer MJ, Colditz GA, *et al.* Folate, methionine, and alcohol intake and risk of colorectal adenoma. *J Natl Cancer Inst* 1993;85(11): 875–84.

56 Lashner BA, Heidenreich PA, Su GL, Kane SV, Hanauer SB. Effect of folate supplementation on the incidence of dysplasia and cancer in chronic ulcerative colitis: a case-control study. *Gastroenterology* 1989; 97(2):255–9.

57 Lashner BA. Red blood cell folate is associated with the development of dysplasia and cancer in ulcerative colitis. *J Cancer Res Clin Oncol* 1993;119(9): 549–54.

58 Lashner BA, Provencher KS, Seidner DL, Knesebeck A, Brzezinski A. The effect of folic acid supplementation on the risk for cancer or dysplasia in ulcerative colitis. *Gastroenterology* 1997;112(1): 29–32.

59 Connell WR, Kamm MA, Dickson M, Balkwill AM, Ritchie JK, Lennard-Jones JE. Long-term neoplasia risk after azathioprine treatment in inflammatory bowel disease. *Lancet* 1994;343(8908):1249–52.

60 Choi PM, Zelig MP. Similarity of colorectal cancer in Crohn's disease and ulcerative colitis: implications for carcinogenesis and prevention. *Gut* 1994;35(7): 950–4.

61 Leijonmarck CE, Persson PG, Hellers G. Factors affecting colectomy rate in ulcerative colitis: an epidemiologic study. *Gut* 1990;31(3):329–33.

62 Gyde S. Screening for colorectal cancer in ulcerative colitis: dubious benefits and high costs. *Gut* 1990;31 (10):1089–92.

63 Morson BC, Pang LS. Rectal biopsy as an aid to cancer control in ulcerative colitis. *Gut* 1967;8(5): 423–34.

64 Riddell RH, Goldman H, Ransohoff DF, *et al.* Dysplasia in inflammatory bowel disease: standardized classification with provisional clinical applications. *Hum Pathol* 1983;14(11):931–68.

65 Rosenstock E, Farmer RG, Petras R, Sivak MV Jr, Rankin GB, Sullivan BH. Surveillance for colonic carcinoma in ulcerative colitis. *Gastroenterology* 1985;89(6):1342–6.

66 Lofberg R, Brostrom O, Karlen P, Tribukait B, Ost A. Colonoscopic surveillance in long-standing total ulcerative colitis – a 15-year follow-up study. *Gastroenterology* 1990;99(4):1021–31.

67 Lennard-Jones JE, Misiewicz JJ, Parrish JA, Ritchie JK, Swarbrick ET, Williams CB. Prospective study of outpatients with extensive colitis. *Lancet* 1974; 1(7866):1065–7.

68 Connell WR, Lennard-Jones JE, Williams CB, Talbot IC, Price AB, Wilkinson KH. Factors affecting the outcome of endoscopic surveillance for cancer in ulcerative colitis. *Gastroenterology* 1994;107(4): 934–44.

69 Taylor BA, Pemberton JH, Carpenter HA, *et al.* Dysplasia in chronic ulcerative colitis: implications for colonoscopic surveillance. *Dis Colon Rectum* 1992; 35(10):950–6.

70 Ransohoff DF, Riddell RH, Levin B. Ulcerative colitis and colonic cancer. Problems in assessing the diagnostic usefulness of mucosal dysplasia. *Dis Colon Rectum* 1985;28(6):383–8.

71 Lynch DA, Lobo AJ, Sobala GM, Dixon MF, Axon AT. Failure of colonoscopic surveillance in ulcerative colitis. *Gut* 1993;34(8):1075–80.

72 Choi PM, Nugent FW, Schoetz DJ Jr, Silverman ML, Haggitt RC. Colonoscopic surveillance reduces mortality from colorectal cancer in ulcerative colitis. *Gastroenterology* 1993;105(2):418–24.

73 Rozen P, Baratz M, Fefer F, Gilat T. Low incidence of significant dysplasia in a successful endoscopic surveillance program of patients with ulcerative colitis. *Gastroenterology* 1995;108(5):1361–70.

74 Jones HW, Grogono J, Hoare AM. Surveillance in ulcerative colitis: burdens and benefit. *Gut* 1988;29 (3):325–31.

75 Axon AT, Lynch DA. Surveillance for ulcerative colitis does not and cannot work. *Gastroenterology* 1994; 106(4):1129–31.

76 Axon AT. Cancer surveillance in ulcerative colitis – a time for reappraisal. *Gut* 1994;35(5):587–9.

77 Collins RH Jr, Feldman M, Fordtran JS. Colon cancer, dysplasia, and surveillance in patients with ulcerative colitis: a critical review. *N Engl J Med* 1987;316(26):1654–8.

78 Karlen P, Kornfeld D, Brostrom O, Lofberg R, Persson PG, Ekbom A. Is colonoscopic surveillance reducing colorectal cancer mortality in ulcerative colitis? A population based case control study. *Gut* 1998;42(5):711–4.

79 Provenzale D, Kowdley KV, Arora S, Wong JB. Prophylactic colectomy or surveillance for chronic ulcerative colitis? A decision analysis. *Gastroenterology* 1995;109(4):1188–96.

80 Brostrom O, Lofberg R, Nordenvall B, Ost A, Hellers G. The risk of colorectal cancer in ulcerative colitis: an epidemiologic study. *Scand J Gastroenterol* 1987; 22(10):1193–9.

81 Gurbuz AK, Giardiello FM, Bayless TM. Colorectal neoplasia in patients with ulcerative colitis and primary sclerosing cholangitis. *Dis Colon Rectum* 1995;38(1):37–41.

82 Vemulapalli R, Lance P. Cancer surveillance in ulcerative colitis: more of the same or progress? *Gastroenterology* 1994;107(4):1196–9.

83 Brostrom O, Ekbom A, Lofberg R, Rutegard J. Great risk of cancer in ulcerative colitis. Colonoscopic monitoring is recommended. *Lakartidningen* 1995;92 (13):1325–6, 1329.

84 Friedman S, Rubin PH, Bodian C, Goldstein E, Harpaz N, Present DH. Screening and surveillance colonoscopy in chronic Crohn's colitis. *Gastroenterology* 2001;120(4):820–6.

85 Greenstein AJ, Sachar DB, Smith H, *et al.* Cancer in universal and left-sided ulcerative colitis: factors determining risk. *Gastroenterology* 1979;77(2): 290–4.

86 Desaint B, Legendre C, Florent C. Dysplasia and cancer in ulcerative colitis. *Hepatogastroenterology* 1989;36(4):219–26.

87 Rubio CA, Befrits R. Colorectal adenocarcinoma in Crohn's disease: a retrospective histologic study. *Dis Colon Rectum* 1997;40(9):1072–8.

88 Lapidus A, Bernell O, Hellers G, Persson PG, Lofberg R. Incidence of Crohn's disease in Stockholm County 1955–1989. *Gut* 1997;41(4):480–6.

89 Yamazaki Y, Ribeiro MB, Sachar DB, Aufses AH,Jr, Greenstein AJ. Malignant colorectal strictures in Crohn's disease. *Am J Gastroenterol* 1991;86(7): 882–5.

90 Gorfine SR, Bauer JJ, Harris MT, Kreel I. Dysplasia complicating chronic ulcerative colitis: is immediate colectomy warranted? *Dis Colon Rectum* 2000;43(11):1575–81.

91 Ullman TA. Making the grade: should patients with UC and low-grade dysplasia graduate to surgery or be held back? *Inflamm Bowel Dis* 2002;8(6):430–1.

92 Ullman TA. Patients with low-grade dysplasia should be advised to undergo colectomy. *Inflamm Bowel Dis* 2003;9(4):267–9; discussion 273–5.

93 Bernstein CN, Shanahan F, Weinstein WM. Are we telling patients the truth about surveillance colonoscopy in ulcerative colitis? *Lancet* 1994; 343(8889):71–4.

94 Befrits R, Ljung T, Jaramillo E, Rubio C. Low-grade dysplasia in extensive, long-standing inflammatory

bowel disease: a follow-up study. *Dis Colon Rectum* 2002;45(5):615–20.

95 Lim CH, Dixon MF, Vail A, Forman D, Lynch DA, Axon AT. Ten year follow up of ulcerative colitis patients with and without low grade dysplasia. *Gut* 2003;52(8):1127–32.

96 von Herbay A, Herfarth C, Otto HF. Cancer and dysplasia in ulcerative colitis: a histologic study of 301 surgical specimen. *Z Gastroenterol* 1994;32(7):382–8.

97 Blackstone MO, Riddell RH, Rogers BH, Levin B. Dysplasia-associated lesion or mass (DALM) detected by colonoscopy in long-standing ulcerative colitis: an indication for colectomy. *Gastroenterology* 1981;80(2):366–74.

98 Rubin PH, Friedman S, Harpaz N, *et al.* Colonoscopic polypectomy in chronic colitis: conservative management after endoscopic resection of dysplastic polyps. *Gastroenterology* 1999;117(6):1295–300.

99 Engelsgjerd M, Farraye FA, Odze RD. Polypectomy may be adequate treatment for adenoma-like dysplastic lesions in chronic ulcerative colitis. *Gastroenterology* 1999;117(6):1288–94; discussion 1488–91.

100 Odze RD, Farraye FA, Hecht JL, Hornick JL. Long-term follow-up after polypectomy treatment for adenoma-like dysplastic lesions in ulcerative colitis. *Clin Gastroenterol Hepatol* 2004;2(7):534–41.

101 Friedman S, Odze RD, Farraye FA. Management of neoplastic polyps in inflammatory bowel disease. *Inflamm Bowel Dis* 2003;9(4):260–6.

23: Cancer: new colonoscopic techniques

Ralf Kiesslich and Markus F. Neurath

Introduction

Patients with longstanding extensive ulcerative colitis are at increased risk of developing colorectal cancer [1]. Colonoscopic surveillance is recommended to reduce associated mortality [2]. Surveillance relies on the detection of pre-malignant dysplastic tissue, and where multi-focal dysplasia is detected, proctocolectomy remains the management of choice, although there is increasing evidence that adenoma-like dysplastic lesions may safely be resected endoscopically [3–5].

Detection of pre-malignant lesions in ulcerative colitis

In patients without ulcerative colitis, the premalignant dysplastic lesion, the adenoma, usually occurs as a clearly delineated macroscopically visible abnormality. However, in ulcerative colitis there is no clear-cut adenoma-carcinoma sequence. Colitis-associated neoplasia can occur in addition to adenomas in patients with long lasting ulcerative colitis. These lesions are triggered by inflammation and the macroscopic appearances are often flat and multifocal [6]. There are no clear-cut endoscopic, histological or immunohistochemical discriminators to permit accurate stratification of mass dysplasia in colitis, and no universally agreed definition. However, the term 'intra-epithelial neoplasia' in accordance with the new Vienna classification was established, which summarises adenomas and colitis-associated neoplasia.

Currently multiple untargeted random biopsies are recommended to diagnose intra-epithelial neoplasia. Four random biopsies per site over nine sites throughout the colon should be undertaken, with increased sampling from the recto-sigmoid and with additional biopsies from raised or suspicious lesions [2]. However this approach is time-consuming and dysplastic lesions might still be overlooked.

Chromoendoscopy can help to identify pre-malignant and malignant lesions. Magnifying endoscopy enables us to analyse surface structure, while confocal laser endomicroscopy enables *in vivo* histology.

Chromoendoscopy

Intravital staining is the oldest and simplest method used to improve the diagnosis of epithelial changes. Chromoendoscopy, vital staining and contrast endoscopy are synonyms for the same technique: dye solutions are applied to the mucosa of the gastrointestinal tract, enhancing the recognition of details in order to uncover mucosal changes not seen by purely optical methods prior to targeted biopsy and histology [7].

In general, there are three classes of dye that can be used for chromoendoscopy [7, 8].

Contrast dyes

These simply coat the colonic mucosal surface, and neither react with nor are absorbed by it. An example is *indigo carmine*. Contrast dyes are effective because the colonic mucosa is covered with tiny pits and whorls of parallel 'innominate' grooves, similar to a fingerprint. When a dye is sprayed onto the surface, this pattern becomes evident, and disruption of these grooves caused by mucosal lesions (which have a different surface topography) is highlighted.

Absorptive dyes

These are absorbed by different cells to different degrees, highlighting particular cell types. An example is *methylene blue,* which after a few minutes, avidly stains non-inflamed mucosa, but is poorly taken up by areas of active inflammation and of dysplasia.

Reactive dyes

The binding of reactive colouring agents with certain mucosal areas is used to identify reactions. Their use is less common and their diagnostic relevance rather low.

In patients with ulcerative colitis the most common dyes are indigo carmine and methylene blue. Chromoendoscopy has two main goals. First, it improves the detection of subtle colonic lesions, raising the sensitivity of the endoscopic examination; this is important in ulcerative colitis, as flat dysplastic lesions can be difficult to detect. Secondly, once a lesion is detected, chromoendoscopy can improve lesion characterisation, increasing the specificity of the examination. This can be further refined with a magnifying colonoscope. Surface analysis of colorectal lesions using magnifying endoscopes is a new optical impression for the endoscopists. Kudo et al. [9] described that some of the regular staining patterns are often seen in hyperplastic polyps or normal mucosa, whereas unstructured surface architecture was associated with malignancy. Also the kind of adenoma (tubular vs villous) can be seen by detailed inspection (Fig 23.1). This experience has lead to a categorisation of the different staining patterns in the colon. The so-called pit-pattern classification [9] differentiated five types and several subtypes. Types 1 and 2 are staining patterns that predict non-neoplastic lesions, whereas types 3–5 predict neoplastic lesions (Fig 23.2). With the help of this classification the endoscopist can predict histology with accuracy [10].

As recently shown in prospective and randomised trials, panchromoendoscopy with methylene blue or indigo carmine-aided biopsies is superior in the detection of intra-epithelial neoplasia as compared to random biopsies [10–12]. Based on the currently available data SURFACE guidelines [13] are proposed for the use and standardisation of this new technique in patients with ulcerative colitis (see Table 23.1).

Ideally, surveillance colonoscopies should be performed in patients whose symptoms are in remission, to aid both macroscopic and histological discrimination between inflammatory changes and dysplasia (Table 23.1, 'Strict patient selection'). Thus, a patient with active symptoms should first have their medical therapy optimised to induce remission, wherever possible. However, as patients with chronic active inflammation are at increased risk of colorectal neoplasia [14], the procedure should not be unduly delayed if they fail to respond to therapy.

Examination technique [8]

A thorough bowel preparation is of crucial importance and a prerequisite for chromoendoscopy. On insertion, all faecal fluid should be aspirated to ensure optimal mucosal views (Table 23.1, 'Unmask the mucosal surface'). When the caecal pole has been reached, meticulous inspection of the colonic mucosa is performed on withdrawal. To reduce spasm and haustral-fold prominence (thus reducing blind spots), intravenous butyl-scopolamine 20 mg, intravenous glucagon 1 mg or other spasmolytic should be given when the caecal pole is reached. Further increments can be given as required (Table 23.1). Adequate air insufflation is necessary, and if the lumen remains collapsed the patient should be turned. Inspection is performed by scouring the mucosa in a spiral fashion. Dye spraying of the entire colorectal mucosa (Panchromoendoscopy) greatly reduces the risk of overlooking subtle abnormalities (see Table 23.1) and adds little to the duration of the procedure. Before the procedure, 100 mL of 0.1% indigo carmine or 0.1% methylene blue is prepared and drawn into 50 mL syringes. A dye-spray catheter is inserted down the instrumentation channel, and the tip protruded 2–3 cm. Under the direction of the endoscopist, an assistant firmly squeezes the syringe, generating a fine mist of dye, which is then painted

CANCER: NEW COLONOSCOPIC TECHNIQUES 295

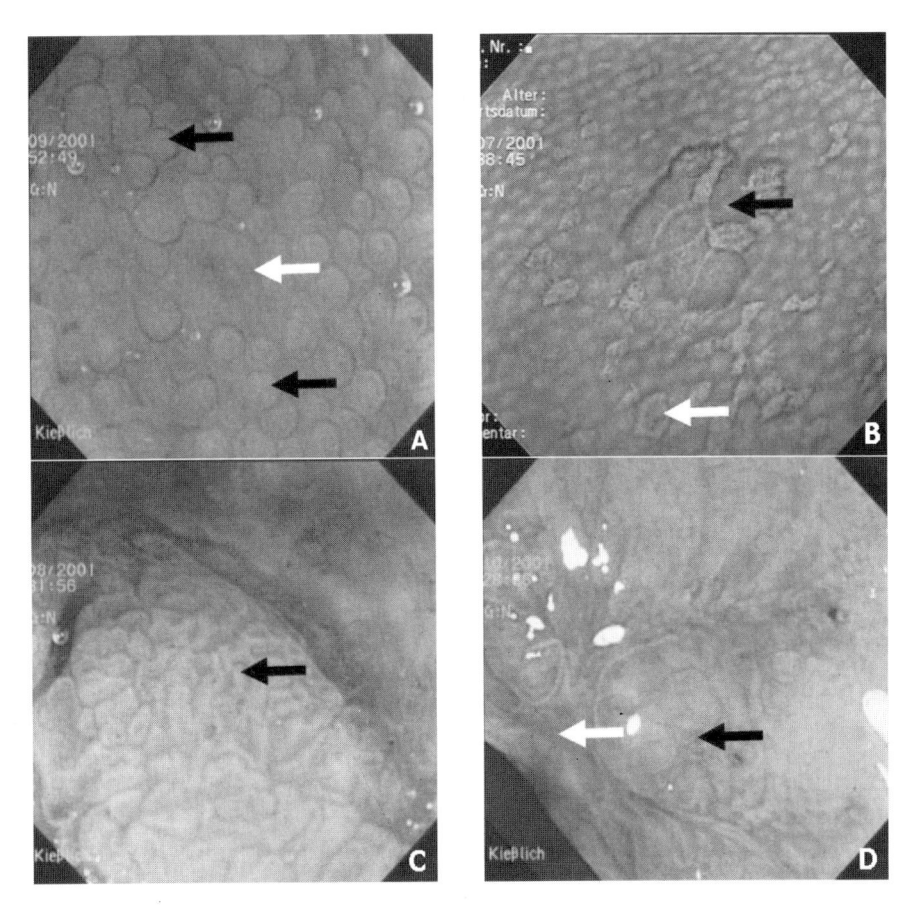

Fig 23.1 (a) Chromo-and magnifying endoscopy of the terminal ileum. Single villi are clearly visible (black arrows). A small erosion (<1 mm) is visible in the centre of the image. (b) Magnification endoscopy after methylene-blue aided chromoendoscopy. Small inflammatory changes are visible (white arrow) surrounded by normal crypt architecture. Chromoendoscopy unmasks an aberrant crypt foci (black arrow). Pit Pattern II. (c) A tubular staining pattern (Type IIIL) is clearly visible after Intravital staining. Targeted biopsy revealed low-grade intra-epithelial neoplasia. (d) A flat-growing cancer with unstructured surface (Pit Pattern V; black arrow) with accompanying ulceration (white arrow) indicates malignancy.

onto the mucosa by withdrawing the colonoscope in a spiral fashion.

Spraying should be done in a segmental fashion (every 20–30 cm). Once a segment has been sprayed, excess dye is suctioned, and the colonoscope re-inserted to the proximal extent of the segment. It is occasionally necessary to wait a few seconds for indigo carmine to settle into the mucosal contours; methylene blue takes about 60 s to be absorbed. Once that segment has been examined, the next segment is sprayed, and so on until the anal margin is reached. On average, 60–100 mL of solution is required to spray the entire colorectal mucosa.

Dye spraying greatly aids the detection of intra-epithelial neoplasia (Table 23.1). Areas of villi-form (velvet-like) mucosa with clear borders (circumscript lesions) are of particular concern. Areas of nodularity or friable mucosa may also indicate intra-epithelial neoplasia (Fig 23.1). Sessile (polypoid) lesions are easier to detect, but careful delineation of the edge of the lesion is required (aided by dye-spraying), and if the lesion is endoscopically

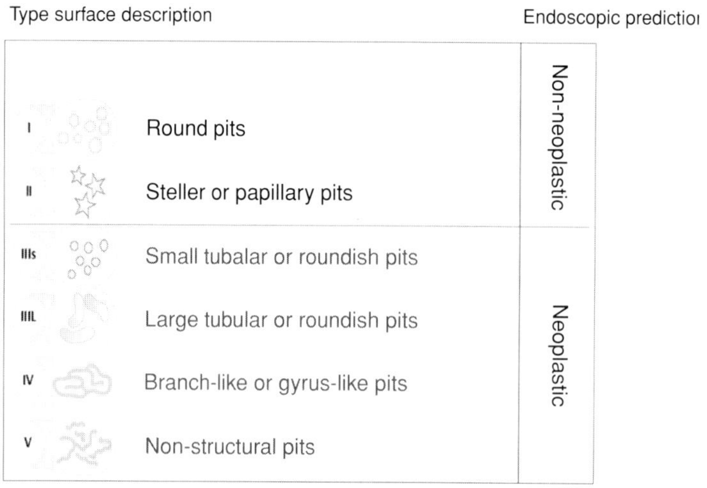

Type surface description			Endoscopic prediction
I	Round pits		Non-neoplastic
II	Steller or papillary pits		
IIIs	Small tubalar or roundish pits		Neoplastic
IIIL	Large tubular or roundish pits		
IV	Branch-like or gyrus-like pits		
V	Non-structural pits		

Fig 23.2 Pit pattern classification.

Table 23.1 SURFACE-guidelines for chromoendoscopy in patients with ulcerative colitis.

Strict patient selection

Patients with histologically proven ulcerative colitis and at least 8 years duration in clinical remission. Avoid patients with active disease

Unmask the mucosal surface

Excellent bowel preparation is needed. Remove mucus and remaining fluid in the colon when necessary

Reduce peristaltic waves

When drawing back the endoscope, a spasmolytic agent should be used (if necessary)

Full length staining of the colon

Perform full length staining of the colon (panchromoendoscopy) in ulcerative colitis rather than local staining

Augmented detection with dyes

Intra-vital staining with 0.4% indigo carmine or 0.1% methylene blue should be used to unmask flat lesions more frequently than with conventional colonoscopy

Crypt architecture analysis

All lesions should be analysed according to the pit pattern classification. Whereas pit pattern types I–II suggest the presence of non-malignant lesions, staining patterns III–V suggest the presence of intra-epithelial neoplasias and carcinomas

Endoscopic targeted biopsies

Perform targeted biopsies of all mucosal alterations, particularly of circumscript lesions with staining patterns indicative of intra-epithelial neoplasias and carcinomas (pit patterns III–V)

resectable, it is essential to take additional biopsies from the surrounding mucosa to ensure there is no residual neoplastic tissue, and to tattoo the site to permit re-inspection later on.

The combination of chromoendoscopy and new-generation magnifying colonoscopes enables detailed mucosal analysis (Table 23.1). Neoplastic changes are characterised by an irregular, tubular or villous crypt architecture staining pattern. Non-neoplastic changes are characterised by stellate or regular round pits. The different staining patterns are categorised using the 'pit pattern' classification [9]. By targeting biopsies towards mucosal abnormalities (Table 23.1), the specificity of each biopsy for dysplasia is increased and the total number of biopsies taken per colonoscopic examination can be reduced in comparison to random biopsies with standard colonoscopy [10–12].

Efficiency of Chromoendoscopy

The first randomised, controlled trial was published in 2003 [10]. This study was designed to test whether chromo- and magnifying endoscopy might facilitate early detection of intra-epithelial neoplasia in patients with ulcerative colitis by using magnifying chromoendoscopy. One hundred and sixty-five patients with long-standing ulcerative colitis were randomised at a 1:1 ratio to undergo conventional colonoscopy or colonoscopy with chromoendoscopy using 0.1% methylene blue. Circumscript lesions in the colon were evaluated according to a modified pit pattern classification. In the chromoendoscopy group, there was a significantly better correlation between the endoscopic assessment of degree and extent of colonic inflammation, and the histopathologic findings compared with the conventional colonoscopy group. More targeted biopsies were possible, and significantly more intra-epithelial neoplasias were detected in the chromoendoscopy group (32 vs 10). Using the modified pit pattern classification, both the sensitivity and specificity for differentiation between non-neoplastic and neoplastic lesions were 93%. The overall sensitivity of magnifying chromoendoscopy to predict neoplasia was 97% with a specificity of 93%, respectively. The ability of the dye technique to identify neoplastic from non-neoplastic lesions to enhance detection of more dysplastic lesions in flat mucosa is a potential major advance in dysplasia surveillance. These first promising data about chromoendoscopy in UC are confirmed by Hurlstone et al. [11]. In a prospective study, 162 patients with long-standing ulcerative colitis and established pan-colitis underwent total colonoscopy by a single endoscopist using a magnifying colonoscope. Subtle mucosal changes such as fold convergence, air-induced deformation, interruption of innominate grooves or focal, discrete colour change were targeted. Intra-vital staining with indigo carmine was used. The macroscopic type and the staining pattern were defined. The control group consisted of 162 disease-matched patients, undergoing conventional colonoscopy. Chromoendoscopy with targeted biopsy significantly increased diagnostic yield for intra-epithelial neoplasia and the number of flat neoplastic changes as opposed to conventional colonoscopy. Intra-epithelial neoplasia in flat mucosal change was observed in 37 lesions of which 31 were detected using chromoendoscopy.

Rutter and colleagues [12] performed a prospective trial in UC on 100 patients with back to back colonoscopy, starting with random and targeted biopsies followed by indigo carmine aided panchromoendoscopy with targeted biopsies only. The diagnostic yield of dysplastic changes was increased in this study by the use of chromoendoscopy from two to seven patients (3.5-fold increase) and from two to nine dysplastic lesions (4.5-fold increase).

In conclusion, magnifying chromoendoscopy is a new and useful tool for improving endoscopic detection of intra-epithelial neoplasia in patients with long-standing ulcerative colitis. Chromoendoscopy increases the diagnostic yield of intra-epithelial neoplasia as compared with conventional colonoscopy and biopsy techniques 3–4.5-fold, which further suggests that more patients with ulcerative colitis could be considered as candidates for colectomy. Differentiation of non-neoplastic from neoplastic lesions is possible with a high overall sensitivity and specificity.

Limitations of chromo- and magnifying endoscopy

At present, there are no severe side effects reported with the local use of indigo carmine. However, Olliver and colleagues [15] recently raised some concerns about the intra-vital dye methylene blue despite a harmless transient discoloration of stool and urine. They found in patients with Barrett oesophagus oxidative DNA damage after chromoendoscopy (as measured by single-cell gel electrophoresis) and argued that methylene blue together with white light during endoscopy could also be a risk for patients because of the possibility that it may drive carcinogenesis. Therefore, the question arises whether methylene blue aided chromoendoscopy may contribute to the carcinogenic process in other diseases like ulcerative colitis leading to an increase of intra-epithelial neoplasia during follow-up. However, in a follow-up report (median follow-up: 23 months) on the safety of methylene blue staining, patients with previous chromoendoscopies showed fewer intra-epithelial neoplasias compared to patients who were screened by colonoscopy. These data suggest that chromoendoscopy with methylene blue is a safe and highly effective approach for the detection of flat colonic lesions in UC. The reported increase of DNA lesions upon methylene blue-light treatment is unlikely to have biologic significance *in vivo*, and unwanted side effects appear to be negligible in view of the advantages of the method [16].

The visual evaluation of minute detail allowed by magnification endoscopy is promising, but some points of criticism must be discussed. Inflammation can cause significant disturbance of the image seen when magnifying endoscopy is used to look for the minute changes indicative of neoplasia, and there is a danger of false-positive results. Inflamed epithelium should be treated prior to final endoscopic evaluation whenever possible. It is not useful or practical to permanently use the zoom mode when screening the lower gastrointestinal tract. The initial evaluation is performed in conventional mode and depends strictly on the knowledge and experience of the endoscopist. After the initial detection of discrete lesions, chromoendoscopy and magnification endoscopy are the tools used to enhance surface mucosal patterns. These techniques disclose a plethora of mucosal detail, the evaluation of which increases the procedure time, at least when the endoscopist is learning the technique.

The proposed classifications for colorectal lesions are too complex relative to their practical clinical value. A simplification is recommended. We are facing the same dilemma as our pathologist colleagues when evaluating dysplasias, with the difference that histological preparation is widely standardised, whereas standardised procedure recommendations are lacking for chromoendoscopy and magnification endoscopy. Another difficulty in the use of magnifying endoscopes is the high magnification levels. The newly developed systems allow enlargement of up to 150 times. A sharp image is focused by manually adjusting the movable lens. Close examination can be difficult due to peristalsis and respiratory movements.

Perspectives and future trends

The limits and concerns surrounding magnifying chromoendoscopy are small and can be overcome by training and increased knowledge of the endoscopists. However, the dream and goal of an ideal colonoscopy is virtual histology, which means 'on-line' *in-vivo* histology. The endoscopists can decide which is the area of interest and can remove the lesion in a targeted fashion without prior biopsy.

Chromoendoscopy can illustrate the surface structure. But what is behind the surface? Many new optical developments are used to try and advance early diagnosis of colorectal cancer. Raman spectroscopy, optical coherence tomography, light scattering spectroscopy, confocal fluorescence endoscopy and immunofluorecence endoscopy are some of the new methods with different advantages and disadvantages [17]. However, the closest step towards virtual histology is confocal laser endoscopy [18].

Confocal laser endomicroscopy

Confocal laser endomicroscopy allows subsurface analysis of the intestinal mucosa and *in vivo* histology during ongoing endoscopy. The components of a confocal laser endoscope are based on integration of a confocal laser microscope in the distal tip of a conventional video endoscope (see Fig 23.3a). During laser endoscopy a single line laser delivers an excitation wavelength of 488 nm and the maximum laser power output is more than or 1mW at the surface of the tissue. Confocal image data are collected at a scan rate of 0.8 frames/s (1024×512 pixels) or 1.6 frames/s (1024×1024 pixels). The optical slice thickness is 7 μm with a lateral resolution of 0.7 μm. The field of view is 500×500 μm). The range of the z-axis was 0–200 μm below the surface layer. Confocal images can be generated simultaneously with endoscopic images (see Fig 23.3).

Technique of confocal laser endomicroscopy

A fluorescent contrast agent is used to achieve high contrast images using confocal endomicroscopy. Potentially suitable agents are fluorescein, acriflavine, tetracycline or cresyl violet. The contrast agent is applied systemically (fluorescein) or topically (all others) by using a spraying catheter. The most common dye used so far is fluorescein.

The confocal endoscope can be handled similarly to a standard endoscope. After the application of a contrast dye (e.g. fluorescein, systemically), the distal tip of the endoscope is placed in gentle contact with the mucosa and the position of the focal plane within the specimen adjusted using the buttons on

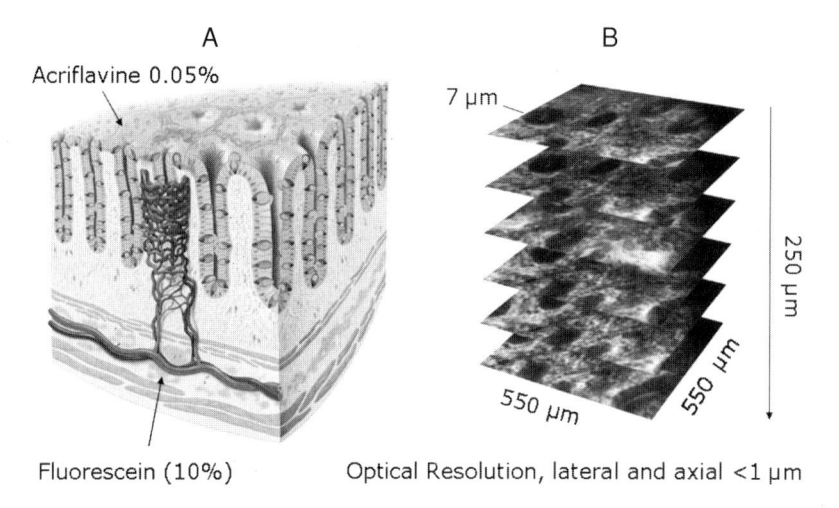

Fig 23.3 Scheme of endomicroscopy. (a) Micro-architecture of the colonic wall. Topical acriflavine or systemic application of fluorescein is mandatory for confocal endomicroscopy. (b) The confocal images are orientated in a horizontal fashion. The optical slice thickness is 7 μm with a lateral resolution of 0.7 μm. The field of view is 500 × 500 μm. The range of the z-axis is 0–250 μm below the surface layer.

the endoscope control body. In every region of interest images from the surface to deeper parts of the mucosal layer can be obtained and stored digitally in a specific folder associated with the site of collection. Targeted biopsies are possible due to the proximity of the working channel and the endomicroscopic window at the distal tip of the endoscope [18], which allows the position of the confocal scanner on the tissue to be seen via the conventional video endoscopic view.

Clinical data

The confocal laser endoscope can be used routinely for screening and surveillance. Suspected lesions can be examined in a targeted fashion by placing the endomicroscopic window onto the lesion. Confocal images can be graduated according to cellular and vascular changes. The images correlated well with conventional histology after targeted biopsies. In the first prospective trial 13,020 confocal images from 390 different locations (256 inconspicuous areas; 134 circumscript lesions) were compared with histologic data from 1038 biopsies. Subsurface analysis during confocal laser endoscopy allowed detailed analysis of cellular structures. The presence of neoplastic changes could be predicted by using the new developed confocal pattern (see Fig 23.3a) classification with high accuracy (Sensitivity: 97.4%; Specificity: 99.4%; Accuracy: 99.2%) [18].

In addition, combination of chromoendoscopy and confocal laser endoscopy facilitates surveillance in ulcerative colitis. Chromoendoscopy unmasks circumscript lesions and confocal laser endomicroscopy can be used to predict intra-epithelial neoplasias with high accuracy. Thus, targeted biopsies of relevant lesions can be performed and rapid prediction of neoplastic changes by confocal laser endoscopy during colonoscopy may lead to significant improvements in the clinical management of UC patients. Different cellular structures (epithelial and blood cells), capillaries and connective tissue limited to the mucosal layer can be identified by confocal microscopy. Due to the pharmacokinetic properties of fluorescein, nuclei cannot be seen. However, the presence of neoplastic changes (Sensitivity: 94.4%; Specificity: 95.6%; Accuracy: 99.3%) and inflammation could be predicted with high accuracy [19] (Figs 23.4 and 23.5).

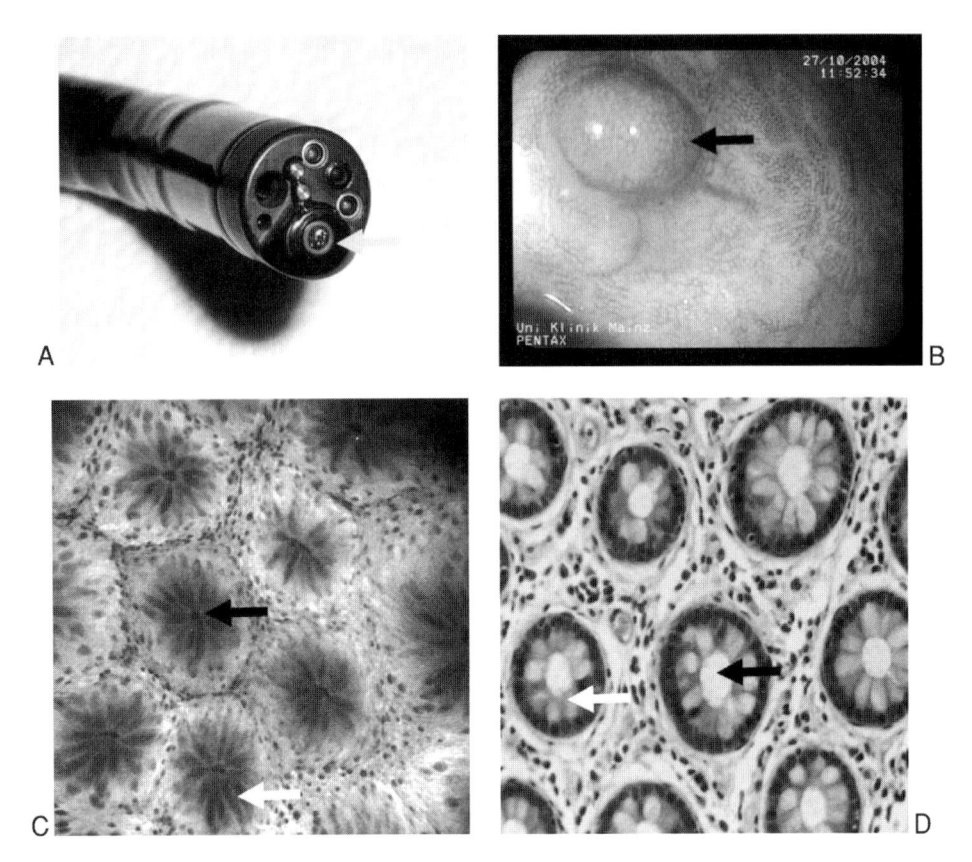

Fig 23.4 Endomicroscopy in ulcerative colitis: non-neoplastic lesion. (a) Confocal laser colonoscope: the confocal microscope is integrated in the distal tip. An additional microscopic window (arrow) enables the emission of blue laser light enabling *in vivo* histology. (b) A small polypoid lesion with regular staining pattern is clearly visible after methylene blue-aided chromoendoscopy. (c) Targeted endomicroscopic imaging shows a normal contribution of crypts and crypt openings (black arrow). The goblet cells within the crypts are displayed black (white arrow). Connective tissue is arranged regularly in a hexagonal fashion. (d) Corresponding histology confirms the endomicroscopic diagnosis. Normal crypts and round openings (black arrow) are visible. In addition mucin in the goblet cells are visible (white arrow).
Note: due to shrinking artefacts the spaces in between the tissue is wider in conventional histology as compared with *in vivo* histology.

Conclusion

The newly developed high-resolution and magnification endoscopes offer features that allow more and new mucosal details to be seen. They are commonly used in conjunction with chromoendoscopy. The analysis of mucosal surface details is beginning to resemble histological examination. More accurate recognition of small flat and depressed neoplastic lesions is possible. Endoscopic prediction of neoplastic and non-neoplastic tissue is possible by analysis surface architecture of the mucosa, which influences the endoscopic management. For the diagnosis of flat adenomas, chromoendoscopy should belong to the endoscopist's armamentarium. In inflammatory bowel disease chromoendoscopy can be used for patients with long-standing ulcerative colitis to unmask flat intra-epithelial neoplasia and is likely to be the new standard method for surveillance colonoscopy in the near future. The new detailed images seen with magnifying chromoendoscopy are the beginning of a new era, where new optical developments like confocal endomicroscopy allow a unique look on detailed cellular structures.

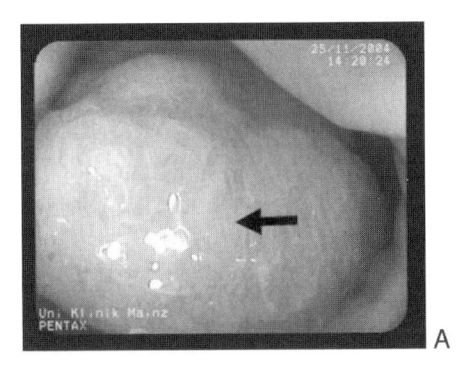

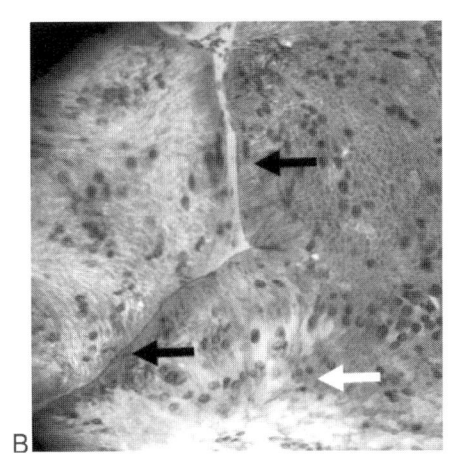

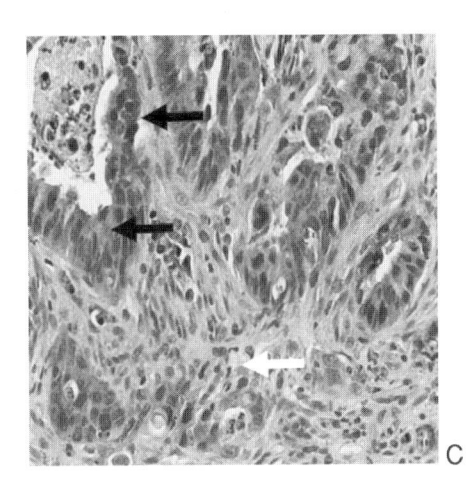

Fig 23.5 Endomicroscopy in ulcerative colitis: neoplastic lesion. (a) A large polypoid lesion is visible in the sigmoid. Chromoendoscopy is not necessary to recognise the lesion. (b) Endomicroscopy shows neoplasia with tubular arranged epithelium with loss of goblet cells (black arrows). In parts vessel and cell architecture is totally irregular (white arrow). (c) Corresponding histology shows high-grade intra-epithelial neoplasia with similar architecture.

References

1 Gilat T, Fireman Z, Grossman A, et al. Colorectal cancer in patients with ulcerative colitis. Gastroenterology 1988;94:870–7.
2 Winawer S, et al. Colorectal cancer screening and surveillance: clinical guidelines and rationale –update based on new evidence. Gastroenterology 2003;124(2):544–60.
3 Odze RD, et al. Long-term follow-up after polypectomy treatment for adenoma-like dysplastic lesions in ulcerative colitis. Clin Gastroenterol Hepatol 2004;2(7):534–41.
4 Sinicrope FA, Wang K. Treating polyps in ulcerative colitis: adenoma-like lesions and dysplasia-associated mass lesions. Clin Gastroenterol Hepatol 2004; 2(7):531–3.
5 Itzkowitz SH, Harpaz N. Diagnosis and management of dysplasia in patients with inflammatory bowel diseases. Gastroenterology 2004;126(6):1634–48.
6 Suzuki K, et al. Differential diagnosis of dysplasia-associated lesion or mass and coincidental adenoma in ulcerative colitis. Dis Colon Rectum 1998;41(3):322–7.
7 Jung M, Kiesslich R. Chromoendoscopy and intravital staining techniques. Baillieres Best Pract Res Clin Gastroenterol 1999;13(1):11–9.
8 Rutter M, Bernstein C, Matsumoto T, Kiesslich R, Neurath M. Endoscopic appearance of dysplasia in ulcerative colitis and the role of staining. Endoscopy 2004;36(12):1109–14.
9 Kudo S, Tamura S, Nakajima T, et al. Diagnosis of colorectal tumorous lesions by magnifying endoscopy. Gastrointest Endosc 1996;44:8–14.

10 Kiesslich R, *et al.* Methylene blue-aided chromoendoscopy for the detection of intraepithelial neoplasia and colon cancer in ulcerative colitis. *Gastroenterology* 2003;124(4):880–8.

11 Hurlstone DP. Further validation of high-magnification-chromoscopic colonoscopy for the detection of intraepithelial neoplasia and colon cancer in ulcerative colitis. *Gastroenterology* 2004;126: 376–8.

12 Rutter MD, Saunders BP, Schofield G, *et al.* Pancolonic indigo carmine dye spraying for the detection of dysplasia in ulcerative colitis. *Gut* 2004; 53: 256–60.

13 Kiesslich R, Neurath MF. Chromoendoscopy: an evolving standard in surveillance for ulcerative colitis. *Inflamm Bowel Dis* 2004;10:695–6.

14 Rutter M, Saunders B, Wilkinson K, *et al.* Severity of inflammation is a risk factor for colorectal neoplasia in ulcerative colitis. *Gastroenterology* 2004;126: 451–9.

15 Olliver JR, Wild CP, Sahay P, *et al.* Chromoendoscopy with methylene blue and associated DNA damage in Barrett's oesophagus. *Lancet* 2003;362:373–4.

16 Kiesslich R, Burg J, Kaina B, *et al.* Safety andefficacy of methylene blue aided chromoendos-copy in ulcerative colitis: a prospective pilotstudy upon previous chromoendoscopies. *Gastrointest Endosc* 2004;59:AB97.

17 Dacosta RS, Wilson BC, Marcon NE. New optical technologies for earlier endoscopic diagnosis of premalignant gastrointestinal lesions. *J Gastroenterol Hepatol* 2002;17:85–104.

18 Kiesslich R, Burg J, Vieth M, *et al.* Confocal laser endoscopy for diagnosing intraepithelial neoplasias and colorectal cancer *in vivo*. *Gastroenterology* 2004; 127:706–13.

19 Kiesslich R, Burg J, Vieth M, *et al. In vivo* fluorescence confocal laser endoscopy for prediction of neoplasia in patients with ulcerative colitis [Abstract]. *Gastrointest Endosc* 2004;59:9.

24: Molecular markers – a realistic hope?

Jacintha N. O'Sullivan and Teresa A. Brentnall

Background

Ulcerative colitis (UC) patients have an elevated risk of developing colorectal cancer (CRC) that rises with increasing duration and extent of the disease[1]. This risk is very difficult to quantify, however the overall absolute risk of CRC in longstanding extensive ulcerative colitis (UC) is estimated to be 10–15%. Recurrent and life-long colonoscopic surveillance is performed with the hope of detecting mucosal dysplasia or early cancer at a surgically curable stage. Despite these intensive efforts, such surveillance programmes have been disappointing and much debate centres on the effectiveness of such screening. There is an urgent need to better identify UC patients that may or may not progress to dysplasia and cancer. Molecular markers hold great promise for refining our ability to establish both early diagnosis and prognosis in UC patients. Understanding the molecular biology of neoplastic progression in UC will allow for the identification of molecular events – candidate neoplastic biomarkers – that occur during the evolution of this disease. Such biomarkers will improve the clinical management of UC patients, enabling us to concentrate our surveillance efforts on those UC patients most likely to benefit from them – in turn surveillance becomes more economical and less invasive for the majority of patients. However, to date, no molecular markers are reliable enough to be used for clinical decision-making.

UC cancer is thought to develop in a stepwise manner with progressive histological changes from negative for dysplasia → indefinite for dysplasia → dysplasia → cancer (Fig 24.1a). Rapid cellular proliferation plays a role in neoplastic progression in UC. Known risk factors for the development of colorectal dysplasia or cancer in UC are total colonic involvement and long duration of the disease. Primary sclerosing cholangitis (PSC) is an independent risk factor for the development of colorectal malignancy in UC [2–5] and highlights patients who need close colonoscopic surveillance with extensive biopsy sampling. Recently, the severity of colonic inflammation has been shown to be an important determinant of the risk of colorectal neoplasia [1] and suggests that endoscopic and histological grading of inflammation could allow better risk stratification for surveillance programmes.

Using dysplasia alone as a useful prognostic marker for subsequent cancer development has many limitations. The large surface area of the colon makes it difficult to detect focal dysplasia and cancer. The histological differentiation of inflammatory atypia from early neoplasia can be difficult, and at times impossible. It is known if 33 biopsies are taken, there is still a 10% chance of missing dysplasia or cancer (90% sensitivity) [6]. The fewer the biopsies taken, the greater the risk of missing neoplasia if it is present. The average number of surveillance biopsies taken at colonoscopy is between 10 and 20, based on surveys of gastroenterologists. This reinforces the limits of current practice and the need for robust and reproducible molecular biomarkers. These biomarkers need to be sufficiently sensitive and specific to separate the small, highest risk group who will progress to dysplasia

(a)

Chronic inflammation, oxidative damage

Shortened telomeres
Anaphase bridges
Loss of 18q telomeric region

Chromosomal instability

p53 LOH and mutation

Expansion of instability

Aneuploidy sialyl-Tn
MSI, Cox2

Loss of Kras and additional tumour suppressor genes

Acquisition of invasive potential

↓ ↓ ↓ ↓

Negative for dysplasia　　**Indefinite for dysplasia**　　**Dysplasia**　**Cancer**

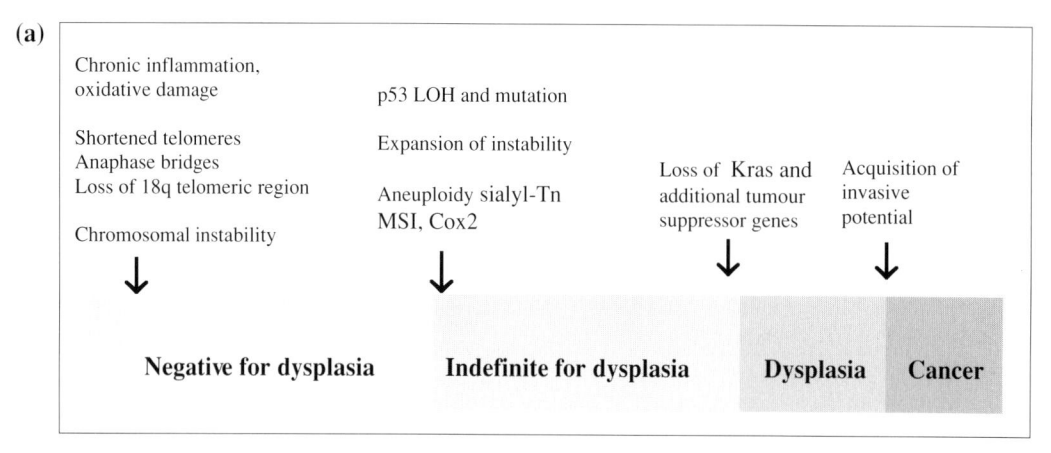

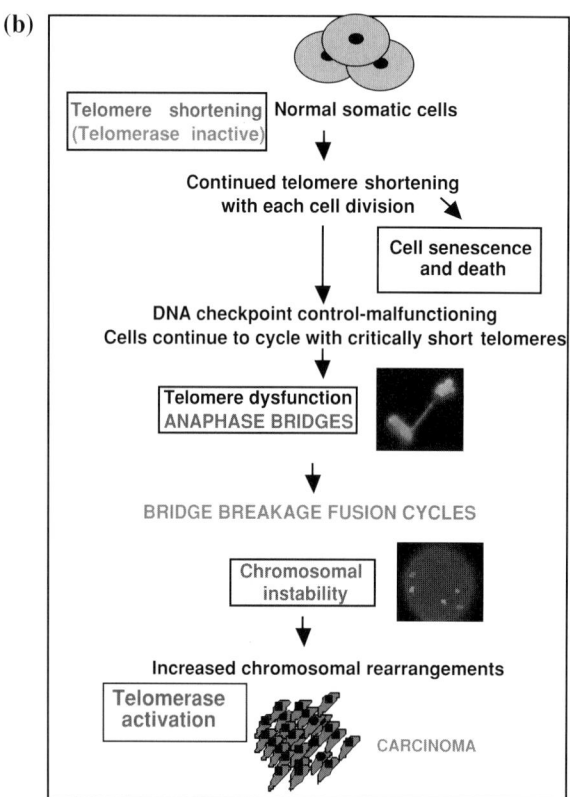

(b)

Telomere shortening (Telomerase inactive) — Normal somatic cells
↓
Continued telomere shortening with each cell division ↘ Cell senescence and death
↓
DNA checkpoint control-malfunctioning
Cells continue to cycle with critically short telomeres
↓
Telomere dysfunction
ANAPHASE BRIDGES
↓
BRIDGE BREAKAGE FUSION CYCLES
↓
Chromosomal instability
↓
Increased chromosomal rearrangements
Telomerase activation
CARCINOMA

Fig 24.1 Proposed pathway of genomic instability leading to UC dyplasia and cancer.

and who require more frequent surveillance, from the majority who will not.

Biomarkers for UC neoplasia could be developed from serum or colonic tissue. A serum biomarker, however, is unlikely to detect dysplasia. Dysplastic epithelial by-products are less likely to present in the blood, yielding fewer or no targets for biomarkers. Therefore, the ideal biomarker would be one that could be detected in colonic tissues, preferably in 1–2 biopsies that are easily obtained (e.g.

rectal biopsies) in an un-prepared colon. The sensitivity and positive predictive value should approach 100%. It is thought that by correlating gene expression profiles in IBD, it might be possible to identify new candidate molecular target genes for IBD therapy and drug discovery [7]. In this chapter we will describe the current knowledge of the different identified markers of dysplasia in UC.

Molecular genetic events in UC tumourigenesis

Although UC-associated cancer and sporadic cancer share several molecular alterations, the frequency and the timing of molecular changes have been shown to differ [8]. The progression of dysplasia to carcinoma in UC are accompanied by mutations in the APC, p53 and K-ras genes [9]. Loss of APC function is a frequent and early event in sporadic colon cancer [10], whereas loss or mutations of APC are infrequent and occur much later in UC in the transition between high grade dysplasia and cancer [11]. Alterations of the β-catenin pathway are important in both UC-related and sporadic colorectal cancers. However, differences in the expression patterns of β-catenin, E-cadherin and APC between UC-related and sporadic colorectal cancers suggest that the specific alterations in this pathway may differ in these two cancer groups [12].

We and others have shown alterations and mutations in p53 during progression in UC [13-17]. Unlike sporadic CRC, p53 alterations occur as an early event in UC tumourigenesis – mutations are present in normal-appearing mucosa adjacent to cancer. One study revealed that the presence of p53 abnormalities increases the relative risk of developing dysplasia by 4.3; moreover, p53 changes preceded the presence of HGD and CRC by 26 and 38 months, respectively, and are associated with cancer-related mortality [18]. Recently, it has been suggested that serum p53 antibody assessment, an indirect marker for p53 gene mutations and abnormally high p53 protein levels, could have potential as a complementary test to improve surveillance programme performance [19].

Over-expression of zinc-binding proteins, metallothioneins, may lead to functional inactivation of the p53 tumour suppressor gene [20] and this is thought to be an independent cancer risk factor in UC. Development of colonic neoplasia in p53-deficient mice with experimental colitis has proven to be an excellent animal model of UC associated neoplasia because its morphological and molecular genetics are similar to those in UCassociated neoplasia in humans [21], further reinforcing the importance of p53 in UC neoplastic progression.

Mutations of the proto-oncogene K-ras that are very common in sporadic CRC, are relatively uncommon in UC neoplasia, and their involvement is thought to be relatively insignificant [10]. No relationship exists between micro-satellite instability (MSI) and K-ras mutations. K-ras mutations are found predominantly in neoplastic mucosa, whereas MSI is found predominantly in regenerative mucosa [22]. Of note, there is a different site distribution of K-ras mutations in UC carcinomas compared to sporadic carcinomas. The incidence of K-ras mutations in rectal carcinomas in UC (9%) is significantly different from levels seen in sporadic rectal carcinomas (72%) [23].

Previous investigations have shown that expression patterns of many cell cycle regulatory genes, like the cyclins may contribute to epithelial cellular turnover and may be implicated in IBD-related dysplasia-carcinoma [24-26]. It is suggested that apoptosis may occur less frequently in UC neoplasia compared to sporadic CRC. This may be due to the high level of instability present in the UC mucosa of Progressors (patients with dysplasia or cancer) – these cells may not die despite the mutational load. UC-associated carcinomas exhibit a lower apoptotic count than their sporadic invasive counterparts, possibly due to elevated levels of surviving expression and/or abnormal Bcl-2 expression [27, 28].

Others have identified abnormal expression of sialosyl-Tn [29], sphingomyelin [30] and Bcl-2 expression [28] in UC dysplasia and associated normal-appearing mucosa. Ki67 has also been assessed as a marker of cellular proliferation to evaluate dysplasia [31]. Restriction of Ki67 staining to the basal third of the crypt appears to exclude a diagnosis of dysplasia, whereas strong intensity p53 staining suggests a diagnosis of dysplasia.

As UC is associated with chronic inflammation, oxidative stress may contribute to the mutator phenotype seen with UC disease progression. It has been shown that oxidative stress can interfere with the normal functioning of mismatch repair enzymes, contributing to MSI [32]. Inflammation associated genes like cycloxygenase-2 are also over-expressed in early stages of UC-associated neoplasia [33, 34]. It remains unknown whether this inflammation is actually causative in the accumulation of the molecular changes.

UC patients with dysplasia/cancer demonstrate global DNA abnormalities in the normal-appearing mucosa adjacent to the cancer, although most UC patients who are dysplasia-free do not have these changes. DNA abnormalities can take the form of chromosomal instability and/or micro-satellite instability. Abnormal epithelial DNA content (aneuploidy) in colonic biopsy specimens from UC patients who are indefinite or negative for dysplasia correlates with future progression to dysplasia [6]. Failure of spindle check-points caused by mutation of the responsible genes may be an important factor for development of aneuploidy [35]. In addition, breakage of chromosomes can occur during anaphase (see anaphase bridges and bridge breakage fusion cycles below) leading to aneuploidy. In UC, aneuploid DNA content is more common than loss of heterozygosity (LOH) where a region of chromosome is deleted, resulting in only one copy remaining. In UC, p53 LOH have been deleted in regions with negative, indefinite or low-grade dysplastic histology [13], suggesting that aneuploidy precedes both p53 LOF and epithelial dysplasia [13]. Another form of genomic instability, micro-satellite instability (MSI), is also common in UC and is present at early stages of neoplastic progression, within mucosa that has no histological evidence of neoplastic change [36, 37]. This MSI may reflect the inability of DNA repair mechanisms to compensate for the stress of chronic inflammation, and may be one mechanism for the heightened neoplastic risk in UC.

Chromosomal instability

Key chromosomes become damaged or unstable during UC tumourigenesis and these unstable chromosomes are pivotal in contributing to the development and progression of tumourigenesis in UC [38, 39]. Using dual colour fluorescence *in situ* hybridisation (FISH) with centromere probes and locus-specific arm probes for chromosome 8, 11, 17 and 18, we have shown that UC non-dysplastic mucosa reveals widespread chromosomal instability (CIN) up to 20–30 cm away from the site of dysplasia or more [39, 40]. The degree of instability in *non-dysplastic* tissue is similar to that of *dysplastic/cancerous* mucosa from the same patient, suggesting that this instability is widespread and reaches the maximum level early in neoplastic progression. In rectal biopsies that were negative for dysplasia, abnormalities in chromosomal arms, especially losses, were most common, whereas centromere gains were most common in dysplasia and cancer. The frequency and type of abnormalities varied between the chromosomes examined; chromosome 8 was the least affected, and 17p loss was found to be an early and frequent event [39]. Other studies have shown that changes in chromosome 17 and p53 copy number directly correlate with CRC risk factors [41]. The DPC4 gene located on the long arm of chromosome 18q21.1 has also been shown to be a target of 18qLOH events in colitis-associated neoplasia [42]. This raises the possibility that a screen for CIN might detect the subset of UC patients who are at greatest risk for development of dysplasia and cancer.

If dysplasia could be predicted in advance of its occurrence, the subset of patients who warrant careful colonoscopic surveillance with biopsies can be selected out from the majority of UC patients who will not develop dysplasia. The question remains how accurate is chromosomal FISH in distinguishing UC Progressors from UC non-Progressors. By using a combination of these chromosomes listed, we have achieved a very high sensitivity and specificity – 94 and 92%, respectively (unpublished data). In addition, we have assessed the used entropy as the measure of aberration rather than just per cent of cells showing aberrations. Entropy is a measure of how 'diverse' the FISH aberrations are among the various possible categories of deviation from the expected count of 2 arm probes per cell. The additive total entropy, using one FISH arm probe per each of the four chromosomes, provides 100% sensitivity and 92% specificity for distinguishing Progressors from non-Progressors in a data set of 26 patients (unpublished data). Of great importance is the fact that this discrimination was made using *only* 1–2 *non-dysplastic* biopsies per patient and inter- and intra-biopsy variability is low (<10%). These instability markers are particularly promising because they are highly sensitive, pan-colonic and are detected in histologically negative rectal biopsies from UC patients with cancer/dysplasia elsewhere in the colon.

Anaphase bridges

A possible cause and indicator of chromosomal instability is the formation of anaphase bridges. These are chromosomes pulled simultaneously to both poles of the micro-tubule spindle during chromosome segregation [43]. When telomeres shorten, the ends of the chromosomes become sticky and the chromosome ends fuse together, altering cytokinesis. These bridges can break under stress from the mitotic apparatus and reform in the next interphase, giving rise to bridge-breakage-fusion (BBF) cycles, known to contribute to chromosomal instability [40, 44, 45]. The aberrant morphology of cells in mitosis leads to changes in metaphase spindles exerting different influences on the final alignment of chromosomes. The correlation between increased numbers of anaphase bridges during tumourigenesis may be due to genetic loss of a particular tumour suppressor and oncogenes. It has been suggested that anaphase bridges may be a new diagnostic tool to distinguish between chromosomally stable and unstable tumours [46], emphasising the importance these mitotic defects may have in predicting UC-associated cancers. We have developed methods for quantifying the anaphase bridges (Fig 24.2c) in UC tissue and demonstrated increasing occurrence of anaphase bridges in normal-appearing mucosa from UC patients with dysplasia elsewhere in their colon (Progressors) and less common in UC patients who are dysplasia-free (non-Progressors) [40].

Telomeres and telomerase

We and others hypothesise that telomere dysfunction and its associated bridge-breakage-fusion cycles may drive chromosomal instability [40, 47–49].

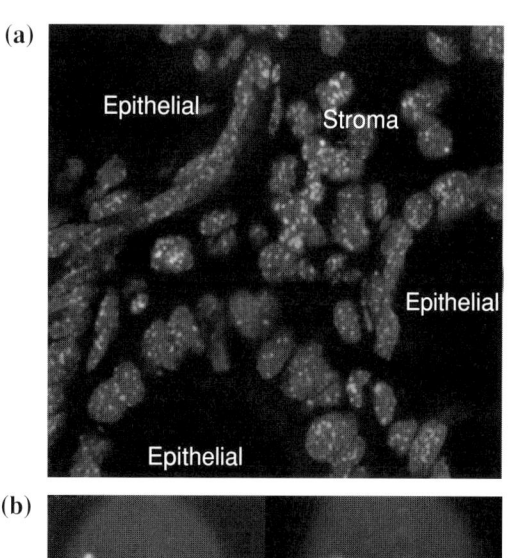

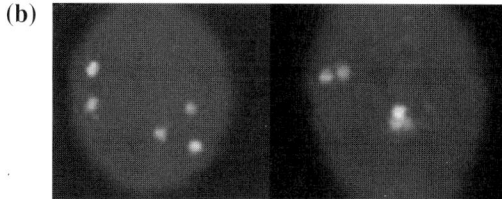

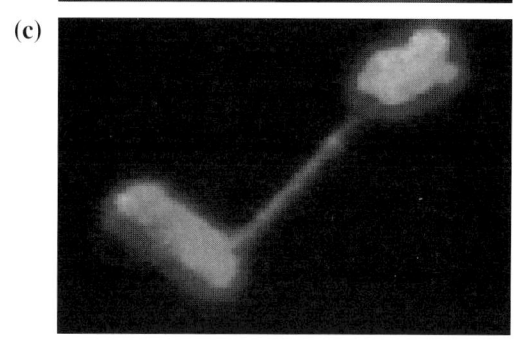

Fig 24.2 (a) Telomere length assay: telomeres (white spots) are present in the stroma, but markedly decreased in the epthalial cells of UC Progressors (b) 17p FISH: the left cell (blue) from a negative rectal biospy from a UC Progessor is abnormal: it shows 3 centrometers (red spots) and 2 chromosomal arms (green dots) (c) Anaphase bridges from a negative biospy of a UC Progessor.

This leads to the accumulation of multiple genetic aberrations needed to form a malignancy and an unstable genome (Fig 24.1b). Telomeres are repetitive DNA sequences (TTAGGG) found at the end of every chromosome [50] that protect the chromosome tips, rather like the glue that prevents the end of shoe-laces from unravelling. Telomere shortening occurs with each round of cell division, ultimately leading to critically short telomeres. These chromosome ends become sticky and, as noted above, the ends can fuse together forming chromosomal bridges. During this time of genetic cell derangement, an enzyme telomerase can be re-activated to *'rescue'* short telomeres; this in turn can allow cancer cells to divide indefinitely. Therefore, telomere shortening acts as a trigger for cells to either senesce, die or up-regulate telomerase and progress into tumour cells. It is widely accepted that one of the most important factors required for indefinite tumour growth is the activation of telomerase [51]. This enzyme is only found in cancer cells and not in most normal dividing cells. This has lead to two hypotheses; telomerase activity is necessary for the proliferation of cancer cells and telomerase inhibitors may be a powerful strategy for cancer therapeutics, acting as a brake on cancer cell growth.

We have demonstrated using *in-situ* histological evaluation of telomere length that telomeres are considerably shorter in the colonocytes of these UC Progressors compared to those of UC non-Progressors [40]. The *in-situ* analysis allows us to assess and control for the admixture of epithelial and non-epithelial cells in the colon. Stromal cells are used as an internal control because they have normal telomere length; we have verified that telomere length shortening is not evident in these cells [40], presumably due to the expression of telomerase in stromal lymphocytes and much slower proliferative rates relative to epithelial cells. Fig 24.2a is a representative image of telomere shortening in a UC biopsy. Images are analysed using a macro developed with Optimas image analysis software (Media Cybernetics, Silver Spring, MD) and image analysis algorithms are used to quantify telomere length measurements [52]. This process of telomere attrition may be accelerated because of the presence of chronic inflammation in UC, which is associated with rapid cell turnover [53], and oxidative injury [54]. Both of these factors are known to accelerate telomere shortening.

We hypothesise that shortened telomeres can elevate the frequency of end-to-end chromosome fusion and result in bridge-breakage-fusion cycles in UC. We have shown that shortened telomere length is directly associated with chromosomal instability in UC [40] using fluorescence *in situ* hybridisation (FISH) (Fig 24.2b). Our finding of high rates of 17p arm loss is consistent with this mechanism, as chromosome 17 has been reported to have the shortest telomeres of any human chromosome [55]. Our unpublished data using BAC array chips reveals statistically significant hot spots on chromosome 5p, 10q, 18q and Xq, each seen as a copy number loss in the UC Progressor negative biopsies, but not in UC non-Progressors biopsies. The regions of these lost BACs are all sub-telomeric in location (at the tip of the chromosome). We speculate that these are the types of losses one would predict with telomere attrition or a bridge-breakage-fusion mechanism associated with shortened telomeres in UC. This evidence provides a mechanism of how these events induce the mutator phenotype that predisposes to loss of tumour suppressor genes and evolution of cancer.

Biomarker performance

The management of UC is challenging but better knowledge of an individual patient's cancer risk in UC would profoundly affect their clinical management. Cancer surveillance in UC is limited by the need to detect small foci of dysplasia – foci that can be endoscopically invisible. There is an urgent need for newer molecular markers to complement the histologic analysis of dysplasia. We need to be able to obtain exceptionally high sensitivity so that a patient with dysplasia or cancer is never missed using a particular bio-marker panel. Despite the overwhelming evidence of molecular markers of dysplasia in UC, many of these are *not colon wide* and/or *not sensitive* enough for regular use as an ideal bio-marker in the clinical setting. To be able to validate a true marker of 'risk' for UC patients, bio-marker data must be extrapolated in a longitudinal manner. To date, this has not been performed and these data are lacking in the field of IBD research. In addition, candidate bio-markers will need to be tested against the best gold standard of care – UC patients undergo colonoscopic surveillance with extensive biopsy procurement to confidently detect dysplasia if it is present. If too few biopsies are obtained when performing a bio-marker clinical trial, then dysplasia could be missed and the bio-marker specificity would be falsely lowered.

It is important to understand the molecular mechanism of genomic instability in UC, as this process is one of the main reasons for cancer therapeutic failures and acquired resistance in cancer therapy. The molecular targeting of pathways responsible for genomic instability, or the selective killing of cells with chromosomal instability, would have a great impact in the clinical management of UC patients. The question remains: what degree of sensitivity and specificity do we need to validate a prognostic marker for UC and be incorporated into surveillance examinations?

We hypothesised that genomic instability underlies cancer formation in UC and that it can distinguish those UC patients with dysplasia or cancer from those who do not have dysplasia. We have exciting preliminary data that suggests that this hypothesis is true. Chromosomal arm loss combining FISH data from all four chromosomes tested showed sensitivity and specificity of (1.00, 0.92) by ROC analysis for distinguishing UC non-Progressors from UC Progressors (unpublished data). Sensitivity and specificity achieved by telomere length and anaphase bridge measures is less, but by adding a combination of telomere length and anaphase bridge assessment to the FISH, the combined bio-markers may be more robust in future samples. As previously discussed, many markers such as aneuploidy, p53 and mucin-associated sialyl-Tn antigen expression also hold promise and have been shown to precede the detection of dysplasia [56]. The successful and efficient clinical validation of such highly promising molecular markers may best be accomplished through the inter-disciplinary collaboration among UC researchers. Finally, molecular diagnostics of dysplasia could change the face of clinical care for UC patients and their providers and save substantial health care dollars. In the future, chemopreventive measures could be undertaken, perhaps even tailored, to rectify the underlying abnormal genetic events.

References

1. Rutter MD, Saunders BP, Wilkinson KH, Rumbles S, Schofield G, Kamm MA, Williams CB, Price AB, Talbot IC, Forbes A. Cancer surveillance in longstanding ulcerative colitis: endoscopic appearances help predict cancer risk. *Gut* 2004;53(12):1813–6.
2. Broome U, Lindberg G, Lofberg R. Primary sclerosing cholangitis in ulcerative colitis – a risk factor for the development of dysplasia and DNA aneuploidy? *Gastroenterology* 1992;102(6):1877–80.
3. Marchesa P, Lashner BA, Lavery IC, Milsom J, Hull TL, Strong SA, Church JM, Navarro G, Fazio VW. The risk of cancer and dysplasia among ulcerative colitis patients with primary sclerosing cholangitis. *Am J Gastroenterol* 1997;92(8):1285–8.
4. Helper DJ. PSC in UC: is it or is it not a risk factor for the development of neoplasia? *Inflamm Bowel Dis* 2000;6(1):61–2.
5. Brentnall TA, Haggitt RC, Rabinovitch PS, Kimmey MB, Bronner MP, Levine DS, Kowdley KV, Stevens AC, Crispin DA, Emond M, Rubin CE. Risk and natural history of colonic neoplasia in patients with primary sclerosing cholangitis and ulcerative colitis. *Gastroenterology* 1996;110(2):331–8.
6. Rubin CE, Haggitt RC, Burmer GC, Brentnall TA, Stevens AC, Levine DS, Dean PJ, Kimmey M, Perera DR, Rabinovitch PS. DNA aneuploidy in colonic biopsies predicts future development of dysplasia in ulcerative colitis. *Gastroenterology* 1992;103:1611–20.
7. Dooley TP, Curto EV, Reddy SP, Davis RL, Lambert GW, Wilborn TW, Elson CO. Regulation of gene expression in inflammatory bowel disease and correlation with IBD drugs: screening by DNA microarrays. *Inflamm Bowel Dis* 2004;10(1):1–14.
8. Itzkowitz S. Colon carcinogenesis in inflammatory bowel disease: applying molecular genetics to clinical practice. *J Clin Gastroenterol* 2003;36(5 Suppl):S70–4; discussion S94–6.
9. Kern SE, Redston M, Seymour AB, Caldas C, Powell SM, Kornacki S, Kinzler KW. Molecular genetic profiles of colitis-associated neoplasms. *Gastroenterology* 1994;107(2):420–8.
10. Umetani N, Sasaki S, Watanabe T, Shinozaki M, Matsuda K, Ishigami H, Ueda E, Muto T. Genetic alterations in ulcerative colitis-associated neoplasia focusing on APC, K-ras gene and microsatellite instability. *Jpn J Cancer Res* 1999;90(10):1081–7.
11. Aust DE, Terdiman JP, Willenbucher RF, Chang CG, Molinaro-Clark A, Baretton GB, Loehrs U, Waldman FM. The APC/beta-catenin pathway in ulcerative colitis-related colorectal carcinomas: a mutational analysis. *Cancer* 2002;94(5):1421–7.
12. Aust DE, Terdiman JP, Willenbucher RF, Chew K, Ferrell L, Florendo C, Molinaro-Clark A, Baretton GB, Lohrs U, Waldman FM. Altered distribution of beta-catenin, and its binding proteins E-cadherin and

APC, in ulcerative colitis-related colorectal cancers. *Mod Pathol* 2001;14(1):29–39.

13 Burmer GC, Rabinovitch PS, Haggitt RC, Crispin DA, Brentnall TA, Kolli VR, Stevens AC, Rubin CE. Neoplastic progression in ulcerative colitis: histology, DNA content, and loss of a p53 allele. *Gastroenterology* 1992;103:1602–10.

14 Harpaz N, Peck AL, Yin J, Fiel I, Hontanosas M, Tong TR, Laurin JN, Abraham JM, Greenwald BD, Meltzer SJ. p53 protein expression in ulcerative colitis-associated colorectal dysplasia and carcinoma. *Hum Pathol* 1994;25(10):1069–74.

15 Hussain SP, Amstad P, Raja K, Ambs S, Nagashima M, Bennett WP, Shields PG, Ham AJ, Swenberg JA, Marrogi AJ, Harris CC. Increased p53 mutation load in noncancerous colon tissue from ulcerative colitis: a cancer-prone chronic inflammatory disease. *Cancer Res* 2000;60(13):3333–7.

16 Fujii S, Fujimori T, Chiba T. Usefulness of analysis of p53 alteration and observation of surface microstructure for diagnosis of ulcerative colitis-associated colorectal neoplasia. *J Exp Clin Cancer Res* 2003;22(1):107–15.

17 Yoshida T, Mikami T, Mitomi H, Okayasu I. Diverse p53 alterations in ulcerative colitis-associated low-grade dysplasia: full-length gene sequencing in microdissected single crypts. *J Pathol* 2003;199(2):166–75.

18 Lashner BA, Shapiro BD, Husain A, Goldblum JR. Evaluation of the usefulness of testing for p53 mutations in colorectal cancer surveillance for ulcerative colitis. *Am J Gastroenterol* 1999;94(2):456–62.

19 Cioffi M, Riegler G, Vietri MT, Pilla P, Caserta L, Carratu R, Sica V, Molinari AM. Serum p53 antibodies in patients affected with ulcerative colitis. *Inflamm Bowel Dis* 2004;10(5):606–11.

20 Bruewer M, Schmid KW, Krieglstein CF, Senninger N, Schuermann G. Metallothionein: early marker in the carcinogenesis of ulcerative colitis-associated colorectal carcinoma. *World J Surg* 2002;26(6):726–31.

21 Fujii S, Fujimori T, Kawamata H, Takeda J, Kitajima K, Omotehara F, Kaihara T, Kusaka T, Ichikawa K, Ohkura Y, Ono Y, Imura J, Yamaoka S, Sakamoto C, Ueda Y, Chiba T. Development of colonic neoplasia in p53 deficient mice with experimental colitis induced by dextran sulphate sodium. *Gut* 2004;53(5):710–6.

22 Lyda MH, Noffsinger A, Belli J, Fenoglio-Preiser CM. Microsatellite instability and K-ras mutations in patients with ulcerative colitis. *Hum Pathol* 2000;31(6):665–71.

23 Bell SM, Kelly SA, Hoyle JA, Lewis FA, Taylor GR, Thompson H, Dixon MF, Quirke P. c-Ki-ras gene mutations in dysplasia and carcinomas complicating ulcerative colitis. *Br J Cancer* 1991;64(1):174–8.

24 Habermann J, Lenander C, Roblick UJ, Kruger S, Ludwig D, Alaiya A, Freitag S, Dumbgen L, Bruch HP, Stange E, Salo S, Tryggvason K, Auer G, Schimmelpenning H. Ulcerative colitis and colorectal carcinoma: DNA-profile, laminin-5 gamma2 chain and cyclin A expression as early markers for risk assessment. *Scand J Gastroenterol* 2001;36(7):751–8.

25 Wong NA, Mayer NJ, Anderson CE, McKenzie HC, Morris RG, Diebold J, Mayr D, Brock IW, Royds JA, Gilmour HM, Harrison DJ. Cyclin D1 and p21 in ulcerative colitis-related inflammation and epithelial neoplasia: a study of aberrant expression and underlying mechanisms. *Hum Pathol* 2003;34(6):580–8.

26 Ioachim EE, Katsanos KH, Michael MC, Tsianos EV, Agnantis NJ. Immunohistochemical expression of cyclin D1, cyclin E, p21/waf1 and p27/kip1 in inflammatory bowel disease: correlation with other cell-cycle-related proteins (Rb, p53, ki-67 and PCNA) and clinicopathological features. *Int J Colorectal Dis* 2004;19(4):325–33.

27 Mikami T, Yoshida T, Akino F, Motoori T, Yajima M, Okayasu I. Apoptosis regulation differs between ulcerative colitis-associated and sporadic colonic tumors. Association with survivin and bcl-2. *Am J Clin Pathol* 2003;119(5):723–30.

28 Itzkowitz SH, Marshall A, Kornbluth A, Harpaz N, McHugh JB, Ahnen D, Sachar DB. Sialosyl-Tn antigen: initial report of a new marker of malignant progression in long-standing ulcerative colitis. *Gastroenterology* 1995;109(2):490–7.

29 Sjoqvist U, Hertervig E, Nilsson A, Duan RD, Ost A, Tribukait B, Lofberg R. Chronic colitis is associated with a reduction of mucosal alkaline sphingomyelinase activity. *Inflamm Bowel Dis* 2002;8(4):258–63.

30 Bronner MP, Culin C, Reed JC, Furth EE. The bcl-2 proto-oncogene and the gastrointestinal epithelial tumor progression model. *Am J Pathol* 1995;146(1):20–6.

31 Andersen S, Rognum T, Bakka A, OP C. Ki-67: a useful marker for the evaluation of dysplasia in ulcerative colitis. *Mol Pathol* 1998;6:327–32.

32 Chang CL, Marra G, Chauhan DP, Ha HT, Chang DK, Ricciardiello L, Randolph A, Carethers JM, Boland CR. Oxidative stress inactivates the human DNA mismatch repair system. *Am J Physiol Cell Physiol* 2002;283(1):C148–54.

33 Agoff SN, Brentnall TA, Crispin DA, Taylor SL, Raaka S, Haggitt RC, Reed MW, Afonina IA, Rabinovitch PS, Stevens AC, Feng Z, Bronner MP. The role of cyclooxygenase 2 in ulcerative colitis-associated neoplasia. *Am J Pathol* 2000;157(3):737–45.

34. Olinski R, Gackowski D, Rozalski R, Foksinski M, Bialkowski K. Oxidative DNA damage in cancer patients: a cause or a consequence of the disease development? *Mutat Res* 2003;531(1–2):177–90.
35. Dey P. Aneuploidy and malignancy: an unsolved equation. *J Clin Pathol* 2004;57(12):1245–49.
36. Brentnall TA, Crispin DA, Bronner MP, Cherian SP, Hueffed M, Rabinovitch PS, Rubin CE, Haggitt RC, Boland CR. Microsatellite instability in nonneoplastic mucosa from patients with chronic ulcerative colitis. *Cancer Res* 1996;56(6):1237–40.
37. Ishitsuka T, Kashiwagi H, Konishi F. Microsatellite instability in inflamed and neoplastic epithelium in ulcerative colitis. *J Clin Pathol* 2001;54(7):526–32.
38. Willenbucher RF, Zelman SJ, Ferrell LD, Moore DHn, Waldman FM. Chromosomal alterations in ulcerative colitis-related neoplastic progression. *Gastroenterology* 1997;113:791–801.
39. Rabinovitch PS, Dziadon S, Brentnall TA, Emond MJ, Crispin DA, Haggitt RC, Bronner MP. Pancolonic chromosomal instability precedes dysplasia and cancer in ulcerative colitis. *Cancer Res* 1999;59(October 15):5148–53.
40. O'Sullivan JN, Bronner MP, Brentnall TA, Finley JC, Shen WT, Emerson S, Emond MJ, Gollahon KA, Moskovitz AH, Crispin DA, Potter JD, Rabinovitch PS. Chromosomal instability in ulcerative colitis is related to telomere shortening. *Nat Genet* 2002;32(2):280–4.
41. Rosman-Urbach M, Niv Y, Birk Y, Smirnoff P, Zusman I, Morgenstern S, Schwartz B. A high degree of aneuploidy, loss of p53 gene, and low soluble p53 protein serum levels are detected in ulcerative colitis patients. *Dis Colon Rectum* 2004;47(3):304–13.
42. Hoque AT, Hahn SA, Schutte M, Kern SE. DPC4 gene mutation in colitis associated neoplasia. *Gut* 1997;40(1):120–2.
43. Lundblad V. Genome instability: McClintock revisited. *Curr Biol* 2001;11(23):R957–60.
44. Fouladi B, Sabatier L, Miller D, Pottier G, Murnane JP. The relationship between spontaneous telomere loss and chromosomal instability in a human tumor cell line. *Neoplasia* 2000;2:540–54.
45. Artandi SE, Chang S, Lee SL, Alson S, Gottlieb GJ, Chin L, DePinho RA. Telomere dysfunction promotes non-reciprocal translocations and epithelial cancers in mice. *Nature* 2000;406(6796):641–5.
46. Saunders W. Bridging mitotic defects and clinical diagnoses. *Cancer Biol Ther* 2003;2(3):253–4.
47. Cottliar A, Fundia A, Boerr L, Sambuelli A, Negreira S, Gill A, Gomez JC, Chopita N, Bernedo A, Slavutsky I. High frequencies of telomeric associations, chromosome aberrations, and sister chromatid exchanges in ulcerative colitis. *Am J Gastroenterology* 2000;95(9):2301–7.
48. Gisselsson D, Pettersson L, Hoglund M, Heidenblad M, Gorunova L, Weigant J, Mertens F, Dal Cin P, Mitelman F, Mandahi N. Chromosomal breakage-fusion-bridge events cause genetic heterogenity. *Proc Acad Natl Acad Sci USA* 2000;97:5357–62.
49. Meeker AK, De Marzo AM. Recent advances in telomere biology: implications for human cancer. *Curr Opin Oncol* 2004;16(1):32–8.
50. Blackburn EH. Structure and function of telomeres. *Nature* 1991;350:569–73.
51. Meyerson M. Role of telomerase in normal and cancer cells. *J Clin Oncol* 2000;18(13):2626–34.
52. O'Sullivan J, Finley J, Risques R, Shen WT, Gollahon K, Moskovitz A, Gryaznov S, Harley C, RP. Telomere length assessment in tissue sections by quantitative FISH: image analysis algorithms. *Cytometry* 2004;58A(2):120–31.
53. Shinozaki M, Watanabe T, Kubota Y, Sawada T, Nagawa H, Muto T. High proliferative activity is associated with dysplasia in ulcerative colitis. *Dis Colon Rectum* 2000;43(10 Suppl):34–9.
54. von Zglinicki T. Oxidative stress shortens telomeres. *Trends Biochem Sci* 2002;27(7):339–44.
55. Martens UM, Zijlmans JM, Poon SS, Dragowska W, Yui J, Chavez EA, Ward RK, Lansdorp PM. Short telomeres on human chromosome 17p. *Nat Genet* 1998;18:76–80.
56. Lofberg R, Brostrom O, Karlen P, Ost A, Tribukait B. DNA aneuploidy in ulcerative colitis: reproducibility, topographic distribution, and relation to dysplasia. *Gastroenterology* 1992;102:1149–54.

25: Adenomas versus dysplasia associated lesion or mass – recognition and management

Maha Guindi and Robert H. Riddell

Classification and terminology

Dysplasia in inflammatory bowel disease (IBD) was defined in 1983 as an unequivocal neoplastic proliferation of the columnar epithelium. Dysplasia may not only be a marker or precursor for carcinoma, but may also itself be malignant and associated with direct invasion into underlying tissue [1, 2]. Although this works well for overt dysplasia in adenomas, and in other inflammatory diseases including colitis, when it is subtle it remains an individual interpretation as some epithelia that are clearly neoplastic (infiltrating) may have very little dysplasia to the point that in isolation it would be virtually impossible to predict the fact that it is neoplastic. This is not unique to colitis and the same holds for diffuse-type gastric carcinomas, and some tumours of the appendix and anal glands, as well as some squamous neoplasms with minimal nuclear changes. The theory of this definition is, therefore, not always as straightforward as the practice, although when originally used it was specifically intended to ensure that anything that could remotely be interpreted as reactive was not included under this rubric.

In the classification and grading system that was proposed for dysplasia in IBD in 1983, dysplasia was classified as being negative, indefinite or positive for dysplasia. If the epithelium was positive for dysplasia, it was further graded into lowgrade dysplasia (LGD) or high grade dysplasia (HGD) [1]. This was later modified to clarify the category of 'indefinite for dysplasia' [3, 4].

More recently, there have been classifications for dysplasia that have tried to be more universal in their international appeal and their applicability to the entire GI tract, as well as having clinical relevance. The Vienna classification falls under this rubric [5], and employs terminology of intra-epithelial neoplasia (NIN), which can be high grade (HGNIN) or low grade (LGNIN), and invasive or non-invasive. It also reintroduces the term 'in situ carcinoma' as a subgroup of HGNIN, acknowledging the growing evidence at the molecular level that this lesion (however defined) bears more similarity to invasive carcinoma than LGNIN. The term intra-epithelial neoplasia (IEN) as a synonym for dysplasia can also be used. The Vienna system also borrows the Japanese term 'suspicious for invasion' for those lesions where one is highly suspicious that a biopsy has really been taken from an invasive carcinoma, but the criteria for invasion are not unequivocally present. The Vienna classification is shown in Table 25.1. Interestingly the Vienna system is now used widely in Europe but less frequently in North America or Japan, although increasingly it is becoming the international gold standard for publication despite the fact that the actual criteria for the grades within this system have never been carefully defined morphologically.

Macroscopic/endoscopic appearance

Dysplasia in IBD may occur in flat mucosa or as a focal lesion. In 1959, Dawson first described polypoid lesions in ulcerative colitis (UC) patients in a retrospective study of carcinoma specimens [6]. Subsequent studies in UC patients described focal dysplastic lesions of variable appearances [7–11].

Table 25.1 Vienna classification of GI epithelial neoplasia.

Category 1	Negative for neoplasia/dysplasia
Category 2	Indefinite for neoplasia/dysplasia
Category 3	Non-invasive low-grade neoplasia (low grade adenoma/dysplasia)
Category 4	Non-invasive high-grade neoplasia
	4.1 High grade adenoma/dysplasia
	4.2 Non-invasive carcinoma (carcinoma *in situ*)*
	4.3 Suspicion of invasive carcinoma
Category 5	Invasive neoplasia
	5.1 Intra-mucosal carcinoma **
	5.2 Submucosal carcinoma or beyond

*Non-invasive indicates absence of evident invasion.
** Intra-mucosal indicates invasion into the lamina propria or muscularis mucosae.
From Schlemper RJ, Riddell RH, Kato Y et al. [5].

In 1981, Blackstone et al. [8] coined the term dysplasia associated lesion or mass (DALM). DALMs are grossly and endoscopically visible, usually elevated, dysplastic lesions that complicate chronic UC. Their gross appearance is heterogeneous in that they may endoscopically appear as plaques, irregular or broad-based masses, strictured lesions, polyps or nodules. Biopsies can only sample the superficial aspects of a DALM showing dysplasia only, even if a malignancy is already present. The underlying carcinoma is not accessible to the biopsy forceps, and cannot be definitively confirmed or excluded without resection.

A subset of DALMs assumes the shape of a discrete, isolated nodule or polyp. These lesions are adenoma-like in appearance (adenoma-like DALM {ALM}), such that it may be endoscopically and histologically impossible to distinguish adenomas in colitic mucosa from DALMs in some cases.

The main problem with DALMs is whether they are really part of a more widespread area of dysplasia that cannot be removed easily endoscopically, or whether they are more adenoma-like, well localised and therefore potentially removable endoscopically. It is the distinction of colitic lesions from sporadic adenomas arising in colitic mucosa that is clinically problematic, as the former cause concern as to whether they are really DALMs, in which case proctocolectomy (and possibly lymphadenectomy in the region of the DALM) should be carried out, or whether the lesion is amenable to local polypectomy.

The issue of the gross appearance of DALMs is further clouded by the increasing use of other techniques to identify areas of dysplasia and DALMs endoscopically. The reason for this search is that although in the original papers [13] dysplasia was widespread and involved the rectum, so that rectal

Problematic aspects of DALMS

The incidence of DALMs and the incidence of carcinoma in DALMs vary between studies (Table 25.2). This variation is likely to be related to the varying definition of DALMs in the different studies, the use of non-standardised criteria for dysplasia, heterogeneous gross appearance of DALMs, evaluation by biopsy as opposed to resection, and possibly, the variable endoscopic features and degree of sensitivity of endoscopic detection.

Table 25.2 Summary of DALM studies.

Series	Percentage (%) DALM	Percentage (%) DALM with cancer
Blackstone (1981) [8]	11	58
Butt (1983) [9]	29	83
Rosenstock (1985) [10]	5	38
Lennard-Jones (1990) [7]	1.5	83
Bernstein (1994) [12]	3.2	43

biopsies alone were thought to be capable of detecting dysplasia if it was present, there was huge selection bias in these patients as most presented clinically with either carcinoma (which could be multiple) or widespread dysplasia, and were therefore a very different subgroup of patients from those seen in clinical practice for surveillance today. Further, in patients undergoing surveillance it was soon appreciated that patients undergoing their first colonoscopy were at much higher risk for having dysplasia, DALMs or carcinoma than those that were past this stage and into regular surveillance colonoscopy. It is the latter group of patients that were problematic as dysplasia in this group was initially detected primarily by random biopsies, so that the likelihood of detecting dysplasia was a function of the number of biopsies taken. Rubin et al. [14] calculated that one would need about 33 biopsies to detect dysplasia with about 90% accuracy. However, simple mathematics in a colon 100 cm long and 10 cm in diameter (i.e. 1000 cm^2) would suggest that if a patch of dysplasia 2 cm in diameter is present (the area πr^2 being 3.142 cm^2), this would require 1000/3.14, or some 320 equally spaced biopsies to be sure of detecting it. This is clearly impractical so a search for better endoscopic markers of dysplasia was required to allow detection and biopsy of lesions that were thought to be dysplastic, or to have an increased risk of being dysplastic. Targeted biopsy of endoscopically visible lesions was much more likely to detect dysplasia provided they could be found. As these could also be dysplasia associated, the line between the DALMs originally described, which were usually overt endoscopically visible masses that gradually gave way to those that were increasingly plaque-like, villous or slightly raised or depressed areas of nodularity. This has led to several major areas of advance to detect these lesions including:

(a) *Chromoendoscopy.* The addition of dye-spray techniques such as methylene blue increased the visibility of subtle lesions that were detected endoscopically, allowing biopsy of such lesions. However, these were used largely to accentuate lesions seen on regular colonoscopy, although when used routinely to examine the entire large bowel it resulted in an increased rate of finding dysplastic lesions [15, 16]. In addition to indigo carmine [16], methylene blue in combination with magnification endoscopy significantly improved the detection of dysplasia, particularly flat lesions, thus allowing for targeted biopsies to be performed. Approximately two-thirds of the dysplastic lesions were identified only after the application of methylene blue [17].

(b) *Magnification endoscopy.* The introduction of the video endoscocope resulted in much better definition of colonoscopic lesions, and this has continued to improve with high resolution, and magnifying colonoscopes now allow recognition of individual crypt orifices [18]. Recently a new generation of high definition colonoscopes in which there is a high intensity chip capable of using all of the pixels of a high definition monitor has resulted in another leap in the quality of the images. Contrary to the previously held view that most dysplasia is endoscopically invisible [19–21] there is some recent evidence that suggests otherwise. In one retrospective study, almost 90% of patients with dysplastic lesions had developed a colonoscopically visible abnormality [22].

(c) *Recognition of pit patterns associated with dysplasia.* The use of high resolution colonoscopes and chromoendoscopy has led to the recognition of pit patterns that can be seen in patients with colitis, and it is clear that some of these are associated with a much greater likelihood of underlying IEN/NIN, and sometimes invasive, neoplasia. These have yet to be fully standardised and are currently descriptive in their terminology. The pit pattern schemes most commonly used are the ones modified by Kudo *et al.* [18] and Kudo [23]. Four of the six pit pattern types described correlate with dysplastic lesions. This does highlight the increasing use of targeted biopsies to detect colonoscopic abnormalities, and the change in the focus of detecting of DALMs as overt lesions to much more subtle lesions, the significance of which remains to be fully elucidated.

Adenomas, adenoma-like masses (ALMS) and DALMS

In the subsequent discussion, the term sporadic adenoma (SA) will be used in its conventional meaning (adenoma as seen in the general population, not related to colitis). DALMs will be used to refer to neoplastic masses of heterogeneous shapes, which may be part of a more widespread area of dysplasia, and are highly associated with the presence of invasive colorectal cancer. Adenoma-like mass (ALM) as used by Bernstein [24] will be used to refer to a subset of smaller and innocuous-looking lesions within the DALM spectrum that, in colitic mucosa, resemble the sporadic adenoma and as such, may be amenable to complete local excision endoscopically.

Although the prevalence of adenomatous/dysplastic polyps appear to be less prevalent in UC patients compared to non-IBD patients [25], there is a major morphological problem in distinguishing polypoid lesions that could well be simple sporadic adenomas developing in colitic mucosa (and sometimes proximal to the colonoscopic limit of disease) from those that are likely to be the result of, or whose growth has been potentiated by, the colitic process. Some have suggested that the architectural distortion typically seen in chronic colitis, when supplemented by dysplasia (IEN/NIN) represents true dysplastic lesions, whereas sporadic adenomas have a regular distribution of crypts [26]. Although this may be good when present, lesions that are otherwise indistinguishable from adenomas occur within colitic mucosa, often at a much younger age than seen in sporadic adenomas (although, increasingly, adenomas in young patients in the non-colitic population are being seen). In Stolte's series [26], 6% of lesions judged by the above criteria to be sporadic adenomas occurred in patients younger than 50 years. When there is no architectural distortion it can be very difficult or impossible to be sure whether these are just sporadic adenomas in patients with colitis, lesions that have been spawned largely as the result of the colitic process and are therefore colitis-associated tumours, or even part of DALMs or more widespread dysplasia. Bernstein has used the term adenoma-like lesions (ALMs) for these [24] – a term which we find quite useful in patient management. When an endoscopic lesion is found within colitic mucosa, the pathologist is often under pressure to distinguish between whether this lesion is an adenoma, in which case local polypectomy may well be adequate, or a DALM, in which case a proctocolectomy will be entertained. The fact that morphologically all of these lesions are dysplastic and there are no good criteria for making such a distinction (unless one uses the criterion of architectural distortion previously mentioned) is not generally appreciated. This is where the use of the term 'ALM' proves of value and allows for the institution of the management algorithm outlined subsequently. Thus, although the incidence of dysplastic polyps per patient year has been variously reported as 0.0046 lesions [25], 0.0023 in the surveillance programme of St. Mark's Hospital, London [27], and 0.0074 in a surveillance study from Stockholm [28], one is never quite sure which of these is being referred to in the older literature.

Distinction between DALMS, ALMS and sporadic adenomas

The tools available to the pathologist to attempt to distinguish these lesions from one another are histological examination, immunohistochemistry and molecular studies. Both immunohistochemistry and molecular studies aim to detect the molecular alterations present, which are presumably responsible for the evolution and development of the lesions. Logically, it is reasonable to expect that neoplasms arising as the result of the colitic process might arise on the basis of a different molecular mechanism, and therefore be distinguishable on this basis. Although there is some truth to this, overall it is also unreliable in any specific lesion and these findings are discussed subsequently (see p. 316).

Histological features

Histological examination of DALMs (and ALMs) reveals features similar to, and in many cases indistinguishable from, a sporadic adenoma, as all lesions are composed of dysplastic glands. Dysplasia (IEN/NIN) may be low grade (LGD, LGNIN) or high grade (HGD, HGNIN). It is generally not possible to distinguish between adenoma-like DALMs and sporadic adenomas on routine histopathological stains. Torres *et al.* [29] found that adenoma-like DALMs (ALMs) in chronic UC patients displayed an admixture of normal and dysplastic epithelium at the surface of the lesion, and a higher degree of lamina propria inflammation. Their chronic UC patients with adenoma-like DALMs (ALMs) had longer disease duration and more polyps with villous architecture. However, these features reflected trends and were far from specific, and so could not be used reliably in a given lesion (we have also found that these features can be seen in sporadic adenomas and in familial adenomatous polyposis). Features such as size, architectural type (tubular, villous or tubulovillous), degree of dysplasia, and nuclear chromatin pattern are not helpful in distinguishing sporadic adenomas from adenoma-like DALMs (ALMS).

Features suggested for distinction between sporadic adenomas and colitis-related dysplastic lesions by Stolte include minimal or absent architectural distortion, regular mucin vacuoles close to the surface, rod-shaped nuclei of regular size and chromatin, the presence of the proliferation zone in the luminal part of the mucosa, and sharp distinction of the dysplastic glands from adjacent normal mucosa in sporadic adenomas [26]. In contrast, in colitis-related dysplastic lesions, architectural distortion is present, the mucin vacuoles are variable in configuration and size and irregular in distribution, nuclei are variable in shape and size and oval to round, the proliferation zone is frequently located in the base of the mucosa and may involve its full thickness, and the dysplastic glands are not clearly demarcated from the surrounding mucosa. The case illustrated in Fig 25.1 demonstrates some of these features. In this study, the distinction between sporadic adenoma and a colitis-related dysplastic lesion was not feasible based on any one criterion, and were made using all the criteria as a whole. Even then, some lesions could not be definitively classified as one or the other.

Molecular features

None of the molecular or genetic alterations known at the present time can reliably distinguish adenoma-like DALM (ALM) from a sporadic adenoma in a given patient. Studies suggest that essentially UC-related colorectal carcinomas (CRCs) develop along a different molecular pathway from that for sporadic adenocarcinomas. The details of these studies are beyond the scope of this chapter, and have been reviewed elsewhere [30] (Table 25.3).

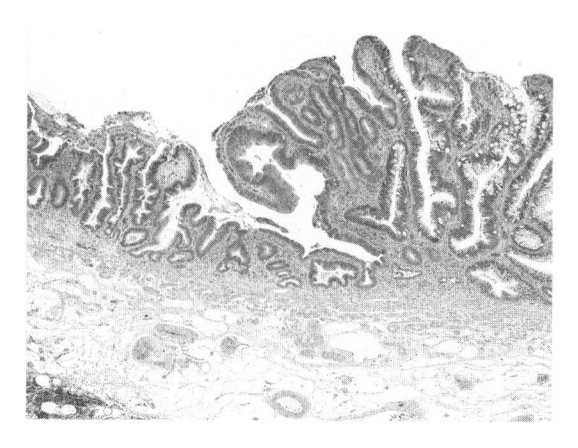

Fig 25.1 Non-adenoma-like DALM lesion. The dysplastic crypts that form the polypoid part of the lesion also show architectural distortion, especially crypt branching (dysplasia superimposed on features of chronic colitis). To the left, the dysplasia extends to involve the adjacent flat mucosa beyond the confines of the polypoid portion of the lesion (this feature is unlike adenoma).

In general, ALMs have genetic alterations similar to sporadic adenomas outside UC [32–34]. Odze et al. [33] showed that UC-associated non-adenoma-like DALMs contained a significantly higher proportion of cases with loss of heterozygosity (LOH) of 3p and p16 in comparison to both UC-associated ALMs and non-UC-related sporadic adenoma. LOH of APC occurred in a similar proportion of cases in all three groups (Table 25.4). The data suggested that there is a difference in frequency and possibly in timing of molecular alterations between UC-associated non-adenoma-like DALMs and UC-associated sporadic adenomas and ALMs.

There have been reports that *ras* proto-oncogene mutations are more common in sporadic adenomas than in DALMs [35]. ß-catenin expression has been reported to be more common in sporadic adenomas than in DALMs [36, 37]. p53 has been found to occur earlier in DALMs than in sporadic adenomas [36–39].

Although the findings of Walsh et al. [36] suggest that the combination of strong p53 expression and weak ß-catenin expression demonstrated

Table 25.3 Comparison of molecular alterations between UC-related and sporadic CRCs ectal.

Molecular aberration	UC-related CRC (%)	Sporadic CRC (%)
p-mutation/LOH*	70–80 (occur at earlier stage – during dysplasia)	70–80
APC mutation/LOH*	10–30	60–90
k-ras mutation	30	50–60
DCC mutation/LOH*	12	65
bcl2 up-regulation	22	50–60
Cyclin D1 over-expression	30	20–64
P21^{waf1} down-regulation	50	25–40
P27^{kip1} down-regulation	100	30
P16^{ink4a} hypermethylation	100	10
β-catenin dysregulation	45–50	70–90
E-cadherin down-regulation	43	30–40
E-cadherin hypermethylation (of gene promoter)	52	36
Significant microsatellite instability	2–9	10–15
MGMT** promoter methylation status	16.7	42.9

* Mutation and/or loss of heterozygosity (LOH).
** MGMT: O6- methylguanine-DNA methyltransferase.
Modified from Wong et al. [30], MGMT data from Matsumura et al. [31].

by immunoperoxidase staining is evidence in favour of ALM (referred to as 'polypoid dysplastic lesion' in this study), the findings lack sensitivity and specificity, limiting their usefulness (Table 25.5).

Further, others could not demonstrate differential ß-catenin and p53 staining between adenoma-like DALMs and sporadic adenoma. ß-catenin and p53, as well as p16 and cyclooxygenase-2 showed similar expression by immunostaining techniques in dysplastic polyps in UC and sporadic adenomas in non-IBD patients, and could not be used to distinguish between the two lesions [25].

Inconsistent terminology makes it difficult to interpret the results of some studies. For instance, in one study of three polymorphic markers that map to the short arm of chromosome 3p were assessed for LOH [34], the terms DALM, 'UC-adenomas lesions', and 'spontaneous adenomas' were used. It is likely that the term 'UC-adenoma' in this study refers to adenoma-like DALM and 'spontaneous adenoma' refers to sporadic adenoma in current terminology. The results of this study provide yet another example that genetic alterations cannot distinguish between adenoma-like DALM and sporadic adenoma.

In summary, none of the molecular or genetic alterations can discriminate definitively between adenoma-like DALM and sporadic adenoma in a given patient.

Molecular events in non-dysplastic mucosa

Early genomic alterations or instability in non-dysplastic-appearing mucosa has received attention in recent years as a tool for stratifying the risk for colorectal neoplasia in UC patients. It would be useful to find abnormalities in the background non-dysplastic mucosa that could predict subsequent development of any form of dysplasia (flat dysplasia, adenomas, ALMs and DALMs) which we propose to refer to collectively as colitis-associated neoplasia (CAN).

CpG island methylator phenotype (CIMP) is a distinct pathway of colorectal carcinogenesis [40]. The CIMP-positive colorectal cancers have a high degree of CpG island methylation of genes compared with normal mucosa. Aberrant methylation of CpG islands in the promoter region of tumour suppressor genes is associated with transcriptional inactivation of the genes and is thought to play

Table 25.4 Genetic alteration in sporadic adenoma, ALMs and DALMs in UC.

Molecular (LOH) marker	Non-CUC adenoma Odze[‡] 2000 [33]	Non-CUC adenoma Fogt[§] 1998 [32]	Non-CUC adenoma Fogt* 2000 [34]	UC adenoma-like DALM (ALM) Within colitis Odze[‡] 2000 [33]	Within colitis Fogt[§] 1998 [32]	Within colitis Fogt* 2000 [34]	Outside colitis Odze[‡] 2000 [33]	Outside colitis Fogt[§] 1998 [32]	Outside colitis Fogt* 2000 [34]	CUC Non-adenoma like DALM Odze[‡] 2000 [33]	Fogt[§] 1998 [32]	Fogt* 2000 [34]
3P	5%	0	5%	30%	Not done	15%	25%	Not done	none	50% (P 0.01)	50%	50%
APC	33%	40%		29%	Not done		38%	Not done		43%	46%	
P16	4%	0		0%	Not done		10%	Not done		56% (P 0.003)	35%	

[§] Fogt et al. 1998 [32] – in this series all ALMs were not evaluated.
* Fogt et al. 2000 [34] – in this series all UC associated ALMs were located within areas of chronic colitis.
[‡] Odze et al. 200c [33].

Table 25.5 p53 and ß-catenin in UC-associated polypoid dysplasia and sporadic adenomas [36].

	CUC-associated		Non-CUC-associated
	Percentage (%) staining positive		
Monoclonal antibody staining by immunoperoxidase technique	PDL (ALM)	SA	(Control) SA
p53	29	5	15
1 + (< 50% cells)	1	1	2
2 + (≥ 50% cells)	4	0	0
ß-catenin	8	40	46
1 + (< 50% cells)	1	6	0
2 + (≥ 50% cells)	0	2	0

an important role in carcinogenesis [41, 42]. The CIMP phenotype is also observed in large colorectal adenomas removed with colorectal cancer [43]. In adenomas unassociated with cancer, CpG island methylation is more common in adenomas with tubulovillous/villous histology, a characteristic associated with more frequent predisposition to invasive carcinoma [44].

There are data to suggest that methylation of several gene-associated CpG islands is substantially higher in dysplastic colorectal epithelium from UC patients when compared with epithelium from UC patients without dysplasia, and non-UC control patients [45]. Importantly, methylation abnormalities are not limited to the neoplastic mucosa but are also present in the non-dysplastic-appearing mucosa of UC patients with HGD/cancer. These findings suggest that the increased levels of methylation are widespread and occur early in the process of tumour development. In UC patients with dysplasia/cancer, hypermethylation appears to be limited to genes that are associated with age-related methylation, but is not present in the genes associated with cancer-related methylation [45].

The finding of widespread methylation abnormalities in non-dysplastic mucosa in patients with HGD could have several implications. It might be used as a tool to predict the development of CAN. Given that dysplasia surveillance can be fraught with sampling error that may only be reduced by exhaustive and time consuming-sampling of the colorectal mucosa (discussed above), a role for testing of easily accessible rectal biopsies for age-related methylation abnormalities can be proposed. If present, they may serve to flag higher risk UC patients, more prone to dysplasia, as requiring extensive mucosal sampling at surveillance. Furthermore, when this genetic background is associated with an ALM, it could help deem it as a colitis-related lesion not a sporadic adenoma especially in the younger patient, serve as a biomarker of mucosal genetic instability, and possibly sway the management decision towards colectomy rather than local excision.

Telomeres are tandem repeated DNA sequences at the ends of every chromosome, which prevent chromosome fusion and instability. Telomere shortening can promote the repeated breakage and fusion of the chromosomes with each cell cycle and result in chromosomal instability [46, 47]. Chromosomal losses have been shown to be greater and telomeres shorter in non-dysplastic biopsy samples from UC patients with cancer or dysplasia (UC progressors) than in those from UC non-progressors (without cancer or dysplasia) or control individuals without ulcerative colitis [48]. There is recent evidence that telomere shortening may be useful in improving the sensitivity and specificity of current dysplasia surveillance in UC patients [49]. The detection of loss of heterozygosity at four sites in the non-dysplastic background mucosa accurately predicted subsequent neoplasia in all 15 patients with cancer.

Telomere shortening may be used to predict dysplasia, guide dysplasia surveillance and the management of ALM lesions in a manner analogous to that proposed for DNA methylation (see above). Telomerase shortening can be evaluated using the quantitative fluorescence *in-situ* hybridisation technique in tissue sections using a few biopsies [48, 50], which makes clinical application quite feasible.

Management

Colectomy has been the practice for the management of DALM for many years [8, 51, 52]. Historically, DALM has been associated with carcinoma in a substantial proportion of patients. Carcinoma was found in 58% of UC patients with DALM at the time of colonic resection in the series of Blackstone *et al.* [8]. Bernstein *et al.* found synchronous carcinoma occurred with a frequency of 19% in patients with flat or polypoid low-grade dysplasia [12]. Given the strong association with cancer, colectomy became the standard of therapy when a DALM was present.

However, colitis-associated neoplasms (adenomas, adenoma-like masses (ALMS) and DALMS) occur in a variety of gross configurations. Adenoma-like DALMs (ALMS) have the appearance of sessile or pedunculated polyps that are well delineated and resemble adenomas in non-colitis. Other DALMs that are not adenoma-like may be broad-based, plaque-like, stricturing, nodular or irregular lesions [8–9, 19] and very subtle lesions are increasingly recognisable colonoscopically as indicated in the previous section.

The earlier reports did not stratify the lesions according to their gross appearance or shape. Blackstone's series [8] had referral bias, so that the percentage of DALMs harbouring carcinomas (58%) in that series is artificially high [29]. It appears that the risk of malignancy correlates with the gross configuration of DALMs.

The findings of two retrospective studies of IBD patients with ALMs identified by, and differentiated from, DALMs by strict endoscopic criteria appear to indicate that ALMs are the ones less likely to harbour a carcinoma.

When ALMs occur within colitic or non-colitic mucosa and there is no synchronous dysplasia in flat mucosa, there is evidence that it is safe to simply perform polypectomy and further endoscopic surveillance [53, 54]. The caveat is that:
(a) the lesion has been completely removed endoscopically; by examination of a stalk if present, or by taking multiple biopsies around the base of the lesion to ensure that dysplastic mucosa has not extended into the adjacent mucosa, when polypectomy would not be curative;
(b) dysplasia should not be demonstrable elsewhere in the large bowel, as this would be an indication for colectomy rather than polypectomy;
(c) ideally the patient should be in the adenoma-bearing age range (>40 years of age).

The length of follow-up evaluation in the previous studies averaged only 42 months [53] and 49 months [54]. During a follow up period of just over 3 years, 58% of the UC patients with adenoma-like DALMs in Engelsgjerd's series [53] developed further adenomas, one patient developed a single focus of LGD and none developed adenocarcinoma.

The significance of the findings of these two series was hampered by the relatively short period of follow up. There are now long-term follow-up data in patients previously reported by Odze *et al.* [55]. UC patients with adenoma-like DALMs treated by polypectomy continued endoscopic surveillance along with reference population of non-colitic patients with sporadic adenomas for a median of 78.1 and 60.4 months respectively. The results are summarised in Table 25.6. 58.8% of UC patients developed at least one further adenoma-like DALM on follow-up evaluation.

One patient had flat low-grade dysplasia present in the colon, which was resected within 6 months of the initial polypectomy, and another patient developed adenocarcinoma 7.5 years after her initial polypectomy. This tumour was not felt to be related to this patient's previous adenoma-like DALM. This patient also had PSC, which is a strong risk factor for the development of adenocarcinoma in UC [56]. There was no significant difference in the incidence of polyp formation on follow-up between UC patients with adenoma-like DALMs, UC patients with dysplastic polyps arising in noncolitic mucosa or in the reference population of non-UC patients. Odze *et al.* concluded that UC patients who develop an adenoma-like DALM may be treated adequately by polypectomy with complete excision and continued endoscopic surveillance.

Management of ALMs, DALMs and adenomas in colitics begins with proper and standardised

Table 25.6 Follow up results after polypectomy for ALMs Odze et al. [55].

Features	UC patient groups Adenoma-like DALM (ALM)	Sporadic adenoma	Non-UC patients Sporadic adenoma
No. of patients	24	10	49
Mean follow-up (months)	82.1	71.8	60.4
Patients developing additional polyps	15 (62.5%)	5 (50%)	24 (49%)
Patients developing flat dysplasia	1 (4%)	0%	0%
Patients developing adenocarcinoma	1 (4%)	0%	0%

dysplasia surveillance. The recommended protocol includes biopsies (3–4 biopsies every 10 cm of the colon) beginning at the caecum. Although it is not unusual to have far fewer biopsies than this, it has to be appreciated that this is a sub-optimal series of biopsies as previously discussed [14]. This also shows the futility of repeating the colonoscopy to try to 'find' the area of dysplasia again – especially if chromoendoscopy is not used to make it easier.

The procedure report should specify the number and locations of biopsies from flat mucosa and the location and endoscopic appearance of any mass or suspicious polypoid lesions that were biopsied or removed (obvious inflammatory {pseudo} polyps need not be biopsied or removed). If there is an adenoma-like polypoid lesion, biopsy or excision of the lesion and then biopsy of the adjacent flat mucosa around it is useful for separating sporadic adenomas from DALMs. Biopsies from the adjacent flat mucosa should be submitted separately to determine if the dysplasia is limited to the polypoid lesion or whether it spills onto the adjacent flat mucosa. If there are abundant inflammatory polyps, a few should be sampled to ensure that these are not dysplastic.

In IBD, designation of a resected dysplastic polypoid lesion as a sporadic adenoma or a DALM should involve consideration of both pathological and clinical factors. Communication between the colonoscopist and pathologist to reach a confident decision regarding DALM versus sporadic adenoma using the criteria enumerated previously is integral to the diagnostic process. If an ALM lesion is completely removed by local endoscopic excision, without dysplasia in the adjacent mucosa or elsewhere in the colon, and the patient is in the adenoma-bearing age, local excision would be adequate. If the lesion does not fulfil the criteria described above (incomplete excision, dysplasia/IEN around polyp or in colorectal mucosa elsewhere) the patient needs either more complete excision of the lesion, or colectomy. However, some endoscopic lesions are irregular and under these circumstances, despite the lack of a diagnosis of infiltrating carcinoma, these patients should be offered total proctocolectomy.

Although prospective studies with longitudinal follow-up are emerging with regard to outcome of conservative treatment of ALMs, there continues to be several outstanding issues. The endoscopic criteria for identifying adenoma-like DALMs, such that they are treated conservatively, are very specifically selected by the authors of the studies that have looked at conservative management of these lesions [53–55]. External validation outside of these referral centres is needed to establish whether other endoscopists are able to apply these criteria with similar reproducibility to identify adenoma-like DALMs endoscopically. The significance of finding HGD in a locally excised adenoma-like DALMs is not clear. A minority of patients in each of the two previous studies by Engelsgjerd et al. [53] and Rubin et al. [54] had HGD in the adenoma-like DALMs (ALMs) removed at the beginning of the studies. A minority of the adenoma-like DALMs (ALMs) found during continued surveillance also exhibited HGD. It is not clear whether the adenoma-like DALMs (ALMs) with HGD found during surveillance occurred in the same patients that had HGD in their locally excised adenoma-like DALMs (ALMs) at the start, or in the patients who developed new adenoma-like DALMs (ALMs) with any grade of dysplasia during the follow-up period. It has been argued that if a presumed adenoma-like DALM (ALM) is removed by polypectomy and found histologically to contain HGD or carcinoma, then colectomy should be performed [57]. Sinicrope and Wang [57] point out that in the recent study by Odze et al. [55], although follow up post-polypectomy for adenoma-like DALM (ALM) was relatively long, the median duration of UC was 9.2 years, which is relatively brief, given that disease duration is the strongest risk factor for development of dysplasia and carcinoma. In the study by Rubin et al. [54], follow-up of UC patients with polypectomy for adenoma-like DALM (ALM) was relatively short, but the average duration of UC was 25.4 years. There are yet no data available as to the outcome of conservative treatment of adenoma-like DALMs in patients with longstanding UC with long follow-up post-polypectomy. Preserving the colon in UC patients for longer periods through conservative treatment of adenoma-like DALMs prolongs duration of disease and may increase the risk for development of dysplasia in flat mucosa and carcinoma, and may lead to some missed cancers.

Colectomy is recommended for all flat dysplasia once the diagnosis is confirmed. Most clinicians recommend colectomy for HGD [58, 59]. However, some still recommend continued surveillance for patients with LGD in flat mucosa [60]. There are several studies that advocate that patients with LGD proceed to colectomy [12, 61, 62]. Ullman and co-workers found that in UC patients, the overall rate of progression of flat LGD to advanced neoplasia was 30% [62]. Of UC patients with flat LGD who did not undergo immediate colectomy, 50% developed HGD, a raised dysplastic lesion or adenocarcinoma in 32 months. The main caveat regarding colectomy for UC with LGD is the poor interobservation in the histological diagnosis of LGD [63].

Adenomas proximal to the upper limit of active disease are not considered to be in colitic mucosa and therefore are treated simply as sporadic adenomas. The caveat is that this is sometimes a problem because mucosa that has been involved previously can return to normal histologically [64] so that it may be impossible to be completely confident that the mucosa has never been involved, and any clinical evidence suggesting that any prior flare was extensive needs to be taken seriously.

Summary

The term 'DALM' was originally coined to draw attention to the possibility that endoscopic lesions that on biopsy showed no indication of invasion could indeed harbour invasive carcinoma (sometimes advanced pathologically). These lesions were usually identified on the initial index colonoscopy rather than subsequent surveillance colonoscopy. Since then it has been increasingly apparent that some endoscopic lesions are virtually indistinguishable from sporadic adenomas, causing clinical confusion about whether these can be handled be simple polypectomy or really do have a high risk of invasion either in the lesion itself or in the remaining colitic mucosa. Such lesions have been called adenoma-like lesions (ALMs). It is increasingly apparent that these lesions can be excised locally provided that local excision can be shown to be complete (stalk free, no dysplasia around the base of the lesion) and that there is no evidence of dysplasia elsewhere in the large bowel when a full surveillance series of biopsies have been examined. The development of new generations of colonoscopes including magnification, high resolution and high definition, usually with chromoendoscopy, allows identification of very subtle dysplastic lesions that might allow targeted biopsies to be taken.

References

1 Riddell RH, Goldman H, Ransohoff DF, et al. Dysplasia in inflammatory bowel disease: standardised classification with provisional clinical applications. *Hum Pathol* 1983;14:931–68.
2 Goldman H. Significance and detection of dysplasia in chronic colitis. *Cancer* 1996;78(11):2261–3.
3 Riddell RH. Premalignant and early malignant lesions of the gastrointestinal tract: definitions, terminology, and problems. *AJG* 1996;91:864–72.

4. Lewin KJ, Riddell RH, Weinstein WM. Inflammatory bowel disease. In: *Gastrointestinal Pathology and its Clinical Implications*. 1st ed. New York: Igaku Shoin; 1992:929–53.

5. Schlemper RJ, Riddell RH, Kato Y, et al. The Vienna classification of gastrointestinal epithelial neoplasia. *Gut* 2000;47:251–5.

6. Dawson IM, Pryse-Davies J. The development of carcinoma of the large intestine in ulcerative colitis. *Br J Surg* 1959;47:113–28.

7. Lennard-Jones JE, Melville DM, Morson BC, Ritchie JK, Williams CB. Precancer and cancer in extensive ulcerative colitis: findings among 401 patients over 22 years. *Gut* 1990;31:800–6.

8. Blackstone MO, Riddell RH, Rogers BH, Levin B. Dysplasia-associated lesion or mass (DALM) detected by colonoscopy in long-standing ulcerative colitis: an indication for colectomy. *Gastroenterology* 1981;80:366–74.

9. Butt JH, Konishi F, Morson BC, Lennard-Jones JE, Ritchie JK. Macroscopic lesions in dysplasia and carcinoma complicating ulcerative colitis. *Dig Dis Sci* 1983;28:18–26.

10. Rosenstock E, Farmer RG, Petras R, Sivak MV, Jr, Rankin GB, Sullivan BH. Surveillance for colonic carcinoma in ulcerative colitis. *Gastroenterology* 1985;89:1342–6.

11. Rubio CA, Johansson C, Slezak P, et al. Villous dysplasia: an ominous histologic sign in colitic patients. *Dis Colon Rectum* 1984;27:283–7.

12. Bernstein CN, Shanahan F, Weinstein WM. Are we telling patients the truth about surveillance colonoscopy in ulcerative colitis? *Lancet* 19948;343(8889):71–4.

13. Morson BC, Pang L. Rectal biopsy as an aid to cancer control in ulcerative colitis. *Gut* 1967;8(5):423–34.

14. Rubin CE, Haggitt RC, Burmer GC, et al. DNA aneuploidy in colonic biopsies predicts future development of dysplasia in ulcerative colitis. *Gastroenterology* 1992;103:1611–20.

15. Jaramillo E, Watanabe M, Slezak P, Rubio C. Flat neoplastic lesions of the colon and rectum detected by high-resolution video endoscopy and chromoscopy. *Gastrointest Endosc* 1995;42(2):114–22.

16. Jaramillo E, Watanabe M, Befrits R, Ponce de Leon E, Rubio C, Slezak P. Small, flat colorectal neoplasias in long-standing ulcerative colitis detected by high-resolution electronic video endoscopy. *Gastrointest Endosc* 1996;44(1):15–22.

17. Kiesslich R, Fritsch J, Holtmann M, et al. Methylene blue-aided chromoendoscopy for the detection of intraepithelial neoplasia and colon cancer in ulcerative colitis. *Gastroenterology* 2003;124(4):880–8.

18. Kudo S, Tamura S, Nakajima T, Yamano H, Kusaka H, Watanabe H. Diagnosis of colorectal tumorous lesions by magnifying endoscopy. *Gastrointest Endosc* 1996;44(1):8–14.

19. Tytgat GN, Dhir V, Gopinath N. Endoscopic appearance of dysplasia and cancer in inflammatory bowel disease. *Eur J Cancer* 1995;31A(7–8):1174–7.

20. Sharan R, Schoen RE. Cancer in inflammatory bowel disease: an evidence-based analysis and guide for physicians and patients. *Gastroenterol Clin North Am* 2002;31(1):237–54.

21. Lewis JD, Deren JJ, Lichtenstein GR. Cancer risk in patients with inflammatory bowel disease. *Gastroenterol Clin North Am* 1999;28(2):459–77.

22. Rutter MD, Saunders BP, Wilkinson KH, Kamm MA, Williams CB, Forbes A. Most dysplasia in ulcerative colitis is visible at colonoscopy. *Gastrointest Endosc* 2004;60(3):334–9.

23. Kudo S. *Early Colorectal Cancer: Detection of Depressed Types of Colorectal Carcinoma*. Tokyo: Igaku-Shoin; 1996:50–2.

24. Bernstein CN. ALMs versus DALMs in ulcerative colitis: polypectomy or colectomy? *Gastroenterology* 1999;117(6):1488–92.

25. Kitiyakara T, Bailey DM, McIntyre AS, Gorard DA. Adenomatous colonic polyps are rare in ulcerative colitis. *Aliment Pharmacol Ther* 200415;19(8):879–87.

26. Schneider A, Stolte M. Differential diagnosis of adenomas and dysplastic lesions in patients with ulcerative colitis. *Z Gastroenterol* 1993;31(11):653–6.

27. Connell WR, Lennard-Jones JE, Williams CB, Talbot IC, Price AB, Wilkinson KH. Factors affecting the outcome of endoscopic surveillance for cancer in ulcerative colitis. *Gastroenterology* 1994;107(4):934–44.

28. Lofberg R, Brostrom O, Karlen P, Tribukait B, Ost A. Colonoscopic surveillance in long-standing total ulcerative colitis – a 15-year follow-up study. *Gastroenterology* 1990;99(4):1021–31.

29. Torres C, Antonioli D, Odze RD. Polypoid dysplasia and adenomas in inflammatory bowel disease: a clinical, pathologic, and follow-up study of 89 polyps from 59 patients. *Am J Surg Pathol* 1998;22:275–84.

30. Wong NACS, Harrison D J. Colorectal neoplasia in ulcerative colitis – recent advances. *Histopathology* 2001;39:221–34.

31. Matsumura S, Oue N, Ito R, et al. The promoter methylation status of the DNA repair gene O6-methylguanine-DNA methyltransferase in ulcerative colitis. *Virchows Arch* 2003;443(4):518–23.

32. Fogt F, Vortmeyer AO, Stolte M, et al. Loss of heterozygosity of the von Hippel Lindau gene locus in

polypoid dysplasia but not flat dysplasia in ulcerative colitis or sporadic adenomas. *Hum Pathol* 1998;29(9): 961–4.

33 Odze RD, Brown CA, Hartmann CJ, Noffsinger AE, Fogt F. Genetic alterations in chronic ulcerative colitis-associated adenoma-like DALMs are similar to non-colitic sporadic adenomas. *Am J Surg Pathol* 2000;24(9):1209–16.

34 Fogt F, Urbanski SJ, Sanders ME, et al. Distinction between dysplasia-associated lesion or mass (DALM) and adenoma in patients with ulcerative colitis. *Hum Pathol* 2000;31(3):288–91.

35 Selaru FM, Xu Y, Yin J, et al. Artificial neural networks distinguish among subtypes of neoplastic colorectal lesions. *Gastroenterology* 2002;122(3): 606–13.

36 Walsh SV, Loda M, Torres CM, Antonioli D, Odze RD. P53 and beta catenin expression in chronic ulcerative colitis-associated polypoid dysplasia and sporadic adenomas: an immunohistochemical study. *Am J Surg Pathol* 1999;23(8):963–9.

37 Odze RD. Adenomas and adenoma-like DALMs in chronic ulcerative colitis: a clinical, pathological, and molecular review. *Am J Gastroenterol* 1999;94(7): 1746–50.

38 Harpaz N, Peck AL, Yin J, et al. p53 protein expression in ulcerative colitis-associated colorectal dysplasia and carcinoma. *Hum Pathol* 1994;25(10): 1069–74.

39 Mueller E, Vieth M, Stolte M, Mueller J. The differentiation of true adenomas from colitis-associated dysplasia in ulcerative colitis: a comparative immunohistochemical study. *Hum Pathol* 1999;30(8):898–905.

40 Toyota M, Ahuja N, Ohe-Toyota M, Herman JG, Baylin SB, Issa JPJ. CpG island methylator phenotype in colorectal cancer. *Proc Natl Acad Sci USA* 1999; 96:8681–6.

41 Baylin SB, Herman JG, Graff JR, Vertino PM, Issa JPJ. Alterations in DNA methylation: a fundamental aspect of neoplasia. *Adv Cancer Res* 1998;72:141–96.

42 Jones PA. DNA methylation errors and cancer. *Cancer Res* 1996;56:2463–7.

43 Toyota M, Ohe-Toyota M, Ahuja N, Issa JPJ. Distinct genetic profiles in colorectal tumors with or without the CpG island methylator phenotype. *Proc Natl Acad Sci USA* 2000;97:710–15.

44 Rashid A, Shen L, Morris JS, Issa JP, Hamilton SR. CpG island methylation in colorectal adenomas. *Am J Pathol* 2001;159(3):1129–35.

45 Issa J-PJ, II, Ahuja N, Toyota M, et al. Accelerated age-related CpG island methylation in ulcerative colitis. *Cancer Res* 2001;61(9):3573–7.

46 Shay JW, Wright WE. Telomeres and telomerase: implications for cancer and aging. *Radiat Res* 2001; 155(1, Pt 2):188–93.

47 Hackett JA, Feldser DM, Greider CW. Telomere dysfunction increases mutation rate and genomic instability. *Cell* 2001;106(3):275–86.

48 O'Sullivan JN, Bronner MP, Brentnall TA, et al. Chromosomal instability in ulcerative colitis is related to telomere shortening. *Nat Genet* 2002;32(2): 280–4.

49 O'Sullivan J, Rabinovitch P, Bronner M, et al. Distinguishing UC patients with dysplasia/cancerfrom those without it using measurements of genomic instability [Abstract]. *Mod Pathol* 2004;17(Suppl 1): 126A.

50 O'Sullivan JN, Finley JC, Risques RA, et al. Telomere length assessment in tissue sections by quantitative FISH: image analysis algorithms. *Cytometry A* 2004; 58(2):120–31.

51 Gage TP. Managing the cancer risk in chronic ulcerative colitis: a decision-analytic approach. *J Clin Gastroenterol* 1986;8(1):50–7.

52 Collins RH Jr, Feldman M, Fordtran JS. Colon cancer, dysplasia, and surveillance in patients with ulcerative colitis: a critical review. *N Engl J Med* 1987;316(26): 1654–8.

53 Engelsgjerd M, Torres C, Odze RD. Adenoma-like polypoid dysplasia in chronic ulcerative colitis: a follow up study of 23 cases. *Gastroenterology* 1999; 117:1288–94.

54 Rubin PH, Friedman S, Harpaz N, et al. Colonoscopic polypectomy in chronic colitis: are we removing adenomas or 'DALMs'. *Gastroenterology* 1999;117: 1295–1300.

55 Odze RD, Farraye FA, Hecht JL, Hornick JL. Long-term follow-up after polypectomy treatment for adenoma-like dysplastic lesions in ulcerative colitis. *Clin Gastroenterol Hepatol* 2004;2(7): 534–41.

56 Shetty K, Rybicki L, Brzezinski A, Carey WD, Lashner BA. The risk for cancer or dysplasia in ulcerative colitis patients with primary sclerosing cholangitis. *Am J Gastroenterol* 1999;94(6):1643–9.

57 Sinicrope FA, Wang K. Treating polyps in ulcerative colitis: adenoma-like lesions and dysplasia-associated mass lesions. *Clin Gastroenterol Hepatol* 2004;2(7): 531–3.

58 Bernstein CN, Weinstein WM, Levine DS, Shanahan F. Physicians' perceptions of dysplasia and approaches to surveillance colonoscopy in ulcerative colitis. *Am J Gastroenterol* 1995;90(12):2106–14.

59 Eaden JA, Ward BA, Mayberry JF. How gastroenterologists screen for colonic cancer in

ulcerative colitis: an analysis of performance. *Gastrointest Endosc* 2000;51(2):123–8.
60. Lim CH, Dixon MF, Vail A, Forman D, Lynch DA, Axon AT. Ten year follow up of ulcerative colitis patients with and without low grade dysplasia. *Gut* 2003;52(8):1127–32.
61. Gorfine SR, Bauer JJ, Harris MT, Kreel I. Dysplasia complicating chronic ulcerative colitis: is immediate colectomy warranted? *Dis Colon Rectum* 2000;43(11):1575–81.
62. Ullman T, Croog V, Harpaz N, Sachar D, Itzkowitz S. Progression of flat low-grade dysplasia to advanced neoplasia in patients with ulcerative colitis. *Gastroenterology* 2003;125(5):1311–9.
63. Axa A, et al. *Gut* 2004.
64. Odze R, Antonioli D, Peppercorn M, Goldman H. Effect of topical 5-aminosalicylic acid (5-ASA) therapy on rectal mucosal biopsy morphology in chronic ulcerative colitis. *Am J Surg Pathol* 1993;17(9):869–75.

V: Special management problems

26: Growth impairment in children

Thomas D. Walters and Anne M. Griffiths

Introduction

Inflammatory bowel disease (IBD) manifests during childhood or adolescence in up to 25% of patients. As among adults, the clinical course, severity and responsiveness to treatments vary greatly among children with Crohn's disease or ulcerative colitis [1, 2]. Unique to paediatric patient populations, however, is the potential for growth impairment as a complication of chronic intestinal inflammation. Therapy of childhood IBD mirrors that of adults, but the challenge in treating each child or adolescent is to employ pharmacological, nutritional and where appropriate, surgical interventions, not only to decrease mucosal inflammation and thereby alleviate symptoms, but also to optimise growth and normalise associated pubertal development. Normal growth is a marker of success of therapy. This chapter reviews the prevalence of growth impairment in paediatric IBD, discusses its pathophysiology and outlines strategies for prevention and management.

Normal growth and pubertal development

'Normal' children grow at very different rates. Patterns of growth and pubertal progression in young patients with IBD can only be accurately recognised as pathologic, if the variations in normal development of healthy children and adolescents are first appreciated.

A child's growth is the result of both genes and environment; it appears to be principally mediated by hormones and nutrition [3]. Linear growth can be represented by stature (attained height) or by the rate of growth (height velocity). A child's attained height represents the culmination of growth in all preceding years; height velocity reflects growth status at a particular point in time.

Growth can be conceptualised as the product of three overlapping biological phases: infancy, childhood and puberty. Final height represents the sum of each of the individual components. The growth hormone/insulin-like growth factor-1 (GH/IGF-1) axis plays a pivotal role in normal post-natal growth. GH produced by the pituitary gland binds to hepatic receptors and induces hepatic release of IGF-1, which stimulates mitosis of epiphyseal chondrocytes resulting in linear bone growth [4]. Thyroxine, cortisol and sex steroids are also implicated in the maintenance of normal linear growth.

Linear growth velocity decreases from birth onwards, punctuated by a short period of growth acceleration (the 'adolescent growth spurt') just prior to completion of growth. As the rapid growth of infancy tails off, the steady growth of childhood predominates. Healthy children grow at a consistent rate in the range of 4–6 cm annually from 6 years of age until the onset of puberty [5].

At puberty there is a rapid alteration in body size, shape and composition; for a year or more height velocity approximately doubles. The age of onset of puberty, and hence of the pubertal growth spurt, vary among normal individuals and between ethnic populations. Puberty begins earlier in girls than in boys; moreover the pubertal growth spurt occurs in mid-puberty (prior to menarche) in girls but in late puberty (after Tanner stage 4) in boys [5]. There is hence quite consistently a 2-year difference in the timing of peak height velocity (PHV) in girls compared to boys [5]. In North American females PHV occurs at a mean age of 11.5 years but in males not until 13.5 years (2SD = 1.8 years) [5]. The occurrence of menarche is an indication that linear growth is nearing completion; usually girls gain only 5–8 cm more in height within the two subsequent years [5].

Monitoring and assessment of growth

Standardised charts are available for graphically recording height, weight and height velocity such that an individual child's growth can be compared to normative values [6–8]. Wherever possible, reference data most appropriate to the child being monitored should be utilised. An individual child's growth measurement can be represented as a percentile or as a standard deviation score, a quantitative expression of distance from the reference population mean (50th percentile) for the same age and gender [9]. Healthy children grow steadily along the same height percentile and hence maintain the same standard deviation score for height from early childhood through until adulthood. Combined parental heights can be used to estimate a child's potential height [9]. Some temporary deviation from the usual growth channel may occur if the pubertal growth spurt occurs particularly early (temporary increase in height velocity and height centile) or late (temporary decrease in height velocity and height centile).

Definitions of impaired growth

Within a large patient group, skewing of (standard deviation score) SDS for height below population reference values is evidence of disease-associated growth impairment. Mean height SDS of a population characterised by normal growth approximates zero. Growth disturbance in an individual child is indicated by an abnormal growth rate [9]. A definition in terms of static height measurement, although sometimes used, may be misleading because it is so influenced by parental heights. An individual child may be normally short; conversely a previously tall child may not have increased his height in 2 years, but still be of average stature. A shift from higher to lower centiles on a growth chart of height attained more sensibly signifies growth faltering. Height velocity expressed either as a centile or as a standard deviation score for age and gender, is the most sensitive parameter by which to recognise impaired growth.

Growth in pediatric IBD

Prevalence of growth impairment in IBD

Inflammatory disease occurring during early adolescence is likely to have a major impact on nutritional status and growth because of the very rapid accumulation of lean body mass that normally occurs at this time. Further, boys are more vulnerable to disturbances in growth than girls because their growth spurt comes later and is ultimately longer and greater [5].

Crohn's disease

Several studies have characterised the growth of children with Crohn's disease as treated in the 1980s and into the 1990s [1, 10–15]. These studies are important as a benchmark of outcomes with traditional therapy. It is to be hoped that the better understanding of the pathogenesis of growth impairment that now exists, together with the greater efficacy of current therapeutic regimens in healing intestinal inflammation, may lead to enhanced growth of young patients diagnosed in the present decade.

As summarised in Table 26.1, the percentage of patients with Crohn's disease, whose growth is affected, varies with the time of assessment, the definition of growth impairment and with the nature of the population under study (tertiary referral centre versus population-based) [1, 10–15]. It has, nevertheless, been consistently observed that impairment of linear growth is common prior to recognition of Crohn's disease as well as during the subsequent years, and that height at maturity has often been compromised [1, 10–15].

At the time of diagnosis mean standard deviation score (SDS) for height is reduced among children with Crohn's disease as a group compared to reference populations, an indication of the growth

Table 26.1 Prevalence of linear growth impairment in paediatric Crohn's disease as treated in the 1980s and into the 1990s.

Study (Reference)	Time of assessment	Patients studied	Definition of linear growth impairment	Percentage with growth impairment
Kanof [11]	At diagnosis	Prepubertal (Tanner I or II) patients ($n = 50$)	Decrease in height velocity	88%
Kirschner [10]	At diagnosis		Decrease in height centile >1 SD	36%
Griffiths [1]	During follow-up	Prepubertal children (Tanner I or II at diagnosis) ($n = 100$)	Height velocity ≤2 SD for age for ≥2 years	49%
Hildebrand [12]	Before diagnosis or during follow-up	Population-based cohort of 46 children	Height velocity ≤2 SD for age for 1 year	65%
Markowitz [13]	At maturity	38 children in tertiary care setting	Failure to reach predicted adult height	37%
Kundhal [15]	During follow-up	Pre-pubertal children (Tanner I or II at diagnosis) ($n = 161$)	Height velocity ≤2 SD for age for ≥2 years	54%

retardation occurring prior to recognition and treatment of intestinal inflammation [1, 12, 14, 15]. During the decade 1990–1999 in Toronto, mean SDS for height at time of diagnosis among 161 Tanner stage 1 or 2 children was -0.74 ± 1.2 [15], indicating overall lesser growth delay in comparison to the earlier decade [1]. Nevertheless, the percentage of children with height less than the fifth centile (SDS < -1.8), based on Center for Disease Control 2000 data, was still 22% [15]. Mean SDS for height among 333 patients aged less than 16 years was -0.54 (95% CI -0.67 to -0.41) in a 1998–1999 population-based surveillance study of incident IBD in the United Kingdom [16]. Thirteen per cent were below the third centile (SDS < -1.96) for height based on data from Child Growth Foundation, London [16]. In Israel SDS for height at diagnosis among a cohort of 93 patients aged less than 18 years was -0.56 ± 1.16, but 20% had SDS less than -2.0 [17]. Taken together these data confirm that growth delay prior to diagnosis still occurs and remains a challenge [15–17].

Delay in epiphyseal closure allows growth to continue longer than normal. Hence mean SDS for height may improve over the course of treatment, when the chronic inflammation can be controlled [1, 12, 15]. No population-based cohort studies have compared pre-illness height centiles with final adult stature in order to determine how often catch-up growth is complete. In spite of gains, mean adult height of patients with pre-pubertal onset of disease remains reduced compared to population reference data [1, 12, 15]. Studies suggesting otherwise have included patients with post-pubertal onset of disease, and therefore not at risk for growth impairment [18, 19].

Ulcerative colitis

Cohort data are sparse in comparison to Crohn's disease, but in general at diagnosis no significant reduction is observed in height-for-age standard deviation scores among young patients with ulcerative colitis compared to the reference population [12, 14, 16]. As an example, SDS for height was not reduced (mean -0.12, 95% CI -0.30–0.05) in 143 children and adolescents with incident UC in the British paediatric surveillance study [16].

During follow-up growth impairment remains a less frequent complication although relatively few studies have carefully described linear growth in ulcerative colitis as compared to the abundance of studies in Crohn's disease. Hildebrand et al. observed that 11 (24%) of 45 children had a height

Table 26.2 Factors contributing to growth impairment in children with Crohn's disease.

Factor	Explanation
Pro-inflammatory cytokines	Direct interference with IGF-1 mediation of linear growth
Decreased food intake	Cytokine-mediated anorexia, fear of worsening gastrointestinal symptoms
Stool losses	Mucosal damage leading to protein-losing enteropathy; diffuse small intestinal disease or resection leading to steatorrhoea
Increased nutritional needs	Fever; required catch-up growth
Corticosteroid treatment	Interference with growth hormone and insulin-like growth factor-1

velocity less than −2.0 SD during at least 1 year [12]. Final attained mean height was comparable to reference population data in this study [12].

Why linear growth impairment is less common in ulcerative colitis than in Crohn's disease is not entirely clear. The usual colitic symptom of bloody diarrhoea is more promptly investigated than the often subtle-presenting symptoms of Crohn's disease, accounting at least in part for the lesser effect on growth prior to diagnosis. Disease-related differences in cytokine production may also be important.

Pathophysiology of growth impairment in IBD

As summarised in Table 26.2, several inter-related factors contribute to linear growth impairment in children with IBD. The fundamental mechanisms have recently been comprehensively reviewed [20].

Chronic caloric insufficiency

Chronic under-nutrition has long been implicated and remains an important and remediable cause of growth retardation [21]. Multiple factors contribute to malnutrition. However, reduced intake, rather than excessive losses or increased needs, is the major cause of the caloric insufficiency. Kirschner *et al.* reported caloric intakes of growth-paired patients to average 54% of that recommended for children of similar height age [22]. Disease-related anorexia may be profound. Cytokines produced by the inflamed bowel are likely to be responsible. Work in a rat model of colitis suggests that tumour necrosis factor alpha (TNF-α) interacts with hypothalamic appetite pathways [23]. Significant intestinal fat malabsorption is uncommon [24], but leakage of protein is frequent [25]. In general resting energy expenditure (REE) does not differ from normal in patients with inactive disease, but can exceed predicted rates in the presence of fever and sepsis. Furthermore, in comparison to comparably malnourished patients with anorexia nervosa, a lack of compensatory reduction in REE has been described in adolescents with Crohn's disease [26]. Reduction in REE is a normal biological response to conserve energy. Production of inflammatory mediators may explain the lack of REE adaptation in patients with Crohn's disease, and further augment the ongoing malnutrition.

Direct cytokine effects

A simple nutritional hypothesis fails to explain all the observations related to growth patterns among children with IBD. Within the past decade the direct growth-inhibiting effects of pro-inflammatory cytokines released from the inflamed intestine have been increasingly recognised and are now the focus of intriguing research [27–30].

IGF-1, produced by the liver in response to growth hormone (GH) stimulation, is the key mediator of GH effects at the growth plate of bones. An association between impaired growth in children with Crohn's disease and low IGF-1 levels is well recognised [31]. Early studies emphasised the role of malnutrition in suppression of IGF-1 production [31]. Recently, transgenic mice with defective growth were found to over-express interleukin-6 (IL-6). Antibody to IL-6 partially corrected the growth defect, whereas administration of IL-6 led to a decrease in IGF-1 before food intake was affected [27]. Further, IGF-1 levels were negatively correlated with IL-6 among children with juvenile rheumatoid arthritis [27]. These findings suggest that an IL-6-mediated decrease in IGF-1 production may represent a major mechanism by which chronic inflammation leads to stunting of growth [27].

The relative contributions of malnutrition and inflammation to linear growth delay have recently been explored by Ballinger et al. using a rat model of TNBS colitis [28]. Two control groups were used: healthy controls with free access to food, and a pair-fed group comprised of healthy animals with daily food intake restricted to match that of colitic rats [28]. In the colitic rats IGF-1 levels were reduced to 35% of control values. Comparison with the healthy but under-nourished pair-fed rats, suggested that malnutrition accounted for 53% of the total depression of IGF-1 in colitic rats, with the remaining 47% attributable to inflammation [28].

There is evidence that inflammatory cytokines also inhibit linear growth through pathways other than IGF-1 production. Animal experiments have shown that TNF-α and interleukin-1 (IL-1) increase chondrocyte death and thus may have a deleterious effect on growth [29]. In an organ culture model of foetal rat parietal bone, marked impairment in osteoblast function and bone growth was observed with addition of serum from children with Crohn's disease, but not from children with ulcerative colitis, nor from healthy controls [30]. Cytokines appear to impair end-organ responsiveness to circulating testosterone, thereby compounding the effects of under-nutrition in delaying progression through puberty [32].

Corticosteroid-suppression of linear growth

Chronic daily corticosteroid administration in children augments the growth impairment associated with inflammatory disease. The growth suppressive effects of glucocorticoids are multi-factorial, and include central suppression of GH release, decreased hepatic transcription of GH receptor, such that production of IGF-1 is decreased, and decreased IGF-1 binding in cartilage [33]. Hence exogenous corticosteroids create a state of functional GH deficiency [33].

Endocrine mediators of growth impairment

It is evident from the above discussion that reduced plasma concentrations of IGF-1, as a result of inflammatory cytokines and/or malnutrition and/or exogenous corticosteroids, play a central role in mediating growth impairment in IBD. GH levels in response to provocative testing are normal [34]. Thyroid gland function is normal. Reduced levels of sex steroids and end-organ resistance may play a role in delayed or abrogated development of secondary sex characteristics and pubertal growth spurt, when inflammation is uncontrolled [33].

Disease susceptibility genes

Comprehensive genotype–phenotype correlation studies in large paediatric patient populations have yet to be performed. Tomer and colleagues suggested that NOD2/CARD15 polymorphisms might be a determinant of growth impairment [35], but analysis did not control for disease location, the phenotypic characteristic clearly influenced by NOD2/CARD15 [36]. A subsequent careful analysis of growth prior to and following diagnosis found no association of growth impairment with the three common Crohn's disease-associated NOD2/CARD15 polymorphisms among children in Israel [17].

Facilitation of normal growth in IBD

The importance of prompt recognition of IBD

The clinical presentation of childhood Crohn's disease may be subtle and varied. Impairment of linear growth and concomitant delay in sexual maturation may precede the development of intestinal symptoms and dominate the presentation. Prompt diagnosis is important in avoiding a long period of growth retardation. The greater the height deficit at diagnosis, the greater is the demand for catch-up growth.

The importance of monitoring growth

In caring for children with IBD, it is important to obtain pre-illness heights, so that the impact of the chronic intestinal inflammation can be fully appreciated. Following diagnosis and institution of treatment, regular measurement and charting of height, together with calculation of height velocity, are central to management. A properly calibrated wall-mounted stadiometer is required for accurate and reproducible serial measurements.

Part of the assessment of response to therapy in children with IBD is a regular analysis of whether rate of growth is normal for age and pubertal stage and whether catch-up growth to pre-illness centiles is being achieved. Height velocity must be appraised in the context of current pubertal stage, because of the variation in normal rates of growth before puberty, during puberty and near the end of puberty. If growth and puberty appear either delayed or very advanced, radiological determination of bone age can be used to indicate the remaining growth potential.

One of the difficulties in evaluating growth in response to a therapy is the relatively long interval of time required for valid assessment. Published normal standards for height velocity throughout childhood are based on height increments during 12-month periods [37]. When growth velocity is calculated over short time- periods, small errors in individual measurements are significantly magnified, and the normal seasonal variation in growth is overlooked. The consensus from paediatric endocrinologists is that height velocity should be calculated over intervals no shorter than 6 months [37]. On a research basis, efforts to reflect growth changes over intervals shorter than 6 months have focused on measuring changes in lower leg length by knemometry and on the determination of circulating levels of markers of collagen metabolism [37]. A valid indicator of anticipated linear growth would allow more timely change in therapy.

Psychosocial impact of impaired growth

Growth impairment and accompanying pubertal delay have a significant psychosocial impact on adolescents, as the physical differences between them and healthy peers become progressively more obvious. In the development process of a disease-specific health-related quality of life instrument for paediatric IBD, body image issues including height and weight were among the concerns most frequently cited by adolescents with Crohn's disease [38].

General principles of management

Prior to recognition of the direct influences of pro-inflammatory cytokines on linear growth, management of growth-impaired children focused on nutritional restitution [21, 22]. Improved growth following supplementary enteral or parenteral nutrition is well documented [39–41], but the relative contribution of improved nutrition versus reduced inflammation is uncertain and may vary between patients. A recent study demonstrated that a decrease in inflammatory parameters and an increase in IGF-1 occurred very early during exclusive enteral nutrition and preceded changes in nutritional parameters [42]. Moreover, a subset of patients fails to grow despite nutritional repletion, because intestinal inflammation remains chronically active. In the management or prevention of growth impairment, attention needs to focus on the treatment of inflammatory disease using the most appropriate pharmacological, nutritional or surgical intervention [43]. Separation of anti-inflammatory and nutritional effects is somewhat artificial, moreover, because of the important interactions between cytokines and nutrition. Nutrition and inflammation constitute a bi-directional pathway [44]. Treatments of paediatric IBD will be briefly discussed with respect to their effects on growth.

Anti-inflammatory treatments and effects on growth

Few interventions have been tested in the randomised controlled trial setting in children, and hence the effects of therapies on growth have seldom been rigorously assessed. The one exception is enteral nutrition as primary therapy of paediatric Crohn's disease. For most other therapies, growth outcomes have been reported only in observational studies.

To date, the key *differences* in management of IBD in children and young adolescents compared to adults have included greater attention to avoidance of long-term corticosteroid therapy, more frequent use of enteral nutrition as an alternate primary therapy in Crohn's disease, and earlier consideration of resection of localised Crohn's disease and steroid-dependent ulcerative colitis [43]. These strategies are all aimed at optimising growth prior to completion of puberty. New biologic therapies, particularly anti-tumour necrosis factor alpha (TNF-α), have brought the management of Crohn's disease into a new era. Children whose disease remains chronically active despite use of immunomodulatory drugs now benefit from such therapy. Ongoing monitoring of long-term safety issues will determine whether infliximab and other biologic agents in future should have a special place in paediatric treatment regimens in order to improve disease-related outcomes including growth and quality of life.

Enteral nutrition

Prior to availability of infliximab, acute treatment options for moderately to severely active Crohn's disease were limited. The appeal of enteral nutrition as primary therapy among paediatric patients, relates to avoidance of steroids, both because of their unwanted cosmetic side effects and their propensity to interfere with growth [43]. Aminoacid based and peptide-based formulae are administered by nocturnal nasogastric infusion, but more palatable polymeric formulae can be consumed orally, and appear comparably efficacious [45]. Open trials in children have documented endoscopic healing and decreased mucosal cytokine production following exclusive enteral nutrition [46]. Some have argued that active Crohn's disease occurring in children is more responsive than that occurring in adults, where corticosteroid therapy more often induces clinical remission [47, 48]. It seems likely, however, that other factors, such as small bowel localisation and recent onset of Crohn's disease, rather than young age *per se*, influence responsiveness of intestinal inflammation to exclusive enteral nutrition [49, 50]. Nevertheless, enteral nutrition does seem to be more feasible in paediatric patients. Children quickly become adept at swallowing the silastic catheter required for nasogastric feeding regimens, and can remove it each morning before school.

If enteral nutrition is to facilitate growth, remission must be maintained. One of the limitations of liquid diet therapy has been the observed tendency for symptoms to recur promptly following its cessation [51]. Chronic intermittent bowel rest with nocturnal infusion of an elemental diet 1 month out of 4 has been reported as a means of sustaining remission and facilitating growth [40]. In a multi-centre Canadian paediatric study, children achieving clinical remission with either prednisone or enteral nutrition, were randomised to receive long-term either low dose (0.3 mg/kg) prednisone on alternate days or exclusive enteral nutrition one month out of four [52]. In the 18-month study, 67% of the children treated with cyclical enteral nutrition remained in continuous clinical remission compared with 47% of those receiving alternate-day prednisone [52]. Although this difference in relapse rate was not statistically significant in the total of 35 patients studied, linear growth was significantly better in the children receiving liquid diet therapy [52]. Another nutritional strategy, continuation of nocturnal nasogastric feeding four to five times weekly as supplement to an unrestricted ad lib daytime diet was also associated with prolonged disease quiescence and improved growth in a historical cohort study [41].

Corticosteroids

Conventional corticosteroids are still the most commonly used drug to treat acute disease exacerbations of paediatric Crohn's disease and ulcerative colitis. Resolution of inflammation, if sustained following a short course of steroids, will be associated with normal linear growth. Chronic daily administration of corticosteroids to control intestinal inflammation is clearly contraindicated in paediatric IBD because of the interference with linear growth in addition to the other unwanted long-term adverse effects common to children and adults. Alternate day administration was long ago advocated as a means of controlling inflammation in Crohn's disease without suppressing IGF-1 [53]. This strategy, inferior to cyclical enteral nutrition [52], has been abandoned in favour of other therapeutic approaches to corticosteroid dependency in children with Crohn's disease. Because of the limited other medical options, it may be reasonable to employ low-dose alternate-day prednisone for a limited time period in some children with steroid-dependent ulcerative colitis, as long as linear growth rate is carefully monitored and found to be maintained.

Children with moderate symptoms of active Crohn's disease localised to the ileum and/or right colon may respond to short-term treatment with controlled ileal release budesonide. Cosmetic effects of steroids are spared in this context, even if efficacy is overall somewhat less than with conventional corticosteroids [54, 55]. Studies in adults demonstrate little benefit in comparison to placebo in maintaining remission. Limited clinical experience with maintenance budesonide in children raised concern that linear growth was impaired during therapy in spite of good weight gain [56].

Azathioprine and 6-mercatopurine

The immunomodulatory drugs, azathioprine and 6-mercaptopurine, are increasingly used to maintain remission in children and adolescents with Crohn's disease, a reflection of the increased body of evidence in support of both their therapeutic efficacy and safety profile. In a multi-centre trial newly diagnosed children with moderately severe Crohn's disease treated with an initial course of prednisone were randomised to receive either concomitant 6-mercaptopurine or placebo [57]. A beneficial effect on linear growth was not clearly apparent in this study in spite of the steroid-sparing effect and improved control of intestinal inflammation, perhaps a function of sample size and difficulties inherent in comparing growth rates among patients of varying ages and pubertal stages [37]. Level one evidence of efficacy of azathioprine/ 6-mercaptopurine in ulcerative colitis is relatively sparse even in adult patients. Nevertheless in clinical practice immunomodulatory drugs are also employed in children whose ulcerative colitis remains steroid-dependent despite optimisation of 5-aminosalicylic acid or sulfasalazine therapy.

Surgery

Optimal management of young patients with IBD includes appropriate and timely referral for intestinal resection. Sustained steroid-dependency and associated impairment of linear growth should not be tolerated in children with ulcerative colitis, where colectomy cures the disease and restores growth [58]. For children with Crohn's disease, the possibility of a significant asymptomatic interval, during which normal growth and pubertal development can resume, makes intestinal resection an attractive therapeutic option, despite the likelihood of eventual disease recrudescence.

In two paediatric studies, anatomic distribution of Crohn's disease was the most important factor influencing duration of post-operative clinical remission [59, 60]. Patients with extensive ileocolonic involvement experienced an excess of early clinical recurrences (50% by 1 year) in comparison to children with pre-operative disease in the terminal ileum +/− right colon or in the more proximal small intestine (50% by 5 years) [59]. Children undergoing resection because of stenosing or fistulising complications (e.g. bowel obstruction or intra-abdominal abscess) had delayed recrudescence of disease in comparison to those operated upon simply for inflammatory symptoms refractory to medical therapy [59]. An early operative approach to localised disease and for complications of chronic inflammation is supported by these data [59, 60]. Significant improvements in height velocity post-operatively compared to pre-operatively are observed in pre-pubertal or early pubertal children [59, 60].

Anti-tumour necrosis factor alpha (anti-TNF-α)

Within the spectrum of paediatric Crohn's disease is a subgroup of patients with chronically active extensive disease not amenable to resection, and refractory to previously available medical therapies. At the Hospital for Sick Children in Toronto, such patients comprised 16–17% of all pre-pubertal children with Crohn's disease diagnosed during each of two decades [1, 15]. These patients, as expected, were also the most likely to have sustained growth impairment [1, 15].

The development of anti-cytokine therapies, such as infliximab, with the potential to achieve mucosal healing, even in otherwise treatment refractory patients constitutes a tremendous advance. The ability of repeated infliximab infusions to sustain clinical remission is well documented in adults. Clinical experience in children is similar; a beneficial effect on linear growth is observed, if treatment is undertaken early enough prior to or during puberty [61, 62]. These observations are cause for optimism that the medical therapy for Crohn's disease available in the present decade will reduce the prevalence of sustained growth impairment in paediatric patients.

Hormonal interventions

Given that corticosteroids interfere with the GH-IGF-1 axis at a number of sites, there is a small experience with the use of exogenous recombinant growth hormone (rGH) therapy for growth failure associated with ongoing steroid therapy in a number of paediatric conditions [32]. Mauras *et al.* reported improvement in IGF-1 levels and height velocity in a pilot study of 10 children with Crohn's disease, whose growth had been impaired in the context of steroid dependency [63]. Three to six months of testosterone therapy, carefully supervised by paediatric endocrinologists, has been used in boys with extreme delay of puberty and has been associated with a growth spurt [33]. It must be emphasised, however, that children requiring consideration of these adjunctive hormonal therapies should be encountered increasingly uncommonly. Treatment of intestinal inflammation and assurance of adequate nutrition are of much greater importance.

Summary

Increased understanding of the mechanisms of linear growth impairment associated with chronic inflammatory disease points the way towards better management. Early recognition of Crohn's disease remains an important challenge. Restoration and maintenance of a child's pre-illness growth pattern indicate success of therapy. Current treatment regimens limit use of the corticosteroids via optimisation of immunomodulatory drugs, use of enteral nutrition in Crohn's disease, and, if necessary, surgery for ulcerative colitis and for intestinal complications of localised Crohn's disease. Biologic agents with the potential for mucosal healing hold promise of growth enhancement even among patients with otherwise refractory disease, whose growth was previously compromised. For all interventions, there is a window of opportunity, which must be taken advantage of before puberty is too advanced.

References

1. Griffiths AM, Nguyen P, Smith C, MacMillan H, Sherman PM. Growth and clinical course of children with Crohn's disease. *Gut* 1993;34:939–43.
2. Hyams JS, Davis P, Grancher K, *et al*. Clinical outcome of ulcerative colitis in children. *J Pediatr* 1996;129:81–8.
3. Karlberg J, Jalil F, Lam B, Low L, Yeung CY. Linear growth retardation in relation to the three phases of growth. *Eur J Clin Nutr* 1994;48:S25–43.
4. Wang J, Zhou J, Cheng CM, Kopchick JJ, Bondy CA. Evidence supporting dual, IGF-I independent and IGF-1-dependent roles for GH in promoting longitudinal bone growth. *J Endocrinol* 2004;180:247–55.
5. Rogol A. Growth at puberty. *J Adolesc Health* 31:192–200.
6. Tanner JM, Whitehouse RH. Clinical longitudinal standard for height, weight, height velocity, weight velocity, and stages of puberty. *Arch Dis Child* 1976;51:170–9.
7. Centers for Disease Control and Prevention, National Center for Health Statistics. CDC growth charts: United States, http://www.cdc.gov/growthcharts/.30-5-2000.
8. Freeman JV, Cole TJ, Chinn S, Jones PRM, White EM, Preece MA. Cross sectional stature and weight reference curves for the UK, 1990. *Arch Dis Child* 1995;73:17–24.
9. Zeferino A, Barros Filho A, Bettiol H, Barbieri M. Monitoring growth. *J Pediatr (Rio J)* 2003; 79(Suppl 1):S23–32.

10. Kirschner BS. Growth and development in chronic inflammatory bowel disease. *Acta Paed Scand* 1990;(Suppl 366):98–104.
11. Kanof ME, Lake AM, Bayless TM. Decreased height velocity in children and adolescents before the diagnosis of Crohn's disease. *Gastroenterology* 1988;95:1523–7.
12. Hildebrand H, Karlberg J, Kristiansson B. Longitudinal growth in children and adolescents with inflammatory bowel disease. *J Pediatr Gastro Nutr* 1994;18:165–73.
13. Markowitz J, Grancher K, Rosa J, Aiges H, Daum F. Growth failure in pediatric inflammatory bowel disease. *J Ped Gastroenterol Nutr* 1993;16:373–80.
14. Motil KJ, Grand RJ, Davis-Kraft L, Ferlic LL, Smith EO. Growth failure in children with inflammatory bowel disease: a prospective study. *Gastroenterology* 1993;105:681–91.
15. Kundhal P, Critch J, Hack C, Griffiths A. Clinical course and growth of children with Crohn's disease. *Can J Gastroenterol* 2002.
16. Sawczendo A, Sandhu KB. Presenting features of inflammatory bowel disease in Great Britain and Ireland. *Arch Dis Child* 2003;88:995–1000.
17. Wine E, Reif SS, Leshinsky-Silver E, et al. Pediatric Crohn's disease and growth retardation: the role of genotype, phenotype, and disease severity. *Pediatrics* 2004;114:1281–6.
18. Ferguson A, Sedgwick DM. Juvenile onset inflammatory bowel disease: height and body mass index in adult life. *Br Med J* 1994;308:1259–63.
19. Alemzadeh N, Redkers-Mombarg LTM, Mearin ML, Wit JM, Lamers CBHW, van Hogezand RA. Adult height in patients with ealy onset of Crohn's disease. *Gut* 2002;51:26–9.
20. Ballinger A. Fundamental mechanisms of growth impairment in inflammatory bowel disease. *Horm Res* 2002:58(Suppl 1):7–10.
21. Kelts DG, Grand RJ, Shen G, Watkins JB, Werlin SL, Boehme C. Nutritional basis of growth failure in children and adolescents with Crohn's disease. *Gastroenterology* 1979;76:720–7.
22. Kirschner BS, Klich JR, Kalman SS, deFavaro MV, Rosenberg IH. Reversal of growth retardation in Crohn's disease with therapy emphasizing oral nutritional restitution. *Gastroenterology* 1981;80:10–15.
23. Ballinger A, El-Haj T, Perrett D, et al. The role of medial hypothalamic serotonin in the suppression of feeding in a rat model of colitis. *Gastroenterology* 2000;118:544–53.
24. Filipsson S, Hulten L, Lindstedt G. Malabsorption of fat and vitamin B12 before and after intestinal resection for Crohn's disease. *Scand J Gastro* 1978;13:529–36.
25. Griffiths AM, Drobnies A, Soldin SJ, Hamilton JR. Enteric protein loss measured by fecal alpha-1-antitrypsin clearance in the assessment of Crohn's disease activity. *J Pediatr Gastro Nutr* 1986;5:907–10.
26. Azcue M, Rashid M, Griffiths A, et al. Energy expenditure and body composition in children with Crohn's disease: effect of enteral nutrition and prednisone treatment. *Gut* 1997;41:203–7.
27. DeBenedetti F, Alonzi T, Moretta A, et al. Interleukin-6 causes growth impairment in transgenic mice through a decrease in insulin-growth factor I. *J Clin Invest* 1997;99:643–50.
28. Ballinger AB, Azooz O, El-Haj T, Poole S, Farthing MJG. Growth failure occurs through a decrease in insulin-like growth factor 1 which is independent of undernutrition in a rat model of colitis. *Gut* 2000;46:1–6.
29. Martensson K, Chrysis D, Savendahl L. Interleukin-1 beta and TNF-alpha act in synergy in inhibit longitudinal growth in fetal rat metatarsal bones. *J Bone Miner Res* 2004;11:1805–12.
30. Varghese S, Wyzga N, Griffiths AM, Sylvester FA. Effects of serum from children newly diagnosed with Crohn's disease on primary cultures of rat osteoblasts. *J Pediatr Gastro Nutr* 2002;35:641–8.
31. Kirschner BS, Sutton MM. Somatomedin-C levels in growth-impaired children and adolescents with chronic inflammatory bowel disease. *Gastroenterology* 1986;91:830–6.
32. Mauras N. Growth hormone therapy in the glucocorticosteroid-dependent child: metabolic and linear growth effects. *Horm Res* 2001;56(Suppl 1):13–18.
33. Ballinger AB, Savage MO, Sanderson IR. Delayed puberty associated with inflammatory bowel disease. *Pediatr Res* 2003;53:205–10.
34. Tenore A, Berman WF, Parks JS, Bongiovannie AM. Basal and stimulated growth hormone concentrations in inflammatory bowel disease. *J Clin Endocrinol Metab* 1977;44:622–8.
35. Tomer G, Ceballos C, Concepcion E, et al. NOD2/CARD15 variants are associated with lower weight at diagnosis in children with Crohn's disease. *Am J Gastroenterol* 2003;98:2479–84.
36. Economour M, Trikalinos TA, Loizou KT, Tsianos EV, Ioannidis JPA. Differential effects of NOD2 variants on Crohn's disease risk and phenotype in diverse populations: a metaanalysis. *Am J Gastroenterol* 2004;99:2393–404.
37. Griffiths AM, Otley AR, Hyams J, et al. A review of activity indices and endpoints for clinical trials in

38. Griffiths AM. Development of a quality of life index for paediatric inflammatory bowel disease: dealing with differences related to age and IBD type. *J Pediatr Gastro Nutr* 1999;28:S46–52.
39. Aiges H, Markowitz J, Rosa J, Daum F. Home nocturnal supplemental nasogastric feedings in growth-retarded adolescents with Crohn's disease. *Gastroenterology* 1989;97:905–10.
40. Belli DC, Seidman E, Bouthillier F, *et al*. Chronic intermittent elemental diet improves growth failure in children with Crohn's disease. *Gastroenterology* 1988;94:603–10.
41. Wilschanski M, Sherman P, Pencharz P, *et al*. Supplementary enteral nutrition maintains remission in paediatric Crohn's disease. *Gut* 1996;38:543–8.
42. Bannerjee K, Camacho-Hubner C, Babinska K, *et al*. Anti-inflammatory and growth-stimulating effects precede nutritional restitution during enteral feeding in Crohn disease. *J Pediatr Gastro Nutr* 2004;38:270–5.
43. Walker-Smith JA. Management of growth failure in Crohn's disease. *Arch Dis Child* 1996;75:351–4.
44. Gassull MA, Stange EF. Nutrition and diet in inflammatory bowel disease. In: Satsangi J, Sutherland LR, eds. *Inflammatory Bowel Diseases*. London, UK: Elsevier; 2003:461–74.
45. Zachos M, Tondeur M, Griffiths AM. A meta-analysis of enteral nutrition as primary therapy of active Crohn's disease: does formula composition influence efficacy? *Cochrane Database Syst Rev* 2001;3:1–24.
46. Fell JME, Paintin M, Arnaud-Battandier F, *et al*. Mucosal healing and a fall in mucosal pro-inflammatory cytokine mRNA induced by specific oral polymeric diet in paediatric Crohn's disease. *Aliment Pharmacol Ther* 14:281–9.
47. Heuschkel RB, Menache CC, Megerian JT, *et al*. Enteral nutrition and corticosteroids in the treatment of acute Crohn's disease in children. *J Pediatr Gastro Nutr* 2000;31:8–15.
48. Griffiths AM, Ohlsson A, Sherman P, Sutherland LR. Meta-analysis of enteral nutrition as primary treatment of active Crohn's disease. *Gastroenterology* 1995;108:1056–67.
49. Seidman E, Griffiths A, Jones A, *et al*. Semi-elemental diet versus prednisone in the treatment of acute Crohn's disease in children and adolescents. *Gastroenterology* 1993;104:A778.
50. Griffiths AM. Enteral nutrition: the neglected primary therapy of active Crohn's disease. *J Pediatr Gastro Nutr* 2000;31:3–5.
51. Rigaud D, Cosnes J, Quintrec Y, *et al*. Controlled trial comparing two types of enteral nutrition in treatment of active Crohn's disease. *Gut* 1991;32:1492–7.
52. Seidman E, Jones A, Issenman R, *et al*. Cyclical exclusive enteral nutrition versus alternate day prednisone in maintaining remission of pediatric Crohn's disease. *J Pediatr Gastro Nutr* 1996;23:A344.
53. Whittington PF, Barnes HV, Bayless TM. Medical management of Crohn's disease in adolescence. *Gastroenterology* 1977;72:1338–45.
54. Escher JC, and the European Collaborative Pediatric IBD Research Group. Budesonide versus prednisolone for the treatment of active Crohn's disease in children: a randomised, double-blind, controlled, multicenter trial. *Eur J Gastroenterol Hepatol* 2004;16:47–54.
55. Papi C, Luchetti R, Gili L, *et al*. Budesonide in the treatment of Crohn disease: a meta-analysis. *Aliment Pharmacol Ther* 2000;14:1419–28.
56. Kundhal P, Zachos M, Smith J, Griffiths AM. Controlled ileal release budesonide in children with Crohn's disease: a retrospective assessment of efficacy and effect on growth. *J Pediatr Gastro Nutr* 2001;33:75–80.
57. Markowitz J. A multicentre trial of 6-mercaptopurine and prednisolone in children with newly diagnosed Crohn's disease. *Gastroenterology* 2000;119:895–902.
58. Nicholls S, Vieira MC, Majrowski WH, *et al*. Linear growth after colectomy for ulcerative colitis in childhood. *J Pediatr Gastro Nutr* 1995;21:82–6.
59. Griffiths AM, *et al*. Factors influencing the postoperative recurrence of Crohn's disease in childhood. *Gut* 1991;32:491–5.
60. Davies G, Evans CM, Shand WS, Walker-Smith JA. Surgery for Crohn's disease in childhood: influence of site of disease and operative procedure on outcome. *Br J Surg* 1990;77:891–4.
61. Borrelli O, Bascietto C, Viola F, *et al*. Infliximab heals intestinal inflammatory lesions and resotres growth in children with Crohn's disease. *Dig Liver Dis* 2004;36:342–7.
62. Walters T, Gilman AR, Griffiths AM. Infliximab restores normal growth in prepubertal patients with chronically active Crohn disease. *Gastroenterology* 2005;A.
63. Mauras N, George D, Evans J, *et al*. Growth hormone has anabolic effects in glucocorticosteroid-dependent children with inflammatory bowel disease: a pilot study. *Metabolism* 2002;51:127–35.

27: Osteopenia

Subrata Ghosh

Introduction

Osteopenia or low bone mineral density (BMD) is a recognised complication of inflammatory bowel disease (IBD). Genant et al. [1] first reported significantly reduced bone mass in adolescents and adults with IBD using spinal and metacarpal radiographs. Availability of more precise and reproducible quantitative measurements of BMD confirmed the earlier finding [2, 3]. The pathogenesis of osteopenia in IBD is multi-factorial and incompletely understood. As expected, vitamin D deficiency in Crohn's disease (CD) and associated osteomalacia has been described [4], but osteopenia with normal vitamin D metabolites [5] is more common. A number of studies established the high prevalence of osteopenia in IBD, both CD and ulcerative colitis (UC) [2, 6, 7]. Decrease in total body calcium has been reported [8] and histomorphometric data are consistent with reduced bone formation [9]. However, with the availability of more sophisticated and sensitive methods of investigating bone metabolism, a more complex and variable effect of IBD on bone metabolism may be appreciated. Osteoporosis, osteomalacia due to vitamin D deficiency and osteonecrosis due to corticosteroids are all known to occur in IBD.

As vitamin D deficiency is no longer common, the two principal factors incriminated in causing osteopenia in IBD are inflammation and iatrogenic, i.e. corticosteroid-induced, bone loss. The relative importance of these two factors are currently debated vigorously, but resolution of this issue is fundamental to rational preventive and therapeutic measures.

Bone physiology

There are two types of bone tissue in adults: cortical or compact bone and spongy or cancellous bone. Eighty per cent of the skeletal mass is cortical. The remaining cancellous bone comprises trabecular plates and rods of tissue, which interconnect with each other [10]. The disposition of trabecular plates and rods is oriented predominantly according to lines of stress. Trabecular bone, the predominant bone at the femoral neck and spine, is metabolically more active and more prone to corticosteroid-induced bone loss.

Bone comprises an organic matrix, a mineral phase and bone cells. The majority of the matrix is composed of collagen. Adult bones contain type 1 collagen laid down by osteoblasts. Each unit of collagen (tropocollagen) comprises a protein heterotrimer consisting of two $\alpha1$ chains and one $\alpha2$ chain. Post-translational modification of synthesised protein consists of hydroxylation of proline and lysine. Hydroxyproline and hydroxylysine release during the metabolism of bone can be utilised as an index of bone break down. Glycosylation and the formation of cross-links with other tropocollagen macromolecules permit their assembly to form collagen fibrils, and evidence of such activity can be measured in serum and urine. Other proteins incorporated within the collagen matrix during or after its formation include proteoglycans, glycoproteins, osteocalcin and osteonectin. Osteocalcin is used to assess the rate of bone turnover in the evaluation of osteoporosis. Hydroxyapatite crystals composed of calcium, phosphate and carbonate form the mineral phase of bone. The crystals also contain other ions such as sodium, magnesium and fluoride.

All bone surfaces are covered by cells with distinct morphological and functional features [10]. These include osteoblasts, osteoclasts and osteocytes. The osteoblast is the cell responsible for the synthesis of collagen and other bone proteins. Osteocytes are osteoblasts that have been trapped within the bone matrix during the process of bone formation. The osteoclast is a multi-nucleated cell, which is responsible for bone resorption. It degrades fully mineralised bone by attaching onto a bone surface and secreting acids and lysosomal enzymes.

Bone remodelling is a constant process in adult bone. Old bone is removed by osteoclasts and replaced by new bone formed by osteoblasts. The term 'coupling' refers to the sequence of bone resorption followed by formation, and the term 'balance' describes the equality of these two processes within individual remodelling units [11]. Mechanical stimuli and endocrine factors such as sex hormones, glucocorticoids, thyroxine, growth hormone and parathyroid hormone exert important effects on bone cells. These effects may be mediated through prostaglandins, nitric oxide, cytokines and growth factors [12]. There are two mechanisms of bone loss in osteoporosis.

1 Increased bone turnover where the number of remodelling units is increased. This results in an increase in the percentage of bone surface occupied by resorption cavities.
2 Negative remodelling imbalance where the bone loss results from bone formation being less than resorption within a remodelling unit.

Increased bone turnover is associated with an increased likelihood of trabecular penetration and erosion, with loss of connectivity of the cancellous bone structure. Remodelling imbalance is associated with trabecular thinning and relatively greater preservation of bone architecture.

Corticosteroids and bone loss

Corticosteroids affect both bone resorption and formation [13]. Resorption is mediated partly by increased parathyroid hormone secretion secondary to calcium malabsorption and increased renal losses. Corticosteroids directly affect osteoblast proliferation, differentiation and activity and also inhibit bone formation by reduced local production of prostaglandin E2 and insulin-like growth factor (IGF)-1. Reduced production of gonadal hormones by the adrenal gland, ovaries and testes may contribute to corticosteroid-induced bone loss [14]. Cancellous bone is metabolically more active than cortical bone and is preferentially affected in corticosteroid-induced bone loss. Thus, the spine and ribs are especially vulnerable. Histomorphometric studies in patients with corticosteroid-induced osteopenia have shown low or normal bone turnover with negative remodelling imbalance due to reduced bone formation [15]. Calcium kinetic studies suggest that increased bone turnover may occur during the early stages of treatment [16].

Physical activity and bone mass

Epidemiological data suggest that lack of physical activity is a risk factor for osteoporotic fracture and exercise can increase BMD both in young adults as well as in post-menopausal women and in elderly people [17, 18]. Although prolonged immobilisation induces bone loss, there is little evidence that normal variations in daily physical activity are responsible for variations in rates of bone loss [10]. Physical exercise improves BMD, but it is difficult to change a habit of a lifetime, the effects are modest and persist only for the duration of exposure to the exercise.

Effect of cytokines on bone metabolism

When leucocytes are exposed to mitogens or antigens *in vitro*, they release bone-resorbing activity into the culture supernatants, which can be detected by bioassay [19]. Like many lymphocyte-monocyte products, this activity has been difficult to purify because of its low abundance in activated leukocyte cultures and the unwieldy bioassay required to detect biological activity. Partially purified preparations of this activity inhibit bone collagen synthesis in organ cultures of foetal rat calvarias

[20]. As both tumour necrosis factor (TNF)-α and TNF-β are likely to be present in activated leucocyte supernatants, purified recombinant preparations were tested for their effects on bone resorption and bone collagen synthesis *in vitro* [21]. Both cytokines at 10^{-7}M to 10^{-9}M caused osteoclastic bone resorption and inhibited bone collagen synthesis. These data suggest that at least part of the bone-resorbing activity present in activated leucocyte culture supernatants may be due to these cytokines. Interleukin (IL)-6 has similar bone-resorbing activity. Experimental colitis induced by instillation of trinitrobenzene-sulphonic acid with ethanol in a rat model results in bone loss [22], providing further evidence of the role of intestinal inflammation in causing osteopenia.

A number of cytokines have been implicated in osteoclast formation. IL-1, TNF and IL-6 have all been shown to affect osteoclast development [23]. It has been recently shown that IL-11 derived from mesenchymal cells provides a more central signal for osteoclast formation [24]. IL-6 increases the recruitment of osteoclast precursors to the osteoclast pool, but IL-6 may not play a role in osteoclast development in physiological conditions, and may only become important in oestrogen-deficient states [25].

Bone resorption mediated by cytokines

Bone-resorbing cytokines are generally active at low concentrations, and IL-1 is the most potent [26]. These act primarily as stimulators of osteoclast formation, although they can affect mature osteoclast function as well [27]. Both IL-1 and TNF-α stimulate multi-nucleated cell formation in long-term bone-marrow culture [28], and these agents act as growth factors for osteoclast precursors, which are of the monocyte-macrophage lineage. Both granulocyte-macrophage colony-stimulating factor (GM-CSF) and macrophage colony-stimulating factor (M-CSF) stimulate multi-nucleated cell formation in long-term bone-marrow cultures [29]. IL-6 has stimulatory effects on haemopoietic stem-cell proliferation *in vitro* [30], and as such may increase the availability of osteoclast precursors. Some cytokines may have permissive effects on bone resorption by maintaining adequate numbers of early osteoclast precursors (GM-CSF, M-CSF and IL-6), whereas others act more locally and quickly to produce large numbers of the relatively more differentiated osteoclast precursors required for osteoclast formation (IL-1 and TNF-α). IL-17 is a recently cloned cytokine that is exclusively produced by activated T cells. IL-17 in combination with TNF-α but not IL-1β increases osteoclastic bone resorption *in vitro*, and IL-17 receptor messenger RNA (mRNA) is expressed by osteoblastic cells in the mouse [31]. Interferon (IFN)-γ may be a candidate factor responsible for termination of osteoclast activity and inhibit basal and cytokine-stimulated bone resorption [32]. IFN-γ decreases the number of osteoclasts and the recruitment of osteoclast precursors rather than having direct calcitonin-like inhibitory effects on mature osteoclasts [33]. IL-4 has also been found to inhibit bone resorption both *in vitro* and *in vivo* [34].

Bone formation mediated by cytokines

Cytokines have effects on both the initial phase of recruitment and differentiation of osteoblast precursors and the later phase of bone matrix production and mineralisation by the mature osteoblasts. Two groups of cytokines with effects on bone formation can be identified. The first group contains those cytokines that stimulate bone-cell proliferation but have inhibitory effects on mature osteoblast function. These agents are generally potent stimulators of bone resorption such as IL-1 and TNF-α. The second group can be categorised as members of the transforming growth factor (TGF)-β family and includes TGF-β, IGFs and bone morphogenetic proteins (BMPs). These agents stimulate both precursor proliferation and mature osteoblast function [35].

Local production of cytokines in bone

Local production of cytokines within the bone micro-environment may be by non-skeletal haematopoietic or immunological cells, or by osteoblasts and osteoclasts. Osteoblasts are capable of secreting most of the osteotropic cytokines *in vitro*.

Synthesis of local cytokines interacts with local cellular events (osteoclast activation or initiation of bone formation) and the effect depends on the stage of development of the skeleton (foetal vs adult) [12]. Cultured osteoblasts from patients with rheumatoid arthritis, osteoarthritis and post-traumatic patients constitutively secrete IL-8, monocyte chemoattractant protein 1 (MCP-1) and growth-related gene product (GRO-a) [36]. However, the cultured osteoblasts do not release IL-1α, IL-1β or TNF-α.

Regulation of cytokine actions in bone

IL-1 has synergistic effects on bone resorption *in vitro* with TNF-α [37] and IL-6 [38]. IL-1 also induces the synthesis and secretion of TNF-α [39]. TGF-β transcription, however, is regulated by osteotropic hormones rather than cytokines, and levels are reduced in vitamin D-deficient animals [40]. Control mechanisms include inhibitory effects of soluble receptors or receptor antagonist proteins such as IL-1 receptor antagonist. Bone metabolism is influenced by the combined effects of a number of cytokines and a high degree of redundancy may exist with no cytokine having a unique role. Interaction with the extra-cellular matrix or modulation of integrin expression may provide further complicated regulation.

The role of cytokines in the pathogenesis of bone disease

Bone destruction in multiple myeloma, rheumatoid arthritis and post-menopausal osteoporosis may result from excess local or generalised production of cytokines. The malignant plasma cells of myeloma release cytokines such as IL-6, TNF-α and IL-1 mediating osteoclast activity and bone destruction. Cytokine levels in the rheumatoid joint favour osteoclast action and juxta-articular osteoporosis and bony erosions. These include high levels of IL-1, TNF-α, IL-6 and M-CSF, but low levels of IFN-γ. It has also been shown that the release of M-CSF and IL-6 by activated cells in the arthroplasty membrane is likely to contribute to pathological bone resorption [41]. In post-menopausal osteoporosis, evidence supports the indirect effect of oestrogen via modulation of cytokine production. Both IL-1 and TNF secretion by peripheral blood monocytes are raised in post-menopausal women [42], and the administration of oestrogen to oophorectomised women is associated with a normalisation of cytokine production [43]. Osteoblast IL-6 production may also be modulated by oestrogen [44].

Measurement of BMD

Osteoporosis is characterised by low bone mass and disruption of bone architecture, leading to reduced bone strength and increased fracture risk. Measurement of BMD provides the best prediction of future fracture risk [45–47] especially in women. Dual-energy X-ray absorptiometry (DEXA) is the most accurate and reproducible method of measuring BMD [11]. It involves a low radiation dose and can measure bone mass in both axial and appendicular skeleton. Dual photon absorptiometry (DPA), single-photon absorptiometry, single X-ray absorptiometry, broadband ultrasonic attenuation and quantitative computed tomography (CT) scanning are also accurate, alternative methods of measuring BMD [11]. Single-photon absorptiometry and single X-ray absorptiometry are suited for BMD measurement at the radius, whereas broadband ultrasonic attenuation is suited for the os calcis. Axial bone mass may be determined by DEXA, DPA and quantitative CT. Prospective studies have demonstrated an increasing fracture risk with decreasing BMD and a reduction of one standard deviation in BMD is associated with a two- to three-fold increase in fracture risk [45–47].

Lateral radiograph of the dorsal and lumbar spine provides evidence of subtle changes in vertebral shape. New generation DEXA-scan images are good enough to be a substitute. Bone biopsy should be considered in severe osteopenia to exclude osteomalacia.

Biochemical markers of bone metabolism

For many years the two markers available were serum alkaline phosphatase (bone formation) and urinary hydroxyproline (bone resorption). Serum alkaline phosphatase may be raised with cholestatic (e.g. sclerosing cholangitis) as well as parenchymal liver disease (e.g. fatty liver), and distinction from bone disease requires clinical details as well as isoenzymes of alkaline phosphatase. Urinary hydroxyproline excretion is influenced by diet and a 24-h collection is necessary. Recently, new biochemical markers of both bone formation and bone resorption have been introduced. Bone-specific alkaline phosphatase (BAP) and plasma osteocalcin specifically reflect osteoblastic activity and are markers of bone formation. Bone resorption is reflected by degradation of collagen type I, which is a major component of bone matrix. After incorporation of collagen into the bone matrix, cross-links are formed to stabilise the collagen fibrils. Bone resorption is characterised by release of pyridinoline (Pyr) and deoxypyridinoline (D-pyr), the mature cross-links that are synthesised by the post-translational modification of collagen molecules, either as the protein-bound (Pyr and D-pyr), free form (DPD), or the cross-linked N-terminal telopeptide of type I collagen (NTX). Pyr, D-Pyr, DPD and NTX all reflect bone resorption. The development of these new, more specific and sensitive non-invasive biochemical markers of bone metabolism in serum or urine has increased the chance of early identification of patients with increased risk of rapid bone loss [48].

Multi-factorial pathogenesis of osteopenia in IBD

Various factors such as small-intestinal resection, vitamin D deficiency [49], smoking, body mass index and height have been correlated with osteopenia in IBD, reflecting the heterogeneous nature of the cohorts studied by various workers. Osteocalcin, bone matrix Gla protein and protein S are involved in bone formation and are vitamin K-dependent. Therefore vitamin K deficiency due to intestinal disease may also affect bone formation and metabolism [50]. It is still not known the extent to which bone mineral loss in IBD occurs as an integral manifestation of the disease as distinct from the secondary osteopenic influences of

Table 27.1 Multi-factorial aetiology of osteopenia in inflammatory bowel disease. Possible contributing factors to osteopenia and their relevance to Crohn's disease (CD) or ulcerative colitis (UC).

Disease-related	CD
Corticosteroid therapy	CD + UC
Calcium, vitamin D deficiency	CD
Inactivity	CD + UC
Hypogonadism/amenorrhoea	CD
Malnutrition	CD + UC
Surgical resection	CD
Vitamin D receptor polymorphism	CD-μ
Smoking	CD

corticosteroid therapy, surgical intervention, inactivity, malabsorption of calcium and vitamin D or the cachexia of inflammation (Table 27.1).

Gender, age and body weight are major determinants of BMD in the normal population as well as the IBD patients [51]. No correlation between bone loss and serum parameters of calcium metabolism has been demonstrated [6]. Although the deleterious effects of corticosteroids on trabecular bone mass are well documented [52], longitudinal studies in patients with IBD have failed to show any significant correlation between the rate of bone loss and prednisolone therapy [7]. Conflicting evidence from cross-sectional studies, however, indicated that cumulative corticosteroid use might be an important or even the sole cause [53] of osteopenia in patients with IBD. This is contradicted by other cross-sectional studies [54, 55]. Increased bone resorption has been described in patients with CD [56] and in IBD patients as a group [57, 58], while bone formation (assessed by bone alkaline phosphatase) is especially suppressed in patients on corticosteroids [58].

Prevalence of osteopenia in IBD

Osteopenia is a common problem in the general population and a 50-year-old Caucasian woman has a 40% chance of fracture in her lifetime and a similar man has a 14% chance of fracture in his lifetime.

OSTEOPENIA

Table 27.2 Estimation of *T*- and *Z*-scores in the measurement of bone mineral density (BMD).

T-Score = Number of SD the BMD is above or below young adult mean.
Z-Score = Number of SD the BMD is above or below age and gender matched mean.

BMD is generally expressed as *T*-scores (to estimate fracture risk) or *Z*-scores (to compare different groups with varying age and sex mix) as shown in Table 27.2.

The World Health Organisation has provided pragmatic definitions of osteopenia and osteoporosis based on BMD measurements as follows: Osteopenia: *T*-score less than or equal to -1; Osteoporosis: *T*-score less than or equal to -2.5.

The risk of fragility fractures based on these *T*-scores are best established for women (especially post-menopausal) and should not be applied to men without further data. The reported prevalence of osteopenia and osteoporosis in IBD is highly variable (Table 27.3) and much of this variation is related to

Table 27.3 Prevalence of osteopenia and osteoporosis in inflammatory bowel disease.

Study (first author, reference)	n	Prevalence
Osteopenia		
Abitbol [97]	84	43%
Roux [98]	23	48%
Dinca [71]	103	32–42%
Vogelsang [85]	30	31%
Schulte [55]	149	33–44%
Bjarnason [57]	79	78%
Osteoporosis		
Motley [99]	70	33%
Roux [98]	23	26%
Vogelsang [85]	30	31%
Bjarnason [57]	79	29%
Dinca [71]	103	6%
Clements [3]	50	10%
Compston [6]	75	30%
Schulte [55]	149	10–16%
Pigot [2]	61	23%

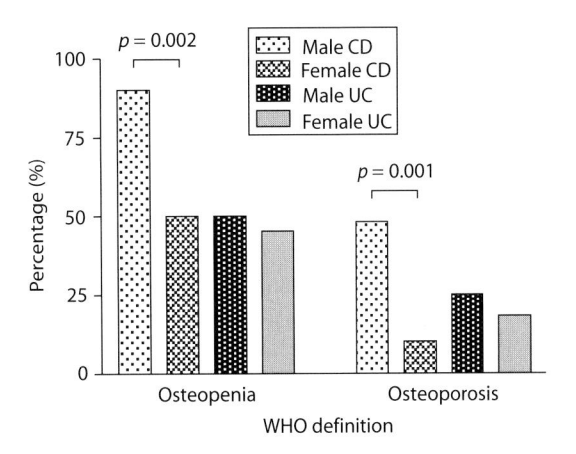

Fig 27.1 Prevalence of osteopenia and osteoporosis according to WHO definition in inflammatory bowel disease patients in Edinburgh. Although osteopenia is very prevalent in male Crohn's disease patients, the validity of the WHO cutoff values for *T*-scores in men is doubtful.

patient selection, proportion of CD and UC patients, referral patterns and type of institution, median duration of disease and treatment preferences. The general prevalence figures conceal important disease and sex differences. It can be seen from Fig 27.1 that out of 94 unselected patients with IBD in our unit, 90% of male CD patients were osteopenic compared with 50% of female CD patients ($c^2 = 9.9$, $P = 0.002$). Osteoporosis was also more common in male CD patients compared with female CD patients (48 vs 10%; $\chi^2 = 11.8$, $P = 0.001$). UC patients, however, showed no such gender differences. Detailed study of gonadal function in men with CD has not been reported, but low free androgen index with normal gonadotrophins may occur and serum testosterone is significantly correlated with plasma osteocalcin [59]. It is not known, however, whether the same cut-off values for BMD are applicable to men, as men achieve a higher peak bone mass than women and have larger bones. Bone loss may be significantly higher in patients on steroids (compared with those not on steroids) at the femoral neck and Ward's triangle, but not at the spine or total body [55]. The greater prevalence of reduced hip BMD as opposed to vertebral BMD has also been described by Bjarnason *et al.* [57]. In patients with ileal pouch-anal anastomosis for UC, low BMD may be reversible after surgery [60]. The current trend is to express lifetime fracture risk rather than *T*-scores in deciding on specific intervention in a patient.

The prevalence of fractures in IBD

Asymptomatic vertebral fractures are common in CD. In the MATRIX multi-centre European/Israeli study investigating budesonide with a focus on bone loss, 25 of 179 steroid-free patients (14%) and 13 of 89 (14.6%) of steroid-dependent patients had asymptomatic vertebral fractures [61]. Even 12.4% of steroid-naïve patients had vertebral fractures and overall, the fracture rate was not correlated with lifetime steroid dose suggesting that the contribution of disease itself to fractures is considerable. The fracture rate was not correlated with bone mineral density, a useful caveat against using BMD as the sole predictive factor for development of fractures.

In a primary care-based nested case-control study based on the General Practice Research Database (GPRD) managed by Medicines Control Agency (MCA) in the United Kingdom, 231,778 fracture cases and an equal number of age-gender matched controls were recruited and the prevalence of CD and UC was 156 and 282 per 100,000 respectively. Patients with IBD had an increased risk of vertebral fracture (OR 1.72, 95% CI 1.13–2.61) and hip fracture (OR 1.59, 95% CI 1.14–2.23). The risk of hip fracture was significantly greater in patients with CD compared with patients with UC [62]. Disease severity predicted fractures even after adjusting for corticosteroid use (Fig 27.2), and this provides estimates of 10-year fracture risks for IBD patients above the age of 50.

In a population-based cohort of UC patients resident in Olmsted County, Minnesota, fracture-risk was not elevated relative to matched community control subjects [63], suggesting that the impact on bones may be less in UC.

The difference between UC and CD

CD may be considered a systemic disease whereas UC is usually limited to colonic mucosal inflammation alone; CD also has important immunological differences from UC [64]. Newly diagnosed patients were studied by us [65] in order to avoid most of the secondary osteopenic influences mentioned previously. The measurement of BMD was repeated about a year after diagnosis to assess progressive bone loss and the effects of therapy. Both spine and forearm BMDs were studied so that trabecular and cortical mineralisation could be assessed, as there are metabolic differences between these two types of bones [66].

At diagnosis, the mean spine Z score in CD patients was significantly lower ($P < 0.01$) than the UC patients (-1.2 ± 0.6 vs 0.1 ± 0.7). The patients were recruited prior to steroid therapy or surgical resection. The mean spine Z-score after 1 year was unchanged despite the majority of patients receiving steroid therapy.

Plasma Ca, PO_4, urinary Ca/creatinine, urinary PO_4/creatinine, urinary hydroxyproline/creatinine, 25-OH vitamin D, alkaline phosphatase, immunoreactive parathormone (iPTH) were all normal at diagnosis. Bone alkaline phosphatase and plasma osteocalcin were similar in CD and UC, but bone resorption markers Dpd/creatinine and Pyd/creatinine were significantly higher in CD than in UC (Fig 27.3a). There was no difference between colonic disease and small-bowel disease in CD patients.

Few of the other previous studies on BMD in IBD patients have documented differences between CD and UC. It is noteworthy that none of these studies had recruited only newly diagnosed patients and scrutiny of the results showed that their cohorts of IBD patients had long-standing disease. It is likely that in such cohorts, many confounding variables will have been present, particularly prolonged steroid therapy and surgical interventions along with complex nutritional deficiencies, so that any primary effect of the disease would be masked. A population-based study from Norway confirmed reduced BMD in 60 patients with CD but not in 60 patients with UC [67], but other studies [57] have found no significant differences between CD and UC. Serum from children with CD-affected osteoblast function and produced osteopenia in foetal rat bone substrate but serum from UC patients produced no effect [68]. In a recently reported Dutch

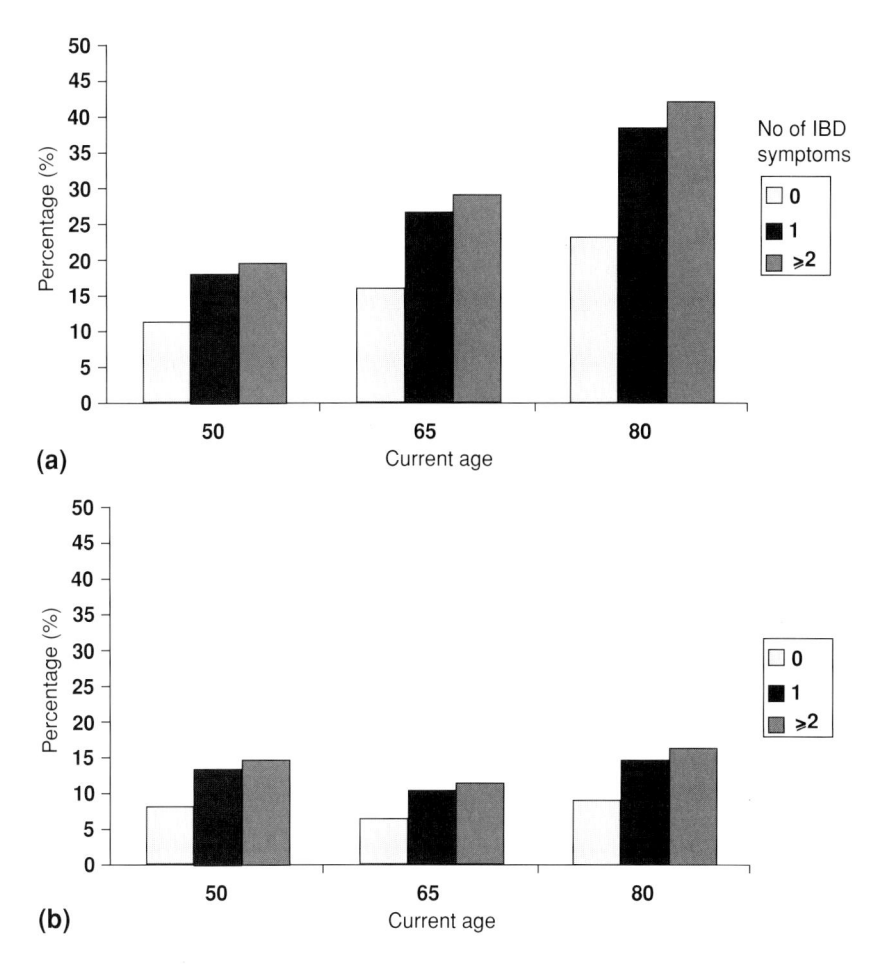

Fig 27.2 Estimated 10-year risk of any fracture (% in Y-axis) in patients with IBD stratified by the number of IBD symptoms, reflecting disease severity. Adapted from data in [62]. Current age given as X-axis: (a) in IBD women; (b) in IBD men.

case-control study, there was no difference in BMD between recently diagnosed CD and UC patients and IBD patients were not osteopenic compared to population controls [69, 70]. However, most of the patients in this cohort had already been treated with steroids and had inactive disease.

In order to resolve this discrepancy we prospectively recruited three groups of IBD patients between the ages of 20 and 75 years. Exclusion criteria were cholestatic liver disease such as primary sclerosing cholangitis, thyroid disorders, renal failure and hormone replacement therapy prescribed specifically for osteoporosis. The three groups were as follows (Fig 27.4a).

Group 1. Newly diagnosed patients. Twenty-one newly diagnosed CD patients and 20 newly diagnosed UC patients were recruited into this study. This was a different cohort from the newly diagnosed patients reported above. BMD measurements were done prior to commencement of any therapy. The mean Z-score for spine BMD was significantly lower in CD ($P < 0.02$) compared with UC (−1.11 (SD 0.57) vs 0.27 (SD 0.54)). The forearm Z-score showed a similar difference between CD and UC (−1.18 (SD 0.67) vs 0.08 (SD 0.74)) ($P < 0.01$). No patient had suffered any pathological fractures within a year of their diagnosis.

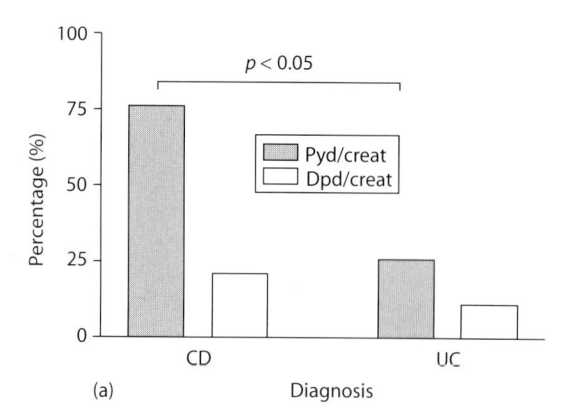

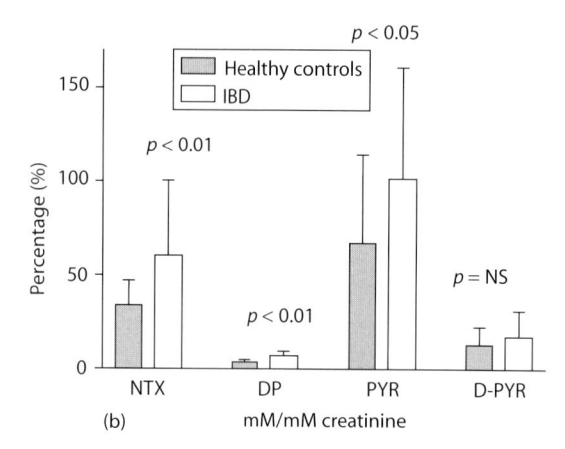

Fig 27.3 (a) Urinary bone resorption markers (indexed against creatinine excretion) in newly diagnosed inflammatory bowel disease (IBD) patients from Edinburgh, separated into Crohn's disease and ulcerative colitis. Pyd: pyridinoline; Dpd: deoxypyridinoline; creat: creatinine. (b) Four urinary bone resorption markers in IBD patients compared with healthy controls. NTX: cross-linked N-terminal telopeptide of type I-collagen; PYR: pyridinoline (Data adapted from Schulte et al. [58]).

Group 2. Patients with intermediate duration of disease. BMD was also measured in 19 patients with CD and 15 patients with UC who did not fulfil the criteria for either group 1 or group 3, i.e. they had disease duration between 6 months and 4 years. The mean Z-score for spine BMD in CD was 1.09 (SD 0.53) and in UC was −0.06 (SD 0.72). This difference is statistically significant ($P < 0.01$). The mean Z-score for forearm BMD in CD was −1.12 (SD 0.78) and in UC was 0.03 (SD 0.72) ($P < 0.01$). No patients had suffered from pathological fractures after diagnosis of IBD.

Group 3. Long-standing disease. The criteria set for patient recruitment were disease duration from diagnosis 35 years and duration of steroid therapy 36 months. Twenty-eight patients with CD and 26 patients with UC were recruited in the study. The mean Z-score for spine BMD in CD was −1.36 (SD 0.81) and in UC was −1.12 (SD 0.57); $P = NS$. The mean Z-score for forearm BMD in CD was −1.24 (SD 1.12) and in UC was −1.18 (SD 0.64), $P = NS$. Following the diagnosis of IBD, two patients with CD had suffered from vertebral collapse and one patient with CD from a fractured humerus after a fall.

In CD, the correlation between the duration of disease and spine or forearm BMD Z-score is weak ($r = −0.18$, $P < 0.05$). There was no significant difference in the spine and forearm Z-scores between the three disease duration groups. In UC there is a significant inverse linear relationship between the duration of disease and spine BMD Z-score ($r = −0.78$, $P < 0.001$) and forearm BMD Z-score ($r = −0.75$, $P < 0.001$). There was no significant difference between newly diagnosed UC and UC of intermediate duration in their mean spine or forearm Z-scores (Fig 27.4a). However, both spine and forearm mean Z-scores (−1.12 (SD 0.57) and −1.18 (SD 0.64)) were significantly lower ($P < 0.05$) in long-standing UC than the corresponding Z-scores in newly diagnosed (0.27 (SD 0.54) and 0.08 (SD 0.74)) or intermediate duration (−0.06 (SD 0.72) and 0.03 (SD 0.72)) UC, respectively. All patients had received systemic steroids, apart from the newly diagnosed IBDs. Cumulative steroid dose was inversely related to spine BMD ($r = −0.66$, $P < 0.001$) and forearm BMD ($r = −0.70$, $P < 0.001$) in UC. In CD, the correlation between cumulative steroid dose and spine and forearm BMD was weaker (spine $r − 0.28$, $P < 0.01$; forearm $r = −0.22$, $P < 0.05$), and more obvious in the patients with long-standing disease.

Therefore, in patients with disease duration between 6 months and 4 years, the difference between CD and UC still persists, with only the former being osteopenic as a group. There was no difference

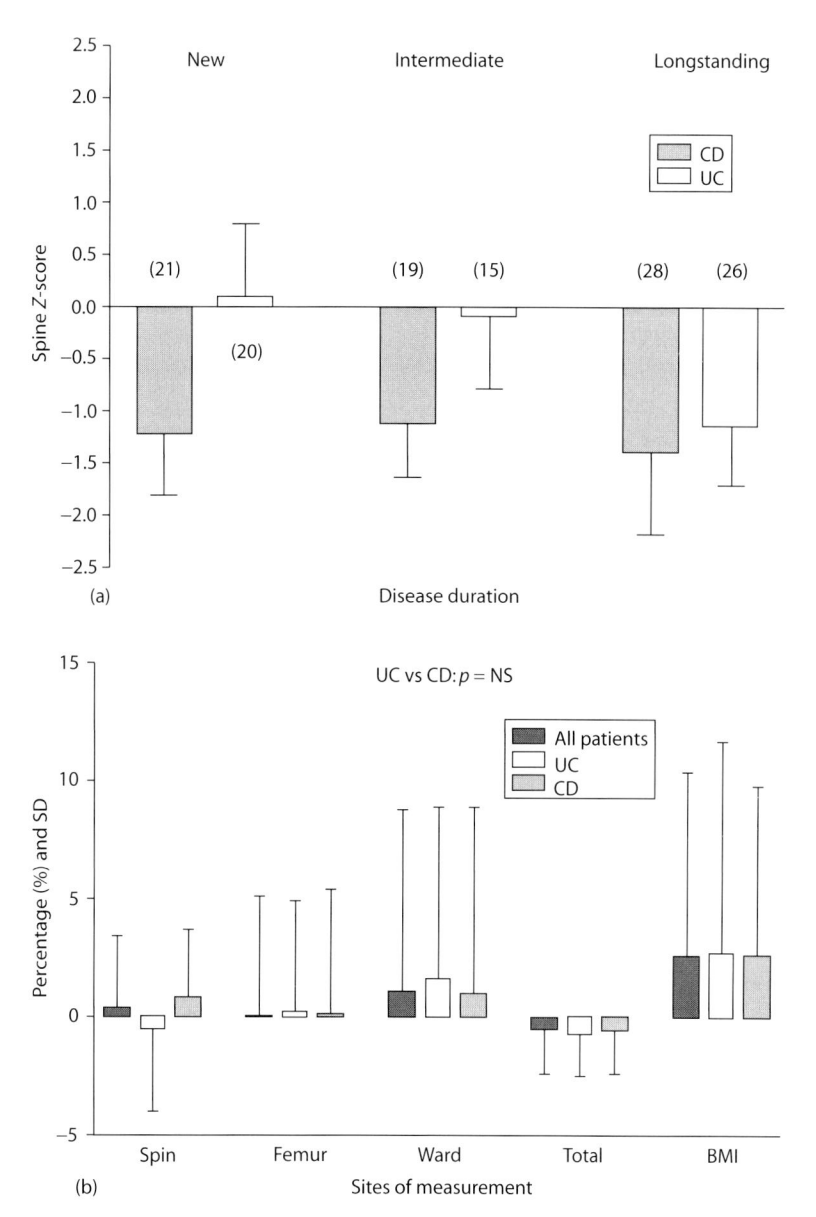

Fig 27.4 (a) Spine Z-scores in inflammatory bowel disease (IBD) cohorts from Edinburgh with different disease durations. New, newly diagnosed, prior to therapy, intermediate and between 6 months and 4 years; Long-standing, 5 years or more with steroid therapy for 6 months or more. Both new and intermediate Crohn's disease (CD) patients had significantly lower mean bone mineral density (BMD) than ulcerative colitis (UC) patients, but no such difference could be detected in long-standing IBD patients. (b) Annual change in BMD as a percentage of baseline at different sites of measurements in IBD patients. A negative percentage indicates net bone loss. (Data adapted from Schulte et al. [55]).

between the mean spine or forearm Z-score between newly diagnosed patients and patients with intermediate disease duration (Fig 27.4a), in spite of the latter group receiving corticosteroid therapy. The median duration of disease in the intermediate disease duration group was 3 years for both CD and UC. In our previous study [65], we had found no significant reduction in BMD following 1 year of systemic corticosteroid therapy. In patients with CD, it is likely that the osteopenic effects of systemic steroid therapy is counter-balanced by the improvement in disease activity upon treatment. In UC, although no significant difference was found between the two groups, the mean spine Z-score had changed from 0.27 to −0.06, with a median cumulative steroid dose of 2.8 g.

In patients with long-standing IBD (median disease duration 8 years for CD and 7 years for UC), there was no significant difference between CD and UC in their mean spine or forearm Z-scores. BMD Z-scores in long-standing UC patients were significantly lower than that in newly diagnosed or intermediate disease-duration UC patients. It is likely that this is the explanation for the lack of significant difference in BMD between CD and UC patients in the previous studies, which had all recruited patients with long-standing disease. In a tertiary referral centre, patient cohorts recruited consecutively from clinics are likely to be biased towards long-standing complicated disease.

In long-standing CD patients, the mean spine or forearm Z-scores were not significantly lower than that observed in newly diagnosed patients. Cumulative steroid dose was the most important factor related to low BMD in UC. Increased duration of disease was associated with increased cumulative steroid dose and was not an independent variable. The lack of significant difference between newly diagnosed and intermediate disease duration IBD patients suggested that the cumulative steroid dose had to exceed a certain threshold before resulting in significant bone loss. In CD, the interplay of factors leading to low BMD is more complex. A primary effect of the disease itself is important, as is evident in the newly diagnosed cohort. However, in a recent report, the BMD in recently diagnosed IBD patients was not significantly decreased compared with age- and gender-matched controls [70]. Our results are in agreement with a prospective Italian study on 54 CD and 49 UC patients with a mean observation period of 21 months. BMD in CD patients was stable, suggesting that low BMD was associated with the pathogenesis of CD. In contrast, BMD in UC patients decreased significantly, suggesting a correlation with corticosteroid therapy [71]. Schulte *et al.* [58] elegantly provided evidence for an increase in bone resorption in IBD patients (see Fig 27.3b) with low bone formation in patients on current corticosteroid therapy.

In a recent study, BMD was confirmed to be reduced at diagnosis prior to corticosteroid therapy in both CD and UC patients as a result of increased bone resorption, illustrating the general point that inflammation *per se* is an important determinant of bone loss [72].

Osteopenia in children with IBD

In children with IBD, retardation of growth and development is a serious problem, intensively investigated especially in patients with CD, but the effects of childhood-onset IBD on bone mineralisation also deserves attention. We have measured BMD in all children and teenagers currently under our care with IBD at this referral centre for IBD management. We compared the results with that in adults with IBD who were well matched as to other aspects of disease characteristics.

Twenty-two children with CD (10 male and 12 female) and 13 children with UC (6 male and 7 female) were included in the study. The median age was 15 (range 12–18) years. During the last 5 years we have measured BMD and collected clinical information in 213 adults with IBD. From this series, each child or adolescent was matched with one adult patient with IBD aged between 21 and 45 years (median age 32 years) of the same sex, who had similar anatomy of disease (ileal, colonic or ileocolonic) and similar disease duration (±2 months) and lifetime steroid use (±0.25g). In none of the adults was the disease onset in childhood. Each patient had their height measured without shoes and weight recorded in light clothes. Each of the patients completed a structured clinical assessment. Smoking status was recorded as non-smoker, ex-smoker or current smoker with the average number of cigarettes per day and duration of smoking quantified. Menstrual history including age of onset of menarche and use of oral contraceptive pill were recorded. Secondary sexual characteristics indicating pubertal status was assessed by genital development and pubic hair in boys (stage 1–5), and breast development and pubic hair in girls (stage 1–5) according to standard ratings. Each patient was then classified as: (i) pre-pubertal; (ii) early puberty; (iii) sexually mature, so that male and female patients could be grouped together. Bone age was assessed from a radiograph of the left wrist and hand (Greulich and

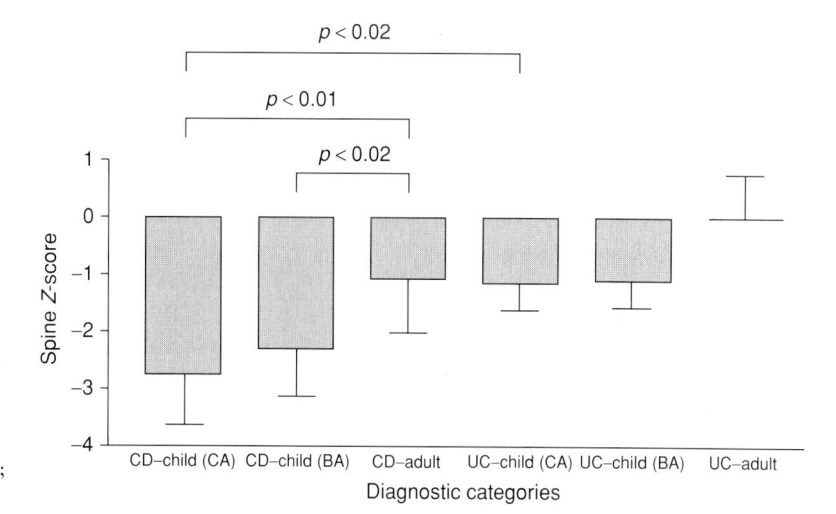

Fig 27.5 Spine Z-score in children and adolescents with inflammatory bowel disease (IBD) from Edinburgh, compared with disease-matched adults. BA: bone age; CA: chronological age.

Pyle). All radiographs were reported by a single, experienced radiologist.

The mean spine Z-score for children with CD was −2.75 (SD 0.87). This was significantly lower than in matched adults with CD (mean Z-score −1.06, SD 0.97; $P < 0.01$). Children with UC had a significantly greater ($P < 0.02$) spine Z-score (mean −1.14, SD 0.47) than children with CD. The mean spine Z-score in matched UC adults was 0.01 (SD 0.75) (Fig 27.5).

Radiological bone age in four patients with CD was 2.1–3 years below; in nine patients was 1.1–2 years below; and in nine patients was 0.6–1 years below chronological ages. All patients with UC had the same radiological bone age as their chronological age. Calculating spine Z-scores by using the radiological bone age instead of the chronological bone age gave a mean Z-score of −2.29 (SD 0.83) in children with CD, still significantly lower than adult patients ($P < 0.02$) (Fig 27.5).

Marked developmental delay was present in 13/22 patients with CD and in none with UC. Prepubertal patients had the lowest spine Z-scores, but the difference between pre-pubertal, early pubertal and sexually mature patients was not statistically significant. However, the 13 patients with marked developmental delay had a significantly lower ($P < 0.05$) mean spine Z-score (−3.44, SD 0.66) compared to the remaining nine patients with CD (mean Z-score −2.58, SD 0.98). When the BMD Z-scores were recalculated using radiological bone age, the difference between those with developmental delay and others was no longer significant.

Height retardation was common in patients with CD, and there was a significant correlation between height centiles and spine Z-scores ($r = 0.75$, $P < 0.001$). Body weight was less than 3rd centile in 6 out of 22, and between 3 and 25 centile in 10 out of 22 patients with CD. There was no correlation between weight centiles and spine Z-scores. When the spine Z-scores were recalculated using radiological bone age instead of chronological age, similar results were obtained. The correlation between height centiles and spine Z-scores calculated by radiological bone age was $r = 0.68$ ($P < 0.01$). None of the patients with UC was height-retarded.

The degree of osteopenia in this cohort of children with IBD, particularly CD recruited from a tertiary care centre, is worrying. Vertebral collapse and loss in height were seen in four out of 35 patients, testifying to the potentially devastating effect of osteopenia in this age group (Fig 27.6a,b). Growing bones are metabolically very active and it is possible that these are susceptible to multiple metabolic influences. Lack of physical activity due

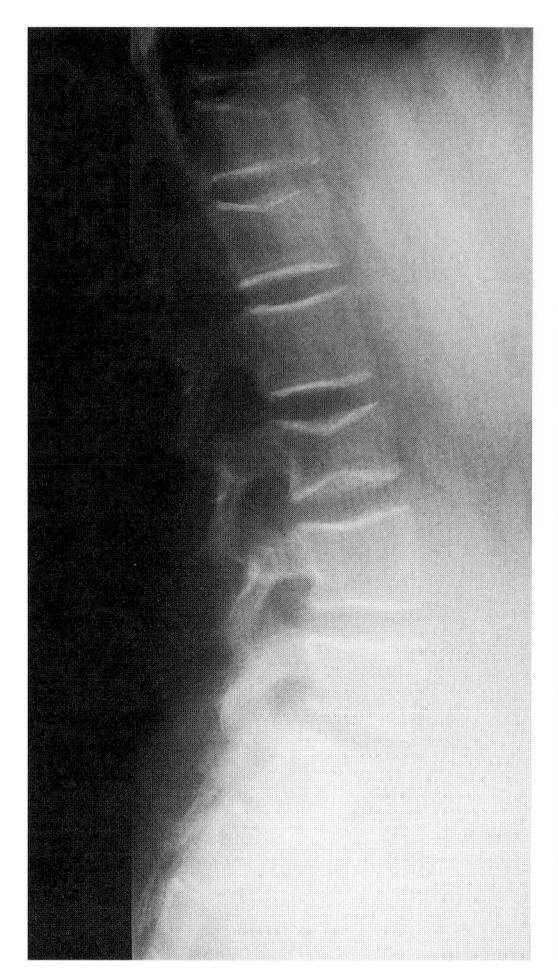

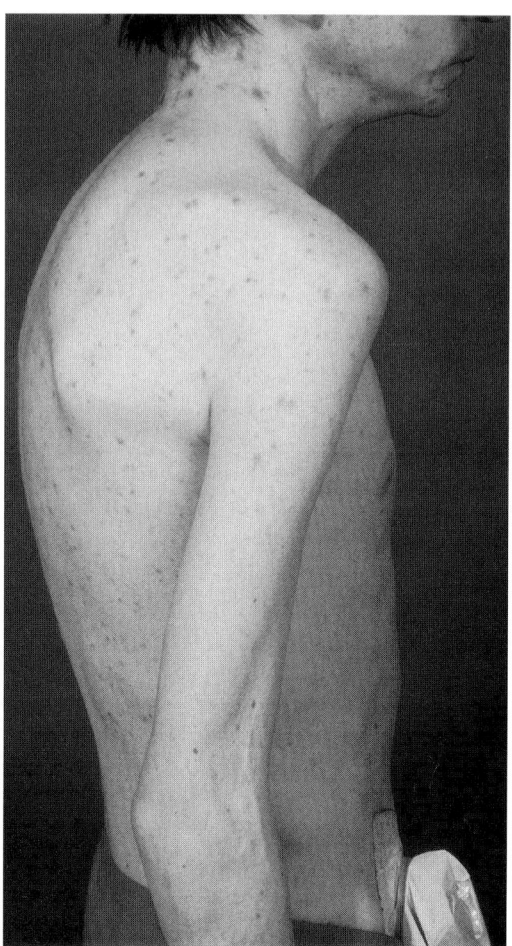

Fig 27.6 (a) Lateral radiograph of the lumbar spine showing vertebral collapse, loss of height and osteopenia in a 15-year-old boy with complicated Crohn's disease. Back pain was a prominent symptom; (b) a photograph of the same patient showing marked lordosis, muscle wasting and an ileostomy.

to hospitalisation and to symptoms of IBD may contribute to low bone density, as there was a marked reduction in physical activity grade at the time of study compared to pre-morbid level of activity. Issenman et al. [73] reported low bone density in paediatric CD compared with normal children, although the difference was less when compared with height-matched controls. Our study shows that osteopenia in children with CD is significantly more severe than in adults with CD even when matched according to other disease characteristics, and the mean spine Z-score is well below 2 SD of normal children data. The degree of osteopenia is very likely to increase pathological fractures, although this was obvious in only two children. Other groups have also reported that low BMD occurs more frequently in children with CD than in UC [74, 75].

Growth and sexual development are obviously important factors related to bone density in children with IBD. Height retardation was significantly related to osteopenia, and was a specific feature of CD. Although it is possible that smaller adolescents require less strong bones to carry their weight, no such effect was detectable for body weight alone.

Height retardation is related to growth delay, but recalculating Z-scores by radiological bone ages still showed a significant relation with height centiles. IGF-1 is a major regulator of bone growth during childhood and influences longitudinal growth. A recent study in healthy white children and adolescents suggests that IGF-I is a major determinant of the cross-sectional properties of bone, but does not influence the BMD [76]. The relationship between IGF-I signalling and bone turnover is complex [77].

Severe osteopenia should now be regarded as another feature of childhood CD, along with growth and developmental delay. In the most severely affected, it may lead to vertebral collapse, chronic back pain and loss in height, further aggravating the considerable morbidity in this group of patients. UC children and adolescents are far less seriously affected. This again highlights the difference between the systemic inflammation in CD and predominantly mucosal inflammation in UC, and a similar difference in morbidity can be seen in growth and developmental delay. For reasons mentioned above, radiological bone age requires monitoring in children and adolescents to fully determine the effect of IBD on the growing bone. Currently, recording of radiological bone age is widely neglected [78].

Management of osteopenia in IBD

Osteoporosis is far better prevented than reversed. Prevention relies on recognition of the problem. Certain general measures have some evidence in favour of improved bone density in the normal population, but usually not in IBD patients. Nevertheless, the following would be sensible advice to follow: (i) regular weight-bearing exercise [79], walking being the easiest, and walking also improves psychological and physical measures in CD [80]; (ii) use of steroids with low systemic availability such as budesonide may not necessarily be safer than conventional steroids; (iii) limitation of corticosteroid use, if necessary by the use of immunosuppressives and anti-TNF therapy; even low doses or short (2-month) courses [81] of corticosteroids are not safe; (iv) encouragement of adequate calcium and vitamin D intake; (v) discouragement of smoking;

Table 27.4 Patients who may be considered to be at high risk of osteopenia.

Oestrogen deficiency before the age of 45
Amenorrhoea for more than 1 year
Long-term use of corticosteroids
7.5 mg prednisolone: 3 months + low BMD
Cumulative steroid dose >10 g
Children <18 years (and below)

and (vi) test for frank vitamin D deficiency, which may occur in CD, regardless of macroscopic site of involvement [82]. However, as progressive bone loss is not the rule, and the rate of bone loss is variable and quite small [55], active pharmacological intervention in all IBD patients is currently not necessary. Certain groups of IBD patients should be considered at high risk of osteopenia and they are listed in Table 27.4. The pharmacological strategies to increase BMD in these patients may be sub-divided into those agents that reduce bone resorption and those agents that stimulate bone formation. The pharmacological agents that reduce bone resorption are: (i) oestrogens; (ii) bisphosphonates; (iii) calcitonin; (iv) vitamin D; and (v) raloxifene, an oestrogen receptor modulator. The pharmacological agents that stimulate bone formation are: (i) fluoride; (ii) PTH peptides; (iii) and strontium. Recently, the British Society of Gastroenterology (BSG) [83] has published the guidelines for the management of osteoporosis in IBD. It recommends 800 units of vitamin D daily in all patients who are on systemic steroids, and bisphosphonates for those with T-score less than or equal to -1.5. All patients with fragility fractures should be considered for hormone replacement therapy (HRT), bisphosphonates or calcitonin. However, the evidence base for many of the recommendations is not derived from IBD patients, and extrapolation from other diseases may not be appropriate. IBD patients with established osteoporosis or patients in high-risk groups may be considered for intervention with medications to improve BMD. Oestrogens in post-menopausal women [84] and low-dose vitamin D [85] have been shown to be effective in IBD patients. Vitamin K deficiency is also associated with osteopenia in IBD [86] but no interventional studies have been performed. The use of bisphosphonates is probably safe, but definitive trials are awaited. In the first published report of the use of 10 mg/day alendronate, lumbar BMD was increased in inactive Crohn's disease patients, and the drug was safe and well-tolerated [87]. In randomised, controlled studies both intravenous ibandronate [88] and pamidronate [89] with vitamin D/calcium administered every 3 months were well tolerated and effective in increasing lumbar and hip BMD. Fluoride may increase BMD, but the resultant bone may be more fragile and prone to fractures [90]. The BSG recommends measurement of serum testosterone in osteoporotic men aged below 55 years and replacement if low; however, treatment of active inflammation effectively alone may restore plasma testosterone to normal. A small study concluded that dihydroepiandrosterone sulfate (DHEAS) deficiency might contribute to bone loss in men with IBD [91]. Men aged above 55 years and post-menopausal women have been specifically targeted in the BSG recommendations, although it is increasingly becoming clear that children and adolescents may be a specific high-risk group. Table 27.5 summarises a pragmatic approach to the investigation of bone disease in IBD.

The therapeutic efficacy of bisphosphonates and calcitonin in glucocorticoid-induced osteoporosis may be in part due to their ability to prevent osteocyte and osteoblast apoptosis [92], caused by glucocorticoids. However, of particular relevance to IBD is the report from early rheumatoid arthritis patients [93] that treatment with alendronate can reduce IL-1, TNF-α, IL-6 and $β_2$-micro-globulin and decrease urinary cross links and urinary hydroxyproline. The use of budesonide in distal ileal CD is associated with less suppression of plasma osteocalcin than prednisolone, but budesonide is associated with bone loss as well. All high-risk patients should be on calcium and vitamin D supplements; post-menopausal women should either have oestrogen as well as, or instead of, these. Recent adverse publicity regarding oestrogen is increasingly making it an unpopular choice. It is associated with increased risk of venous thromboembolic and breast cancer. Strontium ranelate is a new drug recently launched for treatment of post-menopausal osteoporosis. As it increases bone formation (unlike bisphosphonates) and reduces bone resorption, it may be ideally suited for treatment of osteopenia in IBD from a scientific standpoint. It is also relatively inexpensive, safe and easy to use. It is administered orally once daily as a powder mixed with water and is palatable. However, unless studies are carried out specifically in IBD patients its use is unlikely to be accepted by the doctors treating such patients [94]. Teriparatide, recombinant parathyroid hormone, is only used under expert supervision. It is important to realise that bone loss cannot be explained by corticosteroid use alone. Schulte et al. [55] reported only a small change in bone density over 568 ± 60 days follow-up period (Fig 27.4b). Bone loss was significantly higher in patients with steroids than in those without steroids at the femoral neck and Ward triangle, but not at the spine and total body. Genetic factors too may be relevant. However, it is important to control inflammatory activity effectively, as BMD improves during remission in IBD [95].

Currently, only a minority of even high-risk patients are on appropriate therapy for protection of bones and prevention of fractures – in the GPRD fracture study referred to previously [62], only 13% of patients who had already sustained a fracture (and therefore at high risk of suffering from further fractures) were on any form of osteoprotective therapy. Physician and patient education is critically important and in the United Kingdom the National

Table 27.5 Assessment of bone density and metabolism in inflammatory bowel disease.

BMD by DEXA at diagnosis in CD patients, and in a high-risk group (see Table 27.4)

DEXA every 2–3 years in an average risk group (not required in UC patients not requiring systemic steroids and not osteopenic at baseline)

DEXA every year in a high-risk group (see Table 27.4)

Bone formation and resorption markers not routinely necessary

Plasma calcium, alkaline phos, 25-OH-vitamin D at diagnosis and yearly in CD patients

Lumbar spine radiograph only in patients with back pain as a prominent symptom

Record of cumulative steroid use

BMD: bone mineral density; DEXA: dual energy X-ray absorptiometry.

Association of Colitis and Crohn's disease (NACC) have published patient information material specifically related to bone problems in IBD.

Conclusion

Osteopenia in IBD is multi-factorial, with corticosteroid use being the most relevant determinant in UC and inflammatory activity being the most important determinant in CD. The rate of bone loss is variable and quite small in the majority of patients [96] and hence universal treatment with agents that improve BMD may be unnecessary. All patients should be encouraged to take adequate calcium and vitamin D (IBD patients often self-refrain from milk), exercise regularly and stop smoking. Patients at high risk or those with established osteoporosis should receive pharmacological intervention, although the ideal agent is yet to be determined. Bisphosphonates are currently the agent of choice and in patients with significant small intestinal absorption defects, may be administered intravenously. The real challenge is to decide when anti-inflammatory therapy is not enough to halt bone loss and specific pharmacological measures to reduce bone loss are necessary. Patient groups at high risk need to be defined precisely. Children are included in the high-risk group. The recent availability of data regarding fractures in IBD patients would help in the decision-making process. The risk of osteopenia is a major factor in the increasing trend to limit corticosteroid use in IBD patients in favour of a disease-modifying therapy. More powerful and effective anti-inflammatory therapy such as infliximab may reduce the impact of disease on bone loss and early evidence would be in support.

References

1. Genant HK, Mall JC, Wagonfeld JB, Horst JV, Lanzi, LH. Skeletal demineralization and growth retardation in inflammatory bowel disease. *Invest Radiol* 1976; 11:541–9.
2. Pigot F, Roux C, Chaussade S, *et al*. Low bone mineral density in patients with inflammatory bowel disease. *Dig Dis Sci* 1992;37:1396–403.
3. Clements D, Motley RJ, Evans WD, *et al*. Longitudinal study of cortical bone loss in patients with inflammatory bowel disease. *Scand J Gastroenterol* 1992;27:1055–60.
4. Driscoll RHJ, Meredith SC, Sitrin M, Rosenberg IH. Vitamin D deficiency and bone disease in patients with Crohn's disease. *Gastroenterology* 1982;83:1252–8.
5. Hessov I, Mosekilde L, Melsen F, *et al*. Osteopenia with normal vitamin D metabolites after small-bowel resection for Crohn's disease. *Scand J Gastroenterol* 1984;19:691–6.
6. Compston JE, Judd D, Crawley EO, *et al*. Osteoporosis in patients with inflammatory bowel disease. *Gut* 1987;28:410–15.
7. Motley RJ, Crawley EO, Evans C, Rhodes J, Compston JE. Increased rate of spinal trabecular bone loss in patients with inflammatory bowel disease. *Gut* 1988;29:1332–6.
8. Ryde SJ, Clements D, Evans WD, *et al*. Total body calcium in patients with inflammatory bowel disease: a longitudinal study. *Clin Sci* 1991;80:319–24.
9. Croucher PI, Vedi S, Motley RJ, Garrahan NJ, Stanton MR, Compston JE. Reduced bone formation in patients with osteoporosis associated with inflammatory bowel disease *Osteoporosis Int* 1993;3:236–41.
10. Kanis JA. *Osteoporosis*. Oxford: Blackwell Science, 1994.
11. Compston JE, Cooper C, Kanis JA. Bone densitometry in clinical practice [see comments]. *BMJ* 1995;310:1507–10.
12. Macdonald BR, Gowen M. Cytokines and bone. *Br J Rheumatol* 1992;31:149–55.
13. Valentine JF, Sninsky CA. Prevention and treatment of osteoporosis in patients with inflammatory bowel disease. *Am J Gastroenterol* 1999;94:878–83.
14. Compston JE. Review article: osteoporosis, corticosteroids and inflammatory bowel disease. *Aliment Pharmacol Ther* 1995;9:237–50.
15. Bressot C, Meunier PJ, Chapuy MC, Lejeune E, Edouard C, Darby A. Histomorphometric profile, pathophysiology and reversibility of corticosteroid-induced osteoporosis. *Metab Bone Dis Relat Res* 1979;1:303–11.
16. Cannigia A, Nuti R, Lore F, Vattimo A. Pathophysiology of the adverse effects of glucoactive corticosteroids on calcium metabolism in man. *J Steroid Biochem* 1981;15:153–61.
17. Heinonen A, Oja P, Kannus P, *et al*. Bone mineral density in female athletes representing sports with different loading characteristics of the skeleton. *Bone* 1995;17:197–203.

18. McMurdo MET, Mole PA, Paterson CR. Controlled trial of weight bearing exercise in older women in relation to bone density and falls. *Br Med J* 1997;314:569.
19. Mundy GR, Ibbotson KJ, D'Souza SM, Simpson EL, Jacobs JW, Martin TJ. The hypercalcemia of cancer. Clinical implications and pathogenic mechanisms. *N Engl J Med* 1984;310:1718-27.
20. Raisz LG. Local and systemic factors in the pathogenesis of osteoporosis. *N Engl J Med* 1988;318:818-28.
21. Bertolini DR, Nedwin GE, Bringman TS, Smith DD, Mundy GR. Stimulation of bone resorption and inhibition of bone formation *in vitro* by human tumour necrosis factors. *Nature* 1986;319:516-18.
22. Fries W, Giacomin D, Plebani M, Martin A. Effect of experimental colitis on bone metabolism in the rat. *Digestion* 1994;55:229-33.
23. Suda T, Takahashi N, Martin TJ. Modulation of osteoclast differentiation. *Endocr Rev* 1992;13:66-80.
24. Girasole G, Passeri G, Jilka RL, Manolagas SC. Interleukin-11: a new cytokine critical for osteoclast development. *J Clin Invest* 1994;93:1516-24.
25. Jilka RL, Hangoc G, Girasole G, et al. Increased osteoclast development after estrogen loss: mediation by interleukin-6. *Science* 1992;257:88-91.
26. Gowen M, Nedwin GE, Mundy GR. Preferential inhibition of cytokine-stimulated bone resorption by recombinant interferon gamma. *J Bone Min Res* 1986;1:469-74.
27. Thomson BM, Saklatvala J, Chambers TJ. Osteoblasts mediate interleukin-1 stimulation of bone resorption by rat osteoclasts. *J Exp Med* 1986;164:104-12.
28. Pfeilschifter J, Chenu C, Bird A, Mundy GR, Roodman GD. Interleukin-1 and tumour necrosis factor stimulate the formation of human osteoclast-like cells *in vitro*. *J Bone Min Res* 1989;4:113-18.
29. MacDonald BR, Mundy GR, Clark S. Effects of human recombinant CSF-GM and highly purified CSF-1 on the formation of multinucleated cells osteoclast characteristics in long-term bone marrow cultures. *J Bone Min Res* 1986;1:227-35.
30. Brandt J, Srour EF, van Besien K, Bridell RA, Hoffman R. Cytokine-dependent long-term culture of highly enriched precursors of hematopoietic progenitor cells from human bone marrow. *J Clin Invest* 1990;86:932-41.
31. Van Bezooijen RL, Farih-Sips HC, Papapoulos SE, Lowik CW. Interleukin-17: a new bone acting cytokine *in vitro*. *J Bone Min Res* 1999;14:1513-21.
32. Gowen M, Mundy GR. Actions of recombinant interleukin 1, interleukin 2, and interferon gamma on bone resorption *in vitro*. *J Immunol* 1986;136:2478-82.
33. Klaushofer K, Horandner H, Hoffmann O. Interferon gamma and calcitonin induce differential changes in cellular kinetics and morphology of osteoclasts in cultured neonatal mouse calvaria. *J Bone Min Res* 1989;4:585-606.
34. Watanabe K, Sato K, Kasono K, Nakano Y, Eto S. Interleukin 4 inhibits hypercalcemia in parathyroid hormone related protein infused normal mice and tumour bearing nude mice *in vivo*. *J Bone Min Res* 1991;6:S288.
35. Oreffo ROC, Mundy GR, Seyedin SM, Bonewald LM. Activation of bone derived latent TGF beta complex by isolated osteoclasts. *Biochem Biophys Res Commun* 1989;158:817-23.
36. Lisignoli G, Toneguzzi S, Pozzi C. Proinflammatory cytokines and chemokine production and expression by human osteoblasts isolated from patients with rheumatoid arthritis and osteoarthritis. *J Rheumatol* 1999;26:791-9.
37. Gowen M. Actions of IL-1 and TNF on human osteoblast-like cells. In: Kluger M, Oppenheim JJ, Dinarello CA, Powanda M, eds. *Monokines and Other Non-Lymphocytic Cytokines*. New York: Alan R Liss; 1992:266-271.
38. Black KS, Mundy GR, Garrett IR. Interleukin-6 causes hypercalcemia *in vivo* and enhances the bone resorbing potency of interleukin-1 and tumour necrosis factor by two orders of magnitude *in vitro*. *J Bone Min Res* 1990;5(Suppl 2):S271.
39. Gowen M, Chapman K, Littlewood A, Hughes DE, Evans DB, Russel R. Production of tumour necrosis factor by human osteoblasts is modulated by other cytokines, but not by osteotropic hormones. *Endocrinology* 1990;126:1250-5.
40. Finkelman RD, Linkhart TA, Mohan S, Lau KHW, Baylink DJ, Bell NH. Vitamin D deficiency causes a selective reduction in the deposition of transforming growth factor beta in rat bone: possible mechanism for impaired osteoinduction. *Proc Natl Acad Sci USA* 1991;88:3657-60.
41. Neale SD, Sabokbar A, Howie DW, Murray DW, Athanasou NA. Macrophage colony-stimulating factor and interleukin-6 release by periprosthetic cells stimulate osteoclast formation and bone resorption. *J Orthop Res* 1999;17:686-94.
42. Ralston SH, Russell RGG, Gowen M. Estrogen inhibits release of tumour necrosis factor from peripheral blood cells in postmenopausal women. *J Bone Min Res* 1990;5:983-8.
43. Pacifici R, Brown C, Puschek E. Effect of surgical menopause and estrogen replacement on cytokine

44. Girasole G, Sakagami Y, Hustmyer FG. 17-beta estradiol inhibits cytokine induced IL-6 production by bone marrow stromal cells and osteoblasts. *J Bone Min Res* 1990;5(Suppl 2):S273.
45. Cummings SR, Black DM, Nevitt MC, et al. Bone density at various sites for prediction of hip fractures: the study of osteoporotic fractures research group. *Lancet* 1993;341:72–5.
46. Hui SL, Slemenda CW, Johnston CC Jr. Age and bone mass as predictors of fracture in a prospective study. *J Clin Invest* 1988;81:1804–9.
47. Wasnich RD, Ross PD, Heilbrun LK, Vogel JM. Prediction of postmenopausal fracture risk with use of bone mineral measurements. *Am J Obstet Gynecol* 1985;153:745–51.
48. Eastell R, Robins SP, Colwell T, Assiri AMA, Riggs BL, Russell RGG. Evaluation of bone turnover in type I osteoporosis using biochemical markers specific for both bone formation and bone resorption. *Osteoporosis Int* 1993;3:255–60.
49. Vogelsang H, Ferenci P, Woloszczuk W, et al. Bone disease in vitamin D-deficient patients with Crohn's disease. *Dig Dis Sci* 1989;34:1094–9.
50. Buchman AL. Bones and Crohn's: problems and solutions. *Inflamm Bowel Dis* 1999;5: 212–27.
51. Andreassen H, Hylander E, Rix M. Gender, age, and body weight are the major predictive factors for bone mineral density in Crohn's disease: a case-control cross-sectional study of 113 patients. *Am J Gastroenterol* 1999;94:824–8.
52. Smith R. Corticosteroids and osteoporosis. *Thorax* 1990;45:573–8.
53. Bernstein CN, Seeger LL, Sayre JW, Anton PA, Artinian L, Shanahan F. Osteopenia in inflammatory bowel disease (IBD) is related to prednisone use and not disease diagnosis: a prospective study. *Gastroenterology* 1993;105:A541.
54. Bjarnason I, Macpherson A, Buxton-Thomas M, Forgacs I, Moniz C. High prevalence of osteoporosis in patients with inflammatory bowel disease and a low lifetime intake of corticosteroids. *Gastroenterology* 1993;105:A541.
55. Schulte C, Dignass, AU, Mann, K, Goebell H. Bone loss in patients with inflammatory bowel disease is less than expected: a follow-up study. *Scand J Gastroenterol* 1999;34:696–702.
56. Robinson RJ, Iqbal SJ, Abrams K, Al-Azzawi F, Mayberry JF. Increased bone resorption in patients with Crohn's disease. *Aliment Pharmacol Ther* 1998;12:699–705.
57. Bjarnason I, Macpherson A, Mackintosh C, Buxton-Thomas M, Forgacs I, Moniz C. Reduced bone density in patients with inflammatory bowel disease. *Gut* 1997;40:228–33.
58. Schulte C, Dignass AU, Mann K, Goebell H. Reduced bone mineral density and unbalanced bone metabolism in patients with inflammatory bowel disease. *Inflamm Bowel Dis* 1998;4:268–75.
59. Robinson RJ, Iqbal SJ, Al-Azzawi F, Abrams K, Mayberry JF. Sex hormone status and bone metabolism in men with Crohn's disease. *Aliment Pharmacol Ther* 1998;12:21–5.
60. Abitbol V, Roux C, Guillemant S, Valleur P, et al. Bone assessment in patients with ileal pouch-anal anastomosis for inflammatory bowel disease. *Br J Surg* 1997;84:1551–4.
61. Stockbrugger RW, Schoon EJ, Bollani S, Mills PR, et al. Discordance between the degree of osteopenia and the prevalence of spontaneous vertebral fractures in Crohn's disease. *Aliment Pharmacol Ther* 2002;16:1519–27.
62. Van Staa T-P, Cooper C, Brusse LS, Leufkens H, Javaid MK, Arden NK. Inflammatory bowel disease and the risk of fracture. *Gastroenterology* 2003;125:1591–7.
63. Loftus EV, Achenbach SJ, Sandborn WJ, Tremaine WJ, Oberg AL, Melton LJ. Risk of fracture in ulcerative colitis: a population based study from Olmsted County, Minnesota. *Clin Gastroenterol Hepatol* 2003;1:465–73.
64. Shanahan F. Pathogenesis of ulcerative colitis. *Lancet* 1993;342:407–11.
65. Ghosh S, Cowen S, Hannan WJ, Ferguson A. Low bone mineral density in Crohn's disease, but not in ulcerative colitis, at diagnosis. *Gastroenterology* 1994;107:1031–9.
66. Compston JE. Osteoporosis. *Clin Endocrinol* 1990;33:653–82.
67. Jahnsen J, Falch JA, Aadland E, Mowinckel P. Bone mineral density is reduced in patients with Crohn's disease, but not in patients with ulcerative colitis: a population based study. *Gut* 1997;40:313–19.
68. Hyams JS, Wyzg N, Kreutzer DC, Justinich CJ, Gronowicz GA. Alterations in bone metabolism in children with inflammatory bowel disease: an *in vitro* study. *J Pediatr Gastroenterol Nutr* 1997;24:289–95.
69. Schoon EJ, Blok BM, Geerling BJ, Brummer RJ, Stockbrugger RW, Russel MM. Is bone mineral density in patients with inflammatory bowel disease (IBD) low at diagnosis? A case-control study. *Gastroenterology* 1999;116:G3533.
70. Schoon EJ, Blok BM, Geerling BJ, Russel MG, Stockbrugger RW, Brummer RJ. Bone mineral density

71 Dinca M, Fries W, Luisetto G, et al. Evolution of osteopenia in inflammatory bowel disease. *Am J Gastroenterol* 1999;94:1292–7.

72 Lamb EJ, Wong T, Smith DJ, et al. Metabolic bone disease is present at diagnosis in patients with inflammatory bowel disease. *Aliment Pharmacol Ther* 2002;16:1895–1902.

73 Issenman RM. Bone mineral metabolism in pediatric inflammatory bowel disease. *Inflamm Bowel Dis* 1999;5:192–9.

74 Gokhale R, Favus MJ, Karrison T, Sutton MM, Rich B, Kirschner BS. Bone mineral density assessment in children with inflammatory bowel disease. *Gastroenterology* 1998;114:902–11.

75 Boot AM, Bouquet J, Krenning EP, De Muinck K. Bone mineral density and nutritional status in children with chronic inflammatory bowel disease. *Gut* 1998;42:188–94.

76 Mora S, Pitukcheewanont P, Nelson JC, Gilsanz V. Serum levels of insulin-like growth factor I and the density, volume, and cross-sectional area of cortical bone in children. *J Clin Endocrinol Metab* 1999;84:2780–3.

77 Rosen CJ. Serum insulin-like growth factors and insulin-like growth factor-binding proteins: clinical implications. *Clin Chem* 1999;45:1384–90.

78 Ghosh S, Drummond HE, Ferguson A. Neglect of growth and development in the clinical monitoring of children and teenagers with inflammatory bowel disease: review of case records. *BMJ* 1998;317:120–1.

79 Robinson RJ, Krzywicki T, Almond L, et al. Effect of a low-impact exercise program on bone mineral density in Crohn's disease: a randomized controlled trial. *Gastroenterology* 1998;115:36–41.

80 Loudon CP, Corroll V, Butcher J, Rawsthorne P, Bernstein CN. The effects of physical exercise on patients with Crohn's disease. *Am J Gastroenterol* 1999;94:697–703.

81 Tobias JH, Sasi MR, Greenwood R, Probert CSJ. Rapid hip bone loss in active Crohn's disease patients receiving short-term corticosteroid therapy. *Aliment Pharmacol Ther* 2004;20:951–7.

82 Andreassen H, Rix M, Brot C, Eskildsen P. Regulators of calcium homeostasis and bone mineral density in patients with Crohn's disease. *Scand J Gastroenterol* 1998;33:1087–93.

83 British Society of Gastroenterology. Guidelines for osteoporosis in coeliac disease and inflammatory bowel disease. *Gut* 2000;46(Suppl 1):1–8.

84 Clements D, Compston JE, Evans WD, Rhodes J. Hormone replacement therapy prevents bone loss in patients with inflammatory bowel disease. *Gut* 1993;34:1543–6.

85 Vogelsang H, Ferenci P, Resch H, Kiss A, Gangl A. Prevention of bone mineral loss in patients with Crohn's disease by long-term oral vitamin D supplementation. *Eur J Gastroenterol Hepatol* 1995;7:609–14.

86 Duggan P, O'Brien M, Kiely M, McCarthy J, Shanahan F, Cashman KD. Vitamin K status in patients with Crohn's disease and relationship to bone turnover. *Am J Gastroenterol* 2004;99:2178–85.

87 Haderslev KV, Tjellesen L, Sorensen HA, Staun M. Alendronate increases lumbar spine bone mineral density in patients with Crohn's disease. *Gastroenterology* 2000;119:639–46.

88 Von Tirpitz T, Klaus J, Steinkamp M, et al. Therapy of osteoporosis in patients with Crohn's disease: a randomized study comparing sodium fluoride and ibandronate. *Aliment Pharmacol Ther* 2003;17:807–16.

89 Bartram SA, Peaston RT, Rawlings DJ, Francis RM, Thompson NP. A randomized controlled trial of calcium with vitamin D alone or in combination with intravenous pamidronate, for the treatment of low bone mineral density associated with Crohn's disease. *Aliment Pharmacol Ther* 2003;18:1121–7.

90 Adachi JD, Rostom A. Metabolic bone disease in adults with inflammatory bowel disease. *Inflamm Bowel Dis* 1999;5:200–11.

91 Szathmari M, Vaserhelyi B, Treszl A, Tulassay T, Tulassay Z. Association of dihydroepiandrosterone sulfate and testosterone deficiency with bone turnover in men with inflammatory bowel disease. *Int J Colorectal Dis* 2002;17:63–6.

92 Plotkin LI, Weinstein RS, Parfitt AM, Roberson PK, Manolagas SC, Bellido T. Prevention of osteocyte and osteoblast apoptosis by bisphosphonates and calcitonin. *J Clin Invest* 1999;104:1363–74.

93 Cantatore FP, Acquista CA, Pipitone V. Evaluation of bone turnover and osteoclastic cytokines in early rheumatoid arthritis treated with alendronate. *J Rheumatol* 1999;26:2318–23.

94 Meunier PJ, Roux C, Seeman E, et al. The effects of strontium ranelate on the risk of vertebral fractures in women with postmenopausal osteoporosis. *New Engl J Med* 2004;350:459–68.

95 Reffitt DM, Meenan J, Sanderson JD, Jugdaosingh R, Powell JJ, Thompson RPH. Bone density improves with disease remission in patients with inflammatory bowel disease. *Euro J Gastroenterol Hepatol* 2003;15:1267–73.

96 Silvennoinen JA, Karttunen TJ, Niemela SE, Manelius JJ, Lehtola JK. A controlled study of bone mineral density in patients with inflammatory bowel disease. *Gut* 1995;37:71–6.

97 Abitbol V, Roux C, Chaussade S, *et al*. Metabolic bone assessment in patients with inflammatory bowel disease. *Gastroenterology* 1995;108:417–22.

98 Roux C, Abitbol V, Chaussade S. Bone loss in patients with inflammatory bowel disease: a prospective study. *Osteoporosis Int* 1995;5:156–60.

99 Motley R, Clements D, Evans WD. A four-year longitudinal study of bone loss in patients with inflammatory bowel disease. *Bone Mineral* 1993;23:95–104.

28: Pregnancy

Philippe Marteau

Introduction

Inflammatory bowel disease (IBD) often affects young patients who wish to have children. They ask whether IBD will affect their fertility, whether they can transmit the disease to their children, whether there are any specific risks during pregnancy and whether the drugs are safe for the foetus. The clinician has to admit that the answers provided and clinical decisions are usually based on observational studies, which are vulnerable to bias, confounding and of low statistical precision because of the low frequency of adverse birth outcomes.

Fertility

The fertility of subjects with IBD is usually normal [1–3]. However, infertility problems are more frequent in women with active Crohn's disease (CD) and in those who have undergone surgery for IBD, especially proctocolectomy with ileoanal anastomosis (IPAA). Tubal infertility can occur in women with CD who also have extensive adhesions. It is now clear that IPAA significantly reduces fertility in women, although it does not suppress it [4–8]. The two most methodologically sound studies come from Scandinavia [4, 6]. The first study assessed 237 women who had undergone IPAA for ulcerative colitis (UC) and compared the observed number of births with the number expected. The number of births from the onset of UC to colectomy was not significantly decreased; however, during the 12 months after ileostomy closure until data collection the patients reported only 34 deliveries, compared with an expected of 69 ($P < 0.001$) [4]. The second study followed-up 290 women with IPAA and compared them with 66 women in a reference population. Fecundity was found to be normal before IPAA and reduced by 80% after this surgical procedure [6] (Fig 28.1). The mechanism probably involves the formation of adhesion and blockage of the fallopian tubes. Öresland et al. [9] studied 21 women after IPAA and reported that although physical examination was normal in 20, hysterosalpingography was abnormal in 14/21 (67%). Dyspareunia occurs between 20 and 38% after IPAA [1, 6]; however series have shown that sexual desire, coitus frequency and the ability to experience orgasm are maintained or improved [10]. Women with UC who need surgery should be informed of the risk of decreased fecundability after IPAA; some physicians advise ileorectal anastomosis in young women wishing to conceive; research should be carried out to establish preventive treatments, especially if laparoscopic surgery carries a lower risk or if anti-adhesive gels may be effective [8].

Some authors have suggested that the fertility of men with IBD may be reduced, but this is doubtful [1, 2]. Men treated with sulphasalazine have decreased fertility and more than 80% have semen abnormalities [1, 2]. The sulphapyridine moiety of the drug is responsible for this adverse event, and recovery of the sperm characteristics as well as a return to fertility is observed when sulphasalazine is replaced with 5-ASA [1, 2].

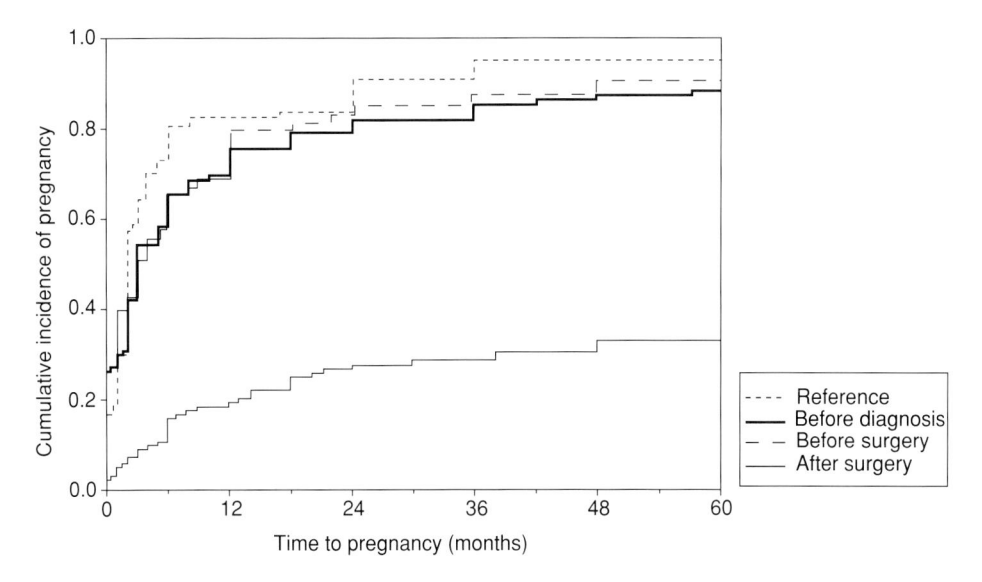

Fig 28.1 Cumulative incidence of pregnancy within 5 years. Patients and reference population.
The fecundability levels of women with UC were equal to or slightly higher than those seen in the reference group up to the time of surgery (before diagnosis, FR 1.46, $P = 0.002$; before colectomy, FR 1.01, $P =$ NS) but very low (FR 0.20, $P < 0.0001$) after IPAA. Taken from Ording Olsen K et al. [6] and reproduced with the permission of the authors and editors.

Transmission of IBD

The risk of IBD among the offspring of patients is 2–13 times higher than the risk within the general population [11]. When only one parent is affected, the risk of transmission of IBD to the child is about 1.5–3.5% [11]. When both parents are affected, the risk was shown to be around 32–36% in two series including 16 and 25 couples (33 and 54 children) [12, 13].

Effect of IBD on pregnancy

Miscarriage and foetal loss

Miscarriage is more frequent in women with IBD, especially when the disease is active (up to 35% of conceptions) [1, 2, 14–17]. The natural risk of foetal loss after 16 weeks is around 1% and it is not demonstrated that this is higher than in the general population. A short series suggested that active CD at the time of conception significantly increased this risk [16]. In a cohort study using registries in Denmark, the risk was increased in patients with UC who received mesalazine and corticosteroids (OR 6.4, CI 95% 1.7–24.9) [17]. The respective role of the disease and of the drug could not be established.

Prematurity and low birth weight

CD and UC increase the risks of pre-term birth [1, 2, 14–22]. The relative risk is usually between 1.5 and 3 and the absolute risk between 7 and 16% [14–22]. CD has repeatedly shown to increase the risk of low birth weight (relative risk 1.5–3.5) [14–20], but this was observed in only one recent study in patients with UC [21]. Fonager et al. [15] conducted a historical registry-based study with linkage between the Danish National Registry of Patients and the Danish Medical Birth Registry. The study included 510 newborns of mothers with CD and 3018 controls. The risk of prematurity was 7.3% versus 4.8% in controls and that of birth weight less than 2500 g was 10.4% versus 4.7%. The average birth weight of the newborns of mothers with CD was 185 g less than expected for primi-paras, and 134 g less than

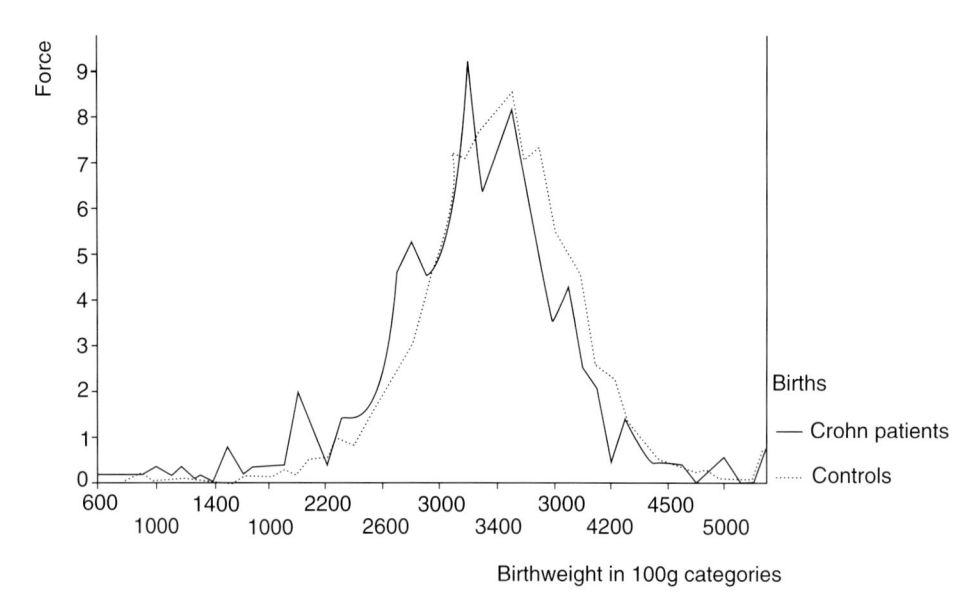

Fig 28.2 Distribution of birth weights of babies born to mothers with Crohn's disease ($n = 510$) and babies born to a control group of healthy mothers ($n = 3018$). Taken from Fonager et al. [15] and reprinted with the permission of the authors and the American College of Gastroenterology.

expected for multi-paras (Fig 28.2). A Canadian series [18] compared the charts of 65 women with quiescent CD at the start of pregnancy with matched controls. Low birth weight was more frequent in CD as well as small-for-gestational-age births. Multivariate analysis showed that ileal CD was a significant independent predictor, and that previous bowel resection was close to statistical significance.

These complications may be multi-factorial. Experts usually advise smoking cessation, careful monitoring of pregnancy, especially in the third trimester, rest and proper treatment of the IBD.

Risk of congenital malformations

The risk of malformations in the general population is between 1 and 4.8%. It has not been found to be increased in patients with IBD [1, 2, 14–19], except in two studies [20, 23]. In the study by Dominitz et al. [20], conducted in Washington State, eight cases of malformation were observed in 107 foetuses born to women with UC (7.9%). In a recent case-control study using the Hungarian case control surveillance of congenital abnormalities register, the risk of having UC was 0.3% ($n = 71$) in the malformation group versus 0.2% in the group without malformations (NS); however limb deficiencies, obstructive urinary congenital abnormalities and multiple congenital abnormalities were more frequent in the UC group [23]. Whether the increase in these rare different malformations is real should be established in future studies.

Influence of pregnancy on the course of IBD

During pregnancy

It seems likely (and is usually accepted) that IBD activity at conception influences the risk of activity during pregnancy [2, 22]. Series have reported that the risk of relapse during pregnancy was about 20–25% when UC or CD is inactive at conception, and at least 50% when the disease is active at conception [2, 18]. Women with IBD should thus be told to avoid conceiving during an acute phase of the disease. Studies assessing the efficacy of treatments for acute IBD during pregnancy are lacking.

After pregnancy

Pregnancy does not seem to significantly influence the clinical course of IBD. Two observational studies suggested that it may decrease the activity of IBD and discussed potential mechanisms [24, 25]. Nwokolo et al. [24] observed that the need for further surgical resection in 88 parous women with CD was reduced with increasing parity. Castiglione et al. [25] studied 18 women with CD (29 pregnancies) and 19 women with UC (25 pregnancies) and reported that their relapse rate was lower during the 3 years after pregnancy than in the 3 years before pregnancy. This might be due to modifications of the immune response induced by pregnancy [1, 25].

Assessment of disease activity in pregnant women

Sigmoidoscopy and colonoscopy do not seem to induce labour or result in congenital malformations. Foetal monitoring is usually not indicated [26]. Their use should only be considered when they are likely to influence an important medical or surgical decision. Non- urgent radiological testing using X-rays should be avoided. The most sensitive period for central nervous system teratogenesis is between 10 and 17 weeks of gestation. Magnetic resonance imaging can be performed.

Safety of drugs

Nearly all the drugs used to treat IBD cross the placenta. Some of them (especially immunosuppressive agents) draw attention as they may be mutagenic and/or fetotoxic at certain doses in pre-clinical studies.

Corticosteroids

Prednisone and prednisolone can be used in pregnant women exactly as in non-pregnant women [2, 27, 28]. High-dose corticosteroids cause cleft palate in rodents [28], and a meta-analysis of human trials suggested that this might also be the case in humans [29]. However, this conclusion of the meta-analysis is not widely accepted as it was based on a subgroup of studies with insufficient quality [1]. The placenta metabolises prednisone, and the foetus is exposed to only 10% of the maternal dose [1]. The placental metabolism of betamethasone and dexamethasone is lower, and these corticosteroids can cause adrenal suppression in the newborn. Inhaled budesonide did not increase the risk of malformations in large series of infants whose mothers had received this treatment for asthma during pregnancy [30]. Budesonide with enteric delivery is probably as safe but has not been assessed in this regard.

Sulphasalazine and 5-aminosalicylic acid (5-ASA)

Numerous studies showed that sulphasalazine and 5-ASA at doses below 3 g/day do not increase the risk of birth defects [2, 22, 28, 31, 32]. Sulphasalazine may induce folate deficiency, which is a well-established cause of neural tube defects. Folate supplementation should, therefore, be taken by women on sulphasalazine, before and during pregnancy. In a prospective study [31] in Toronto, 165 women with IBD exposed to 5-ASA during pregnancy were compared with a control group without IBD. There was no increase in major malformations (0.8% on 5-ASA vs 3.8% among controls). However, there was a significant increase in the rate of pre-term deliveries (13% in the IBD group vs 4.7% in controls), lesser mean maternal weight gain during pregnancy, and a lower mean birth weight. This effect is likely to be due to the disease, although a role for the drug cannot be excluded. Norgard et al. conducted a Danish cohort study based on Prescription, Birth, and Hospital Discharge Registries [17]. Outcomes of 88 pregnancies exposed during the entire pregnancy were compared with those of 19,418 pregnancies in which no drugs were prescribed. Odds ratios for stillbirth and pre-term birth in women who were prescribed 5-ASA were 6.4 (1.7–24.9), 1.9 (0.9–3.9), respectively. They were increased only in patients with UC. It was not possible to distinguish the specific effects of disease activity and drugs. The risk of malformation was not increased. The safety of large doses of 5-ASA during pregnancy is poorly known, but was questioned in 1994 when Colombel et al. reported a case of severe foetal nephropathy [33] in which the mother had taken 4 g/day 5-ASA during the period corresponding to foetal nephrogenesis. The boy recovered and no other case has been reported since. In our series of 37 women receiving at least 3 g/day 5-ASA, we observed no renal toxicity [1].

It is thus usually recommended that alternative treatments should be used preferentially to high doses of 5-ASA and to use sonographic monitoring of the foetal kidneys if high doses are nonetheless administered.

Antibiotics and probiotics

Short-course metronidazole (7–10 days) has been shown to be safe in pregnant women [34], but the safety of longer treatments is unknown. The quinolones are contraindicated in pregnancy, given the musculo-skeletual aformalities associated with these medications in immature animals [35].

Azathioprine and 6-mercaptopurine (6-MP)

Azathioprine and 6-MP at doses 10–30 times higher than the dose usually used to treat IBD have been found to cause malformations, foetal loss, and immunosuppression in animals [2, 27, 36, 37]. A decreased number of live births was observed in three successive generations of mice that had been exposed to 6-MP [38]. Chromosomal aberrations have been noted in three infants exposed to azathioprine *in utero*. Infantile immunosuppression has also been reported in humans. The most severe cases consisted of foetal athymia, lymphopenia and immune deficiency. Two of five such children were stillborn, another two died after a few days of life, and the fifth had lymphopenia and low immunoglobulin levels, which resolved after 15 weeks of life (see [37]).

Nevertheless, azathioprine has been used by many pregnant women with renal allografts or to treat systemic lupus erythematosus or IBD [28, 61]. From 700 published case reports, Roubenoff *et al.* [27] calculated that the rate of congenital malformations in foetuses exposed to azathioprine was 4.3%. The outcome of pregnancy in series of patients who had received azathioprine for IBD is usually unremarkable. The largest series included 79 women and 76 men (325 pregnancies) [39]. There was no statistical difference in spontaneous abortion, malformations, infections or neoplasia among patients taking 6-MP before or during pregnancy compared with controls not taking 6-MP. In a Danish cohort study based on data from a population-based prescription registry, 11 women exposed to purine analogues were compared to 19,418 pregnancies in which no drugs were prescribed [40]. The risks of malformations and peri-natal mortality were increased (OR 6.7 and 20.0 respectively). The low number of cases limits the interpretation of these results. A group from New York assessed the complications of pregnancy and child development when mothers had stopped 6-MP before conception [36]. Patients who were taking 6-MP at the time of conception and those who took 6-MP after conception were excluded. Twenty-nine patients had 72 pregnancies after 6-MP cessation and results were compared to that of a historical group of 75 women with IBD who had not received 6-MP and had 140 pregnancies. There was greater foetal loss in the 6-MP cessation group (29.2% vs 14.3%) and 2 chromosomal aberrations (trisomy 22 and mosaicism). The authors speculated that 6-MP given prior to pregnancy might have caused chromosomal aberrations in ova leading to increased incidence of abortion. The evidence from this study is, however, limited by comparison to a historical group [36]. One interpretation could be that stopping the drug does not affect a risk.

In summary, the risks associated with azathioprine and 6-MP are low and statistically not certain. If a women receiving azathioprine becomes pregnant, azathioprine can be maintained (if the indication is correct), but foetal growth and the maternal leukocyte count should be monitored. Davison *et al.* [41] reported that maternal leukocyte counts at week 32 of pregnancy correlated with leukocyte suppression in the neonate and proposed to half the azathioprine dose at 32 weeks of pregnancy whenever the maternal leukocyte count was below the 1SD band for normal pregnancy.

Methotrexate and mycophenolate mofetil

Methotrexate is strictly contra-indicated both for men and women who plan parenthood as it is highly teratogenic in animals and humans, and causes chromosomal damage and miscarriage [28]. Analysis of series involving more than 350 patients shows that the risk of foetal malformation is not increased when methotrexate is stopped more than 1 year before conception [28]. Mycophenolate is also teratogenic and contra-indicated [42].

Ciclosporine

Ciclosporine can be used to treat fulminant colitis during pregnancy [43]. It is not teratogenic. However, a high dose of 25 mg/kg day caused renal tubule damage in the foetal rat [44]. Close monitoring of arterial pressure, serum creatinine and ciclosporine blood levels is needed.

Anti-TNF antibodies

Information is still very limited and found only in abstracts. Katz *et al.* [45] reported cases mentioning pregnancy in the safety database for infliximab. One hundred and thirty-three pregnancies were identified in women with CD or rheumatoid arthritis treated with infliximab; 74 cases were exposed in the 3 months before conception and 33 both before and in the 3 months after conception. Among the 65 documented pregnancies, live births occurred in 65%, miscarriages in 17% and therapeutic termination in 22%. Of the 26 live births, 2 infants were delivered with complications to mothers with CD. The authors considered that these results were consistent with those in a national cohort of healthy women and that inadvertent exposure to infliximab during pregnancy was safe. Six cases of intentional use of regular infusions of infliximab in pregnant women for maintenance of acute CD confirmed this safety [46].

Other drugs

Thalidomide is strictly contra-indicated in patients of both genders wishing to conceive, as it is highly teratogenic in humans [28].

Delivery

The question is whether subgroups of women with IBD need a caesarean section to prevent the occurrence or aggravation of perineal disease and/or anal incontinence general population elective.

Mode of delivery in women with perineal CD

Post-episiotomy rectovaginal fistulae have been described in patients with CD [1]. Active perianal disease at delivery is an indication for caesarean section. In contrast, for women with either no history of perianal disease or inactive perianal disease, the risk of perianal disease relapse and the need for preventive caesarean section are controversial. A questionnaire-based series from New York series [47] involved 80 women with CD who were free of pre-existing perineal involvement and who had had a total of 179 pregnancies. The rate of perineal involvement after vaginal delivery, usually with episiotomy, was 17.9%. In other series [48] the mode of delivery did not influence the risk of perineal disease. In a series from Manitoba, perianal symptoms always worsened post-partum in the 15 women who had active perianal disease before delivery [49]. In contrast, the 11 women with inactive perianal disease at delivery had no relapse of perianal disease during 1 year of follow-up post-partum, and in the 39 vaginal deliveries of women without perianal disease, only one case of perianal disease occurred during 1 year of post-partum follow-up [49].

Delivery in women with IPAA

Several consecutive studies in the large series women with IPAA followed at the Mayo Clinic in Rochester concluded that vaginal delivery, multiple births, the length of labour and birth weight had no permanent adverse effects on subsequent pouch function [50–52]. The method of delivery should be dictated by obstetrical considerations.

Invasive treatments: surgery and artificial nutrition

Surgery may be needed during pregnancy for the acute complications of IBD, such as intestinal obstruction and fulminant colitis. There is an increased risk of miscarriage and foetal loss. Abscesses occurring in pregnant patients with CD should be treated as in non-pregnant women, i.e. by removal of the source of the sepsis and exteriorisation of the bowel ends [53, 54]. Blowhole colostomy and ileostomy may be recommended to avoid the specific difficulties of managing a rectosigmoid stump and of the dissection below the retroperitoneal reflexion [54].

Short series suggest that enteral feeding is safe during pregnancy [55]. If total parenteral nutrition is indicated, the use of fat emulsions should be limited, as they can theoretically cause fat embolisation to the placenta [1].

Breastfeeding

Breastfeeding is recommended in the general population and studies suggested that subjects who were breastfed have a decreased risk of CD [56–58], although data on UC are contradictory [56–58]. However, nearly all drugs used to treat IBD are excreted in breast milk.

It is usually considered that prednisone and prednisolone can be used during breastfeeding [37]. Some physicians recommend that mothers on doses above 20 mg/day wait at least 4 h before nursing [37, 59]. Some clinicians do not use immunosuppressants during the period of breastfeeding, because of the theoretical risk of immune suppression in the baby (cytopenia and carcinogenesis) [57]. Quinolones are contraindicated because of their toxic effects on joints when given to young animals [60]. As only very low doses of loperamide are secreted in milk, this drug can be used by breastfeeding mothers [61].

Drugs for fathers with IBD at the time of conception

Little is known about the safety of drugs in men who are planning to have children, and small series may probably be biased. Sulphasalazine may decrease fertility due to semen abnormalities but 5-ASA does not [1, 2]. The safety of azathioprine and 6-MP for fathers has recently been questioned, but the evidence is still minimal. A series from New York including 13 pregnancies conceived within 3 months of 6-MP use by the father versus controls suggested that pregnancy-related complications might be significantly increased by the treatment (2 spontaneous abortions and 2 malformations) [62]. No significant increase in the risk of congenital abnormalities was found in a Danish population-based cohort study on 54 exposed pregnancies [63]. No increase in the risk was also noticed in the series by Francella from New York [39].

References

1 Couve S, Seksik P, Elefant E, et al. Maladie inflammatoires de l'intestin et grossesse. *Gastroenterol Clin Biol* 2003;27:618–26.
2 Steinlauf AF, Present DH. Medical management of the pregnant patient with inflammatory bowel disease. *Gastroenterol Clin North Am* 2004;33:361–85.
3 Hudson M, Flett G, Sinclair TS, et al. Fertility and pregnancy in inflammatory bowel disease. *Int J Gynaecol Obstet* 1997;58:229–37.
4 Olsen KO, Joelsson M, Laurberg S, et al. Fertility after ileal pouch-anal anastomosis in women with ulcerative colitis. *Br J Surg* 1999;86:493–5.
5 Tiainen J, Matikainen M, Hiltunen KM. Ileal J-pouch-anal anastomosis, sexual dysfunction, and fertility. *Scand J Gastroenterol* 1999;34:185–8.
6 Ording Olsen K, Juul S, Berndtsson I, et al. Ulcerative colitis: female fecundity before diagnosis, during disease, and after surgery compared with a population sample. *Gastroenterology* 2002;122:15–9.
7 Johnson P, Richard C, Ravid A, et al. Female infertility after ileal pouch-anal anastomosis for ulcerative colitis. *Dis Colon Rectum* 2004;47:1119–26.
8 Wolf JL. The impact of surgery for ulcerative colitis on fertility and sexual function in women. *Gastroenterology* 2002;122:226–7.
9 Oresland T, Palmblad S, Ellstrom M, et al. Gynaecological and sexual function related to anatomical changes in the female pelvis after restorative proctocolectomy. *Int J Colorectal Dis* 1994;9:77–81.
10 Wax JR, Pinette MG, Cartin A, et al. Female reproductive health after ileal pouch anal anastomosis for ulcerative colitis. *Obstet Gynecol Surv* 2003;58:270–4.
11 Binder V. Genetic epidemiology in inflammatory bowel disease. *Dig Dis* 1998;16:351–5.
12 Bennett RA, Rubin PH, Present DH. Frequency of inflammatory bowel disease in offspring of couples both presenting with inflammatory bowel disease. *Gastroenterology* 1991;100:1638–43.
13 Laharie D, Debeugny S, Peeters M, et al. Inflammatory bowel disease in spouses and their offspring. *Gastroenterology* 2001;120:816–9.

14. Baird DD, Narendranathan M, Sandler RS. Increased risk of preterm birth for women with inflammatory bowel disease. *Gastroenterology* 1990;9:987–94.
15. Fonager K, Sorensen HT, Olsen J, et al. Pregnancy outcome for women with Crohn's disease: a follow-up study based on linkage between national registries. *Am J Gastroenterol* 1998;93:2426–30.
16. Morales M, Berney T, Jenny A, et al. Crohn's disease as a risk factor for the outcome of pregnancy. *Hepatogastroenterology* 2000;47:1595–8.
17. Norgard B, Fonager K, Pedersen L, et al. Birth outcome in women exposed to 5-aminosalicylic acid during pregnancy: a Danish cohort study. *Gut* 2003;52:243–7.
18. Moser MA, Okun NB, Mayes DC, et al. Crohn's disease, pregnancy, and birth weight. *Am J Gastroenterol* 2000;95:1021–6.
19. Khosla R, Willoughby CP, Jewell DP. Crohn's disease and pregnancy. *Gut* 1984;25:52–6.
20. Dominitz JA, Young JC, Boyko EJ. Outcomes of infants born to mothers with inflammatory bowel disease: a population-based cohort study. *Am J Gastroenterol* 2002;97:641–8.
21. Ludvigsson JF, Ludvigsson J. Inflammatory bowel disease in mother or father and neonatal outcome. *Acta Paediatr* 2002;91:145–51.
22. Mogadam M, Dobbins WO, Korelitz BI, et al. Pregnancy in inflammatory bowel disease: effect of sulfasalazine and corticosteroids on fetal outcome. *Gastroenterology* 1981;80:72–6.
23. Norgard B, Puho E, Pedersen L, et al. Risk of congenital abnormalities in children born to women with ulcerative colitis: a population-based, case-control study. *Am J Gastroenterol* 2003;98:2006–10.
24. Nwokolo CU, Tan WC, Andrews Ha, et al. Surgical resections in parous patients with distal ileal and colonic Crohn's disease. *Gut* 1994;35:220–3.
25. Castiglione F, Pignata S, Morace F, et al. Effect of pregnancy on the clinical course of a cohort of women with inflammatory bowel disease. *Ital J Gastroenterol* 1996;28:199–204.
26. Katz JA. Endoscopy in the pregnant patient with inflammatory bowel disease. *Gastrointest Endosc Clin N Am* 2002;12:635–46.
27. Roubenoff R, Hoyt J, Petri M, et al. Effects of antiinflammatory and immunosuppressive drugs on pregnancy and fertility. *Semin Arthr Rheum* 1988;18:88–110.
28. Koren G, Pastuszak A, Ito S. Drugs in pregnancy. *N Eng J Med* 1998;338:1128–37.
29. Park-Wyllie L, Mazzotta P, Pastuszak A, et al. Birth defects after maternal exposure to corticosteroids: prospective cohort study and meta-analysis of epidemiological studies. *Teratology* 2000;62:385–92.
30. Norjavaara E, de Verdier MG. Normal pregnancy outcomes in a population-based study including 2,968 pregnant women exposed to budesonide. *J Allergy Clin Immunol* 2003;111:736–42.
31. Diav-Citrin O, Park YH, Veerasuntharam G, et al. The safety of mesalamine in human pregnancy: a prospective controlled cohort study. *Gastroenterology* 1998;114:23–8.
32. Marteau P, Tennenbaum R, Elefant E, et al. Fœtal outcome in women with inflammatory bowel disease treated during pregnancy with oral mesalazine microgranules. *Alim Pharmacol Ther* 1998;12:1101–8.
33. Colombel JF, Brabant G, Gubler MC, et al. Renal insufficiency in infant: side-effect of prenatal exposure to mesalazine? *Lancet* 1994;344:620–1.
34. Burtin P, Taddio A, Ariburnu O, et al. Safety of metronidazole in pregnancy: a metanalysis. *Am J Obstet Gynecol* 1995;172:525–9.
35. Berkovitch M, Pastuszak A, Gazarian M, et al. Safety of the new quinolones in pregnancy. *Obstet Gynecol* 1994;84:535–8.
36. Zlatanic J, Korelitz BI, Rajapakse R, et al. Complications of pregnancy and child development after cessation of treatment with 6-mercaptopurine for inflammatory bowel disease. *J Clin Gastroenterol* 2003;36:303–9.
37. Ramsey-Goldman R, Schilling E. Immunosuppressive drug use during pregnancy. *Rheum Dis Clin North Am* 1997;23:149–69.
38. Reimers TJ, Sluss PM. 6-mercaptopurine treatment of pregnant mice: effects on second and third generations. *Science* 1978;201:65–7.
39. Francella A, Dyan A, Bodian C, et al. The safety of 6-mercaptopurine for childbearing patients with inflammatory bowel disease: a retrospective cohort study. *Gastroenterology* 2003;124:9–17.
40. Norgard B, Pedersen L, Fonager K, et al. Azathioprine, mercaptopurine and birth outcome: a population-based cohort study. *Aliment Pharmacol Ther* 2003;17:827–34.
41. Davison JM, Dellagrammatikas H, Partkin JM. Maternal azathioprine therapy and depressed haematopoiesis in the babies of renal allograft patients. *Br J Obstet Gynaecol* 1985;92:233–9.
42. EBPG Expert Group on Renal Transplantation. European best practice guidelines for renal transplantation. Section IV: long-term management of the transplant recipient. IV.10. Pregnancy in renal transplant recipients. *Nephrol Dial Transplant* 2002;17(Suppl 4):50–5.

43 Bertschinger P, Himmelmann A, Risti B, et al. Cyclosporine treatment of severe ulcerative colitis during pregnancy. *Am J Gastroenterol* 1995;90:330.

44 Bar Oz B, Hackman R, Einarson T, et al. Pregnancy outcome after cyclosporine therapy during pregnancy: a meta-analysis. *Transplantation* 2001;71:1051–5.

45 Katz J, Keenan G, Snith D, et al. Outcome of pregnancy in patients receiving infliximab for the treatment of Crohn's disease and rheumatoid arthritis [Abstract]. *Gastroenterology* 2003;124:A63.

46 Mahadevan U, Kane S, Sandborn W, et al. Intentional infliximab use for maintenance of acute Crohn's disease flare in pregnancy [Abstract]. *Gastroenterology* 2004;126:1402.

47 Brandt LJ, Estabrook SG, Reinus JF. Vaginal delivery and episiotomy lead to perineal involvement in women with Crohn's disease. *Am J Gastroenterol* 1995;90:1918–22.

48 Rogers RG, Katz VL. Course of Crohn's disease during pregnancy and its effect on pregnancy outcome: a retrospective review. *Am J Perinatol* 1995;12:262–4.

49 Ilnyckyji A, Blanchard JF, Rawsthorne P, et al. Perianal Crohn's disease and pregnancy: role of the mode of delivery. *Am J Gastroenterol* 1999;94:3274–8.

50 Juhasz ES, Fozard B, Dozois RR, et al. Ileal pouch-anal anastomosis function following childbirth: an extended evaluation. *Dis Colon Rectum* 1995;38:159–65.

51 Farouk R, Pemberton JH, Wolff BG, et al. Functional outcomes after ileal pouch-anal anastomosis for chronic ulcerative colitis. *Ann Surg* 2000;231:919–26.

52 Hahnloser D, Pemberton JH, Wolff BG, et al. Pregnancy and delivery before and after ileal pouch-anal anastomosis for inflammatory bowel disease: immediate and long-term consequences and outcomes. *Dis Colon Rectum* 2004;47:1127–35.

53 Hill J, Clark A, Scott NA. Surgical treatment of acute manifestations of Crohn's disease during pregnancy. *J R Soc Med* 1997;90:64–6.

54 Ooi BS, Remzi FH, Fazio VW. Turnbull-Blowhole colostomy for toxic ulcerative colitis in pregnancy: report of two cases. *Dis Colon Rectum* 2003;46:111–5.

55 Teahon K, Pearson M, Levi AJ, et al. Elemental diet in the management of Crohn's disease during pregnancy. *Gut* 1991;32:1079–81.

56 Rigas A, Rigas B, Glassman M, et al. Breast-feeding and maternal smoking in the etiology of Crohn's disease and ulcerative colitis in childhood. *Ann Epidemiol* 1993;3:387–92.

57 Corrao G, Tragnone A, Caprilli R, et al. Risk of inflammatory bowel disease attributable to smoking, oral contraception and breastfeeding in Italy: a nationwide case-control study. Cooperative investigators of the Italian group for the study of the colon and the rectum (GISC). *Int J Epidemiol* 1998;27:397–404.

58 Thompson NP, Montgomery SM, Wadsworth ME, et al. Early determinants of inflammatory bowel disease: use of two national longitudinal birth cohorts. *Eur J Gastroenterol Hepatol* 2000;12:25–30.

59 Ost L, Wettrell G, Bjorkhem I, et al. Prednisolone excretion in human milk. *J Pediatr* 1985;106:1008–11.

60 Giamarellou H, Kolokythas E, Petrikkos G, et al. Pharmacokinetics of three newer quinolones in pregnant and lactating women. *Am J Med* 1989;87:49S–51S.

61 Hagemann TM. Gastrointestinal medications and breastfeeding. *J Hum Lact* 1998;14:259–62.

62 Rajapakse RO, Korelitz BI, Zlatanic J, et al. Outcome of pregnancies when fathers are treated with 6-mercaptopurine for inflammatory bowel disease. *Am J Gastroenterol* 2000;95:684–8.

63 Norgard B, Pedersen L, Jacobsen J, et al. The risk of congenital abnormalities in children fathered by men treated with azathioprine or mercaptopurine before conception. *Aliment Pharmacol Ther* 2004;19:679–85.

29: Can prognosis of ulcerative colitis be predicted?

Robert Hilsden and Lloyd Sutherland

Introduction

Experienced clinicians will be able to predict the clinical course of many patients. They will recognise that patients with limited disease do better than those with extensive colitis. They will recognise that many patients will eventually come to colectomy, but only rarely will a patient die from their ulcerative colitis. Prognostic studies seek to codify these clinical impressions, such that they can provide useful information to guide care of those with ulcerative colitis and inform those suffering from the disease. Table 29.1 provides an overview of the prognosis of ulcerative colitis based on findings consistently reportedly by well-designed, population-based studies.

Natural history

The natural history of untreated ulcerative colitis has not been systematically studied. Inferences about the natural history of ulcerative colitis have been made based on the experiences of patients allocated to the placebo arm of randomised clinical trials [1–4]. However, placebo-treated patients are likely to be a poor proxy for establishing the natural history of ulcerative colitis for several reasons. First, those recruited into clinical trials are a select group and are unlikely to be representative of all those with ulcerative colitis. Second, the natural history of the disease is only one component of the response seen in placebo-treated patients. The 'placebo-response' and the effects of other components of a clinical trial (frequent clinic visits) also play a role. Third, patients in clinical trials are usually not newly diagnosed patients, but include patients with different durations of disease and nearly all have received medical treatment at some time prior to their entrance into the study.

In an analysis of 38 placebo-controlled treatment studies of active UC, Ilnyckyj et al. found the clinical remission rate was 9.1% (95% CI 6.6–11.6) and the clinical benefit rate was 26.7% (95% CI 21.1–29.2) [2]. Arguing against these rates being purely the result of the natural history of the disease was the finding that the placebo response rate varied depending on the number of study visits. In an earlier study, Meyer and Janowitz reported that 51% (95% CI 36–66%) of patients on placebo in maintenance trials remained in remission at 6 months. Those who had been in remission over the preceding year were more likely to stay in remission. Patients with proctitis or proctosigmoiditis were more likely to stay in remission than those with pan-colitis.

Prognosis

Common questions about prognosis in someone first diagnosed with ulcerative colitis includes (1) what is the likelihood of entering remission or requiring surgery with the first attack, (2) how active will the disease be in the future and (3) will the extent of the disease increase?

Prognosis of the first attack

Early prognosis studies are at great risk for bias as they are usually retrospective studies of non-population-based cohorts. They also provide little

Table 29.1 Prognosis of ulcerative colitis – key points.

First attack
>85% enter remission
Colectomy with first attack   <5%
Minority have no further episodes
   (? Misdiagnosed infectious colitis)

Clinical course of UC
Transient   25–30%
Intermittent   65–70%
Continuous   5%

Predictors of relapse
Prior relapse history

Risk of colectomy
Colectomy within 1 year   <10%
Colectomy by 10 years   12–25%
Increased risk: first years after
   diagnosis, extensive disease
Predictors of failure of IV
   corticosteroids: frequency of bowel
   motions, C-reactive protein

Mortality
Unaffected or slightly increased

---

relevant information for today's patients given the dramatic changes in the medical and surgical management of ulcerative colitis. However, they do provide an important and sobering historical context. Edwards and Truelove studied the prognosis of 624 patients with ulcerative colitis, including 250 experiencing their first attack, admitted to the Radcliffe Infirmary or Churchill Hospital, Oxford, from 1938 to 1962 [5]. In the 1930s and 1940s, mortality rates over 20% were seen during first attacks and around 10% for relapses. Mortality rates were highest in those with more severe disease, a finding confirmed in two other early series [6, 7].

There are limited high-quality, population-based data on the prognosis of a first attack of ulcerative colitis. Sinclair et al. studied 537 patients newly diagnosed with ulcerative colitis between 1967 and 1976 in northeastern Scotland [8]. Eighty-eight per cent of patients entered remission after the first attack. Fifteen patients (3%) required colectomy. Only 17 patients (3%) died and the majority of these were older than age 70 and only one-half of the deaths were attributed to ulcerative colitis. Severity of disease was a prognostic factor for entering remission.

Of those with mild, moderate or severe disease activity, 92, 82 and 40% entered remission, respectively. No one with mild disease required surgery compared with 4% of those with moderate disease and 31% of those with severe disease. The extent of the disease was associated with disease severity. The limitations of this study are significant and include its retrospective design and the reliance on barium enema to determine extent of disease. In addition, some therapies commonly used now for the treatment of ulcerative colitis would have been unavailable to these patients, and there is no description of the medical treatment that they did receive. Therefore, it is difficult to extrapolate the results from this cohort to patients being diagnosed in the 2000s.

Other studies have reported that 18–28% of patients diagnosed with ulcerative colitis during their first attack do not experience a subsequent relapse [5, 8, 9]. However, it is likely that this group includes many patients with misdiagnosed infectious colitis. Moum et al. found that 12% of patients originally diagnosed with ulcerative colitis could not have that diagnosis confirmed on re-evaluation 1–2 years after the initial diagnosis [10]. Schumacher et al. suggest that historical and clinical features may help distinguish non-relapsing colitis from ulcerative colitis [11]. They followed 42 patients for at least 5 years. Fever, shorter duration of symptoms and more bowel movements were more frequently seen in patients with infectious non-relapsing colitis. Ulcerative colitis patients reported a longer prodrome of symptoms. When a variety of symptoms were analysed using logistic regression, a history of gradually increasing diarrhoea could successfully identify ulcerative colitis patients. Endoscopic findings could not separate the two entities. Rectal biopsies demonstrating basal plasmacytosis and crypt distortion were seen more often in ulcerative colitis patients.

Subsequent disease course

Good data on the clinical course of ulcerative colitis during the first year after diagnosis are available from a prospective, population-based study of 496 ulcerative colitis patients in south-eastern Norway with a mean follow-up of 16.2 months [12]. Fifty per cent entered remission and remained relapse-free at 1 year. One to two relapses were experienced by 36% of patients and approximately 5% suffered a chronic relapsing course with more than 5 relapses. The only prognostic factor predicting disease relapse was age, with those under age 50 more likely to experience a relapse than older patients. Only 20 (4%) patients underwent a colectomy. Patients with pancolitis were more likely to undergo colectomy than those with left-sided disease (8% vs 2%).

Data from a Danish cohort of 1169 incident cases of ulcerative colitis accrued prospectively between 1962 and 1987 with a median follow-up of 11.7 years provides information on the longer term course of ulcerative colitis [13]. At any time 50% of patients were in clinical remission. Approximately 20% of patients were suffering from moderately to severely active disease. Intermittent episodes of disease activity were seen most commonly, although 25% of patients had no episodes of disease activity over a 5-year period and 18% suffered yearly relapses. The number of episodes of disease activity in the first 2 years after diagnosis was a significant predictor of the subsequent disease course.

Based on evidence from placebo-controlled therapeutic trials of oral mesalamine and sulfasalazine, 58–89% of patients receiving placebo will suffer a relapse within 1 year [14]. Several retrospective studies examined potential risk factors. Implicated risk factors have included seasonality, psychological stress, viral illness, non-steroidal anti-inflammatory drugs and *Clostridium difficile* infections [15–24].

Three prospective studies have examined clinical risk factors for relapse. Leo *et al.* examined factors predicting relapse in a prospective cohort of 72 patients with ulcerative colitis [25]. Three factors were found to be predictive in a logistic regression model: fibre-poor diet, number of previous episodes of relapse and history of extra-intestinal manifestations. In a prospective study of 92 patients with ulcerative colitis in remission who were followed for over 48 weeks, Riley *et al.* examined the influence of several factors including infections, dietary changes, episodes of non-bloody diarrhoea, seasonality and life stress, on the risk of relapse [26]. Only previous relapse history and seasonality were significantly associated with relapse with most relapses occurring from August to January. Bitton *et al.* recruited 74 patients with clinically and endoscopically inactive ulcerative colitis and followed them for up to 1 year [27]. Younger age and multiple previous relapses in women were independent predictors of relapse.

Therefore, to date consistent clinical risk factors for disease relapse, apart from prior relapse history, have not been identified. Other potential risk factors identified in the above studies need to be validated in larger studies prior to being accepted. Most patients in the three prospective studies quoted above were on maintenance therapy during the course of the study. Therefore, the impact of the identified risk factors on the management of ulcerative colitis in remission is likely to be negligible as most of the risk factors are not amenable to intervention.

Disease extension

The extent of the colon affected in ulcerative colitis has several implications, including the use of topical therapy, likelihood of undergoing a colectomy and need for cancer surveillance. Establishing the extent of the disease requires accurate delineation of the proximal extent. Early studies suggested that 30–50% of patients would have extension of their disease [28–31]. However, early studies demonstrating extension may be affected by information bias as these studies relied on rigid proctosigmoidoscopy and barium enema to define the extent of disease. Barium enema has been shown to underestimate the extent of the disease [32, 33]. However, even with the use of colonoscopy there can be disagreements between the endoscopic and histologic assessment of the extent of disease [34]. In a small study of 31 ulcerative colitis patients who underwent at least two colonoscopies, Niv *et al.* found that only 23% of patients had no change in the extent of their disease [35]. Of the remaining patients, one-half had a greater extent and one-half had a lesser extent of disease on their second colonoscopy. Moum *et al.* examined changes in disease extent in a population-based cohort of 399 patients who had undergone at least two colonoscopies: one at the time of diagnosis, the second 12–23 months later. Overall, 34% of patients showed no change in the colonoscopic extent of their disease. Of the remainder 14% showed disease progression, 22% had disease regression and 30% had normal appearing mucosa at their second colonoscopy. It is not readily apparent, what proportion of patients were on medical therapy at the time of their second colonoscopy and what effect this had on the extent of the disease. The combination of relatively poor agreement between endoscopic and histological assessment of disease extent and the variation in disease extent on two different exams has led some to question the practice of basing cancer surveillance practices on disease extent [36].

Mortality

Mortality rates in early series of ulcerative colitis patients were very high. Edwards and Truelove found that the 20-year mortality rate for those with ulcerative colitis diagnosed between 1938 and 1962 was 35% compared to an expected rate of only 5% [37]. Even accounting for the potential of selection bias influencing these results, given that Oxford was a tertiary referral centre, this series demonstrates the high mortality rates experienced by those with ulcerative colitis prior to the introduction of effective therapies. In Oxford, the mortality rates fell dramatically after the introduction of steroid treatment. For those recruited suffering their first attack, the 7-year mortality rate decreased from 24% in the period 1938–1952 to 9% in the period 1953–1962. Truelove and Witt's pivotal clinical trial of cortisone in ulcerative colitis also found a lower, though not quite statistically significant, death rate in those receiving cortisone (4.6% vs 10.9%) [38].

When comparing death rates between a cohort of patients with ulcerative colitis and the general population adjustment is required to take into account the different age and sex distribution of the two groups. Many studies report standardised mortality ratios (SMR). The SMR is the ratio of the observed number of deaths in the ulcerative colitis group to the number of deaths that would have been expected if this group suffered from the same age-sex specific mortality rates occurring in the general population. SMRs can also be expressed as percentages, with an SMR of 100 indicating that number of observed and expected deaths were equivalent. SMRs greater than 100 indicate excess risk of death and less than 100 reduced risk of death. Table 29.2 shows SMRs for ulcerative colitis and different disease subtypes reported in population-based studies.

The overall trend in studies examining mortality in ulcerative colitis is a decrease in the risk of excess mortality over time [42]. Modern studies reveal that those with ulcerative colitis enjoy a life expectancy little different from the general public [8, 39–42]. In the Danish inception cohort of 1161 ulcerative colitis patients followed from diagnosis to end of 1987 no overall excess mortality was noted [40]. However, there was excess mortality in the first year after diagnosis with a relative risk of death of 2.4. Similarly, the north-eastern Scotland cohort also found excess mortality within the first years of diagnosis and in those with extensive disease at onset but no significant long-term differences between the observed and expected mortality in all 537 patients [8]. Two Swedish population-based studies found modestly decreased survival for those with ulcerative colitis. Persson *et al.* included 1547 subjects with ulcerative colitis diagnosed in Stockholm between 1955 and 1984 [41]. The observed versus expected survival rate after 15 years was 94.2% (95%

Table 29.2 Standardised mortality ratios of ulcerative colitis.

Author	Country	Year of diagnosis	End of follow-up	Subgroup	SMR
Ekbom [39]	Sweden	1965–83	1986	All UC	140 (120–150)
				Proctitis	100 (90–120)
				Left-sided	120 (100–140)
				Pancolitis	190 (170–220)
Langholz [40]	Denmark	1962–87	1987	All UC	106 (NS)
				First year	235 ($P < 0.001$)
Persson [41]	Sweden	1955–90	1990	All UC	137 (120–154)

CI 92.4–96.1%). Ekbom *et al.* studied 2509 patients diagnosed with ulcerative colitis within the Uppsala Region of Sweden from 1965 to 1983 with follow-up to the end of 1986 [42]. The 10-year survival of those with ulcerative colitis was 95.9% (95% CI 94.3–97.5) relative to that of the general population. Decreased survival was not seen in those with proctitis.

Predictors of risk of colectomy

Colectomy rates after 1 year of disease were 10% in two series from Sweden and Denmark [43, 44]. In the earlier series from Copenhagen, Hendriksen *et al.* found a cumulative colectomy rate at 1 year of 10%, 3% in the second year and thereafter approximately 1% per year in patients diagnosed between 1960 and 1978 [44]. The cumulative 10- and 18-year colectomy rate was 23 and 31%, respectively. The Swedish study included patients diagnosed with ulcerative colitis in Stockholm County from 1955 to 1984 [43]. In this series, the colectomy rate was 28% at 10 years and 45% at 25 years. In contrast, Sinclair *et al.* reported a cumulative colectomy rate at 10 years of approximately 12% or about half of the rate reported in the above two studies [8]. A more recent series of patients diagnosed between 1991 and 1993 in 20 European sites reported that after 4 years of follow-up 4% of ulcerative colitis patients had undergone surgery [45].

As discussed earlier, extensive and severely active disease are markers of poor prognosis. Therefore, one would expect colectomy rates in reported series to vary based on the proportion of patients with these features. However, colectomy rates vary greatly across different surgical series. Therefore other factors must also affect colectomy rates. These may include regional definitions of medical failure, degree of use of immunosuppressants and cyclosporine (although most series pre-date the use of cyclosporine for severe flares) and surgical practice patterns. New surgical techniques, including the ileoanal pouch, are better accepted by patients, but their impact on surgical rates is unclear.

Leijonmarck found that those with proctitis and left-sided colitis had similar colectomy rates, though even for those with proctitis the 10-year colectomy rate was approximately 15%. For those with pan-colitis, the 10-year colectomy rate was 40%. Comparable 10-year colectomy rates from the northeastern Scotland cohort are 6, 12 and 35% for those with distal, left-sided and pan-colitis, respectively [8]. Therefore, although colectomy rates are similar for those with pan-colitis, there appears to be marked differences in the rates for limited disease between studies, probably reflecting local surgical practice patterns rather than characteristics of the disease.

Several investigators have examined factors that could predict the need for colectomy in patients admitted with an exacerbation of ulcerative colitis. Chakravarty examined 89 patients at Auckland Hospital to determine predictors of medical treatment failure [46]. Surgery was required in 28% of patients. In a multivariate model, severity of diarrhoea and low albumen level were the only predictors of surgery. Travis *et al.* examined predictors of response to medical therapy in a series of 49 patients with 51 consecutive severe attacks of colitis [47]. Complete response, defined as three or fewer bowel motions without visible blood, was seen in 21 episodes. Fifteen had an incomplete response, defined as more than three bowel motions or visible blood on day 7 but no colectomy. Fifteen (29%) failed medical therapy and underwent colectomy during the admission. Complete responders remained in remission for a median of 9 months and had a 5% chance of eventual colectomy. Incomplete responders had a 60% chance of continuous symptoms and a 40% chance of colectomy. During the first 5 days, stool frequency and C-reactive protein (CRP) could distinguish between treatment failures and successes. On day 3, patients with either (1) three to eight bowel motions with a CRP more than 45 mg/L or (2) eight or more bowel motions had an 85% chance of colectomy.

Lindgren *et al.* conducted a retrospective analysis of 97 patients with acute attacks of ulcerative colitis admitted to four Swedish university hospitals and treated with intravenous corticosteroids [48]. They found that c-reactive protein levels greater than or equal to 25 mg/L and more than 4 bowel movements/day on day 3 of hospitalisation independently predicted a high risk for colectomy.

Table 29.3 Ho et al. failure of medical therapy risk index [49].

Factor	Score
3-day mean stool frequency	
<4	0
4–7	1
7–9	2
>9	4
Colonic dilation within 3 days	4
Hypoalbuminemia (<30 g/L) on day 1	1

Index (range 0–9) = Mean stool frequency + colonic dilation + hypoalbuminemia.

Score	Risk category	Failure rate
0–1	Low risk	11%
2–3	Intermediate risk	45%
≥ 4	High risk	85%

Ho et al. developed an index to allow the early identification of patients at risk of not responding to intravenous corticosteroid therapy to facilitate second-line treatment with ciclosporine or colectomy [49]. They recruited 167 consecutive patients with severe ulcerative colitis from 1995–2002. They used multiple logistic regression to analyse parameters within the first 3 days of medical therapy that were associated with failure of first-line medical therapy. Their final index included mean stool frequency, presence of colonic dilation and hypoalbuminemia on day 1 (<30 g/L) and was scored from 0 to 9 (Table 29.3). All those with a score of six or higher failed medical therapy.

However, all of these studies are at risk of information bias. Those caring for the patients and making the decision regarding the outcome (medical failure, colectomy) were not blinded as to the results of the putative predictive variables. CRP has been reported as a predictor of colectomy [50]. Therefore, it is possible that patients were selected for colectomy based on their CRP level or other clinical features, meaning that knowledge of the predictive factors may have influenced the 'measurement' of the outcome. The greatest risk would have been in those with a partial or incomplete response to medical therapy. Therefore, the results in these studies may reflect local practice patterns as well as the true biological refractoriness of the disease.

Genetic factors may, in the future, play a role in determining susceptibility and predicting behaviour of ulcerative colitis. Human leukocyte antigen (HLA) class II genes regulate immune responses and have been studied as markers of disease behaviour in ulcerative colitis. HLA-DRB1*01303 has been shown to predict the need for surgery and HLA-DR3-DQ2 haplotype is more common in extensive disease [51]. Susceptibility to ulcerative colitis, particularly extensive disease, has been associated with an allele in the second intron of the gene encoding the interleukin (IL)-1 receptor antagonist (IL-1Ra), which is a potent anti-inflammatory protein [52]. Roussomoustakaki et al. examined HLA-DRB1*0103 and allele 2 of the IL-1Ra gene in 107 ulcerative colitis patients undergoing colectomy compared to 482 healthy controls [53]. The HLA-DRB1*103 allele was more common in ulcerative colitis patients compared to controls (14.1% vs 3.2%). It was also more common in patients with extensive disease (15.8% vs 8.7% in distal colitis) and in those with extra-intestinal manifestations (EIMs) (22.8% vs 2.4% in those with no EIMs). In this study the frequency of the IL-1Ra allele was not different than controls. It was, however, seen less frequently in patients with distal disease and may provide a marker for patients at risk for developing extensive colitis. HLA-DRB1*0102 was found to be more common in patients requiring colectomy in a French series of 91 ulcerative colitis patients [54].

References

1. Meyers S, Janowitz HD. The 'natural history' of ulcerative colitis: an analysis of the placebo response [Review] [19 refs]. *J Clin Gastroenterol* 1989; 11:33–7.
2. Ilnyckyj A, Shanahan F, Anton PA, Cheang M, Bernstein CN. Quantification of the placebo response in ulcerative colitis. *Gastroenterology* 1997;112: 1854–8.
3. Janowitz HD, Bodian C. The placebo response and the 'natural history' of inflammatory bowel disease. *Inflamm Bowel Dis* 2001;7:64–6.

4 Kornbluth AA, Salomon P, Sacks HS, Mitty R, Janowitz HD. Meta-analysis of the effectiveness of current drug therapy of ulcerative colitis. *J Clin Gastroenterol* 1993;16:215–18.

5 Edwards F, Truelove SC. The course and prognosis of ulcerative colitis: I. Short-term prognosis. *Gut* 1963;4:299–308.

6 Jalan KN, Prescott RJ, Sircus W, et al. An experience of ulcerative colitis: II. Short term outcome. *Gastroenterology* 1970;59:589–97.

7 Watts JM, De Dombal FT, Watkinson G, Goligher JC. Early course of ulcerative colitis. *Gut* 1966;7:16–31.

8 Sinclair TS, Brunt PW, Mowat NA. Nonspecific proctocolitis in northeastern Scotland: a community study. *Gastroenterology* 1983;85:1–11.

9 Stonnington CM, Phillips SF, Zinsmeister AR, Melton LJ III. Prognosis of chronic ulcerative colitis in a community. *Gut* 1987;28:1261–6.

10 Moum B, Ekbom A, Vatn MH, et al. Inflammatory bowel disease: re-evaluation of the diagnosis in a prospective population based study in south eastern Norway. *Gut* 1997;40:328–32.

11 Schumacher G, Sandstedt B, Mollby R, Kollberg B. Clinical and histologic features differentiating non-relapsing colitis from first attacks of inflammatory bowel disease. *Scand J Gastroenterol* 1991;26:151–61.

12 Moum B, Ekbom A, Vatn MH, et al. Clinical course during the 1st year after diagnosis in ulcerative colitis and Crohn's disease. Results of a large, prospective population-based study in southeastern Norway, 1990-93. *Scand J Gastroenterol* 1997;32:1005–12.

13 Langholz E, Munkholm P, Davidsen M, Binder V. Course of ulcerative colitis: analysis of changes in disease activity over years. *Gastroenterology* 1994;107:3–11.

14 Sutherland L, Roth D, Beck P, May G, Makiyama K. Oral 5-aminosalicylic acid for maintenance of remission in ulcerative colitis. *Cochrane Database of Sys Rev* 2004;2004.

15 Kangro HO, Chong SK, Hardiman A, Heath RB, Walker-smith JA. A prospective study of viral and mycoplasma infections in chronic inflammatory bowel disease. *Gastroenterology* 1990;98:549–53.

16 Myszor M, Calam J. Seasonality of ulcerative colitis. *Lancet* 1984;2:522–3.

17 Rampton DS, McNeil NI, Sarner M. Food intolerance, prostaglandins, and irritable bowel syndrome. *Lancet* 1983;1:123–4.

18 Bartlett JG. *Clostridium difficile* and inflammatory bowel disease. *Gastroenterology* 1981;80:863–5.

19 Meyers S, Mayer L, Bottone E, Desmond E, Janowitz HD. Occurrence of *Clostridium difficile* toxin during the course of inflammatory bowel disease. *Gastroenterology* 1981;80:697–70.

20 Trnka YM, LaMont JT. Association of *Clostridium difficile* toxin with symptomatic relapse of chronic inflammatory bowel disease. *Gastroenterology* 1981;80:693–6.

21 LaMont JT, Trnka YM. Therapeutic implications of *Clostridium difficile* toxin during relapse of chronic inflammatory bowel disease. *Lancet* 1980;1:381–3.

22 Burke DA, Axon AT. *Clostridium difficile*, sulphasalazine, and ulcerative colitis. *Postgrad Med J* 1987;63:955–7.

23 Sellu DP. Seasonal variation in onset of exacerbations of ulcerative proctocolitis. *J R Coll Surg Edinb* 1986;31:158–60.

24 Isgar B, Harman M, Whorwell PJ. Factors preceding relapse of ulcerative colitis. *Digestion* 1983;26:236–8.

25 Leo S, Leandro G, Di Matteo G, Caruso ML, Lorusso D. Ulcerative colitis in remission: is it possible to predict the risk of relapse. *Digestion* 1989;44:217–21.

26 Riley SA, Mani V, Goodman MJ, Lucas S. Why do patients with ulcerative colitis relapse? *Gut* 1990;31:179–83.

27 Bitton A, Peppercorn MA, Antonioli DA, et al. Clinical, biological, and histologic parameters as predictors of relapse in ulcerative colitis. *Gastroenterology* 2001;120:13–20.

28 Farmer RG, Brown CH. Emerging concepts of proctosigmoiditis. *Dis Colon Rectum* 1972;15:142–6.

29 Powell-Tuck J, Ritchie JK, Lennard-Jones JE. The prognosis of idiopathic proctitis. *Scand J Gastroenterol* 1977;12:727–32.

30 Lennard-Jones JE. The clinical outcome of ulcerative colitis depends on how much of the colonic mucosa is involved. *Scand J Gastroenterol* 1983;88(Suppl):48–53.

31 Langholz E, Munkholm P, Davidsen M, Nielsen OH, Binder V. Changes in extent of ulcerative colitis: a study on the course and prognostic factors. *Scand J Gastroenterol* 1996;31:260–6.

32 Gabrielsson N, Granqvist S, Sundelin P, Thorgeirsson T. Extent of inflammatory lesions in ulcerative colitis assessed by radiology, colonoscopy, and endoscopic biopsies. *Gastrointest Radiol* 1979;4:395–400.

33 Williams C. Symposium: evaluation of the colonoscopic examination: results of three studies. *Dis Colon Rectum* 1975;18:366–8.

34 Moum B, Ekbom A, Vatn MH, Elgjo K. Change in the extent of colonoscopic and histological involvement in ulcerative colitis over time. *Am J Gastroenterol* 1999;94:1564–9.

35 Niv Y, Bat L, Ron E, Theodor E. Change in the extent of colonic involvement in ulcerative colitis: a

colonoscopic study. *Am J Gastroenterol* 1987;82: 1046–51.

36 Rhodes JM. Ulcerative colitis extent varies with time but endoscopic appearances may be deceptive. *Gut* 2001;49:322–3.

37 Edwards F, Truelove SC. The course and prognosis of ulcerative colitis: II. Long-term prognosis. *Gut* 1963; 4:309–15.

38 Truelove SC, Witts LJ. Cortisone in ulcerative colitis: final report of a therapeutic trial. *BMJ* 1955;ii: 1041–8.

39 Ekbom A, Helmick CG, Zack M, Holmberg L, Adami HO. Survival and causes of death in patients with inflammatory bowel disease: a population-based study. *Gastroenterology* 1992;103:954–60.

40 Langholz E, Munkholm P, Davidsen M, Binder V. Colorectal cancer risk and mortality in patients with ulcerative colitis. *Gastroenterology* 1992;103: 1444–51.

41 Persson PG, Bernell O, Leijonmarck CE, Farahmand BY, Hellers G, Ahlbom A. Survival and cause-specific mortality in inflammatory bowel disease: a population-based cohort study. *Gastroenterology* 1996;110:1339–45.

42 Farrokhyar F, Swarbrick E, Grace R, Hellier MD, Gent A, Irvine EJ. Low mortality in ulcerative colitis and Crohn's disease in three regional centers in England. *Am J Gastroenterol* 2001;96:501–7.

43 Leijonmarck CE, Persson PG, Hellers G. Factors affecting colectomy rate in ulcerative-colitis: an epidemiologic-study. *Gut* 1990;31:329–33.

44 Hendriksen C, Kreiner S, Binder V. Long-term prognosis in ulcerative-colitis: based on results from a regional patient group from the County of Copenhagen. *Gut* 1985;26:158–63.

45 Witte J, Shivananda S, Lennard-Jones JE, *et al.* Disease outcome in inflammatory bowel disease: mortality, morbidity and therapeutic management of a 796-person inception cohort in the European collaborative study on inflammatory bowel disease (EC-IBD). *Scand J Gastroenterol* 2000;35:1272–7.

46 Chakravarty BJ. Predictors and the rate of medical treatment failure in ulcerative colitis. *Am J Gastroenterol* 1993;88:852–5.

47 Travis SP, Farrant JM, Ricketts C, *et al.* Predicting outcome in severe ulcerative colitis. *Gut* 1996;38: 905–10.

48 Lindgren SC, Flood LM, Kilander AF, Lofberg R, Persson TB, Sjodahl RI. Early predictors of glucocorticosteroid treatment failure in severe and moderately severe attacks of ulcerative colitis. *Eur J Gastroenterol Hepatol* 1998;10:831–5.

49 Ho GT, Mowat C, Goddard CJR, *et al.* Predicting the outcome of severe ulcerative colitis: development of a novel risk score to aid early selection of patients for second-line medical therapy or surgery. *Aliment Pharmacol Ther* 2004;19:1079–87.

50 Buckell NA, Lennard-Jones JE, Hernandez MA, Kohn J, Riches PG, Wadsworth J. Measurement of serum proteins during attacks of ulcerative colitis as a guide to patient management. *Gut* 1920;20:22–7.

51 Satsangi J, Welsh KI, Bunce M, *et al.* Contribution of genes of the major histocompatibility complex to susceptibility and disease phenotype in inflammatory bowel disease. *Lancet* 1996;347:1212–17.

52 Mansfield JC, Holden H, Tarlow JK, *et al.* Novel genetic association between ulcerative-colitis and the antiinflammatory cytokine interleukin-1 receptor antagonist. *Gastroenterology* 1994;106:637–42.

53 Roussomoustakaki M, Satsangi J, Welsh K, *et al.* Genetic markers may predict disease behavior in patients with ulcerative colitis. *Gastroenterology* 1997;112:1845–53.

54 Heresbach D, Alizadeh M, Reumaux D, *et al.* Are HLA-DR or TAP genes genetic markers of severity in ulcerative colitis? *J Autoimmun* 1996;9:777–84.

Index

Notes: page numbers in *italics* refer to figures and those in **bold** refer to tables. Please note that as the subject of this book is inflammatory bowel disease all entries refer to this subject unless otherwise stated.

Abdominal bloating, refractory distal colitis, 129
Abdominal pain, refractory distal colitis, 129
Abdominal surgery, delayed capsule transit, 96
Abscess(es), 100, 106, *107*
   computed tomography, 106, *107*
   crypt, 67, 72
   examination under anaesthetic (EUA), 251, *251*, 255, 261
   magnetic resonance imaging (MRI), 109
   perianal *see* Perianal abscess(es)
   pregnancy and, 365
   ultrasound, 251–2, *252*
Absorptive dyes/stains, chromoendoscopy, 294
ACCENT trials, 224
   ACCENT-1 trial, 213–14
   ACCENT-2 trial, 214, 236–7
Adalimumab (Humira™), 224
Adenoma(s), 293
   carcinoma formation and, 267
   dysplasia-associated lesions *vs.*, 78–9, 274, 287–8
     see also Adenoma-like mass (ALM)
   incidence in ulcerative colitis, 315
   molecular features, 316–20, **319**
   staining patterns, 294
Adenoma–carcinoma pathway, 267–8
Adenoma-like mass (ALM), 269, 271, 314–15
   definition, 313, 314
   management, 320–2
     follow-up, 320, *321*
     outcome, 321
     see also Colonoscopic surveillance
   sporadic adenoma *vs.*, 315–20
     histology, 315–16
     molecular features, 316–20, **318**, **319**
Adenomatous polyposis coli (APC) gene, dysplasia/neoplasia, 267–8, 305, 316

Adolescents
   growth spurt, 329
   IBD in *see* Juvenile-onset IBD
   puberty, 329–30
Adrenal suppression, steroid-induced, 194
Aetiology, 1–64
   appendix and, 57–65
   bacteria, role, 44–56, 206
   environmental factors *see* Environmental factors
   genetics *see* Genetics of IBD
   osteopenia, **344**, 344–6
   perinatal/early infancy, 9
Alendronate, 354
Alkaline phosphatase, 343–4
Allopurinol, pouchitis treatment, 174
ALMs *see* Adenoma-like mass (ALM)
American Gastroenterological Association, fistulae treatment algorithm, 238–9
5-Aminosalicylate *see* Mesalazine (5-ASA; mesalamine)
Aminosalicylates
   adherence/compliance, 122, 126–7, 133
   cancer risk reduction, 121, 283
   colitis due to, 130
   failure, 216–17
   fistulae, 236
   formulations, 119, 127
   induction therapy, 119–20
   maintenance therapy, 119–23, 132–4
     dose, 119–21
     duration, 121–2
     patient adherence, 122
   male fertility and, 366
   mechanism of action, 119
   pharmacogenetics, 25
   pouchitis treatment, 174
   pregnancy and, 363–4

Aminosalicylates (*Continued*)
  refractoriness and
    adherence/compliance, 126–7
    drug choice, 126
    pharmacokinetics, 127–8
    tissue concentrations, 127
  in refractory distal colitis, 128, 130–1
    corticosteroids *vs.*, 129
    maintaining remission, 132–4, *133*
  topical (rectal), 120–1
    pharmacokinetics, 127–8
    refractory distal colitis, 130–1, 133–4
    steroids *vs.*, 130
    tissue concentrations, 127
  see also specific drugs/formulations
Amoebic colitis, CIBD *vs.*, 67, 69
Anaerobic bacteria, 45
Anaesthetic gel, refractory distal colitis, **135**
Anal canal
  Crohn's disease lesions, 246, 248–9
  rectal dissection and, 159
Anal fissures, Crohn's disease, 248–9
Anal flap advancement, perianal fistula management, 259, 260
Anal stenosis, Crohn's disease, 249
Anal transitional zone (ATZ; residual epithelial cuff), pouchitis and, 171
Anaphase bridges, 307, *307*
Anastomosis
  ileoanal (IPAA), 158, 167, 360, 365
  ileorectal, 155–6, 158
  stapled *vs.* handsewn, 160, 168, 241
  see also Ileal pouch(es)
Aneuploidy, dysplasia/neoplasia, 267, 268, 306, 309
Animal models
  pathogenic effects of bacteria, 46–7
  pattern recognition receptors, 33
  ulcerative colitis, 62
Anorectal inflammation, mucosectomy and, 160
Anorexia, 332
Antibiotics, 48
  breastfeeding and, 366
  commensal micro-flora and, 46
  Crohn's disease, 48, 206–12
    antimycobacterial agents, 209–11, *210*
    bridging therapy, 209
    broad spectrum, 209
    ciprofloxacin, 208–9
    fistulae management, 236
    metronidazole, 207–8, 211
    perianal abscess, 254
  pouchitis, 170, 173–4

  pregnancy and, 208, 364
  resistance, 207
  see also specific drugs/drug types
Antibodies to infliximab (ATIs), 214, 215–16, 223, 226
Anti-inflammatory drugs
  growth impairment treatment/prevention, 334–7
  pouchitis, 174
  see also Immunomodulators; *specific drugs*
Antimycobacterial agents, 209–11
Anti-OmpC antibody, 226, 227
Anti-*Saccharomyces cerevisiae* antibodies (ASCA), 226
Anti-tumour necrosis factor-α therapies, 213, 223–4
  in children, 336–7
  growth impairment prevention/treatment, 336–7
  infliximab *see* Infliximab
  pregnancy and, 365
APC (adenomatous polyposis coli) gene, dysplasia/neoplasia, 267–8, 305, 316
Aphthous ulcers, Crohn's disease, 75, 95
Appendectomy
  clinical studies in ulcerative colitis, 62–63
  negative association with ulcerative colitis, 57–60
    cohort studies, 57–8
    mechanism, 62
    meta-analysis, 58
    natural history effects, 59–60
    primary *vs.* incidental surgery, 57–8
    as protective factor, 59
  neonatal, effects of, 61
  rates of, 61
  refractory distal colitis, 138
Appendicitis
  incidence, 60–1
  ulcerative, 63
  ulcerative colitis susceptibility and, 59
Appendix, 60–1
  Crohn's disease pathology, skip lesions, 71
  history, 60
  immune functions, 60, 61
  ulcerative colitis pathogenesis and, 59, 60, 61–2
  ulcerative colitis pathology, 62, 63
  ulcerative colitis susceptibility and, 57–64
    epidemiological observations, 57–60
Arsenic, refractory distal colitis, **135**
Asacol®, 119, 120, **182**
  placebo-controlled RCTs in active Crohn's disease, 184
  refractory distal colitis, 128, 133
  tissue concentrations, 127
ASCA (anti-*Saccharomyces cerevisiae* antibodies), 226
Aspirin, colorectal cancer and, 283
Assessment, 66–116
Association studies, 14
Attained height, 329

Autoimmune response, appendix and, 61
Azathioprine (AZA), 196
   colorectal cancer prevention, 284
   Crohn's disease
      fistulae management, 236, 255
      post-operative prophylaxis, 241
   growth impairment treatment/prevention, 336
   male fertility and, 366
   pregnancy and, 364
   refractory distal colitis, 128, 134
   TPMT polymorphism and, 24

Backwash ileitis
   Crohn's disease *vs.*, 74
   pouchitis and, 170
Bacteria (intestinal), 33, 144
   alterations in IBD, 47–8
      Crohn's disease, 206
   commensal *see* Commensal micro-flora
   host–flora interactions, 145–6
      bacterial recognition *see* Pattern recognition receptors (PRRs)
   IBD pathogenesis and, 44–56, 146, 206, 222, 222
      alterations in microbial flora in, 47–8
      animal models, 46–7
      dose–response relationship, 44, 46
      pathogenic bacteria, 45, **45**
      systemic immune response, 47–8
      therapeutic manipulation, 48–50, **49**
         see also Pharmabiotics
   tolerance of, 44
   variation, 147
   see also individual species
Bacterial overgrowth, Crohn's disease, 206
Balsalazide, 119, **182**
Barium small bowel radiography
   capsule endoscopy *vs.*, 91
   Crohn's disease, 85–6
Basiliximab, 225
B-cell development, appendix and, 61
Bcl-2 gene, dysplasia/neoplasia, 269, 305
Bifidobacterium
   as prebiotic, 49
   as probiotic, 144, 147
Biological therapies, 196, 221, 223–5
   children, 335
   cytokine manipulation, 224, 225
   GM-CSF, 225
   immunophenotype and, 226–8
   leukocyte adhesion molecule modulation, 224
   subgroup analysis and, 225–6
   Th1 inhibitors, 224–5
   TNF inhibition *see* Anti-tumour necrosis factor-α therapies
   see also specific agents
Biomarkers
   bone metabolism, 343–4
   cancer *see* Cancer biomarkers
Biopsy
   cancer biomarkers, 304–5
   colonoscopic, 76, 284–5
   Crohn's disease appearance, 67, 68
   in dysplasia, 79, 271, **271**, 284–5, 293, 319
      DALMs, 313, 314
   indeterminate colitis diagnosis, 69–71
   sampling error, 271, 286, 319
   scoring systems, 77
   ulcerative colitis appearance, 67, 68
Bismuth compounds, refractory distal colitis, 135
Bisphosphonates, 353, 354
Blood vessel density, ultrasound, 112
Bone, 340–1
   age, radiographic, 351
   fractures, 194, 346
   metabolism
      biochemical markers, 343–4
      cytokines and, 341–3
      remodelling/resorption, 341, 342
   types, 340
Bone mineral density (BMD), 340
   IBD-induced loss, 194
   importance of, 201
   juvenile-onset IBD and, 195, 346, 350–3, *351*
   measurement, 343
   mechanisms of maintenance, 341
   physical activity and, 341
   steroid-induced loss, 194–6, **195**, 340, 341, 344
   T-scores, 344, **345**
   Z-scores, 344, **345**, 351
   see also Osteopenia; Osteoporosis
Bone morphogenetic proteins (BMPs), 342
Bone-specific alkaline phosphatase (BAP), 344
Bovine colostrum, refractory distal colitis, 135
Bowel preparation, capsule transit time and, 98
'Bowel rest,' 197, 199, 335
Bowel wall thickness, 111–12
   computed tomography, 106
   magnetic resonance imaging, 108–9, 110
   ultrasound, 111
Breastfeeding, 366
   see also Pregnancy
Bridge-breakage-fusion (BBF) cycles, 307
Bridging therapy
   antibiotics, 209
   infliximab, 217

380 INDEX

Brisbane Inflammatory Bowel Disease database, appendectomy effects on UC, 59
British Society of Gastroenterology (BSG) guidelines
   colonoscopic biopsy, 76
   osteoporosis prevention/management, 353
   'tick box' system, 77
Broad spectrum antibiotics, Crohn's disease, 209
Budesonide
   Crohn's disease
      in children, 336
         mesalazine *vs.* in active disease, 184
         post-operative prophylaxis, 241
   fracture prevention, 346
   osteopenia prevention/management, 346, 354
   pouchitis management, 174
   pregnancy and, 363
'Bugs to drugs,' 144, 148
Bursa of Fabricius, 57, 61
Butyrate production, Crohn's disease, 196–7

Caecal patch lesion
   Crohn's disease, 70
   refractory distal colitis, 132
Caesarean section, indications, 365
Calcitonin, osteopenia and, 353, 354
Calcium supplements, 354
Campylobacter spp.
   Campylobacter jejuni colitis, CIBD *vs.*, 67
   treatment in pouchitis, 173
Cancellous (spongy) bone, 340
Cancer
   colorectal *see* Colorectal carcinoma
   endoscopic diagnosis, 293–302
   individual risk in IBD, 308–9
   molecular markers *see* Cancer biomarkers
   overall risk in IBD, 281–6, 289
   pouch mucosa, 80, 162, 171
   precancerous lesions *see* Dysplasia
   small bowel, 281
   surveillance *see* Colonoscopic surveillance
Cancer biomarkers, 303–11, 316–20, **317, 318, 319**
   chromosome instability, 306–8, 307
   DNA methylation, 317, 319
   need for, 303–4
   non-dysplastic mucosa, 317–20
   performance, 308–9
   serum markers, 304
   telomere shortening, 307, 307–8
   tissue (biopsy) markers, 304–5
   see also specific markers
Capsule endoscopy, 85–104
   advantages, 87–8
   case studies, 88

   clinical studies, 88–92, **89**
      obstruction and, 90
   disadvantages/problems, 92, 97–100
      capsule retention, 88, 97–8
      delayed transit, 98–9
      image quality, 99
      inability to biopsy, 99–100
      incomplete examination, 98–9
      inter-observer variability/image interpretation, 100
      mucosal healing, 99
      transmural disease, 100
   economic decision model, 101
   indeterminate colitis and, 96
   lesion appearance, 93–4, 95, 99
   lesion distribution, 93
   methodology/technology, 87–8
      patency capsule, 95–7
      PillCam™ capsule, 87, 87
      RAPID™ workstation, 87
   other diagnostic modalities *vs.*, 92–3
      colonoscopy, 91, 92
      CT, 90–1, 92, 93
      double-balloon enteroscopy, 92–3
      ileoscopy, 92
      MR enterography, 93
      push enteroscopy, 91, 93
      SBFT, 90–1, 92–3, 96
      small bowel enteroclysis, 91
   paediatric patients, 94–5
   safety, 100–1
      pacemakers/defibrillators and, 100–1
      paediatric patients, 94
      pregnant patients, 100
   scoring, 94, 99
   treatment decisions and, 91–2
   ulcerative colitis and, 95–6
Carbohydrate metabolism, Crohn's disease, 196–7
Carcinoembryonic antigen (CEA), dysplasia and, 273
Carcinogenesis, 303
   adenoma-carcinoma sequence, 267–8
   molecular mechanism, 268, 268–9, 304, 305–6
   non-dysplastic mucosa, 317–20
   oxidative stress and, 306
Carcinoma *in situ*, 271
CARD (caspase activation and recruitment domain), 37
CARD4 (NOD1), 16, 37
   cellular distribution, 38
   domain structure, 37
   function, 38
CARD15 (NOD2), 15, 16, 19, 37–9, 47, 146, 222
   cellular distribution, 38
   domain structure, 37
   drug design and, 226

function, 38
growth impairment and, 333
intracellular signalling, 19–20, 20, 34, 37–8
knockout mice, 20, 21
ligand, 19, 38
polymorphism, 15, 16, 25
  clinical practice and, 23, 39
  Crohn's pathogenesis and, 19–21, 38–9
  ethnic heterogeneity, 18–19
  IBD5 and, 17
  IBD8 and, 17–18
  phenotype–genotype relationship, 19
Caspase activation and recruitment domain (CARD), 37
β-Catenin, dysplasia/neoplasia, 269, 305, 316–17
CD4-CD8-B220+ αβ T-cells, 61
CD19, appendiceal expression in UC, 62
CD62L+CD4+ T-cells, experimental chronic colitis, 62
CD138, appendiceal expression in UC, 62
CDP870, 223, 225–6
CDP571, 66, 223
Cell adhesion molecules
  dysplasia/neoplasia, 224, 269
  genetics of IBD, 17
Cell cycle, dysplasia/neoplasia, 269, 305
Cell structure genes, dysplasia/neoplasia, 269
Celsus, Aulus Cornelius, 60
Chromoendoscopy, 269, 293–8, 295
  confocal endomicroscopy and, 299, 300
  DALM (dysplasia associated lesion/mass), 314
  diagnostic yield, 297
  dyes/stains, 293–4
  efficiency, 296–8
  false-positives, 298
  goals, 294
  lesions visualised, 294, 295–6
  limitations, 297–8
  magnifying, 269, 295, 296–8, 300
  panchromoendoscopy, 294, 297
  pit-pattern classification, 294, 296, 296
    complexity, 298
    DALMs, 314
  safety issues, 297
  SURFACE guidelines, **296**
  technique, 294–6
Chromosomal instability (CIN), dysplasia/neoplasia, 267, 306–8
Chronic idiopathic inflammatory bowel disease (CIBD)
  acute self-limiting (infective) colitis vs., 67, 68, 69
    sequelae vs., 68–9
  effect of treatment on histopathology, 75–6
Churg–Strauss syndrome, 74
Ciprofloxacin, 48
  activity, 208

Crohn's disease, 208–9
  fistulae management, 236
  mesalazine vs., 208
  pouchitis, 173–4
  side effects, 209
Clarithromycin, Crohn's disease, 209, 210
Claversal, refractory distal colitis, 131
Clinical diagnosis, pouchitis, 79
Clostridium difficile, treatment in pouchitis, 173
Colazide (balsalazide), 119, **182**
Colectomy
  DALMs management, 320, 322
  emergency, 154, 234
  with ileorectal anastomosis, 155–6
    female fertility and, 158
    intermediate colitis, 156
  with ileostomy
    defunctioning ileostomy, need, 160
    emergency surgery, 154
  prediction of risk in ulcerative colitis, 370, 373–4, **374**
  total, refractory distal colitis, 138
Colitis
  acute self-limiting (infective) see Infective colitis
  aminosalicylate-induced, 130
  Campylobacter jejuni, 67
  carcinogenesis and, 268
  Crohn's disease
    cancer risk, 281, 282, 286
    misdiagnosis, 132
  differential diagnosis, 67–9, 68, 69
  distal see Distal colitis
  diversion, 71
  diverticular, 71, 73, 74, 75
  fulminant, 154–5, 365
  indeterminate see Indeterminate colitis
  secondary, 129
  ulcerative see Ulcerative colitis
Colitis–dysplasia–carcinoma pathway, 268
Collagen, bone structure, 340
Colon
  commensal micro-flora, 45–7
  dilation, treatment failure prediction, 374
  physiology, proximal vs. distal, 125
Colonoscopic surveillance, 281–92
  aims/prerequisites, 285–6
  chromoendoscopy see Chromoendoscopy
  confocal imaging, 298–9, 299, 300
  in Crohn's disease, 286
  DALMs/ALMs, 221
  impact on cancer morbidity/mortality, 285
  multiple biopsy, 284, 285, 286, 319, 321
  new techniques, 293–302
  patient selection, 294, **296**

Colonoscopic surveillance (*Continued*)
   schedule, 286–8
   timing, 285–6, 286–7
   in ulcerative colitis, 155, 284–5
   see also Dysplasia
Colonoscopy
   biopsy, 76, 284–5
   capsule endoscopy *vs.*, 91, 92
   difficulty in Crohn's disease, 286
   disease extent in ulcerative colitis, 371
   incidence effects, 6
   pregnancy and, 363
   pre-operative decision making, 234
   screening, 286–7
   surveillance *see* Colonoscopic surveillance
   value of biopsy series in diagnosis, 76
   virtual CT, 107–8
   see also specific techniques
Colorectal carcinoma
   carcinogenesis, 303, 316
      adenoma–carcinoma sequence, 267–8
      molecular mechanism, **268**, 268–9, 305–6
   Crohn's disease association, 269, 286
      overall risk, 282
   Crohn's disease *vs.*, 73–5
   management strategies, 284–6
   molecular markers *see* Cancer biomarkers
   precancerous lesions *see* Dysplasia
   primary sclerosing cholangitis and, 283, 285, 286, 303, 320
   protective factors, 283–4
      5-Aminosalicylates (5-ASAs), 121, 283
      folic acid, 283–4
      immunomodulating drugs, 284
      ursodeoxycholic acid, 283
   restorative proctocolectomy and, 157, 162
   risk, 268, 281–4
   surveillance *see* Colonoscopic surveillance
   ulcerative colitis association, 155, 266, 268, 289, 293, 303
      clinical risk factors, 282–3
      individual risk, 308–9
      overall risk, 281–2
Colostomy
   blowhole in pregnancy, 366
   fistulae management, 261
Colostrum (bovine), refractory distal colitis, 135
Columnar cuff disorders, pouchitis and, 171
Commensal micro-flora, 45–7, 144
   anaerobic, 45
   factors affecting, 46
   host–flora interactions, 145–6
      recognition *see* Pattern recognition receptors (PRRs)
   IBD pathogenesis, 45, **45**, 206
      animal models, 46–7
   normal functions, 45
   variation, 147
Compact (cortical) bone, 340
Computed tomography (CT), 104–7
   abscess(es), 107, *108*
   advantages/disadvantages, 107
   BMD measurement, 343
   capsule endoscopy *vs.*, 90–1, 92, 93
   contrast agents, 105
   diagnosis, 106
   disease activity, 107
   enteroclysis, 106
      capsule endoscopy *vs.*, 90
   extra-luminal disease assessment, 105, 106, *107*
   MRI *vs.*, 109
   multi-slice, 105
   perianal fistulae, 251
   standard techniques, 105–6
   ultrasound *vs.*, 111
   virtual colonoscopy, 107–8
Conception, 360, *361*
   paternal drugs at time of, 366
   see also Fertility
Confocal endoscope, 298, *300*
Confocal laser endomicroscopy, 298–9, *299*, *300*
Congenital malformation
   effect of drug therapy on, 364
   effect of IBD on risk, 362
Congestive heart failure, infliximab and, 215, 216
Connective tissue changes, Crohn's disease, 74, 75
Contrast agents
   chromoendoscopy dyes/stains, 293–4
   computed tomography, 105
   confocal laser endomicroscopy, 298
   magnetic resonance imaging, 108
Contrast radiography, Crohn's disease diagnosis, 85–6
Controlled-release drugs, aminosalicylates, 119
Cortical (compact) bone, 340
Corticosteroids, 194–6, 200
   active Crohn's disease
      in children, 335–6
      sulphasalazine *vs.*, 181–2
   adverse effects, 129, 194–6, **195**
      adrenal suppression, 194
      bone mineral loss, 194–6, **195**, 340, 341, 344
         see also Osteopenia
      growth suppression, 333
      metabolic dysfunction, 194
   alternatives to, 196, 200
   breastfeeding and, 366
   colorectal cancer prevention, 284

dependence, 196, 201, 336
fistulae, 236
growth impairment treatment/prevention, 335–6
intravenous, refractory distal colitis, 131–2
nutritional therapy vs., 194–205
oral, refractory distal colitis, 128–9
osteopenia treatment/prevention, 353
pouchitis management, 174
pregnancy and, 363
probiotics vs., 150
refractory distal colitis, 128–9
  aminosalicylates vs., 130
  ciclosporin and, 131–2
topical (rectal) therapy
  pharmacokinetics, 127–8
  refractory distal colitis, 128–9, 130
as treatment of choice, 194
see also specific drugs
Counselling, female fertility following surgery, 158
COX-2 expression, TLR$_9$-associated, 36
CpG island methylator phenotype (CIMP), 317, 319
C-reactive protein (CRP), prediction of medical failure, 373, 374
Crohn's disease, 281
  abscess(es), 100, 106, 107
    perianal see Perianal abscess(es)
  animal models, 47
  appendectomy and, 59
  assessment/scoring
    Crohn's disease activity index (CDAI), 110, 182, 183, 184
    endoscopic, 94, 99
    histopathological, 77
    MRI, 253–4, 254
    perianal disease, 246–8, 247, 248, 253–4, 254
  bone mineral density loss, 340, 344
    prevalence, 345, 345
    ulcerative colitis vs., 346–50, 348, 349
    see also Osteopenia
  cancer risk
    colorectal cancer, 269, 282
    small bowel carcinoma, 281
    surveillance, 286
    see also Cancer; Colonoscopic surveillance; Dysplasia
  children see Juvenile-onset IBD
  colitis
    cancer risk, 281, 282, 286
    misdiagnosis, 132
  diagnostic imaging, 85–6
    capsule endoscopy see Capsule endoscopy
    computed tomography, 106
    economic decision model, 101
    inadequacy/problems, 86–7
    MRI, 108–9
    ultrasound, 111
    see also specific modalities
  differential diagnosis
    backwash ileitis vs., 73
    colorectal carcinoma vs., 74–5
    diversion colitis vs., 71
    diverticular colitis vs., 71, 73, 74, 75
    granulomatous vasculitis vs., 74
    infective colitis vs., 67, 68, 69
    NSAID-induced lesions vs., 94
    sarcoidosis vs., 73
    tuberculosis vs., 73, 73–4
    ulcerative colitis vs., 70–72, 85, 95–6
  endoscopic appearance, 91–2, 93, 97
  extra-intestinal see Extra-intestinal manifestation (EIMs)
  fertility issues, 360
  fistulating, 100, 106, 235–6
    children, 336
    management, 214–15, 218, 235–9, 238
    perianal see Perianal fistulae
    pouchitis and, 172
  genetics
    CARD15 polymorphism see CARD15 (NOD2)
    familial clustering, 14
    see also Genetics of IBD
  global changes in incidence, 3
    geographical trends, 7
    morbidity data, 4
    time trends, 5, 5–6
  histopathological diagnosis, 67, 68, 70–72, 233–5
    aphthous ulcers, 75
    caecal patch lesion, 70
    connective tissue changes, 74, 75
    cyst abscess rupture, 72
    depth of inflammation, 72
    fat-wrapping, 74
    fissuring ulcers, 74
    focal inflammatory infiltrate, 71
    gastro-duodenal disease, 81
    granulomas/microgranulomas, 71, 71–72, 72–3
    inflammatory cell type, 72
    scoring, 77
    skip lesions, 70, 78
    specific diagnostic features, 73–5
    transmural inflammation, 74–5
    ulcer-associated cell lineage, 75
  ileoanal pouches, 168–9, 232–3
  juvenile-onset see Juvenile-onset IBD
  malnutrition in, 197
  management, 179–326
    adults vs. children, 335
    antibiotics, 48, 206–12

Crohn's disease (*Continued*)
   'bowel rest,' 197, 199
   children, 334–7
   corticosteroids, 194–6
   designer drugs, 221–31
   induction therapy, 181–6, **185**
   infliximab, 196, 213–20
   maintenance therapy, 186–7, **187**, 200, 201
   mesalazine, 181–93
   nutritional, 196–201
   post-operative prophylaxis, 189–91, **190**, 240–1
   probiotic therapy, **149**, 197
   refractory disease, 213–14
   surgical *see* Surgical management
   see also specific drugs/treatments
  mortality, 4
  nutritional deficiency, 196
  obstructions/stenosis, 88, 94, 97–8
   in pregnancy, 365
  pathogenesis, 44, 206, 209, 213
  perianal *see* Perianal Crohn's disease
  phenotypic overlap with ulcerative colitis, 15
  pregnancy *see* Pregnancy
  proctitis, refractory distal colitis *vs.*, 129
  refractory disease, 227
   infliximab, 213–14
  remission, prognosis and, 189
  restorative proctocolectomy contraindication, 157
  serologic associations, 226–8
  small intestine, 85
  transmural disease, 100
  upper GI tract involvement, 81
Crohn's disease activity index (CDAI)
  magnetic resonance imaging correlation, 110
  mesalazine trials, 182, 183, 184
Crohn's disease endoscopic index of severity, capsule endoscopy, 95
Crohn's proctitis, refractory distal colitis *vs.*, 129
Crypt abscesses
  granuloma formation, 72
  histopathological diagnosis and, 67
Crypt architecture, 67, 68
  dysplasia, 271–2, 273, 316, *316*
  restitution, 275
Cryptolytic granulomas, Crohn's disease, 71, *71*–72
Cutaneous advancement flap, 237–8
Cyclin D1 gene, dysplasia/neoplasia, 269
Cyclo-oxygenase 2 (COX-2), dysplasia/neoplasia, 269, 317
Cyclosporin, 196
  fistulae management, 236, 255–6, 261
  fulminant colitis, 154
  pregnancy and, 365

  'pseudodysplasia' induction, 75–6
  refractory distal colitis, 131–2, **135**
Cytokeratins, dysplasia/neoplasia, 269
Cytokines
  biological therapies, 224–5
  bone metabolism and, 341–3
   regulation, 343
  growth impairment and, **332**, 332–3
  IBD pathogenesis, 223
  see also individual molecules
Cytology, dysplasia diagnosis, 272–3, 275
Cytomegalovirus, treatment in pouchitis, 173

Daclizumab, 225
DALM (dysplasia associated lesion/mass), 269, 271
  adenoma-like *see* Adenoma-like mass (ALM)
  chromoendoscopy, 314
  colonoscopic surveillance, 284, 320
   schedule, 287
  definition, 313
  follow-up, 320
  high-grade dysplasia in, 321–2
  incidence, 313
  low-grade dysplasia in, 322
  macroscopic appearance, 313
  management, 320–2
  multiple biopsy, 313, 314
  problematic aspects, **313**, 313–14
  sporadic adenomas *vs.*, 78–9, 274, 287–8, 312–25
   histologic features, 315–16, *316*
   molecular features, 316–20, **317**, **319**
Danish National Patient Registry, effects of appendectomy on UC natural history, 59
da Vinci, Leonardo, 59
DCC (deleted in colorectal cancer) gene, dysplasia/neoplasia, 268
Defaecation
  pouch dysfunction and, 167–8
   pouchitis, 170
  pouch volume and, 159
  see also Stool frequency
Defensins, 38, 39
Defibrillators, capsule endoscopy and, 100–1
Delayed-release drugs, aminosalicylates, 119
Deleted in colorectal cancer (DCC) gene, dysplasia/neoplasia, 268
Demyelinating disease, infliximab and, 215, 216
Deoxypyridinoline (D-Pyr), 344
Designer drugs, 221–31
Dextran sodium sulphate (DSS) mutant mice, 20–1
Diabetes mellitus, delayed capsule transit, 98
Diagnosis, 66–116
  accurate coding, 4
  histopathological *see* Histopathological diagnosis

imaging *see* Imaging studies, *specific modalities*
intra-operative, 77–8
pouchitis, 79–80
Diet
commensal micro-flora and, 45, 46
Crohn's disease and, 196, 197
see also Nutritional therapy
Dihydroepiandrosterone (DHEAS), osteopenia in men, 354
Dipentum *see* Olsalazine
Disease activity assessment
computed tomography (CT), 107
Crohn's disease *see* Crohn's disease, assessment/scoring
magnetic resonance imaging (MRI), 110
ultrasound, 111–12
Distal colitis
definition, 125–6
neuroimmune factors, 126
proximal extension, 132
refractory *see* Refractory distal colitis
threshold phenomenon, 126
Distal colon, proximal *vs.*, 125
Diversion colitis, Crohn's disease *vs.*, 71
Diversion proctitis, 74
Diverticular colitis, Crohn's disease *vs.*, 71, 73, 74, 75
DLG5 gene, 15, 16
DNA content, dysplasia/cancer, 267, 268, 306
DNA methylation, 317, 319
DNA repair genes, dysplasia/cancer, 306
Doppler ultrasound, 111, 112
Double-balloon enteroscopy
capsule endoscopy *vs.*, 92–3
Crohn's disease diagnosis, 86
Drains, 237, 257
Drug adherence/compliance, aminosalicylates, 122, 126–7
Drug development, 221–31
Drug therapy *see* Medical management
Dual-energy X-ray absorptiometry (DEXA), 343
Dual photon absorptiometry (DPA), 343
Duodenum, Crohn's disease, 81
Dysplasia, 155, 266–80, 293
biopsy, 79, 271, **271**, 284–5, 293, 313
carcinogenesis and, 267–8
ciclosporin-induced 'pseudodysplasia,' 75–6
classification/grading, 271, **271**, 312
histopathology, 78, 315
Vienna classification, 312, **313**
colonoscopic surveillance, 284–5, 287
DALMs *see* DALM (dysplasia associated lesion/mass)
definition, 266–7, 312
diagnosis, 269–73
DALMs, 78–9, 269, 271
difficulty/problems, 273

endoscopic, 293–302
macroscopic, 269, 271, 312–13
microscopic *see histopathological diagnosis (below)*
differential diagnosis, 274–5, **277**
colonoscopic surveillance and, 287–8
hyperplastic polyps *vs.*, 274
inflammatory pseudopolyps *vs.*, 274
reparative phenomena *vs.*, 273, 274–5, **276**
sporadic adenomas *vs.*, 78–9, 274, 287–8, 312–25
double reporting, 79
high-grade, 271, 275, 312
in DALMs, 321–2
surveillance schedule, 287
histopathological diagnosis, 270, 271–3
ancillary studies, 273–4
crypt architecture, 271–2, **273**
DALMs, 315–16, **316**
differential diagnosis, 75–6, 274–5, **276**, **277**, 315–20
double reporting, 79
grading, 78, 315
low-grade, 272
pouch mucosa, 78
'indefinite,' 78, 312
low-grade, 271, 272, 275, 312
cancer risk and, 285
DALMs, 322
surveillance schedule, 287
molecular features/mechanisms, 267–9, **268**, 273–4, 305–6, **319**
chromosome instability, 267, 306–8, **307**
DALMs, 316–20, **317**
see also Cancer biomarkers
morphology, 267
natural history, 275, **277**
polypoid, 270, 274, 312, **319**
see also Adenoma-like mass (ALM)
pouch mucosa, 80, 162, 171
as prognostic factor, 303
rectal dissection and, 158
retained rectal mucosa, 171
Dysplasia-associated lesion/mass *see* DALM (dysplasia associated lesion/mass)

Ecabet sodium enema, refractory distal colitis, 135
Efferent limb obstruction, 175
Elective surgery, ulcerative colitis, 155–62
Elemental diets, Crohn's disease, 198, *198*
Emergency surgery
surgical decision making, 234
ulcerative colitis, 154–5
Endocrine cells, dysplasia and, 272

Endorectal ultrasound (EUS), perianal abscess/fistula, 251–2, 252
Endoscopy
　Crohn's disease
　　capsule see Capsule endoscopy
　　traditional, 86
　dysplasia/cancer, 293–302, 312–13
　pouchitis, 79
　upper GI tract, 81
　see also specific techniques
Enteral nutrition
　children/adolescents, 197, 200, 201, 335
　Crohn's disease, 197–201
　elemental diets, 198, 198, 199, 200
　fat content and, 198, 199, 199, 200
　as maintenance therapy, 200, 201
　patient characteristics and, 199–200
　polymeric diets, 198, 199
　in pregnancy, 366
　as primary treatment, 197, 201
　RCTs, 197–8, 200
　soluble oligosaccharides, 201
Enteroclysis
　computed tomography, 106
　　capsule endoscopy vs., 91
　magnetic resonance, 109
Enteroscopy
　capsule endoscopy vs., 91, 92–3, 93
　Crohn's disease diagnosis, 86
　see also specific techniques
Environmental factors, 10, 57
　commensal micro-flora and, 44, 46
Epidermal growth factor enemas, refractory distal colitis, 135
Escherichia coli, Crohn's disease and, 206–7
Etanercept, 213, 223
Ethnic/racial variation
　CARD15 polymorphism, 18–19
　diet and Crohn's disease, 197
　IBD5 and, 23
European collaborative study on IBD (EC-IBD), 3
European Co-operative Crohn's Disease Study (ECCDS), sulphasalazine vs. steroids in active disease, 181–2
Examination under anaesthetic (EUA), perianal abscess/fistula, 251, 251, 255, 261
Exercise, bone mineral density and, 341
　juvenile-onset IBD, 352
　osteopenia prevention, 353
Extra-intestinal manifestation (EIMs)
　computed tomography (CT), 105, 106, 106
　HLA haplotype and, 23, 374
　magnetic resonance imaging (MRI), 109

pouchitis risk, 170
treatment failure prediction, 374
ultrasound, 111
see also Abscess(es); Fistulae

Fabricius, Hieronymus, 61
Faecal diversion, effects on CIBD diagnosis, 76
Faecal stasis, pouchitis, 170
Familial clustering, 14
Familial polyposis, pouchitis, 170
Far East, incidence, 8, 10
Fat, dietary in Crohn's disease, 197, 198, 199, 200
Fat-wrapping, Crohn's disease, 74
Fecundability, following surgery, 158
Fertility
　female, 360, 361
　　following surgery, 158, 360
　　ulcerative colitis and, 158
　male, 360, 366
　see also Pregnancy
Fetus
　congenital malformation, 364
　miscarriage/loss, 361
　renal toxicity, 364, 365
　see also Pregnancy
Fibrin glue, fistula management, 237
Fibrofatty proliferation
　computed tomography, 107
　magnetic resonance imaging, 110
Fissuring ulcers, Crohn's disease, 74
Fistulae
　computed tomography, 106
　Crohn's disease, 100, 106, 214–15, 218, 235–6, 235–9, 238
　ileal pouch dysfunction, 172, 175
　magnetic resonance imaging, 109, 109, 252–4, 253, 254
　management, 175, 214–15, 218, 235–9, 238
　mucous, as emergency procedure, 154–5
　perianal see Perianal fistulae
Fistula-in-ano, 249, 250
Fistulography, 251
Fistulotomy, 254–5, 258, 258, 260
Flagellins
　antibodies to, 227–8
　function, 228
　systemic immune response, 47
　TLR$_5$ binding, 36
Fluorescence in situ hybridisation (FISH), dysplasia/neoplasia, 306–7, 307, 309
Fluoride, osteopenia, 353, 354
Folic acid
　colorectal cancer and, 283–4
　sulphasalazine effects, 363

Folypolyglutamase hydrolase (FPGH) gene, methotrexate toxicity and, 24
Fractures, 194, 346
   see also Osteopenia; Osteoporosis
Frozen sections, histopathological diagnosis, 77–8, 234–5
Fulminant colitis
   ciclosporin, 154
   emergency surgery, 154–5
   pregnancy and, 365
Functional foods, 145
Functional genomics, 14

Gastritis, Crohn's disease, 81
Gastro-duodenal Crohn's disease, 81
Gene identification strategies, 14
General Practice Research Database (GPRD), fracture frequency, 346
Genetically modified organisms (GMOs), probiotics, 150
Genetics of IBD, 14–32, 222, 222, 226
   bacterial pathogens and, 44, 46
   clinical practice and, 23–5
   drug design and, 226
   dysplasia/neoplasia and, 267–8
   familial clustering, 14
   growth impairment and, 333
   linkage areas/susceptibility loci, 15, 15–23
      see also specific genes/loci
   osteopenia and, 354
   pharmacogenetics, 24–5
   phenotype and *see* Phenotype-genotype relationship
   treatment failure and, 374
Genomic instability, 267, 269, 306–8
Genotype, phenotype and *see* Phenotype-genotype relationship
Geographic trends in incidence, 7, 7–8
   commensal micro-flora and, 46
Germ-free animal models, 46
Glucocorticoids, pharmacogenetics, 24
GM-tri$_{DAP}$ peptidoglycan, 38
Goblet cells, dysplasia and, 271–2
Graft-versus-host disease (GvHD), CARD15 and, 21
Granulocyte-macrophage colony stimulating factor (GM-CSF), 225
   bone metabolism and, 342
Granulomas
   Crohn's disease, 71, 71–72, 73–4
   cryptolytic, 71, 71–73
   micro-, 71
   mucosal, 71, 71–72
   sarcoidosis, 72
   tuberculous, 73, 73–4
Granulomatous vasculitis, 74

Growth
   impaired *see* Growth impairment
   monitoring/assessment, 330, 334
   normal patterns, 329–30
Growth hormone (GH), 329
   growth impairment and, 333
   recombinant, 337
Growth impairment, 329–39, 350, 351, 352–3
   Crohn's disease, 330–1, 331, 332
   definition, 330
   incidence/prevalence, 330, 331
   pathophysiology, 332, 332–3
   psychosocial impact, 334
   steroid-induced, 333
   treatment effects, 331, 333
   treatment/prevention, 333–7
      anti-inflammatory agents, 334–7
         see also specific drugs
      early diagnosis and, 333
      enteral nutrition, 335
      general principles, 334
      monitoring/assessment, 334
      recombinant growth hormone, 337
      surgery, 336
   ulcerative colitis, 331–2

Haemorrhoids, Crohn's disease, 249
Heidleberg pouchitis index, 80
Height percentiles, 330
Height velocity, 329, 334
   males *vs.* females, 229–330
   peak, 330
Histopathological diagnosis
   biopsy *see* Biopsy
   CIBD *vs.* infective colitis
      acute early infective colitis, 67, 68, 69
      chronic infections, 68–9
   controversies, 67–84
   Crohn's disease *see under* Crohn's disease
   dysplasia *see under* Dysplasia
   effect of treatment on CIBD pathology, 75–6
      ciclosporin-induced 'pseudodysplasia,' 75–6
      diversion effects, 76
   frozen sections, 77–8, 234–5
   indeterminate colitis, 69–70, 74
   intra-operative, 234
   neoplastic transformation, pouch mucosa, 80
   pathologist's role, 81
   pouch mucosa
      dysplasia, 81
      follow-up, 80–81
      neoplastic transformation, 80
      pouchitis in, 79–80, 80

Histopathological diagnosis (*Continued*)
 pre-operative decision making and, 233–4
 reparative lesions, 274–5, 276
 reporting, 77
 scoring systems, 77
 specialists *vs.* generalists, 78
 ulcerative colitis *see under* Ulcerative colitis
 upper GI endoscopy, 81
Histopathological scoring, 77
HLADQB haplotype, 16
HLADR3 locus, 23, 374
HLADRB1 locus, 16, 22, 374
HLA system *see* Human leukocyte antigen (HLA) system
Hospital admission, morbidity data, 4
Hospital episode statistics, 4
Human leukocyte antigen (HLA) system, 16, 21–2
 association studies, 21–2
 DQB haplotype, 16
 DR3 locus, 23, 374
 DRB1 locus, 16, 22, 374
 linkage analysis, 16
 phenotypic variation and, 22–3
 treatment failure prediction, 374
Humoral immune response, appendix and, 61
Humira™ (adalimumab), 224
Hydroxyproline, 340
 urinary analysis, 343–4
Hydroxyserine, 340
Hygiene, IBD and, 57
Hyperglycaemia, steroid-induced, 194
Hyperplastic polyps, dysplasia *vs.*, 274
Hypoalbuminaemia, treatment failure prediction, 374, **374**
Hypocalcaemia, steroid-induced, 194

IBD1 locus, 15, *15*, 16
IBD2 locus, 15, *15*, 16
IBD3 locus, 15, *15*, 16, 21–2
 phenotype and, 22–3
IBD4 locus, 15, *15*, 16–17
IBD5 locus, 15, *15*, 17
 ethnic variations, 23
IBD6 locus, 15, *15*, 17
IBD7 locus, 15, *15*, 17
IBD8 locus, 15, *15*, 17–18
IBD9 locus, 15, *15*, 18
IBD International Genetics Consortium, 16
ICAM-1, 17
 antisense therapy, 224
Ileal disease, CARD15 polymorphism, 19
Ileal pouch(es)
 capacity/compliance, 160, 173
 Crohn's disease and, 168–9, 232–3
 design, 159
 dysfunction, 161, 167–78
  efferent limb obstruction, 175
  evacuation disorders, 170, 171–2, 174–5
  fistulae, 172, 175
  incontinence, 172
  increased stool frequency, 167–8
  motility disorders, 168
  natural history, 1
  pelvic sepsis, 161, 169, 173
  pouchitis *see* Pouchitis
  salvage surgery, 161–2
  specific infections, 168–70, 173
  strictures, 171–2, 174
  treatment, 172–5
  underlying Crohn's disease, 168–9, 172
 dysplasia/neoplasia, 80, 162, 171
 evacuation, 170
 failure, 161, 233
 female fertility and, 158, 360
 follow-up, 80–1
 function, determinants, 167
 inflammation *see* Pouchitis
 mobility, 160
 pregnancy and delivery issues, 360, 365
 refractory distal colitis, 138
 volume, 159, 167–8
 see also specific techniques
Ileal pouch-anal anastomosis (IPAA), 167
 fertility after, 158, 360
 pregnancy and delivery issues, 365
 see also Ileal pouch(es)
Ileoanal pouches *see* Ileal pouch(es)
Ileocolonoscopy, capsule endoscopy *vs.*, 91
Ileostomy
 blowhole in pregnancy, 366
 defunctioning, 160
 perianal fistula management, 258, 261
 pouch dysfunction management, 173, 174
Imaging studies
 Crohn's disease, 85–6
  capsule endoscopy *see* Capsule endoscopy
  economic decision model, 101
  inadequacy/problems, 86–7
 cross-sectional, 105–16
 see also specific modalities
Immune cells, toll-like receptors, 35
Immune dysregulation, 222, **222**
 bacteria and, 46–7, 47–8, 145–6
 genetics, 16
 ulcerative colitis pathogenesis, 61–2
Immune response
 activators, 225
 appendectomy effects, 60
 appendix role, 60, 61

immunophenotype and, 227
microbial flora and, 47–8, 145–6
Immunoglobulin G enemas, refractory distal colitis, 136
Immunohistochemistry, dysplasia diagnosis, 271, 273, 273, 275
Immunomodulators
colorectal cancer prevention, 284
Crohn's disease, fistulae management, 236
growth impairment treatment/prevention, 336
pregnancy and, 364–5
refractory distal colitis, 134
Immunophenotypes
drug design and, 226–8, 228
genetic associations, 226
see also Genetics of IBD
serologic associations, 226–8
Immunosuppressants, infliximab and, 214, 217
Incidence
appendicitis, 59–60
global changes in, 3–13
geographic trends, 7, 7–8
juvenile-onset Crohn's disease, 8–10, 9, 10
morbidity data, 3–5
mortality data, 3–4
north-south gradient, 7
outside of Europe/N. America, 8
time trends, 5, 5–7, 6
refractory distal colitis, 124–5
Incontinence, pouch dysfunction, 172
'Indefinite for dysplasia,' 78, 312
Indeterminate colitis
capsule endoscopy, 96
fistulae, pouchitis and, 172
histopathological diagnosis, 69–70, 76
pouchitis, 172, 233
surgical management, 233
colectomy with ileorectal anastomosis, 156
diversion effects, 76
restorative proctocolectomy, 69, 157
Indigo carmine, 293–4
Induction therapy
Crohn's disease
infliximab, 217–18
mesalazine, 181–6, 185
ulcerative colitis
aminosalicylates, 119–20
mesalazine, 120
see also specific drugs/treatments
Infective colitis
histopathological differential diagnosis, 67, 68, 68–9, 69
refractory distal colitis vs., 129
sequelae, 68–9
see also specific infections

Infective proctitis, refractory distal colitis vs., 129–30
Infertility, 360
Inflammation
cytokines, 223
depth of, histopathological diagnosis, 72
pouchitis, causes, 79
therapeutic targets, 222–3
TLR_9-associated down-regulation, 36–7
transmural, Crohn's disease, 74–5
Inflammatory infiltrates
focality in Crohn's disease, 71
histopathological diagnosis, 72
Inflammatory modulators, 22
Inflammatory pseudopolyps, dysplasia vs., 274
Infliximab, 25, 223
antibodies to (ATIs), 214, 215–16, 223, 226
bridging therapy, 217
Crohn's disease, 196, 213–20, 223
as first-line therapy, 216–17
fistulae management, 214–15, 218, 236–7, 256–7, 259, 261
growth impairment prevention/treatment, 337
immunosuppressants and, 214, 217
induction therapy, 217–18
maintenance therapy, 214, 217–18, 236–7
pre-operative, 218
pretreatment measures, 218–19
refractory disease, 213–14
response markers, 219
loss of response, 214, 218
pharmacogenetics, 25
safety issues, 215–19, 237, 257
children, 337
congestive heart failure, 215, 216
demyelinating disease, 215, 216
infusion reactions, 215–16, 218
pregnancy and, 365
pretreatment measures, 218–19
tuberculosis reactivation, 215, 218–19
Insulin-like growth factor-1 (IGF-1)
growth impairment and, 332, 333
normal growth, 329
Interferon-γ, 223
bone metabolism and, 342, 343
inhibitors, 225
Interleukin(s), 223
bone metabolism and, 342
see also specific molecules
Interleukin-1 (IL-1)
bone metabolism and, 342, 343
growth impairment and, 333
Interleukin-2 (IL-2), 223
receptor antagonists, 225

Interleukin-4 (IL-4)
  bone metabolism and, 342
  TCRα knockout mice, 62
Interleukin-6 (IL-6)
  bone metabolism and, 342, 343
  growth impairment and, 332–3
Interleukin-8 (IL-8), bone metabolism and, 343
Interleukin-10 (IL-10), 224
  enemas, refractory distal colitis, 136
Interleukin-11 (IL-11)
  as biological therapy, 224
  bone metabolism and, 342
Interleukin-12 (IL-12), inhibition, 225
Interleukin-17 (IL-17), bone metabolism and, 342
International Organisation for IBD, follow-up of pouch patients, 80–1
Intersphincteric fistula, 249, 250
Intestinal dendritic cells, host–flora interactions, 146
Intestinal epithelial cells (IECs)
  CARD15 and, 20, 20, 38
  normal vs. dysplastic, 267
  pattern recognition receptors, 33
Intestinal flora see Bacteria (intestinal)
Intestinal morphology, 267
Intra-epithelial neoplasia see Dysplasia
Intra-operative diagnosis
  enteroscopy, Crohn's disease, 86
  frozen sections, 77–8, 234–5
Inulin, Crohn's disease, 196–7
Irritable bowel syndrome (IBS)
  ileal pouch dysfunction, 168
  refractory distal colitis vs., 129
Ischiorectal fistula, 249, 250
ISIS, 2302, 224

Japan, incidence, 8, 10
Jejunum, Crohn's disease, 95
J-reservoirs, 159
  stool frequency and, 168
Juvenile-onset IBD
  bone mass in, 195, 346, 350–3, 351
  Crohn's disease
    capsule endoscopy, 94–5
    enteral nutrition in, 197, 200, 201, 335
    global changes in incidence, 8–10, 10
    growth effects, 330–1
    upper GI tract involvement, 81
  early diagnosis, importance, 333
  growth impairment see Growth impairment
  growth monitoring in, 330, 334
  incidence, 329
    global changes in, 8–10, 9, 10
  management
    adults vs., 335
    anti-inflammatory drugs, 334–7
    enteral nutrition, 197, 200, 201, 335
  ulcerative colitis
    global changes in incidence, 9
    growth effects, 331–2

Knockout mice
  CARD15, 20, 21
  TCRα, 59
Koch's postulates, 46–7
Kock's continent ileostomy, 159
  dysplasia/neoplasia, 80
Korea, incidence, 8
K-ras oncogene, dysplasia/neoplasia, 268, 305

Lactobacillus
  as prebiotic, 49
  as probiotic, 144, 147
    genetically modified, 150
Lamina propria, oedema, 67, 69
Laparoscopic surgery
  Crohn's disease management, 239–40
  ulcerative colitis management, 161
Laxatives, refractory distal colitis, 131
Leucocyte adhesion molecules, 224
Lewis scoring system, capsule endoscopy, 94, 99
Linkage analysis, 14, 15, 15–16
Linkage disequilibrium, 17
Lipopolysaccharide (LPS), TLR$_4$ binding, 35–6
Listeria monocytogenes, effect on CARD15 knockout mice, 21
Long-draining seton, 237
Loop ileostomy
  perianal fistula management, 258, 261
  pouch dysfunction management, 173, 174
Lordosis, juvenile-onset IBD, 352
Loss of heterozygosity (LOH), dysplasia/neoplasia, 267, 269, 306, 316, 317, 319
Low-birth weight, IBD effects, 361–2, 362
Lymphadenopathy, magnetic resonance imaging (MRI), 110
Lymphoid aggregates, CIBD differential diagnosis, 67

Macrophage colony stimulating factor (M-CSF), bone metabolism and, 342, 343
Magnetic resonance imaging (MRI), 108–10
  advantages, 108
  capsule endoscopy vs., 93
  contrast agents, 108
  CT vs., 109
  diagnostic, 108–9

disease activity assessment, 110
enteroclysis, 109
extra-luminal complications, 109
gadolinium enhancement, 108, 110
HASTE, 108
perianal disease, *109*, 109–10, 252–4, *253*
   scoring, 253–4, **254**
pregnancy and, 363
T1-weighted, 108, *109*
T2-weighted, 108
   perianal fistulae, 253, *253*
technique, 108
True FISP, 108
ultrasound *vs.*, 111
Magnifying endoscopy, 269, 295, 296, 300
   DALM (dysplasia associated lesion/mass), 314
   efficiency, 296–8
   limitations, 297–8
Maintenance therapy
   Crohn's disease
      enteral nutrition, 200, 201
      infliximab, 214, 217–18, 236–7
      mesalazine, 186–9, **187**
   ulcerative colitis
      aminosalicylates, 119–23, 132–4, *133*
      mesalazine, 119–23
      refractory distal colitis, 132–4, *133*
   see also specific drugs/treatments
Malignancy *see* Cancer
Malnutrition
   Crohn's disease, 197
   growth impairment, 332
Management
   adults *vs.* children, 335
   appendectomy and, 61–2
   bacterial management (pharmabiotics), 48–50, **49**, 144–53
   Crohn's disease *see* Crohn's disease
   IBD subtype-specific, 228, *228*
   imaging and
      capsule endoscopy, 91–92
      cross-sectional, 111
      see also specific modalities
   lack of specific treatment, 221
   medical *see* Medical management
   nutritional, 196–201
   special problems in, 327–76
      children, 329–39
      osteopenia, 340–59
      pregnancy and conception, 360–8
   surgical *see* Surgical management
   ulcerative colitis *see* Ulcerative colitis
   see also specific drugs/treatments

M cells, host–flora interactions, 146
Medical management
   aminosalicylates *see* Aminosalicylates
   antibiotics *see* Antibiotics
   commensal micro-flora and, 44, 46
   Crohn's disease *see* Crohn's disease, management
   designer drugs, 221–31
   drug development, 221–31
   failure
      prediction, 373–4, **374**
      surgery indication, 155
   perianal fistulae, 236–7, 255–7, 259, 261
   pouchitis, 173–4
   pregnancy and, 208, 363–5
   safety during pregnancy, 208, 363–5
   steroids *see* Corticosteroids
   ulcerative colitis *see* Ulcerative colitis, management
   see also specific drugs/drug types
6-Mercaptopurine (6-MP), 196
   colorectal cancer prevention, 284
   Crohn's disease
      fistulae management, 236, 255
      post-operative prophylaxis, 241
   growth impairment treatment/prevention, 336
   male fertility and, 366
   pregnancy and, 364
   refractory distal colitis, 134
   TPMT polymorphism and, 24
Mesalamine *see* Mesalazine (5-ASA; mesalamine)
Mesalazine (5-ASA; mesalamine)
   cancer risk reduction, 121, 283
   Crohn's disease, 181–93
      active disease, 181–6, **185**
      budesonide *vs.*, 184
      ciprofloxacin *vs.*, 208
      efficacy/effectiveness, 184–6, 187, 190–1
      fistulae management, 236
      formulation effects, 186, 188–9
      maintenance therapy, 186–9, **187**
      placebo-controlled trials, 183–4
      post-operative prophylaxis, 189–91, *190*, 240–1
   formulations, 119, 181, **182**
   induction therapy/active disease
      Crohn's disease, 181–6, **185**
      ulcerative colitis, 120
   maintenance therapy
      Crohn's disease, 186–9, **187**
      dose issues, 119–21
      duration issues, 121–2
      patient adherence, 122
      ulcerative colitis, 119–23
   male fertility and, 366
   pregnancy and, 363–4

Mesalazine (5-ASA; mesalamine) (*Continued*)
  safety, 120, 186
  topical (rectal), 120–1
    pharmacokinetics, 127–8
    tissue concentrations, 127
  ulcerative colitis
    active disease, 120
    maintenance therapy, 119–23
    rectal steroids and, 128
    refractory distal colitis, 128
  see also specific formulations
Mesasal, 182
Mesenteric lymph node, host–flora interactions, 146
Meta-analysis
  appendectomy and ulcerative colitis, 57
  mesalazine in Crohn's disease
    in medically-induced remission, 187–9
    post-operative prevention, 189–90
  nutritional therapy in Crohn's disease, 198–9
Metabolic dysfunction, steroid-induced, 194
Methotrexate, 196
  Crohn's disease, post-operative prophylaxis, 241
  pharmacogenetics, 24
  pregnancy and, 364–5
  refractory distal colitis, 134
Methylene blue, 294, 297
Methylenetetrahydrofolate reductase (MTHFR) gene, methotrexate toxicity and, 24
Methylprednisolone, active Crohn's disease
  mesalazine *vs.*, 184
  sulphasalazine *vs.*, 181–2
Metronidazole, 48, 49
  activity, 207
  Crohn's disease, 182, 207–8, 211
    ciprofloxacin combinations, 208–9
    fistulae management, 236, 255
    post-operative prophylaxis, 241
    recurrence prevention, 207–8
  pouchitis, 173
  pregnancy and, 208, 364
  resistance, 207
  side effects, 208
  sulphasalazine *vs.*, 182, 207
MIC gene family, 22
Micro-array technology, 14
Microbe-(pathogen)-associated molecular patterns (MAMPs), 33
Microbial sensing, 33–41
  see also Pattern recognition receptors (PRRs)
Micro-granulomas, 71
Micronutrient deficiency, Crohn's disease, 196
Micro-satellite instability (MSI), dysplasia/neoplasia, 267, 269, 306

Minerals, bone, 340
Miscarriage/foetal loss, IBD effects, 361
Mismatch repair genes, dysplasia/cancer, 306
Mitotic figures, dysplasia and, 272, 273
MLN-02, 224
Molecular biology, dysplasia/neoplasia, 267–9, **268**, 273–4, 304, 305–6
  DALMs, 316–20, **317**
  see also Cancer biomarkers
Molecular markers *see* Biomarkers
Monocyte chemoattractant protein I (MCP-I), bone metabolism and, 343
Morbidity data, 3–5
Mortality data, 3–4, 370, **370**, 372, **372**–3
Motility disorders
  pouch dysfunction, 168
  refractory distal colitis, 131
6-MP *see* 6-Mercaptopurine (6-MP)
Mucin depletion, 67
  Crohn's *vs.* ulcerative colitis, 70–1
Mucosal advancement flap, 238, **238**
Mucosal immune cells, 222, **222**
  appendectomy and, 59
  pattern recognition receptors, 33
  response to bacteria, 44
Mucosal injury, 222, **222**
Mucosectomy, 159–60
Mucous fistula
  complications, 155
  emergency surgery, 154–5
Multi-drug resistance 1 (MDR1) gene, glucocorticoid efficacy and, 24
Muramyl dipeptide (MDP), 19, 38, 44
  receptor *see* CARD15 (NOD2)
Mycobacteria, Crohn's disease and, 206, 209–11
Mycobacterium paratuberculosis, 209
Mycophenolate mofetil, 196
  fistulae management, 236
  pregnancy and, 364–5

N-acetyl transferases (NATs), pharmacogenetics, 25
Natalizumab, 224
National Co-operative Crohn's Disease Study (NCCDS), sulphasalazine *vs.* steroids in active disease, 181
Neoplasia *see* Cancer
Neuroimmune factors, distal colitis, 126
Neutrophils, histopathological diagnosis, 70
Nicotine, refractory distal colitis, **136**
NOD1 (nucleotide oligomerisation domain 1) *see* CARD4 (NOD1)
NOD2 (nucleotide oligomerisation domain 2) *see* CARD15 (NOD2)

Non-steroidal anti-inflammatory drugs (NSAIDs)
  colorectal cancer prevention, 283
  NSAID-induced lesions, Crohn's disease *vs.*, 94
North America
  CARD15 polymorphism, 18–19
  incidence, 7–8, 10
    morbidity data, 4
North–south gradient, 7
Nuclear changes, dysplasia and, 272
Nuclear factor-κB (NFκB) signalling, 19, 20, 20, 37–8, 44, 146
Nucleotide oligomerisation domain (NOD) proteins, 16, 37–9
  cellular distribution, 38
  domain structure, 37
  functions, 38
  ligands, **35**, 38, 145
  NOD1 *see* CARD4 (NOD1)
  NOD2 *see* CARD15 (NOD2)
  signalling pathways, 34
Nutritional deficiency
  Crohn's disease, 196
  growth impairment pathophysiology, 332
Nutritional therapy
  corticosteroids *vs.*, 194–205
  Crohn's disease, 196–201
    as primary treatment, 201
  enteral diets *see* Enteral nutrition
  pouchitis and, 174

Obstructions/obstructive disease
  capsule endoscopy and, 90
  computed tomography, 106
  Crohn's disease, 88, 95, 97–8
    in pregnancy, 365
    in pouch dysfunction, 175
  pouchitis, 171–2, 174
OCTN gene, 226
Oesophagogastroduodenoscopic examination, Crohn's disease, 86
Oestrogens, osteopenia, 353
Oligosaccharides, Crohn's disease, 201
Olsalazine, 119, **182**
  refractory distal colitis, 133
Onercept, 223–4
Organic cationic transporter (OCTN) gene, 226
Ornidazole, Crohn's disease, 208
Osteoblasts, 340
  cytokine production, 342–3
Osteocalcin, 340
Osteoclasts, 340
Osteocytes, 340
Osteonecrosis, 194

Osteopenia, 340–59
  aetiopathogenesis, **344**, 344–6
  BMD measurement, 343
  Crohn's disease *vs.* ulcerative colitis, 346–50, 348, 349
    intermediate disease duration, 348–9, 349
    long-standing disease, 348, 349, 350
    newly diagnosed patients, 346, 347, 349
    prospective study, 347–50
    steroid dose effects, 349, 350
  fracture risk, 194, 346
    males *vs.* females, 347
  genetic factors, 354
  high risk patients, 353, **353**
  IBD-induced loss, 194
  juvenile-onset IBD, 195, 346, 350–3
  management in IBD, 353–5
  prevalence, 340, 344–6, **345**, 345
  prevention, 353
  steroid-induced loss, 194–6, **195**, 340, 341, 344
  vitamin D deficiency, 340
  WHO definition, 345
  see also Bone mineral density (BMD); Osteoporosis
Osteoporosis
  BMD measurement, 343
  fractures, 194
  mechanism of bone loss, 340
  prevalence, 345, **345**, 345
  prevention/management, 353–5
  WHO definition, 345
  see also Bone mineral density (BMD); Osteopenia
Oxidative stress, carcinogenesis role, 306

p16 gene, dysplasia/neoplasia and, 317
p53 gene
  dysplasia diagnosis, 270, 273, 274, 309, 316–17
  tumourigenesis and, 268, 305
Pacemakers, capsule endoscopy and, 100–2
Paediatric IBD *see* Juvenile-onset IBD
pANCA (perinuclear antineutrophil cytoplasmic antibody), 226–7
Panchromoendoscopy, 294, 297
Paneth cells
  CARD15 expression, 21, 38, 39
  dysplasia and, 272
Parathyroid peptides, osteopenia, 353
Parenteral nutrition, Crohn's disease, 197
Parks classification, 249, 250
PASSCLAIM, 145
Patency capsule, 97–8
Pathogenesis, 1–65
  appendix and, 57–64, 59, 60, 61–2
  bacteria and *see* Bacteria (intestinal)
  genetics and *see* Genetics of IBD

Pathogenesis (*Continued*)
  growth impairment, 332, 332–3
  immune function *see* Immune dysregulation
  osteopenia, **344**, 344–6
  therapeutic targets, 222, 222–3
Pattern recognition receptors (PRRs), 33–41, 44, 145
  animal models, 33
  ligands, **35**, 145
  NODs *see* Nucleotide oligomerisation domain (NOD) proteins
  signalling pathways, 34, 145, 146
  TLRs *see* Toll-like receptors (TLRs)
Peak height velocity, 330
Pentasa®, 119, 120, **182**
  in active Crohn's disease
    budesonide *vs.*, 184
    placebo-controlled RCTs, 183
  refractory distal colitis, 133–4
  tissue concentrations, 127
Perianal abscess(es), 249–61
  assessment, **248**
  clinical evaluation, 250–4, 259–60
    endorectal ultrasound, 251–2, *252*
    examination under anaesthetic, 251
  diagnosis/classification, 249, *250*
    MRI scores, 253–4, **254**
  management, 259–61
  prevention, 257
  treatment options, 254
Perianal Crohn's disease, 246–65
  abscess *see* Perianal abscess(es)
  anal canal lesions, 246
    fissures, 248–9
    haemorrhoids, 249
    stenosis, 249
    ulcers, 248
  classification, 246, 249, *250*, 253–4, **254**
  fistulae *see* Perianal fistulae
  frequency, 246
  magnetic resonance imaging, *109*, 109–10
  measurement of disease severity, 246–8, **247**, **248**
  'neglected,' 255
  pregnancy and delivery in, 365
  pre-operative decision making, 234
  skin lesions, 246
Perianal Crohn's Disease Activity Index (PCDAI), **247**, **248**
Perianal Disease Activity Index (PDAI), 246–7, **247**
Perianal fistulae, *109*, 110–11, 235–6, 246, 249–61, 251, *258*
  abscess formation, 257
    see also Perianal abscess(es)
  activity index (drainage assessment), 247–8, **248**
  clinical evaluation, 250–4, 259–60

computed tomography, 251
endorectal ultrasound, 251–2, *252*
examination under anaesthetic, 251, *251*, 255, 261
fistulography, 251
MRI, 252–4, *253*
  complex, 255, 257
diagnosis/classification, 249, *250*
  MRI scores, 253–4, **254**
natural history, 257
recto-vaginal, 259, *260*, 261
simple, 254–5
treatment, 254–61
  clinical remission *vs.* healing, 257
  complex fistula, 255
  fistulotomy, 254–5, *258*, 258, 260
  high fistulae, 235–6
  laying open, 235–6
  low fistulae, 235
  medical therapy, 236–7, 255–7, 259, 261
  observation, 236
  options, 254–9
  recto-vaginal fistula, 259, *260*, 261
  simple fistula, 254–5
  surgical therapy, 237–8, **238**, 257–9, *258*, *260*
  treatment algorithm, 238–9
  see also specific therapies/procedures
Perianal salvage surgery, 161–2
Perineum
  pouch–perineal fistulae, 175
  sepsis, 261
Perinuclear antineutrophil cytoplasmic antibody (pANCA), 226–7
Peyer's patches, 61
Pharmabiotics, 48–50, 144–53
  'bugs to drugs,' 144, **148**
  definitions/terminology, 144–5
  genetically-modified organisms, 150
  prebiotics, 49
  probiotics *see* Probiotic therapy
  promise, 150
Pharmacogenetics, 24–5
Pharmacological therapy *see* Medical management
Phenotype–genotype relationship, 15
  CARD15 polymorphism and, 19, 39
  IBD3 and HLA polymorphism, 22–3
  IBD5 and, 23
Phenotype, sero-reactivity and, 48
PillCam™ capsule, 87, *87*
Pit-pattern chromoendoscopy classification, 294, 296, *296*
  complexity, 298
  DALMs, 314
Placebo-controlled trials, mesalazine in Crohn's disease, 183–4

Placebo-response, in ulcerative colitis, 369, 371
Polymeric diets, Crohn's disease, 198, 199
Polypectomy, ALMs management, 320, 321
Polyps
  APC gene, 267–8, 305, 316
  dysplasia vs., 274
  familial polyposis coli, 170
  hyperplastic, 274
  pseudopolyps, 274
  see also Adenoma(s)
Polyunsaturated fatty acids (PUFA), Crohn's disease and, 197
Positron emission tomography (PET), FDG-PET, 112
Post-operative prophylaxis, Crohn's disease, 240–1
  azathioprine, 241
  budesonide, 241
  6-mercaptopurine, 241
  mesalazine, 189–91, 190, 240–1
  methotrexate, 241
  metronidazole, 241
Pouchitis, 80, 169–70
  aetiology/risk factors, 170–3
    columnar cuff disorders, 171
    evacuation disorders, 170, 171–2
    fistula formation, 172, 175
    strictures, 171–2
  antibiotics, 48
  diagnosis, 79–80
  histology, 170–1
  implications of, 169–70
  incidence, 169
  indeterminate colitis, 172, 233
  natural history, 174
  probiotic therapy, 144, 148, 149
  scoring systems, 79–80
  short-chain fatty acids and, 170
  treatment, 173–4
    allopurinol, 174
    antibiotics, 170, 173–4
    anti-inflammatories, 174
    loop ileostomy, 173, 174
    nutritional agents, 174
    pouch dysfunction, 172–3
    strictures, 174
  ulcerative colitis vs. familial polyposis, 170
Pouch–perineal fistulae, 175
Pouch–vaginal fistulae, 175
Prebiotic therapy, 49
  definition, 49, 145
  probiotic therapy and (synbiotics), 145
Prednisolone
  breastfeeding and, 366
  pregnancy and, 363
  refractory distal colitis, 128–9
Prednisone
  active Crohn's disease, sulphasalazine vs., 181
  breastfeeding and, 366
  pregnancy and, 363
Pregnancy, 360–8
  assessment of disease activity in, 363
  capsule endoscopy and, 100
  delivery issues, 365
  effect of IBD on pregnancy, 361–2
    congenital malformation, 362
    miscarriage/foetal loss, 361
    prematurity/low birth weight, 361–2, 362
  effect of pregnancy on IBD, 362–3
    during, 362
    after, 363
  enteral feeding during, 366
  IBD transmission to offspring, 361
    see also Genetics of IBD
  medical therapy during, 363–5
    aminosalicylates, 363–4
    antibiotics, 208, 364
    corticosteroids, 363
    immunomodulators, 364–5
  surgical therapy during, 365–6
Prematurity, IBD effects, 361–2, 362
Presacral nerves, rectal dissection and, 159
Primary sclerosing cholangitis (PSC)
  colorectal carcinoma and, 283, 285, 286, 303, 320
  pouchitis risk, 170
  restorative proctocolectomy contraindication, 158
  ulcerative colitis phenotype in, 58, 63
Probiotic therapy, 48, 197
  biologic effects, 49
  definition, 144
  dosimetry, 147
  efficacy, 148, 148, 149
  impact on intestinal ecosystem, 147
  prebiotic therapy and (synbiotics), 145
  pregnancy and, 364
  strain selection, 146–50
    guidelines, 146
    single vs. combination, 147–8
  turbo probiotics (genetically modified organisms), 150
Process for the assessment of scientific support for claims on foods (PASSCLAIM), 145
Proctectomy, perianal fistula management, 258–9, 261
Proctitis
  Crohn's disease, refractory distal colitis vs., 129
  infective, refractory distal colitis vs., 129–30
  radiation, refractory distal colitis vs., 129
  ulcerative colitis, colectomy risk, 373

Proctocolectomy, 155
    age and, 156–7
    conventional *vs.* restorative, 155–7, 160
    defunctioning ileostomy, need, 160
    fertility and, 158, 360
    laparoscopic, 161
    rectal dissection, 158–9
    restorative *see* Restorative proctocolectomy (RPC)
Pro-drugs, aminosalicylates, 119
PROGID trial, 148
Pro-inflammatory cytokines, 223
    bone metabolism and, 341–3
    growth impairment and, **332**, 332–3
Prokinetic agents, capsule transit time and, 98
Proliferation markers, dysplasia and, 273, 305
Propionyl-L-carnitine (PLC) enemas, refractory distal colitis, **136**
Prostaglandins, TLR$_9$-associated induction, 36
Protein hyper-catabolism, steroid-induced, 194
Proteomics, drug design, 228
Proximal colon
    constipation, refractory distal colitis, 131
    physiology, distal *vs.*, 125
'Pseudodysplasia,' ciclosporin-induced, 75–6
Pseudopolyps, dysplasia *vs.*, 274
Pubertal development
    IBD, 350
    normal, 329–30
Push enteroscopy
    capsule endoscopy *vs.*, 91, 93
    Crohn's disease diagnosis, 86
Pyridinoline (Pyr), 344

Qebehsenuef, 60
Quality of life, restorative proctocolectomy and, 155
Quinolones
    breastfeeding and, 366
    pregnancy and, 364

Radiation proctitis, refractory distal colitis *vs.*, 129
Raloxifene, osteopenia prevention/management, 353
RAPID™ workstation, 87
Reactive dyes/stains, chromoendoscopy, 294
Rectal advancement flap, 238, **238**
Rectal compliance, 127–8
Rectal dissection, 158–9
Rectal diversion, effects on CIBD diagnosis, 76
Rectal excision, fulminant colitis, 154
Rectal mucosa
    changes in ulcerative colitis, 76–7
    prolapse (solitary rectal ulcer syndrome), refractory distal colitis *vs.*, 129

Rectal stump
    length of, 155
    pouch dysfunction and, 175
    preservation, 154
Recto-vaginal fistula, management, 259, 260, 261
Reduced folate carrier gene (RFC1), methotrexate toxicity and, 24
Refractoriness, definition, 124
Refractory distal colitis, 124–43
    caecal patch lesion, 132
    definition, 124–5
    differential diagnosis, **129**, 129–30
    disease extent assessment, 132
    management, 128–9
        algorithm, *125*
        alternative therapies, 134–8, **135–7**
        aminosalicylates, 128, 130–1, 132–4
        ciclosporin, 131–2
        conventional, 128–9
        immunomodulators, 134
        intensive, 131–2
        intravenous steroids, 131–2
        maintenance therapy, 132–4, *133*
        proximal constipation, 131
        steroids, 128–9, 130
        strategy, 128
        surgical, 138
        topical therapy *see below*
        see also specific drugs/formulations
    pathophysiology, 125–8
        distal *vs.* proximal colon, 126
        environmental causes, 126–7
        physiological causes, 127–8
    prevalence, 124–5
    relapse, 131
    topical (rectal) therapy
        aminosalicylates, 130–1, 133–4
        dose and delivery, 130–1
        pharmacokinetics, 127–8
        steroids, 128–9, 130
Renal toxicity, foetal
    aminosalicylates, 364
    ciclosporin, 365
Resection specimens, indeterminate colitis diagnosis, 69–70
Residual epithelial cuff (anal transitional zone; ATZ), pouchitis and, 171
Resting energy expenditure (REE), 332
Restitution, dysplasia *vs.*, 273, 274–5, 276
Restorative proctocolectomy (RPC), 155
    age and, 156–7
    complications, 156
    contraindications, 157–8
    conventional *vs.*, 155–7, 160

failure rate, 156
female fertility and, 158, 360
follow-up, 162
indeterminate colitis and, 69, 157
indications, 156
laparoscopic, 161
rectal dissection, 158–9
see also Ileal pouch(es)
Riddell's dysplasia grading system, 78
Ridogrel, refractory distal colitis, 136
Rifabutin, Crohn's disease, 210–11
Risk factors, 57
colorectal carcinoma, 282–3
environmental *see* Environmental factors
genetic *see* Genetics of IBD
perinatal/early infancy, 9
pouchitis, 170–3
relapse, 371
'Rosary' of colorectal cancer, 74–5

Salazopyrine *see* Sulphasalazine
Salmonella, treatment in pouchitis, 173
Salofalk, 182
Salvage surgery, 160–1
Sarcoidosis, 73
Scoring systems, 77
capsule endoscopy, 94, 99
chronic IBD, 77
Crohn's disease *see* Crohn's disease
dysplasia, 78, 271, 312, 313, 315
magnetic resonance imaging correlation, 110
perianal disease, 246–8, **247**, **248**, 253–4, **254**
pouchitis, 79–80
Scotland, juvenile-onset IBD, 8–9, 10
Secondary colitis, refractory distal colitis *vs.*, 129
Segregation studies, 14–15
Sepsis
perianal disease and, 261
pouch dysfunction and, 169
pouch surgery and, 161
Serologic associations, 226–8
Setons, 237, 257
Sexual dysfunction, rectal dissection and, 158
Shigella infections
chronic, CIBD *vs.*, 68–9
treatment in pouchitis, 173
Short-chain fatty acids
pouchitis and, 170, 174
refractory distal colitis, 136
Sialyl-Tn antigen (STn), dysplasia and, 273, 305, 309
Sigmoidoscopy
perianal disease, 260
pregnancy and, 363

Single nucleotide polymorphisms (SNPs), 14
Single photon absorptiometry, 343
Single X-ray absorptiometry, 343
Skip lesions, 70
frozen sections, 78
Small bowel (intestine)
commensal micro-flora, 43
Crohn's disease, 85
appearance in, 95
carcinoma, 281
imaging, 85–6
see also specific modalities
Small bowel carcinoma, Crohn's disease, 281
Small bowel enteroclysis, capsule endoscopy *vs.*, 91
Small bowel follow-through (SBFT)
capsule endoscopy *vs.*, 90–1, 92–3, 96
Crohn's disease diagnosis, 85–6
Small bowel radiography
capsule endoscopy *vs.*, 90–1, 92–3
Crohn's disease diagnosis, 85–6
see also specific techniques
Social factors, juvenile-onset Crohn's disease, 10
Solitary rectal ulcer syndrome (rectal mucosal prolapse), refractory distal colitis *vs.*, 129
Sonde enteroscopy, Crohn's disease diagnosis, 86
South Africa, IBD incidence, 8
Spasmolytics, chromoendoscopy, 294
Sphincterotomy, Crohn's disease, 249
Spine, osteopenia and, 346, 351, *351*, 352
Split ileostomy, perianal fistula management, 258
Spongy (cancellous) bone, 340
S-pouch, 159
efferent limb obstruction, 175
evacuation disorders, 171
stool frequency and, 168
stricture formation, 171, 174
Stapled anastomosis, 160, 168, 241
Stenosis, Crohn's disease, 88, 95, 97–8
anal, 249
children, 336
Steroid drugs *see* Corticosteroids
Steroid receptor expression, 127
St. Mark's scoring system, pouchitis, 79–80
Stomach, commensal micro-flora, 43
Stomas, 138
Stomatherapist, 138
Stool frequency
pouch dysfunction and, 167–8
prediction of medical failure, 373, **374**
Strictures
Crohn's disease, 88, 95, 97–8
pouchitis, 171–2, 174
Strontium, osteopenia, 353

Sucralfate, refractory distal colitis, 137
Sulphasalazine, 119, 120, 181, **182**
   in active disease, 181–3
   cancer risk reduction, 121, 283
   male fertility and, 366
   metronidazole *vs.*, 182, 207
   pregnancy and, 363–4
   refractory distal colitis, 128, 132–3
   steroids *vs.*, 181–2
Superior mesenteric artery (SMA), ultrasound examination, 111
Supralevator fistula, 249, 250
SURFACE chromoendoscopy guidelines, **296**
Surgical management
   appendectomy and, 62–3
   Crohn's disease
      anal fistulae, 235–6, 237–8
      in children, 336
      controversies, 232–45
      laparoscopic, 239–40
      outcomes, 233
      post-surgical prophylaxis, 189–91, **190**, 240–1
      pouch surgery, 168–9, 232–3
      stapled anastomoses, 241
   fertility and, 158, 360
   growth impairment treatment/prevention, 336
   indeterminate colitis, 233
      colectomy with ileorectal anastomosis, 156
      diversion effects, 76
      restorative proctocolectomy, 69, 157
   pouchitis, 174
   preoperative decision making, 233–5
      non-commital pathology reports, 233–4
      staging surgery, 234–5
      see also Histopathological diagnosis
   ulcerative colitis
      choice of procedure, 155–8
      controversies, 154–66
      elective surgery, 155–62
      emergency surgery, 154–5
      indications, 155
      laparoscopic, 161
      number of stages, 160–1
      prognostic indicators, 370, 373–4, **374**
      salvage surgery, 160–1
      technical aspects, 158–62
   see also specific techniques/procedures
Sweden, IBD incidence
   juvenile-onset IBD, 9–10
   time trends, 5
Swedish Inpatient Register, appendectomy, protection against UC, 59

Synbiotics, 145
Systemic immune response, microbial flora and, 42–8

Tacrolimus, 196
   fistulae management, 236, 256, 261
T-cells, appendix and, 61
TCRα knockout mice, 62
Telomerase, 307–8
Telomere shortening, 307, 307–8, 319–20
Thalidomide, pregnancy contraindication, 365
T helper (Th)-1 response, 223
   inhibitors, 224–5
Thiopurine S-methyltransferase (TPMT) polymorphism, 24
Threshold phenomenon, distal colitis, 126
Thromboxane A_2 inhibitor, refractory distal colitis, 137
Time trends in incidence, 5, 5–7, 6
TLR_1, 35
TLR_2, 35, **35**
   mutation/polymorphism, 37
TLR_3, 35
TLR_4, 35, 35–6
   mutation/polymorphism, 37, 42
TLR_5, 35, **35**, 36
   mutation/polymorphism, 37
TLR_6, 35
TLR_7, 35
TLR_8, 35
TLR_9, **35**, 36–7
   mutation/polymorphism, 37, 42–3
TLRs *see* Toll-like receptors (TLRs)
Toll-like receptors (TLRs), 33, 35–7, 42–3, 145, 146
   CARD15 regulation, 39
   expression patterns
      inflamed intestine, 33, 35
      normal intestine, 33
   ligands, **35**, 145
   mutation/polymorphism in IBD, 37
   signalling pathways, 34, 145, 146
   see also specific types
Topical (rectal) therapy
   aminosalicylates, 120–1
      pharmacokinetics, 127–8
      tissue concentrations, 127
   corticosteroids, pharmacokinetics, 127–8
   see also specific drugs/formulations
Total colectomy, refractory distal colitis, 138
Total enteral nutrition (TEN), Crohn's disease, 197
Total parenteral nutrition (TPN), Crohn's disease, 197
Toxic megacolon, mucin depletion, 71
Transforming growth factor-β (TGF-β), bone metabolism and, 342, 343
Transmission disequilibrium tests (TDTs), 15, 18

Transmural inflammation, Crohn's disease, 74–5
Transporter of antigenic peptide 2 (TAP2) gene, glucocorticoid efficacy and, 24
TREAT registry, 216
T-scores, 344, **345**
Tuberculosis
　granulomas, 73, 73–4
　infliximab reactivation, 215, 218–19
Tumour necrosis factor-α (TNF-α), 22, 23, 213, 223
　bone metabolism and, 342, 343
　growth impairment and, 332, 333
　inhibition see Anti-tumour necrosis factor-α therapies
Tumour necrosis factor-β (TNF-β), bone metabolism and, 342
Tumours see Cancer
Turbo probiotics (genetically modified organisms), 150
Twin studies, 15

Ulcer-associated cell lineage (UACL), Crohn's disease, 75
Ulcerative colitis
　animal models, 62
　appendicitis and, 59
　backwash ileitis, 73
　bone mineral density loss, 340
　　Crohn's disease vs., 346–50, **348**, **349**
　　prevalence, 345, **345**
　　see also Osteopenia
　caecal patch lesion, 132
　cancer association, 155, 266, 268, 281, 289, 293
　　clinical risk factors, 282–3
　　overall risk, 281–2, 303
　　surveillance and see Colonoscopic surveillance
　　see also Colorectal carcinoma; Dysplasia
　capsule endoscopy, 94–6
　clinical course
　　disease extension, 371–2
　　predicting, **370**, 370–1
　diagnostic imaging
　　CT, 106
　　MRI, 108–9
　　ultrasound, 111
　differential diagnosis
　　Crohn's disease vs., 70–2, 85, 95–6
　　infective colitis vs., 67, **68**, **69**
　　sporadic adenomas vs. DALM, 78–9
　disease extent
　　histopathological diagnosis, 371
　　prognosis and, 370
　distal disease see Distal colitis
　diversion proctitis, 74
　familial clustering, 14
　　see also Genetics of IBD
　fertility and, 158, 360
　global changes in incidence, 3
　　geographical trends, 7
　　morbidity data, 4
　　time trends, 6, 6–7
　histopathological diagnosis, 67, **68**, 70–2
　　depth of inflammation, 72
　　disease extent, 371
　　inflammatory cell type, 72
　　mucin depletion, 67, 70–1
　　rectal mucosa changes, 76–7
　　scoring, 77
　management, 117–79
　　induction therapy, 119–20
　　left-sided disease, 120–1, 131
　　maintenance therapy, 119–23, 132–4
　　predicting medical therapy failure, 373–4, **374**
　　probiotics, 48, **148**
　　refractory distal colitis, 124–43
　　surgical see Surgical management
　　see also specific drugs/treatments
　mortality, 4, 370, **370**, 372, 372–3
　natural history, 369
　　appendectomy effects, 59–60
　pathogenesis, 42
　　appendix role, 59, 60, 61–2
　　see also Appendix
　phenotypic overlap with Crohn's disease, 15
　placebo-response, 369, 371
　pregnancy and see Pregnancy
　primary sclerosing cholangitis and see Primary sclerosing cholangitis (PSC)
　prodrome, 370
　prognosis, 369–76
　　clinical course and, **370**, 370–1
　　colectomy risk, 370, 373–4, **374**
　　common questions, 369
　　disease extension, 371–2
　　first attack, 369–70, **370**
　　mortality, 370, **370**, 372, 372–3
　　relapse prediction, 370, **370**, 371
　　remission prediction, 370, 371
　protection against, appendectomy, 56–8
　refractory
　　definition, 124
　　distal see Refractory distal colitis
　　prevalence, 124–5
　regression, 372
　relapses, 131
　　clinical risk factors, 371
　　predicting, 370, **370**, 371
　remission, predicting, 370, 371

Ulcers/ulceration
  appendicitis, 63
  in Crohn's disease, 75, 95
    anal canal, 248
  ulcerative colitis see Ulcerative colitis
Ultrasound, 110–12
  CT vs., 111
  diagnosis, 111
  disease activity, 111–12
  Doppler flow analysis, 111
  endorectal (EUS), perianal abscess/fistula, 251–2, 252
  extra-luminal complications, 111
  MRI vs., 111
  technique, 110–11
United Kingdom, incidence
  hospital admission data, 4
  juvenile-onset IBD, 8–9
  time trends, 5–6
Urine analysis, bone metabolism, 343–4
Ursodeoxycholic acid (UDCA), colorectal carcinoma prevention, 283

Vaginal fistulae
  pouch–vaginal, 175
  recto-vaginal, 259, 260, 261
Verheyen, Phillipe, 60
Vertebral collapse, juvenile-onset IBD, 351, 352
Vertebral fractures, 346
Vesalius, Andreas, 60
Vienna dysplasia classification, 312, 313
Virtual CT colonoscopy, 107–8
Virtual histology, 298
Visilizumab, 225
Vitamin D
  deficiency, 340, 353
  supplements, 353, 354
Vitamin K deficiency, 344, 353

Wheat grass juice, refractory distal colitis, 137
World Health Organisation (WHO), osteopenia/osteoporosis definitions, 345
W-reservoirs, 159
  stool frequency and, 168

Zinc-binding proteins, tumourigenesis and, 305
Z-scores, 344, **345**, 351